Respiratory Care
Clinical Competency
LAB MANUAL

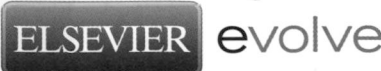

YOU'VE JUST PURCHASED MORE THAN A TEXTBOOK!

Evolve Student Resources for *Hinski: Respiratory Care Clinical Competency Lab Manual*, include the following:

- NBRC Correlation Guide (for the combined CRT/RRT Exam matrices)

- Procedural Assessment forms

- Tests and Reference Ranges

- Answer Key—Lab Activities

- Answer Key—Self Assessment Questions

- Answer Key—Case Studies

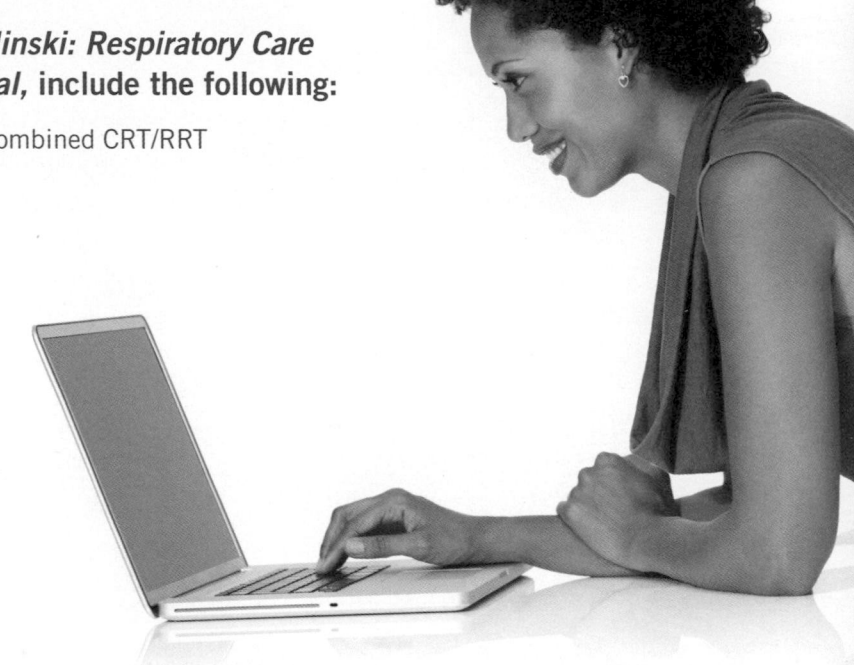

Activate the complete learning experience that comes with each *NEW* textbook purchase by registering at

http://evolve.elsevier.com/Hinski/respcarelabmanual/

REGISTER TODAY!

Respiratory Care Clinical Competency LAB MANUAL

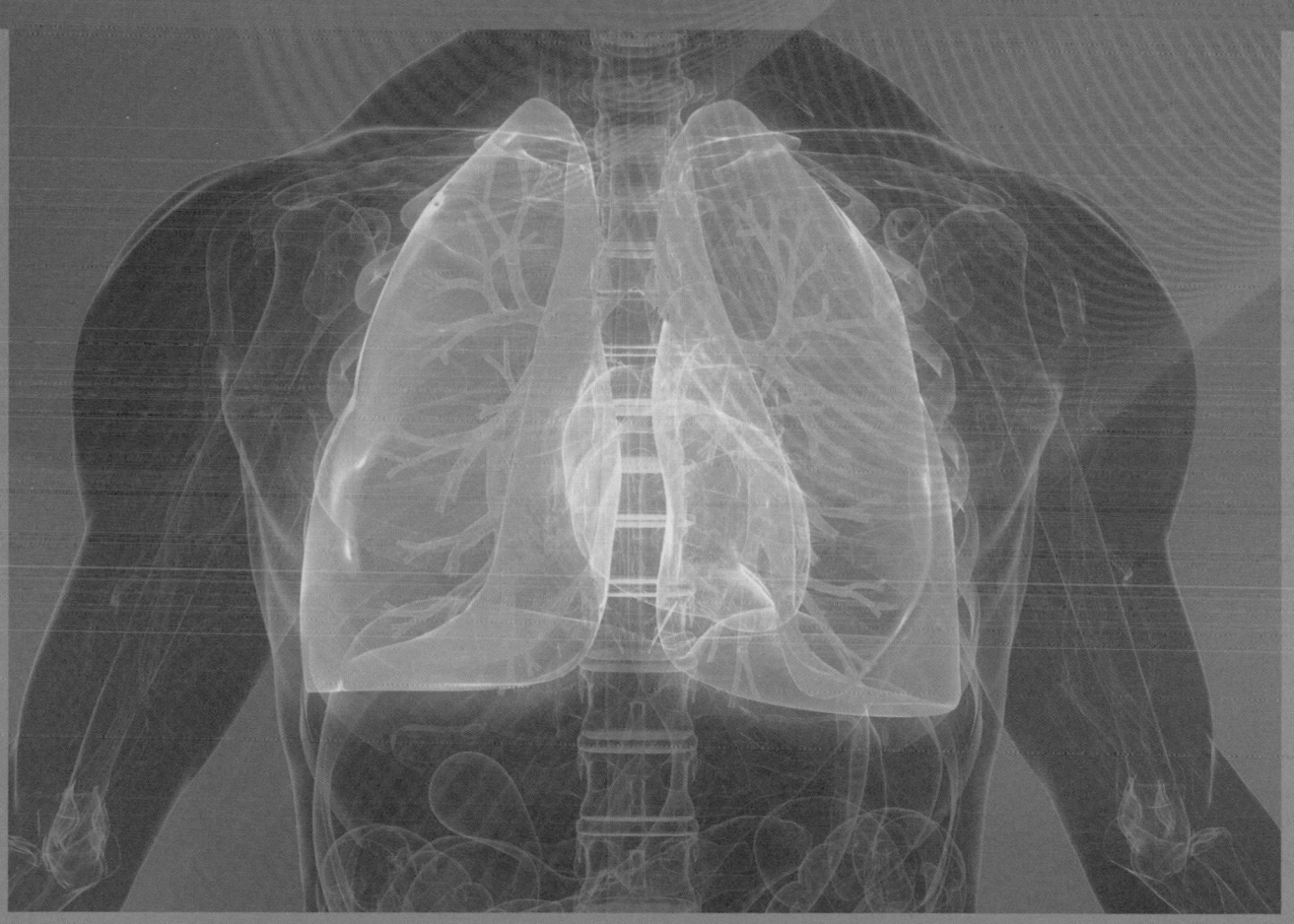

Sandra T. Hinski, MS, RRT-NPS

Faculty
Respiratory Care Division
Gateway Community College
Phoenix, Arizona

ELSEVIER

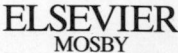

3251 Riverport Lane
St. Louis, Missouri 63043

RESPIRATORY CARE CLINICAL COMPETENCY LAB MANUAL   ISBN: 978-0-323-10057-1

ISBN: **978-0-323-10057-1**

Content Manager: Billie Sharp
Content Development Specialist: Kathleen Sartori
Publishing Services Manager: Catherine Albright Jackson
Project Manager: Sara Alsup
Design Direction: Karen Pauls

Printed in India

Last digit is the print number: 9   8   7   6

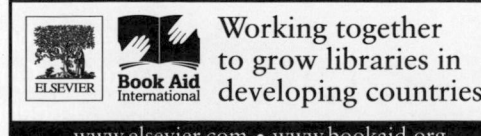

Working together
to grow libraries in
developing countries

www.elsevier.com • www.bookaid.org

For my dad.
His memory gives me purpose.

Contributors

Douglas S. Gardenhire, EdD, RRT-NPS, FAARC
Director of Clinical Education
Department of Respiratory Therapy
Byrdine F. Lewis School of Nursing and Health Professions
Georgia State University
Atlanta, Georgia

Edward Hoskins, MEd, RRT
Division Chair and Faculty
Gateway Community College
Phoenix, Arizona

Jonathan R. Marino, BS, RRT
Respiratory Care Practitioner
Phoenix, Arizona

Wendi M. Nugent, MBA, RPSGT, R. EEG T.
Director PSG Technology Program
Director EEG/END Technology Program
Gateway Community College
Phoenix, Arizona

Kathryn Patterson, BS, RRT
Respiratory Care Faculty
Gateway Community College
Phoenix, Arizona

Toni L. Rodriguez, EdD, RRT, FAARC
Program Director
Respiratory Care Program
Gateway Community College
Phoenix, Arizona

Susan Townsley, RRT, RPFT, RPSGT
Midwest Chest Consultants
St. Charles, Missouri

Brigham C. Willis, MD
Associate Professor of Pediatrics
University of Arizona College of Medicine—Phoenix
Co-Medical Director
Gateway Community College Respiratory Care Program
Phoenix, Arizona

Reviewers

Elaine K. Allen, RRT-NPS, RPFT, RPSGT
Respiratory Care Program Director
Laurel Technical Institute
Sharon, Pennsylvania

Allen W. Barbaro, MS, RRT
Department Chair
Respiratory Care Education
St. Luke's College–UnityPoint Health
Sioux City, Iowa

Susan Blonshine, BS, RRT, RPFT, FAARC, AE-C
President/CEO
TechEd Consultants,Inc.
Mason, Michigan

Margaret-Ann Carno, PhD, MBA, RN, CPNP, D,ABSM, FNAP, FAAN
Associate Professor of Clinical Nursing and Pediatrics
University of Rochester
School of Nursing
Rochester, New York

Christine A. Hamilton, DHSc, RRT, PD
Cardio-Respiratory Care Program Director and Assistant Professor
College of Health Sciences
Tennessee State University
Nashville, Tennessee

Chris Kallus, MEd., RRT
Professor and Program Director
Victoria College
Victoria, Texas

Jennifer L. Keely, MEd, RRT-ACCS
Assistant Clinical Professor
Respiratory Therapy Program
School of Health Professions
University of Missouri
Columbia, Missouri

Shane Keene, DHSc, MBA, RRT-NPS, CPFT, RPSGT, RST
Department Head, Department of Analytical and Diagnostic Sciences
Associate Professor, Director Respiratory Therapy Program
College of Allied Health Sciences
University of Cincinnati
Cincinnati, Ohio

J. Kenneth LeJeune, MS, RRT, CPFT
Program Director
Respiratory Education
University of Arkansas Community College–Hope
Hope, Arkansas

Joel S. Livesay, MS, RRT
Department Chair, Respiratory Care
Spartanburg Community College
Spartanburg, South Carolina

Cory E. Martin, EdS, RRT
Program Director and Associate Professor
Volunteer State Community College
Gallatin, Tennessee

Kerry J. McNiven, MS, RRT
Professor and Director of Clinical Education
Manchester Community College
Manchester, Connecticut

Ronald P. Mlcak, PhD, RRT, FAARC
Director
Respiratory Care
Shriners Hospital for Children
Galveston, Texas

Jill Sand, MEd, RRT
Program Director Respiratory Care
Southeast Community College
Lincoln, Nebraska

Paula Denise Silver, BS Biology, PharmD.
Medical Instructor
ECPI University
Newport News, Virginia

Shawna Strickland, PhD, RRT-NPS, AE-C, FAARC
Clinical Associate Professor
Director, Respiratory Therapy Program
School of Health Professions
University of Missouri
Columbia, Missouri

Michael D. Werner, MS, RRT, CPFT
Respiratory Therapy Program Director
Concorde Career College–North Hollywood
Los Angeles, California

James R. Woods, MS, RRT, RPFT
Program Chair
Respiratory Care
Florida State College at Jacksonville
Jacksonville, Florida

Foreword

I am honored to write the forward for this first edition of *Respiratory Care Clinical Competency Lab Manual*. I am honored because after 23 years of teaching, I see a new generation of leaders in respiratory therapy education beginning to take their place. Sandra Hinski was among a group of shining stars in our first integrated master's-entry class at Georgia State University a few years ago and now, as she continues to excel, she serves on the faculty at Gateway Community College. I am honored to write the forward for this text because this is an opportunity to introduce new students in our profession to the importance of technical problem solving and critical thinking in respiratory care. The acuity of patients in acute care settings, particularly the intensive care units, requires respiratory therapists to perform at the highest practice level. Sandra, with her vast knowledge of emergency medical care and respiratory care, has provided a text that offers students a clear pathway to laboratory competencies that must be rendered competently at the patient's bedside. And finally, I am honored because a former student has done something that I have not done!! Sandra has written a textbook so that future students may benefit from her experience!

To use a cliché, a new lab manual is needed for clinical competency and is well overdue. Not that the one or two texts we've had in the past have been poorly written, but there has been a limited variety of lab competency manuals for educators to choose from. Students in our classrooms today are part of what has been coined "digital natives"[1] or the "Net generation[2]" due to their familiarity with information and communication technology. From my "analog" or "digital immigrant" perspective as one who has had to adapt to technology my entire career, I see where students today think and process information fundamentally differently from the way my school classmates and I learned. Today's "digital natives" are described as receiving and processing information rapidly and with an uncanny ability to multitask. This will bode well for students entering the health care arena today with the fast-paced, monitor-driven, complex ICUs in which they will practice in the future. The exercises used in this laboratory manual will assist students in becoming competent in technical modalities that are essential for quality patient care. I also believe that mastery of these procedures will reveal that the analog term "team" is to be replaced with the digital "integrative care" concept that is necessary in the delivery of patient services for the 21st century.

Lynda T. Goodfellow
Professor of Respiratory Therapy
Georgia State University

[1]Prensky, M. "Digital Natives, Digital Immigrants" *On the Horizon,* NCB University Press, Vol. 9 No. 5, October2001. Accessed at: http://www.nnstoy.org/download/technology/Digital%20Natives%20-%20Digital%20Immigrants.pdf on October 10, 2013.

[2]Oblinger, DG & Oblinger JL. Educating the Net Generation, Educause. ISBN 0-9672853-2-1 Accessed at: https://net.educause.edu/ir/library/pdf/pub7101.pdf on October 10, 2013.

A Note to Students

I feel like it was just yesterday I sat in my very first respiratory therapy class. My professors captivated me with every word, the field of respiratory therapy intrigued me, and the future the profession was offering was limitless. I reminisced about all of those feelings while writing this book. My intentions for this book are to offer you, the student, a practical learning tool to help aid in your transition from the classroom and lab setting to the clinical world, as well as to support educators with meaningful lab activities. Clinical experience cannot be taught,

but a strong foundation that begins in the lab setting is a great way to start. Deliberate practice can develop into the skilled performance of procedural assessments with motivation by you as a student and guidance from an instructor. I hope you will use this book as your starting point for a life of learning in the field of respiratory care.

—**Sandra T. Hinski**

Preface

Current trends in the respiratory therapy profession are advancing, requiring students to attain a larger knowledge base. The expanding scope of practice of the respiratory therapist presents a challenge to the educational process in preparing students with the skills, knowledge, and competencies necessary to meet the demands of the profession and provide the best patient care. *Respiratory Care Clinical Competency Lab Manual* provides the practical skills an RT student will need to bridge classroom theory with clinical practice.

Respiratory Care Clinical Competency Lab Manual is not intended to be all-inclusive of every task and every piece of respiratory equipment that may be encountered in the profession, nor is it intended to be used as a replacement for theoretical knowledge found in the respiratory care texts. We have chosen to follow the content coverage in *Egan's Fundamentals of Respiratory Care*, 10th edition, as it is comprehensive in its coverage of topics for respiratory therapy competencies; however, *Respiratory Care Clinical Competency Lab Manual* has the flexibility to be used in conjunction with other respiratory care titles. Special attention has been given to the National Board for Respiratory Care (NBRC) content outlines and the Committee on Accreditation for Respiratory Care (CoARC) competencies. All procedures are in compliance with the American Association for Respiratory Care (AARC) Clinical Practice Guidelines (CPGs).

Organization

Laboratory skills are an essential part of the educational process for the respiratory therapist. To enable the student to practice and assess cognitive and psychomotor skills in relation to the knowledge acquired in their text, *Respiratory Care Clinical Competency Lab Manual* includes detailed step-by-step procedures, supporting procedural illustrations, hands-on lab exercises, case studies, and critical thinking questions. Chapters follow the developing therapist's skill base, beginning with simple procedures and progressing to the most advanced skills. Special care has been placed in ordering the chapters in a way to aid the novice learner through a likely progression of their respiratory therapy curriculum.

Evaluation and assessment of a student's ability to understand and apply theoretical knowledge by demonstrating a specific skill is also an important element in the process of teaching and learning. To this end, *Respiratory Care Clinical Competency Lab Manual* includes clinical performance and procedural competency evaluation forms called Procedure Assessments. Most of these helpful assessment tools are included in the text and all are on Evolve (**http://evolve.elsevier.com/Hinski/respcarelabmanual/**) for multiple student assessment opportunities. Students can assess their progress and educators can measure performance.

Features

Objectives

Each chapter begins with a clearly stated set of learning objectives. This becomes your "learning checklist."

Key Terms

This is a list of terms you might encounter as you review topics for the skills covered in a particular chapter. All terms are defined in the Glossary located in the back of the book.

Content Review Topics

Content Review Topics list the content you will want to review using a comprehensive fundamentals text, such as *Egan's Fundamentals of Respiratory Care*. Other resources such as the NBRC Therapist Content Outline and CoARC's Respiratory Therapy Competencies can also be used.

Procedural Checklists

Step-by-step procedural competencies, from procedure preparation and evaluation, through implementation and documentation, cover the RT competency areas established by the American Association of Respiratory Care (AARC) and meet the national practice standards for patient care.

Reality Check Boxes

Reality Checks = Practical knowledge you're going to need in real practice!

Tip Boxes

Tips = Instructional theory-based information

Positive patient outcomes are reliant on the respiratory therapist's level of competence in not only theoretical knowledge, but cognitive and psychomotor skills. Interpersonal skills and specific behavioral attributes must be developed to become competent in the profession and provide optimal care for patients. Knowing how to communicate with other professionals, as well as with patients, is equally important for the respiratory professional to succeed in providing the best possible patient care. Although each chapter contains elements of successful patient communication, Chapter 30 provides specific content on preparing for clinical rotations that will help you get ready for this important aspect of your education.

Answer Keys for the Lab Activities, Self-Assessment Questions, and the Case Studies can be found on (**http://evolve.elsevier.com/Hinski/respcarelabmanual/**).

It is also important for you to know that you won't always be "just a student..." The profession is just around the corner! The final section in this text, Preparing to Enter the Respiratory Care Profession, will help to lead you toward the final step on your journey.

Acknowledgments

Many people go through life without a mentor or a person that truly guides them. I have two. I owe everything I have learned, intend to learn, where I am, and where I want to be to Lynda Goodfellow and Toni Rodriguez. I explain to people that I have had the pedigree of respiratory care education and career because I studied under Dr. Goodfellow and work with Dr. Rodriguez. How could it get any better than that? I cannot thank them enough for their profound influence on the instructor, professional, and person I am. I am blessed. I also want to thank my instructors Bob, Doug, Chip, Mcryl, Larry, and Arzu for opening my mind and making me love the field of respiratory care. Their philosophies and styles have influenced how I teach.

I need to thank Billie Sharp, Elsevier Content Manager, who, two years ago, asked me the question "Would you be interested in writing a book?", for having faith in me that I could do it, even when I was a bit unsure. I could not have accomplished this endeavor without Kathleen Sartori, Elsevier Content Development Specialist, or as I refer to her "my editor, Kathy the Great." Her guidance and support has been fundamental to the completion of this first edition.

I would like to thank Toni, Ed, Kathy, Doug, Jon, Wendi, Brig, and Susan for their contributions to this text. I could not have done it without them. Also, thank you to all the reviewers for their insight and advice during revisions.

I would like to thank my friend Alison for the life-long friendship we formed during respiratory therapy school and Diane for showing me what a true professional is.

Last, but not least, none of this would have been possible without the love and support from my husband, Bill, our two children Charlie and Stella, and my mom.

—Sandra T. Hinski

Contents

Contents

Preparing for Clinical Rotations

▪ OBJECTIVES

Upon the completion of the chapter activities and content review topics, the student should be able to:

1. Identify lab and clinical policies, procedures, and safety guidelines.
2. Identify the incident reporting process.
3. Identify all requirements for clinical placement.
4. Identify the role of the respiratory care student in the lab and clinical setting.

▪ KEY TERMS

- Incident
- Rapid response team
- Vaccines

▪ CONTENT REVIEW TOPICS

- Joint Commission
- Professionalism

▪ PROCEDURAL ASSESSMENT

1-1 Incident Reporting

▪ EQUIPMENT

- Program policy manual
- Clinical schedule

The idea of taking care of a "real" patient is an exciting idea to some students but completely terrifying to others. Your time in the controlled setting of the lab must be optimized as to prepare you for your first patient encounters as a respiratory care student. The clinical experience is, first and foremost, your chance to hone your skills and learn as much as you possibly can. But it is also the longest job interview you will ever have. Respect should be given to all staff you encounter, from nurses, to medical students, to the cleaning staff. Bad impressions could come back to haunt you.

During your time as a student at a clinical site, it is the staff's job to evaluate you as a student. But they are also looking at you as a potential employee. Attitude, professionalism, appearance, punctuality, and preparedness are all qualities the clinical site faculty will be assessing in you when you are a student at their facility. You should be eager to learn and respectfully communicate your needs as a student. Although it is true that your clinical rotations are your opportunity to see firsthand how disease affects patients, you should always be aware that the diseases you find interesting may be horrifying for the patient. On the one hand, try not to act overexcited when learning or seeing a procedure. On the other hand, standing in the corner of a patient's room surfing the net on your cell phone is not acceptable. You must maintain a level of professionalism at all times.

This chapter will cover the basic steps you should take as a student to make the most out of your laboratory instruction and how to most effectively apply these practices directly into your clinical rotations. Remember, you never get a second chance to make a first impression.

> ✳ **Tip** Some clinical affiliates require the student to have a site-specific background check or a Level One Fingerprint Clearance Card, which requires a higher eligibility standard to receive than a regular Clearance Card.*

*Law specific to the state of Arizona, but most facilities require background checks.

⟫ SKILL CHECK LIST

1-1 Incident Reporting

Incident reporting is a very important part of the health care system. An incident is any event not consistent with the routine operation of a health care unit or routine care of a patient. As a student, you must be aware of the steps an educational institution or a clinical site requires you to follow regarding an incident in which harm was caused, a near-miss incident, or an incident that caused no harm. Although not a part of the patient's permanent medical record, incident reports are used by risk management and other similar departments as a source of data. They may be used to identify the source of errors and how to prevent future incidents. Examples of incident report entries can be found in Table 1-1. The following is the step-by-step process for incident reporting.

Procedural Preparation

1. Review the patient chart.
2. Verify the physician's order or the facility's protocol for standard of care.

TABLE 1-1 Examples of Respiratory Care Incident Entries

Correct Entry	Incorrect Entry
6 PM Patient found on floor at foot of bed with oxygen tubing tangled around the left ankle; able to respond to name when called. 2-cm abrasion noted across left forehead. Vital signs stable. Dr. Smith notified and arrived on floor at 6:15 PM. Nurse placed patient on fall-prevention protocol.	Patient found on floor at foot of bed, probably fell on way to bathroom. Small abrasion over left forehead. Dr. Smith notified. Patient instructed to use call light when needing to go to bathroom.
Administered albuterol sulfate 2.5 mL via nebulization. 2.5 mg ordered. Monitored vital signs q 15 minutes; called Dr. Jones; vital signs remain stable.	Administered 2.5 mL morphine sulfate at 4 PM without checking vial for concentration before administering. 2.5 mg albuterol sulfate ordered.
Needlestick to right index finger; caused minimal bleeding. Notified employee health department.	Needlestick to right index finger, likely from needle left in bed linen after blood drawing. Notified employee health.

Modified from Perry AG, Potter PA: *Clinical nursing skills and techniques*, ed 7, St. Louis, MO, 2010, Mosby.

3. Obtain, clean, and inspect the appropriate equipment prior to entering the patient's room.
4. Follow personal protective equipment (PPE) requirements, and observe standard precautions for any transmission-based isolation procedure.
5. Identify the patient using two patient identifiers.
6. Introduce yourself to the patient and to the family.
7. Explain the procedure to the patient and to the family, and acknowledge the patient's understanding.
8. Perform proper hand hygiene, and put on gloves, mask, and protective eyewear, as appropriate for procedure.

Implementation

1. Report accurate, objective information in chronological order.
2. Restore the patient's safety.
3. Assess the extent of injury.
4. Notify the proper medical personnel needed to treat the patient if he or she is injured.
5. If the injured party is not a patient of the facility, refer him or her to the appropriate location for evaluation.
6. If the injured party is a patient, assess and implement any ordered therapies.

Documentation and Reporting

1. Complete an incident report promptly.
2. Document the events of the incident in the patient's chart, if applicable.
3. Deliver the report to the appropriate designated department.

Bibliography

Kacmarek RM, Stoller JK, Heuer AJ: *Egan's fundamentals of respiratory care*, ed 10, St. Louis, MO, 2013, Mosby.

Rapid Response Teams: http://www.aarc.org/resources/rapid _response. Accessed March 2012.

The Joint Commission: http://www.jointcommission.org. Accessed March 2012.

Vaccines.gov: http://www.vaccines.gov/more_info/glossary/ index.html. Accessed April 2012.

1. Use your program's policy and procedure manual or course syllabus to answer the following questions:

    a. What time is the lab open for extra practice?

_____

    b. What is the policy regarding lab attire?

_____

    c. What is the dress code and hygiene code for students in the clinical setting?

_____

    d. What is the policy regarding the use of perfumes and colognes by students?

_____

    e. Is eating or drinking allowed in the lab or clinical settings?

_____

    f. What is the cell phone policy in the lab and at clinical sites?

_____

    g. As a student, are you allowed to access the Internet using the computers at your clinical site?

_____

    h. What is the attendance policy for the lab and for clinicals?

_____

    i. What are the clinical requirements and procedural assessments that must be completed after graduation?

_____

    j. What should you do if you are injured during lab or clinical time?

_____

    k. What should you do if you have an accidental needlestick or exposure to a body substance?

_____

    l. What is the smoking policy at your clinical site?

_____

    m. Are you allowed to take equipment home or outside the lab?

_____

n. How are you required to report absences from a clinical shift?

_____

o. Are you required to take a drug test before attending clinicals?

_____

p. What are the "for cause" drug testing policies in your program?

_____

q. What is the name of the medical director for your program?

_____

2. Have your lab partner simulate a fall injury. Using the incident reporting checklist, write an incident report, and present it to your instructor.

> ✳ **Tip** Facilities are transitioning into electronic medical records for all patients. At times, they have policies in place regarding the charting of persons other than patients who are involved in an incident requiring attention from hospital staff.

3. Review all of the requirements for clinical placement for your educational institution (Box 1-1). Respiratory programs as well as clinical affiliates often require numerous vaccines. Vaccines are defined as products that produce immunity thereby protecting the body from the disease (Box 1-2). Vaccines are administered through injections, by mouth, and by aerosol. Make a check list to ensure that you meet all criteria.

> → **Reality Check** Vaccines, drug testing, and background checks are costly, and the financial responsibility may fall on the student.

> → **Reality Check** It is important to understand that hospitals, long-term acute care centers, and other clinical affiliates may use different "lingo" when referring to locations within their facilities. It is imperative that you know what terms are used at a particular facility.

BOX 1-1	Additional Facility Requirements for Clinical Placement

- Healthcare cardiopulmonary resuscitation (CPR) card (American Heart Association)
- Department of Public Safety (DPS) fingerprint Clearance Card
- Health care physical examination
- Facility-specific background checks
- Drug screening
- Nicotine testing

BOX 1-2	Common Vaccine Requirements

- MMR (measles, mumps, rubella): 2 doses, or positive titer for all three diseases
- Varicella (chicken pox): 2 doses, or positive titer
- Tetanus (Td or TDap): 1 dose within past 10 years
- Annual influenza vaccination
- Hepatitis B: 3 doses, or positive titer
- Two-step tuberculosis (TB) testing, annual test, or both
  - Chest x-ray, if positive protein purified derivative (PPD)
  - TB symptom form

4. Define the following acronyms:

a. ACLS_____

b. BLS_____

c. CPG_____

d. CPR_____

e. HIPAA_____

f. ICU_____

g. JCAHO_____

h. MICU_____

i. OSHA_____

j. SICU_____

k. CVICU_____

l. NICU_____

m. PICU_____

5. If you will be treating patients on mechanical ventilators, find out which ventilator(s) your clinical site uses. If you have that ventilator at your educational institution, become familiar with it. If not, use any textbook or online tools available to help you familiarize yourself with that particular ventilator.

> → **Reality Check** It is important to understand the objectives you have at different clinical sites (i.e., NICU/PICU rotation, floorcare, ICU). You should begin each rotation with a clear sense of the goals you need to accomplish while attending a specific site.

6. To ensure your timely arrival on your first day of clinical, do a test run to the site. Drive there, and make sure you know where to go and how long it will take you during specific times of the day, traffic, and so on. Confirm the location of the respiratory care department, where you need to check in, and the designated parking location for students.

7. Go to the American Association of Respiratory Care website (www.AARC.org) and locate information on "Rapid Response." Read the information relating to rapid response teams. Write a synopsis for your instructor that answers the following questions:

a. Why were rapid response teams started?

_____

b. Who organized this effort, and what is the key part of the original plan?

_____

c. Why is it important for a respiratory therapist (RT) to be part of a rapid response team?

_____

Self-Assessment Questions

1. What is the primary purpose for HIPAA standards?
   A. To provide a medical record number for each patient
   B. To allow for charts to be organized easily
   C. To provide patients with more control over the use and disclosure of their medical information
   D. To protect the medical information of politicians

2. Where is protected health information located?
   A. In paper charts
   B. In computer charts
   C. In conversations between health care workers
   D. All of the above

3. Which of the following are patient safety goals of the Joint Commission?
   1. To ensure that all patients spend 1 week or less hospitalized
   2. To improve accuracy of patient identification
   3. To decrease the cost of medications to facilities
   4. To improve the effectiveness of communicating critical test values among caregivers

   A. 1, 2, and 3 only
   B. 1 and 2 only
   C. 2 and 4 only
   D. 1, 2, 3, and 4

4. Which of the following situations are examples of incidents?
   1. Patient falls
   2. PRN (as needed) medication administration
   3. A needlestick injury
   4. Medication error

   A. 1 and 2 only
   B. 2 and 3 only
   C. 1, 3, and 4 only
   D. 1, 2, 3, and 4

5. A needlestick injury incident report involving a respiratory therapist is part of the patient's permanent medical record.
   A. True
   B. False

>> **CASE STUDY 1-1**

You are a student on the first day of your clinical rotation on the general floor when your preceptor gets a call from a nurse regarding a patient's status. You follow your preceptor to the patient's room. During your initial patient assessment, you determine that the patient's vital signs are failing and that the patient is in severe respiratory distress.

1. What should you do?

_____

_____

2. What is the purpose of a rapid response team?

_____

_____

>> **CASE STUDY 1-2**

You are a respiratory care student completing your last rotation before graduation. You still need to observe a patient receiving high-frequency ventilation. You and another student, Sherry, are assigned to the same preceptor. It is the first clinical rotation for Sherry, who is very pushy and wants to take all the treatments assigned for the first part of the shift. You say nothing and let it happen. Later that morning, the shift supervisor approaches your preceptor and asks which student wants to assist in transitioning a patient from conventional ventilation to the oscillator. Sherry quickly speaks up and requests to assist.

1. What should you do?

_____

_____

>> **CASE STUDY 1-3**

It is your first day at a clinical site. The lead RT assigns you a preceptor to follow for the day. The preceptor is very reluctant to have a student and tells you, "I don't like working with students. They slow me down."

1. What should you do?

_____

_____

Procedural Assessment forms are available online at http://evolve.elsevier.com/Hinski/respcarelabmanual/

Quality and Evidence-based Respiratory Care

■ OBJECTIVES

Upon the completion of the chapter activities and content review topics, the student should be able to:

1. Describe the role and responsibilities of a respiratory care medical director.
2. Identify American Association for Respiratory Care's (AARC) Clinical Practice Guidelines (CPGs) as a respiratory care information source.
3. Explain how protocols are used.
4. Read and comment on a peer-reviewed piece of literature.
5. Define quality assurance in respiratory care.
6. Define evidence-based medicine.
7. Present a case study.

■ KEY TERMS

- Algorithms
- CPGs
- Evidence-based medicine
- Peer-reviewed literature
- Respiratory care protocols

■ CONTENT REVIEW TOPICS

- AARC's CPGs
- Committee on Accreditation for Respiratory Care (CoARC)
- Respiratory therapist competencies
- Respiratory disease management
- Institutional Review Board (IRB)

■ PROCEDURAL ASSESSMENTS

2-1 Case study Presentation

■ EQUIPMENT

- Access to a computer with word processing, PowerPoint, and Internet capabilities.

The field of respiratory care is continuously evolving. As a respiratory care student, you must be able to use peer-reviewed research papers to understand clinical practice and as references for papers and case study presentations. Once you graduate, you will be expected to apply these skills in your daily professional life and maintain current evidence-based practice.

This chapter directs you to describe the role a respiratory care medical director fills in a hospital and in an educational institution. Understanding peer-reviewed literature through article critiquing as well as issues relating to quality assurance in respiratory care will be discussed.

❯❯ SKILLS CHECK LIST

2-1 Case Study Presentation

Whether at a professional conference or on rounds with the health care team in the intensive care unit (ICU), comprehensible and purposeful patient presentation is important for conveying information in a conference lecture format or for providing care in the hospital setting. The following is the step-by-step process for a case study presentation.

During your academic career, you may be asked to present a patient in a case study format. Mastery of patient presentation in the oral form takes time and practice.

> → **Reality Check** Case presentation to faculty and other students can be practice for doing rounds with physicians and other health care team members when you are a licensed practitioner.

This does not happen overnight. Find a patient to present to the class. Gather the information listed in Box 2-1. You will need to gather all information necessary to discuss the patient's overall care in a comprehensive manner, focusing on the respiratory treatments provided. A format for case study presentations with an example can be found in Box 2-2. Your oral presentation can be reinforced by an accompanying PowerPoint presentation. Box 2-3 provides you with some very important tips when preparing and presenting your case study.

> ✳ **Tip** The purpose of the presentation is to provide the big picture to other clinicians. You are the one that saw the patient. You must tell the story in a coherent and inclusive way.

Procedural Preparation

Please note that patient interaction may not be a part of this skill. Presenting a patient from a chart review is also possible. Steps 1 through 3 will not be necessary if no patient interaction takes place.

1. Choose a patient with whom contact and respiratory assessment was performed.
2. Follow all facility protocols for patient interaction; interview the patient, and collect all pertinent data for presentation.
3. Follow PPE and observe standard precautions for any transmission-based isolation procedure, and perform a physical assessment of the patient.
4. Prepare a PowerPoint presentation to aid in oral case study presentation.

BOX 2-1	Information Required for Case Study Presentation of a Patient with Respiratory Illness

- Patient's age
- Patient's gender
- Chief complaint
- History of present illness
- Admission diagnosis
- Past medical history
- Relevant pulmonary history
- Social and environmental histories
- Physical assessment
- Vital Signs
- Laboratory tests, including arterial blood gases (ABGs), complete blood cell count (CBC), electrolytes, brain natriuretic peptide (BNP), albumin, and specific tests relating to medical history (e.g., liver or kidney function tests)
- Radiologic tests
- Medications
- If patient is on noninvasive or invasive mechanical ventilation, identify the apparatus being used to deliver treatment, get the set parameters and mode along with actual values

5. Prepare any materials that will be needed by your audience.

Implementation

1. Dress professionally on the day of the presentation.
2. Identify yourself to your audience.
3. State the patient's age, gender, and pertinent demographic information.
4. State the chief complaint.
5. State the history of the patient's present illness.
6. State the admitting diagnosis.
7. State the past medical history, and identify the relevant pulmonary history.
8. State the patient's social and environmental histories.
9. Provide a well-ordered explanation of the physical assessment and a relevant review of systems information.
10. Provide and explain all laboratory data and radiologic test results.
11. List the patient's medications, with focus on the respiratory medications.
12. Describe the effect of the medications on the patient's respiratory condition.
13. Clearly describe all respiratory care modalities performed.

Evaluation of Procedure

1. Compare the actual management of the patient with textbook management.
2. Develop appropriate respiratory care plan based on information, and evaluate current care using CPGs.
3. Give a patient update.

Documentation and Reporting

1. Ensure that the PowerPoint or other media presentation material is easy to read with no misspellings and no inappropriate use of acronyms.
2. Do not use patient identifiers during presentation.
3. Do not criticize the care given by any of the health care providers involved in the care of the patient.
4. Present the case study in a timely manner.
5. Submit the corresponding case study written paper according to rubric.

BOX 2-2	Format for Oral Case Study Presentation

Chief Complaint (CC)

Only one complaint answers the question, "What is the patient's reason for seeking a medical evaluation?" It should also set the tone for the rest of the presentation. It is not a laundry list of all the patient's problems, that is, it should not be too inclusive. It needs to be direct and focused to one main issue.

   Example: "Mr. T is a 59-year-old male with COPD (chronic obstructive pulmonary disease), who presented in the emergency department with a chief complaint of shortness of breath."

History of Present Illness (HPI)

The history of present illness needs to be presented as a chronologic description of the patient's symptoms and should be centered on the patient's chief complaint. Very often, a patient with pulmonary disease has more than one problem. This overlapping

of problems and how these problems relate to the pulmonary issue need to be linked together when presenting

 Reality Check Interpreting which past information is important and which is nonessential depends on clinical experience and a keen understanding of pathophysiology. Mastering this will take time, a lot of examination of patients, and a lot of patience.

Depending on how progressed you are in your respiratory care education, your ability to link all this together may be quite limited.
   Example: "Mr. T was diagnosed with COPD in 1992 and has been leading a relatively active life until recently. Mr. T had been

BOX 2-2 Format for Oral Case Study Presentation—cont'd

able to walk unassisted to his shed and gather gardening equipment without feeling short of breath until approximately 3 week ago when this activity began to cause dyspnea. This dyspnea on exertion progressed to dyspnea at rest. About 2 days ago, he developed a fever along with a wet cough, which produced yellow-colored sputum. He has spent the last 24 hours in bed. He denies chest pain, headache, hemoptysis, abdominal pain, and diarrhea. He denies any history of asthma, myocardial infarction, or congestive heart failure."

Past Medical History (PMH)

This includes all of the patient's past medical problems. Although all are listed, focus should be on the past medical problems that are related to the patient's current complaint. Information in this section should also include immunizations, allergies, medication, habits, and a description of the patient's general health.

> → **Reality Check** Patients may lie about parts of their history because they are embarrassed or are intentionally trying to hide the truth.

Example: "The patient's PMH includes the following:
1. *COPD*
2. *Hypertension*
3. *Gastroesophageal reflux disease*
4. *Cholecystectomy in 1985*

The patient denies any alcohol or illicit drug use. He is compliant with his medications and up to date with his flu vaccination. He did not receive a pneumonia vaccine this year. He smoked 2 packs a day for 20 years and quit in 1992, which gives him a 40-pack year history. The patient takes the following medications: Lopressor 50 mg, PO, bid Combivent: ipratropium 18 micrograms per puff (mcg/puff) and albuterol 90 mcg/puff, qid and prn.

He has no allergies to medications that he is aware of."

Family History

The family history should emphasize the identification of illnesses within the family, especially among first-degree relatives (e.g., mother, father, grandmother, grandfather, siblings). Examples include history of coronary artery disease, diabetes, certain cancers, and so on.

Example: "Both of the patient's parents were killed in a motor vehicle collision 3 years ago. He is an only child."

Social and Environmental Histories

This section should include a brief description of the patient's work history, living arrangements, home environment, marital history, and history of hobbies and recreational. Special attention should be paid if the patient has a history of working in an environment that has known pulmonary pathologies that can be caused because of work-related exposure. An example of this would be coal mining.

Example: "Mr. T works as a bank manager a large financial institution in Phoenix, Arizona. He lives with his wife in a large house in the city. He likes to garden."

Physical Examination and Review of Systems

This section of the presentation should begin with a short description of the patient's appearance along with his vital signs.

Example: "Mr. T was sitting upright on the bed in the emergency room (ER), tripodding, breathing through a simple face
mask oxygen delivery system running at 7 liters per minute (LPM). His breathing was labored with accessory muscles use. Wheezing was audible to the naked ear.

Vital signs: Temp. 102°F, HR 122, BP 150/90; RR 28, SpO_2 89% on SFM at 7 LPM.

Head, Eyes, Ears, Nose, Throat (HEENT): Pupils equal, round and reactive to light; no drainage from ears; airway patent; mucosa dry.

Lungs: Inspiratory and expiratory wheezing during auscultation throughout lung fields, with breath sounds diminished in the right lower lobe. Dullness to percussion and increased fremitus were also appreciated at the right lower lobe.

Heart (cardiac): Rhythm was sinus tachycardia.

Abdomen: Symmetric appearing; soft, non-tender; no palpable masses; well healed incisions at sites of prior cholecystectomy.

Extremities: No evidence of clubbing, cyanosis, or edema.

Skin: No skin abnormalities identified.

Neurologic: Awake, alert, and appropriately oriented to person, place, and time.

Laboratory Results, Radiologic Studies, Electrocardiograms (ECGs)

You should try to limit the information presented in this section to the laboratory values pertinent to your differential diagnosis, as well as values that are abnormal. Likewise, if the interpretations of any radiologic studies are directly relevant to the case, they most certainly should be discussed.

Example: "Mr. T's laboratory work was remarkable for white blood cell (WBC) count of 19,000 with 12% bands; a sputum culture is pending; room air arterial blood gas: pH of 7.46, $PaCO_2$ of 59, $PaHCO_3^-$ 33, PaO_2 49. Chest x-ray showed a dense right lower lobe infiltrate without effusion and hyperinflation consistent with acute exacerbation of COPD."

Impression and Plan

A summary of the important features of the history, physical examination, and laboratory tests should be presented to devise a differential diagnosis for your patient. A respiratory care plan should be implemented and must include the physician's findings and corroboration.

Example: "Mr. T is a patient with COPD, who presents with an exacerbation of his COPD along with an acute pulmonary process. The sputum culture needs follow-up to determine proper antibiotic therapy. The rapid progression of his dyspnea, coupled with findings on lung examination and chest radiography, suggest an infection. The respiratory care plan is as follows:
1. *Follow up on cultures of sputum.*
2. *Establish an appropriate oxygen therapy modality with the goal to keep saturation between 88% and 92%.*
3. *Add patient education on coughing technique.*
4. *Ensure that an advanced directive is in place.*
5. *If the patient does not show improvement (or his condition worsens), consider suggesting bronchoscopy to the physician."*

Question-and-Answer Time

Allow an ample amount of time for the audience to ask questions.

BOX 2-3	Important Tips for Preparing and Presenting a Case Study

- Remember, no one else saw this patient. You must be able to present it in a storylike way so the audience can follow along and understand all the aspects of the case.
- Practice, practice, practice. Do not be afraid to use notes if not following a PowerPoint presentation format.
- Watch how the physicians at a clinical site present a patient to other clinicians. Learn from their expertise.
- Do not get "caught up" in a patient's medical problems. Remember, your main audience is respiratory care students, faculty, and other practitioners. Focus on the respiratory care modalities. Try to be thorough about the respiratory procedures.

- Beware of the patient with renal problems. These patients and the way they present can be very confusing to a first-year student.
- Try a "dry run" with some fellow students. Ask for feedback from them. This will allow you to correct errors and improve after presentation of the case.
- *Never* use any information that could compromise patient confidentiality! This includes the patient's name, medical record number, photograph, or name of facility where the patient is being treated. This is a Health Insurance Portability and Accountability Act (HIPAA) violation. HIPAA is a federal law to protect the privacy and security of health information.

Kacmarek RM, Stoller JK, Heuer AJ: *Egan's fundamentals of respiratory care*, ed 10, St. Louis, MO, 2013, Mosby.

1. List the responsibilities of a respiratory care medical director.

_____

_____

_____

_____

_____

_____

2. Form groups of two or three fellow students, and pick a CPGs from the American Association for Respiratory Care (AARC) website to make a PowerPoint presentation to the class.

3. List six elements of a respiratory care protocol as described by the American College of Chest Physicians (ACCP). The protocol is available on ACCP's website.

_____

_____

_____

_____

_____

4. Complete a critique of an article from a peer-reviewed journal using the following rubric (Box 2-4). The topic should be related to some aspect of respiratory care.

BOX 2-4	Rubric Critique

Criteria Points = 100

Summary

Briefly summarize the main points of the article. What were the objectives, main findings, conclusions, and recommendations provided by the article? Was the main topic communicated effectively?

Summarized main points of article	15 pts
Summarized objectives, main findings, conclusions, and/or recommendations	15 pts

Critique

Presented strengths of the article, including examples	10 pts
Presented weaknesses of the article, including examples	10 pts
Identified contributions to the literature	10 pts
Addressed importance of article to the field, including why other health care providers would read the article	10 pts
Provided personal reactions to the article	10 pts
Critiqued article is refereed and/or research based and is related to the selected topic	10 pts
Followed the format (e.g., copy of article is attached, article critique is double-spaced, 12 point font, one-inch margins, no more than 2 pages)	10 pts
TOTAL	100 pts

5. List the nine steps for a quality assurance plan.

_____

_____

_____

_____

_____

_____

_____

_____

6. What are cohort studies?

_____

7. What is evidence-based medicine?

_____

_____

_____

Self-Assessment Questions

1. Who is the medical professional in charge of the clinical function of a respiratory care department?
   A. Medical director
   B. Attending pulmonologist
   C. Clinical educator
   D. Lead respiratory therapist

2. Which committee ensures the quality of a respiratory care education program?
   A. IRB
   B. AARC
   C. The National Board for Respiratory Care
   D. Committee for Accreditation of Respiratory Care

3. Which term is used to describe treatment based on careful review of available literature?
   A. Protocols
   B. Evidence-based medicine
   C. Physician orders
   D. Reviewed medicine

4. Which of the following are levels of general practice credentialing in respiratory care?
   A. Certified respiratory therapists (CRTs)
   B. Registered respiratory therapists (RRTs)
   C. Student respiratory therapist (RTS)
   D. A and B

5. The term used to describe guided pathways used to help direct specific aspects of a patient's treatment regimen is:
   A. Protocols
   B. Evidence-based medicine
   C. Physician orders
   D. Reviewed medicine

▶▶ CASE STUDY 2-1

A 72-year-old male patient is admitted to the general floor of a small community hospital with a diagnosis of asthma exacerbation. The patient has had no recent hospitalizations relating to his asthma, does not smoke cigarettes, and is generally in good health. His physical examination reveals a well-nourished male, semi-alert, with a respiratory rate of 34 breaths per minute and shallow breathing, and a heart rate of 102 beats per minute. Auscultation reveals inspiratory and expiratory wheezing anteriorly in the apices and bases.

1. Using the aerosol therapy protocol algorithm (see Figure 2-1), describe how you should deliver bronchodilator therapy to this patient.

_____

_____

2. This patient has Medicare as his primary insurance. What system has the federal government developed to evaluate the quality of care given to Medicare beneficiaries?

_____

_____

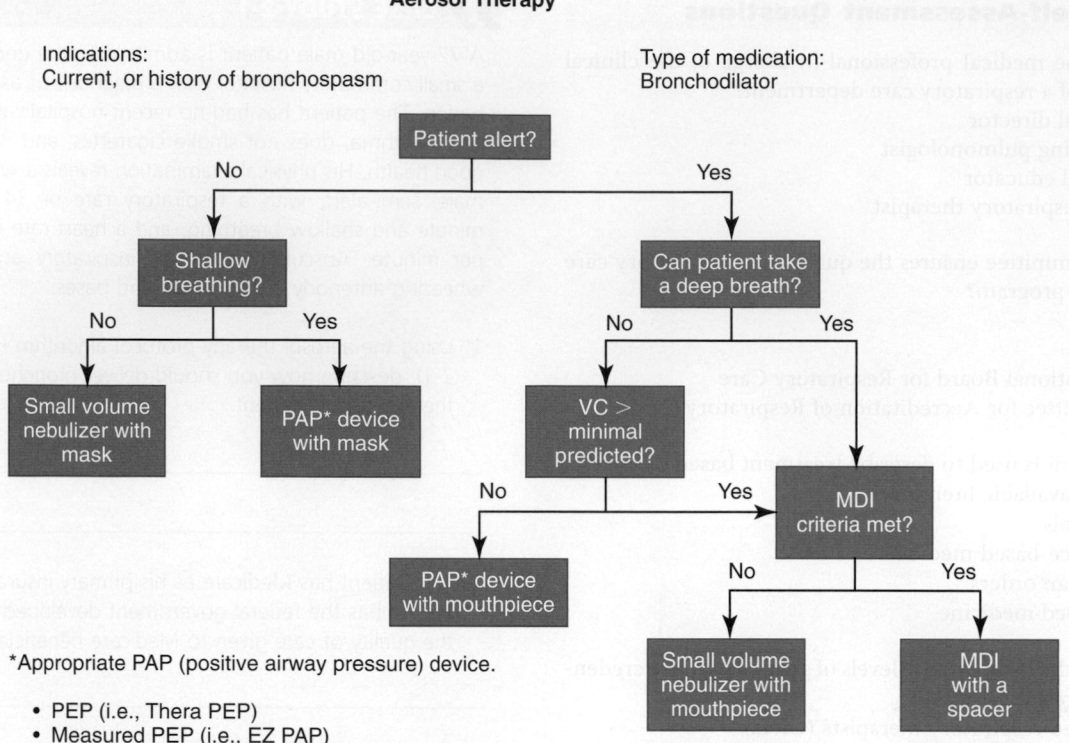

Figure 2-1 Respiratory care protocol. Aerosolized bronchodilator therapy algorithm for current or history of bronchospasm. (From Kacmarek, RM, Stoller, JK and Heuer AJ: *Egan's fundamentals of respiratory care*, ed 10, St. Louis, MO, 2013, Mosby.)

Procedural Assessment forms are available online at http://evolve.elsevier.com/Hinski/respcarelabmanual/

Patient Safety, Communication, and Medical Records

▪ OBJECTIVES

Upon the completion of the chapter activities and content review topics, the student should be able to:

1. Document a respiratory care progress note.
2. Give a verbal change-of-shift report.
3. Identify the proper body mechanics involved in safely moving a patient.
4. Identify the read-back and verified process.

▪ KEY TERMS

- Ambulation
- Health Insurance Portability and Accountability Act (HIPAA)

▪ CONTENT REVIEW TOPICS

- Problem-oriented medical record (POMR)
- SOAP format
- Two-patient identifier system

▪ PROCEDURAL ASSESSMENTS

3-1 Documenting Respiratory Care Progress Notes
3-2 Giving a Change-of-Shift Report
3-3 Safe Patient Transfer

▪ EQUIPMENT

- Patient transfer board
- Draw sheet
- Hospital bed(s)
- Stretcher

The health care team has the responsibility to provide patients with a safe environment that promotes the best possible medical care. As part of that team, the respiratory care student has the duty to make every effort to prepare for the clinical setting by understanding procedures that promote safety and excellent patient care. These procedures start in the lab and may be conveyed into the clinical setting.

This chapter will focus on ways to practice safely and reinforce the skills needed to effectively communicate in both the laboratory and clinical settings. Safety and communication go hand in hand in the hospital realm. Practical application in the laboratory setting will help strengthen good practice habits.

≫ SKILL CHECK LISTS

3-1 Documenting Respiratory Care Progress Notes

Charting is one of the most important tasks that a respiratory therapist (RT) performs.

> **✱ Tip** Remember the saying, "If you didn't chart it, you didn't do it."

> → **Reality Check** Each facility has its own way of setting up patient charts. You will need to get used to the method of charting at many different facilities as a student. Some facilities do not let you chart as a student.

Consistency in charting helps ensure that a patient's care follows a plan and that everyone is "on the same page." The hopes of the U.S. government are that by 2014, all medical records and charting will be electronic. Medical records are legal documents, and the information they contain is protected under the Health Insurance Portability and Accountability Act (HIPAA). Respiratory care usually has a specialized therapy portion of the patent's chart, which is used to record information. However, the entire chart is essential to you as an RT, and you should be utilizing the information in it throughout your patient's hospitalization to ensure that all body systems are taken into account when managing pulmonary problems (Box 3-1). The following is the step-by-step process for documenting respiratory care progress notes.

Procedural Preparation
Note that the following eight steps are basic preparation steps that should be observed before any patient interaction:
1. Review the patient's chart.
2. Verify the physician's order or the facility's protocol for standard of care.

BOX 3-1   General Sections Found in a Patient's Medical Record

Admission Sheet
Records pertinent patient information (e.g., name, address, religion, nearest of kin), admitting physician, and admission diagnosis

History and Physical Examination
Records the patient's admitting history and physical examination findings, as performed by the attending physician or resident

Health Maintenance and Immunizations
Records the dates of administration

Physician's Orders
Records the physician's orders and prescriptions

Progress Sheet
Keeps a continuing account of the patient's progress for the physician

Nurses' Notes
Describes the nursing care given to the patient, including the patient's complaints (subjective symptoms), the nurses' observations (objective signs), and the patient's response to therapy

Medication Record
Notes drugs and intravenous fluids that are given to the patient

Allergies
Notes reaction, severity, type, and date observed

Vital Signs Graphic Sheet
Records the patient's temperature, pulse, respirations, and blood pressure over time

I/O Sheet
Records patient's fluid intake (I) and output (O) over time

Laboratory Sheet
Summarizes the results of laboratory tests

Consultation Sheet
Records notes by physicians who are called in to examine a patient to make a diagnosis

Surgical or Treatment Consent
Records the patient's authorization for surgery or treatment

Anesthesia and Surgical Record
Notes key events before, during, and immediately after surgery

Specialized Therapy Records or Progress Notes
Records specialized treatments or treatment plans and patient progress for various specialized therapeutic services (e.g., respiratory care, physical therapy)

Specialized Flow Sheets
Records measurement made over time during specialized procedures (e.g., mechanical ventilation, kidney dialysis)

Advanced Directives
Records wishes and documents regarding living wills, power of attorney and Do Not Resuscitate (DNR) orders

From Kacmarek RM, Stoller JK, Heuer AJ: *Egan's fundamentals of respiratory care*, ed 10 , St. Louis, MO, 2013, Mosby.

---

3. Obtain, clean, and inspect appropriate equipment prior to entering the patient's room.
4. Follow personal protective equipment (PPE) requirements, and observe standard precautions for any transmission-based isolation procedure.
5. Identify the patient using two patient identifiers.
6. Introduce yourself to the patient and to the family.
7. Explain the procedure to the patient and to the family and acknowledge patient understanding.
8. Perform proper hand hygiene, and put on gloves, mask, and protective eyewear, as appropriate for procedure.

Implementation

1. Complete a patient assessment and any interventions necessary, and note the patient's responses.
2. Remove supplies from the patient's room, and clean the area, as needed.
3. Remove PPE, and observe standard precautions prior to leaving the patient's room.
4. Use appropriate forms, and maintain these in their proper locations in the chart.
5. Document information in a timely manner. If you are using paper charting, ensure that these forms are legible.
6. Include significant patient status changes, findings, and progress toward any goals set.
7. Sign the note according to policy.

Documentation and Reporting

1. Report any abnormal findings to the appropriate health care provider, and document the provider's name and credentials.

3-2 Giving a Change-of-Shift Report

Although documentation is important when recording information in a patient's chart, effectively handing over care to the RT on the next shift is crucial to your patient's care and well-being. Prioritizing patients, prioritizing any tasks that need to be completed, any immediate concerns regarding patients, and upcoming tests or procedures requiring patient transport are all topics that should all be communicated in the change-of-shift report.

> ✳ **Tip** If you have a heavy patient load, make small notes on a piece of paper to ensure that no vital information is omitted from your report to the oncoming therapist. But remember to dispose of that paper in the proper container to ensure that no protected patient information is exposed.

The following is the step-by-step process for giving a change-of-shift report.

Procedural Preparation

1. Review the patient's chart.
2. Verify the physician's order or the facility's protocol for standard of care.
3. Obtain, clean, and inspect appropriate equipment prior to entering the patient's room.
4. Follow PPE requirements, and observe standard precautions for any transmission-based isolation procedure.
5. Identify the patient using two patient identifiers.
6. Introduce yourself to the patient and to the family.

7. Explain the procedure to the patient and to the family, and acknowledge the patient's understanding.
8. Perform proper hand hygiene, and put on gloves, mask, and protective eyewear, as appropriate for the procedure.
9. Assess the patient for risk of injury and determine the need for special transfer equipment.
10. Assess the patient for the presence of weakness, dizziness, or postural hypotension.
11. Determine the number of people needed to safely transfer the patient.

Implementation

1. Gather pertinent information regarding the patient and his or her condition.
2. Prioritize information.
3. Prepare a detailed description of the patient's current status.
4. Report any significant needs or changes.
5. Report the patient's postoperative, postdiagnostic, or post–therapeutic procedure status.
6. Make a clear verbal report to oncoming staff.
7. Respect the patient's privacy. Give the report in the appropriate location.

3-3 Safe Patient Transfer

Whether delivering medications, performing invasive procedures, or assisting a physician with bronchoscopy, patient safety is the RT's top priority. Patient movement from location to location requires planning to ensure patient safety. Ambulation, or walking, helps a patient take deep breaths, prevents problems associated with immobilization, and maintains normal activities of daily living. The following is the step-by-step process for the implementation portion procedural assessment for safe patient transfer techniques.

Procedural Preparation

1. Review the patient's chart.
2. Verify the physician's order or the facility's protocol for standard of care.
3. Obtain, clean, and inspect appropriate equipment prior to entering the patient's room.
4. Follow PPE requirements, and observe standard precautions for any transmission-based isolation procedure.
5. Identify the patient using two patient identifiers.
6. Introduce yourself to the patient and to the family.
7. Explain the procedure to the patient and to the family, and acknowledge the patient's understanding.
8. Perform proper hand hygiene, and put on gloves, mask, and protective eyewear, as appropriate for the procedure.
9. Assess the patient for risk of injury, and determine the need for special transfer equipment.
10. Assess the patient for the presence of weakness, dizziness, or postural hypotension.
11. Determine the number of people needed to safely transfer the patient.

Implementation

1. Instruct the patient to breathe normally.
2. Position the bed into the low position.
3. Ensure that all equipment (intravenous lines, oxygen tubing, etc.) is close to the patient, so that it will not get dislodged.

4. Assist the patient to the sitting position:
   a. Place the patient in the supine position; remove pillows.
   b. Place your feet apart to improve balance.
   c. Place one hand under the patient's shoulders and the other on the bed surface.
   d. Raise the patient to the sitting position.
   e. Have the patient push against the bed with your hand on the bed surface.
5. Assist the patient to the sitting position, using an electrical bed:
   a. Raise the head of the bed to 30 degrees.
   b. Place the patient on his or her side.
   c. Stand and turn diagonally to face the patient and the far corner of the bed.
   d. Place your feet apart to improve balance.
   e. Place your arm near the bed under the patient's shoulders.
   f. Place the other arm over the patient's thighs.
   g. Move the patient's lower legs and feet over the side of the bed.
   h. Shift your weight to elevate the patient, and remain in front of the patient until he or she has regained balance.
6. Assist the patient from the bed to the chair:
   a. Assist the patient to the sitting position on the side of the bed, with a chair placed in the appropriate spot.
   b. Apply the transfer belt or other aids, if needed.
   c. Ensure that the patient's footwear is nonskid.
   d. Keep your weight-bearing foot forward.
   e. Place your feet apart to improve balance.
   f. Flex your knees and hips and align your knees with the patient's knees.
   g. Grasp the transfer belt or the patient at sides.
   h. Rock the patient to the standing position on a count of three.
   i. Use your knees to maintain stability.
   j. Pivot on your foot that was farthest from chair.
   k. Instruct the patient to use the arm rests of the chair for support.
   l. Flex your hips and knees while lowering the patient into the chair.
   m. Ensure that the patient is sitting in the proper position.
7. Assist the patient in a horizontal transfer from the bed to the stretcher (or to a different bed):
   a. Determine the number of staff required for the transfer.
   b. Lock the bed brakes.
   c. Lower the head of the bed as tolerated by patient.
   d. Lower the side rails.
   e. Cross the patient's arms on his or her chest.
   f. Place the slide board under the patient with help from staff on the other side of the bed.
   g. Place the drawsheet on either side of the bed.
   h. Working together, turn the patient onto the side.
   i. Place the slide board under the drawsheet.
   j. Roll the patient back onto the slide board, gently.
   k. Line up the stretcher with the patient's bed. Lock the stretcher brakes.
   l. Both you and the other staff should position yourselves along the sides of the stretcher and the bed.
   m. Pull the drawsheet with the patient on it onto the stretcher while the other staff holds the slide board in place.
   n. Ensure that the patient is placed in the center of the stretcher. Raise the side rails. Cover the patient.

8. Remove supplies from the patient's room, and clean the area, as needed.
9. Remove PPE, and observe standard precautions prior to leaving the patient's room.

> → **Reality Check** Many facilities have special lift devices to assist with patient transfer.

Evaluation of Procedure
1. Assess the patient's vital signs.
2. Ask the patient if he or she is feeling dizzy or experiencing any pain during transfer.
3. Identify any unexpected outcomes.

Documentation and Reporting
1. Record the transfer procedure in the patient's chart.
2. Report any abnormal findings to the appropriate health care provider.

Bibliography
Gardenhire DS: *Rau's respiratory care pharmacology*, ed 8, St. Louis, MO, 2012, Mosby.
Kacmarek RM, Stoller JK, Heuer AJ: *Egan's fundamentals of respiratory care*, ed 10, St. Louis, MO, 2013, Mosby.

1. Write a progress report for the three patients below using the charts that follow. Have a lab partner review your notes to make certain that all pertinent information is included. Have lab partner sign below when the report is completed.

   a. A 62-year-old man has a long history of cough and shortness of breath (SOB) with multiple hospitalizations. He was admitted because of severe, worsening dyspnea. His vital signs were BP 156/110 mm Hg, HR 95 beats/min, RR 25 breaths/min, and oral temperature 38.3°C. He was using his accessory muscles of inspiration and pursed-lip breathing. An enlarged anteroposterior (AP) diameter of the chest could easily be seen. Expiration was prolonged, and auscultation revealed mild inspiratory and expiratory wheezing in the apices anteriorly. Following two puffs of Combivent via a metered dose inhaler (MDI) and holding chamber, the patients states his breathing is much better; his vital signs are BP 136/90 mm Hg, HR 85 beat/min, RR 16 breaths/min, and the wheezing has lessened.

Subjective →	Objective →	Assessment →	Plan →
Respiratory Assessment Flow Chart	Vital signs: RR ____ HR ____ BP ____ Temp. ____ On antipyretic agent? ☐ Yes ☐ No Chest assessment: Insp. _____ Palp. _____ Perc. _____ Ausc. _____ Radiography _____ Bedside spir.: PEFR $\bar{a}$____ $\bar{p}$____Tx SVC ____ FVC ____ NIF ____ Cough: ☐ Strong ☐ Weak Sputum production: ☐ Yes ☐ No Sputum char. _____		PRESENT PLAN PLAN MODIFICATIONS
Anterior R L Posterior L R			
Pt. name			
Age	Male	Female	ABG: pH____ Paco$_2$____HCO$_3^-$____ PaO$_2$____ Sao$_2$____ SpO$_2$____ Neg. O$_2$ transport factors _____		
Date	Time			
Admitting diagnosis			
Therapist	Other: _____		
Hospital			

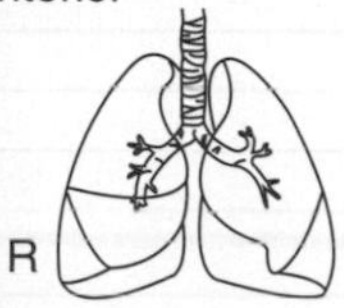

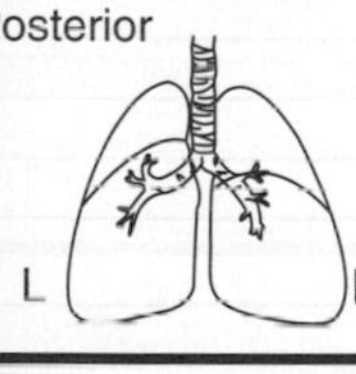

Figure 3-1 Respiratory care progress note. (From Des Jardins T, Burton GG: *Clinical manifestations and assessment of respiratory disease*, ed 6, St. Louis, MO, 2011, Mosby.)

Lab partner's signature for scenario a:_____

b. You are called to the emergency department (ED) to treat an 18-year-old female, who has been admitted with an acute asthma attack. She received two albuterol treatments prior to entering the ED. Her breath sounds reveal wheezes bilaterally in the apices and bases posteriorly, and she is unable to perform a peak expiratory flow rate (PEFR) test. Vital signs are BP 130/90 mm Hg, HR 120 beats/min, RR 26 breaths/min, SpO$_2$ 94%. Following an small-volume nebulizer (SVN) containing 5 mg of albuterol, her vital signs are BP 120/84 mm Hg, HR 80 beats/min, and RR 16 breaths/min, and lung sounds have improved, with no wheezing detected on auscultation.

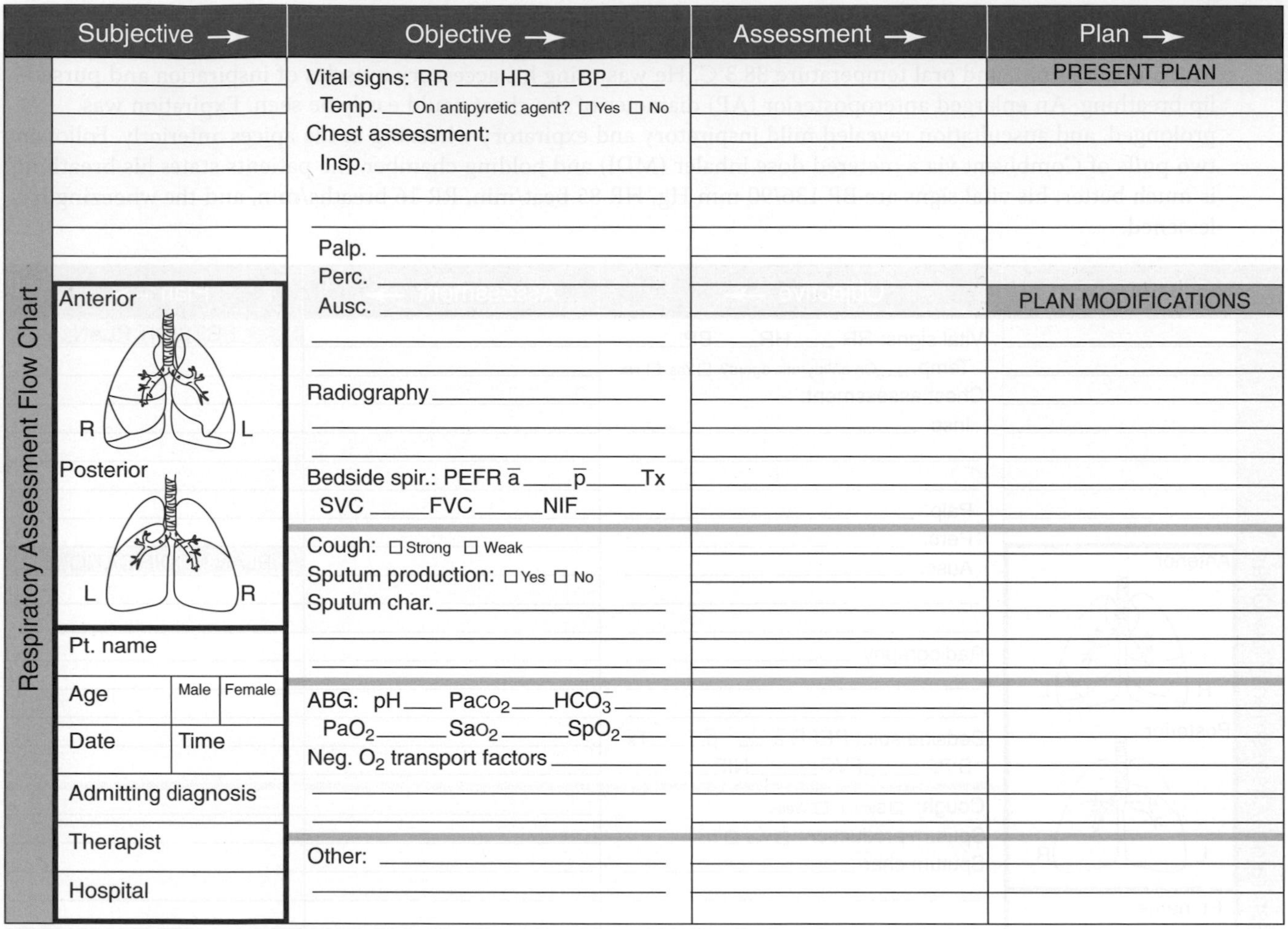

Subjective →	Objective →	Assessment →	Plan →

Respiratory Assessment Flow Chart	Vital signs: RR ____ HR ____ BP ____
	  Temp. ____ On antipyretic agent? ☐ Yes ☐ No
	Chest assessment:
	  Insp. _____
	
	  Palp. _____
	  Perc. _____
	  Ausc. _____
	
	Radiography _____
	
	Bedside spir.: PEFR ā____ p̄____ Tx
	  SVC ____ FVC ____ NIF ____
	Cough: ☐ Strong ☐ Weak
	Sputum production: ☐ Yes ☐ No
	Sputum char. _____
	
	ABG: pH ____ Paco$_2$ ____ HCO$_3^-$ ____
	  PaO$_2$ ____ Sao$_2$ ____ SpO$_2$ ____
	Neg. O$_2$ transport factors ____
	
	Other: _____
			PRESENT PLAN
			
			PLAN MODIFICATIONS

Anterior
R   L
Posterior
L   R

Pt. name
Age — Male | Female
Date | Time
Admitting diagnosis
Therapist
Hospital

Figure 3-2 Respiratory care progress note. (From Des Jardins T, Burton GG: *Clinical manifestations and assessment of respiratory disease*, ed 6, St. Louis, MO, 2011, Mosby.)

Lab partner's signature for scenario b: _____

c. A 29 weeks' gestation, 2-hour old infant is in the ED in an oxyhood with an F_1O_2 of 0.5. Physical examination reveals intercostal and substernal retractions; vital signs are RR 68 breaths/min and HR 145 beats/min. The arterial blood gas (ABG) values are as follows: pH = 7.19, $PaCO_2$ = 70 mm Hg, HCO_3^- of 21 mEq/L PaO_2 = 41 mm Hg. Manual ventilation of this patient demonstrates bilateral chest movement and aeration at 25 cm H_2O. The patient is about to be transported via helicopter to a hospital with a neonatal intensive care unit (NICU).

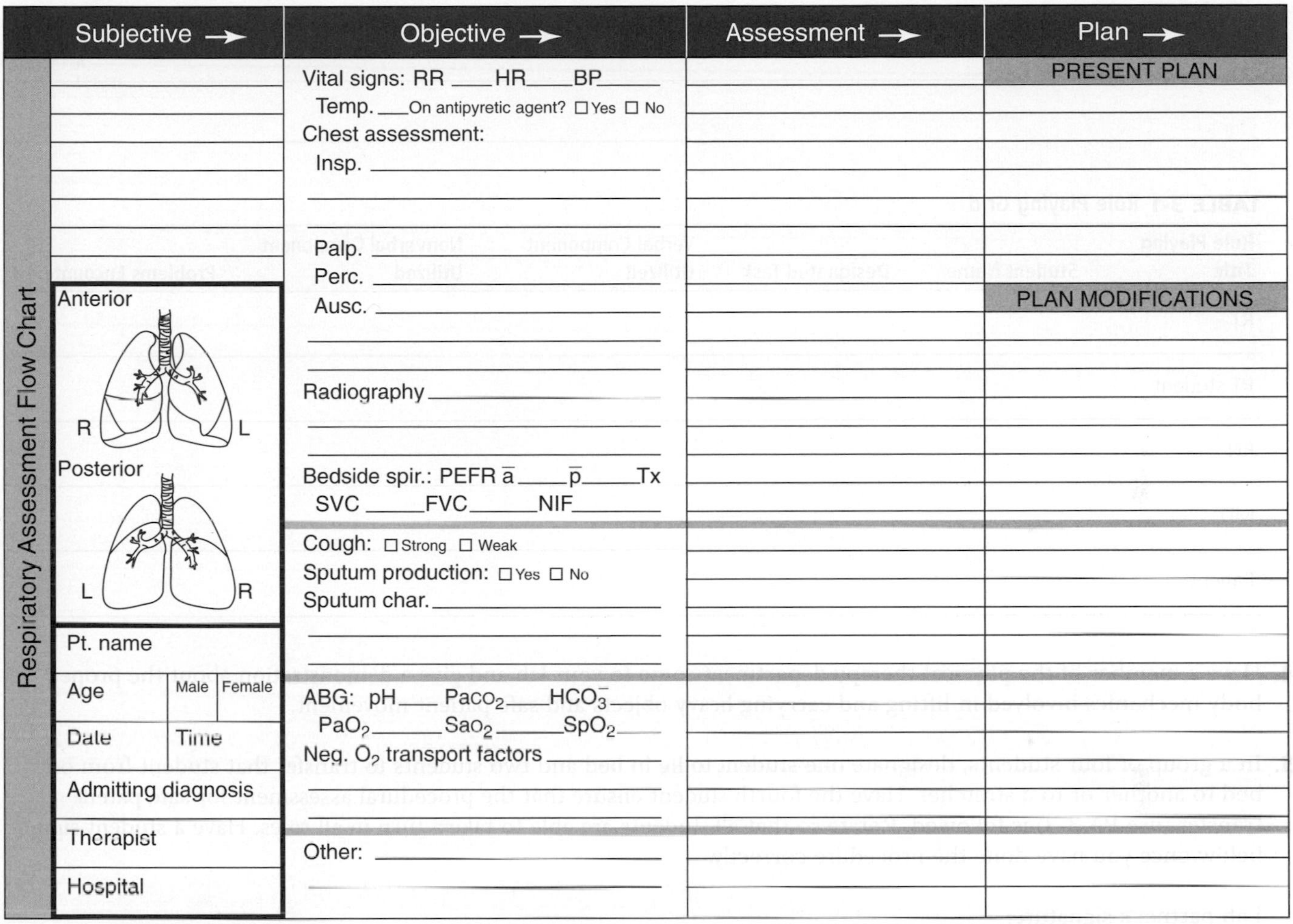

Subjective →	Objective →	Assessment →	Plan →
	Vital signs: RR ___ HR ___ BP ___		PRESENT PLAN
	Temp. ___ On antipyretic agent? ☐ Yes ☐ No		
	Chest assessment:		
	Insp. _____		
	Palp. _____		
	Perc. _____		
Anterior	Ausc. _____		PLAN MODIFICATIONS
R L			
Posterior	Radiography _____		
L R	Bedside spir.: PEFR ā ___ p̄ ___ Tx		
	SVC ___ FVC ___ NIF ___		
Pt. name	Cough: ☐ Strong ☐ Weak		
	Sputum production: ☐ Yes ☐ No		
	Sputum char. _____		
Age	Male	Female	ABG: pH ___ $PaCO_2$ ___ HCO_3^- ___		
Date	Time	PaO_2 ___ SaO_2 ___ SpO_2 ___		
	Neg. O_2 transport factors _____		
Admitting diagnosis			
Therapist	Other: _____		
Hospital			

Respiratory Assessment Flow Chart

Figure 3-3 Respiratory care progress note. (From Des Jardins T, Burton GG: *Clinical manifestations and assessment of respiratory disease*, ed 6, St. Louis, MO, 2011, Mosby.)

Lab partner's signature for scenario c: _____

2. Using the three patient scenarios from question #1, give a verbal change-of-shift report to a lab partner for each of the patients (use PA 3-2). If all information is correctly conveyed, have your partner sign below. Multiple attempts may be required until your skills are honed.

Lab partner's signature for scenario a: _____

Lab partner's signature for scenario b: _____

Lab partner's signature for scenario c: _____

3. Set up a role-playing, patient care scenario using the scenario provided below where the students are designated as: RT, RT student, registered nurse (RN), physician (MD), and patient. Using Table 3-1, discuss the different roles each person plays and how important effective communication is among health care professionals.

A 58-year-old male patient with severe emphysema is brought into the ED in cardiopulmonary arrest. The patient's wife was driving him to see his primary care physician when he began having severe trouble breathing and slumped over in the passenger seat of their car just outside the hospital. His wife is frantic. Discuss how to treat this patient as a team.

_____

_____

TABLE 3-1 Role Playing Grid

Role Playing Title	Student Name	Designated Task	Verbal Component Utilized	Nonverbal Component Utilized	Problems Encountered
RT					
RT student					
RN					
MD					
Patient					

4. Have a member of the physical therapy department come to your lab and give a demonstration about the proper body mechanics involved in lifting and carrying heavy objects and safe patient movement.

5. In a group of four students, designate one student to lie in bed and two students to transfer that student from one bed to another or to a stretcher. Have the fourth student ensure that the procedural assessment for safe patent transfer (use PA 3-3) is followed. Rotate so that all students are able to take a turn in all roles. Have a student sign below once you have done the procedure correctly.

Lab partner's signature: _____

6. Using a piece of heavy respiratory equipment (e.g., Vest© Airway Clearance System) demonstrate to a lab partner correct body mechanics (Figure 3-4) for lifting a heavy object. Have lab partner sign off that you performed the lift correctly using a straight spine and leg muscles to lift the object.

Lab partner's signature: _____

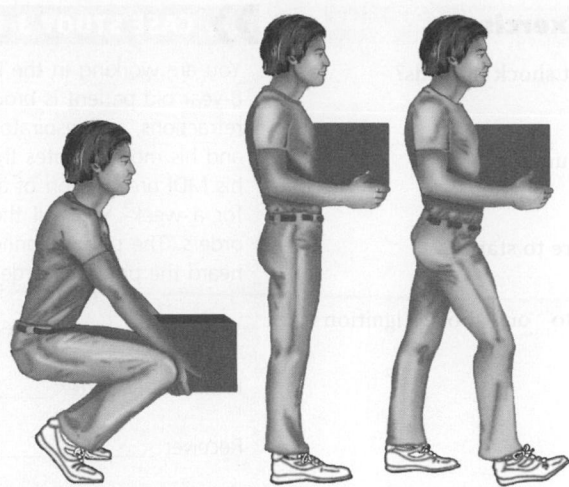

Figure 3-4 Body mechanics of lifting and carrying objects. (From Kacmarek RM, Stoller JK, Heuer AJ: *Egan's fundamentals of respiratory care*, ed 10, St. Louis, MO, 2013, Mosby.)

7. List three patient identifiers that health care personnel can use to correctly identify a patient.

_____

Self-Assessment Exercises

1. Which of the following causes most shock hazards?
A. Frayed electrical cords
B. Defibrillators
C. Inappropriate or inadequate grounding
D. Lightning

2. What conditions must exist for a fire to start?

1. Flammable material present
2. Flammable material heated to or above ignition temperature
3. Oxygen
4. Nitric oxide

A. 1 and 4 only
B. 1, 2, and 3 only
C. 3 only
D. 1 and 2 only

3. How can you identify which outlets function in the hospital's backup generator?
A. All hospital outlets function on the backup generator
B. Hospitals do not utilize backup generators
C. The outlet may be red or have a red dot on it
D. Hospital equipment functions on batter backup only

4. The term used to describe the power potential behind electrical energy is:
A. Voltage
B. Current
C. Resistance
D. Ohm

5. Which are examples of nonverbal communication?

1. Written message
2. Facial expressions
3. Voice tone
4. Eye contact

A. 1 only
B. 2, 3, and 4 only
C. 3 only
D. 1, 2, 3, and 4

6. What does the acronym RACE stand for?

_____

_____

7. List the five basic components of communication.

_____

_____

8. What is the "read back" process, and why is it important?

_____

_____

▶▶ CASE STUDY 3-1

You are working in the ED of a small, rural hospital when an 8-year old patient is brought in with complaints of wheezing, retractions, and respiratory distress. He has a history of asthma and his mother states that she has not had a chance to refill his MDI prescription of albuterol and that he has not taken it for a week. You call the pediatrician on call for medication orders. The phone connection is scratchy, and you think you heard the physician order "2.5 mills of albuterol via SVN."

1. How should you proceed?

Prescriber/Reporter:_____

Receiver:_____

2. Explain the responsibilities of the prescriber, or reporter and those of the receiver in the "read back" process.

_____

_____

▶▶ CASE STUDY 3-2

You are an RT working the night shift in a busy urban trauma center. Your patient is currently being treated for pneumonia on the general floor. She has been in the hospital for 7 days. Her past medical history includes chronic obstructive pulmonary disease (COPD), hypertension, and myocardial infarction. Her oxygen requirements have been steady at 2 liters per minute (L/min) via nasal cannula for the duration of her stay, but an overnight exacerbation of her COPD has necessitated an increase in her oxygen therapy to 4 L/min to maintain her oxygen saturations.

1. What pertinent information regarding the patient's condition should be conveyed during your change-of-shift report?

_____

_____

2. What information should be a priority during your report?

_____

_____

3. Chart an entry as you would in the patient's chart (Figure 3-5). Have your instructor review it to ensure that all information is reported correctly. If it is a paper chart, it must be legible.

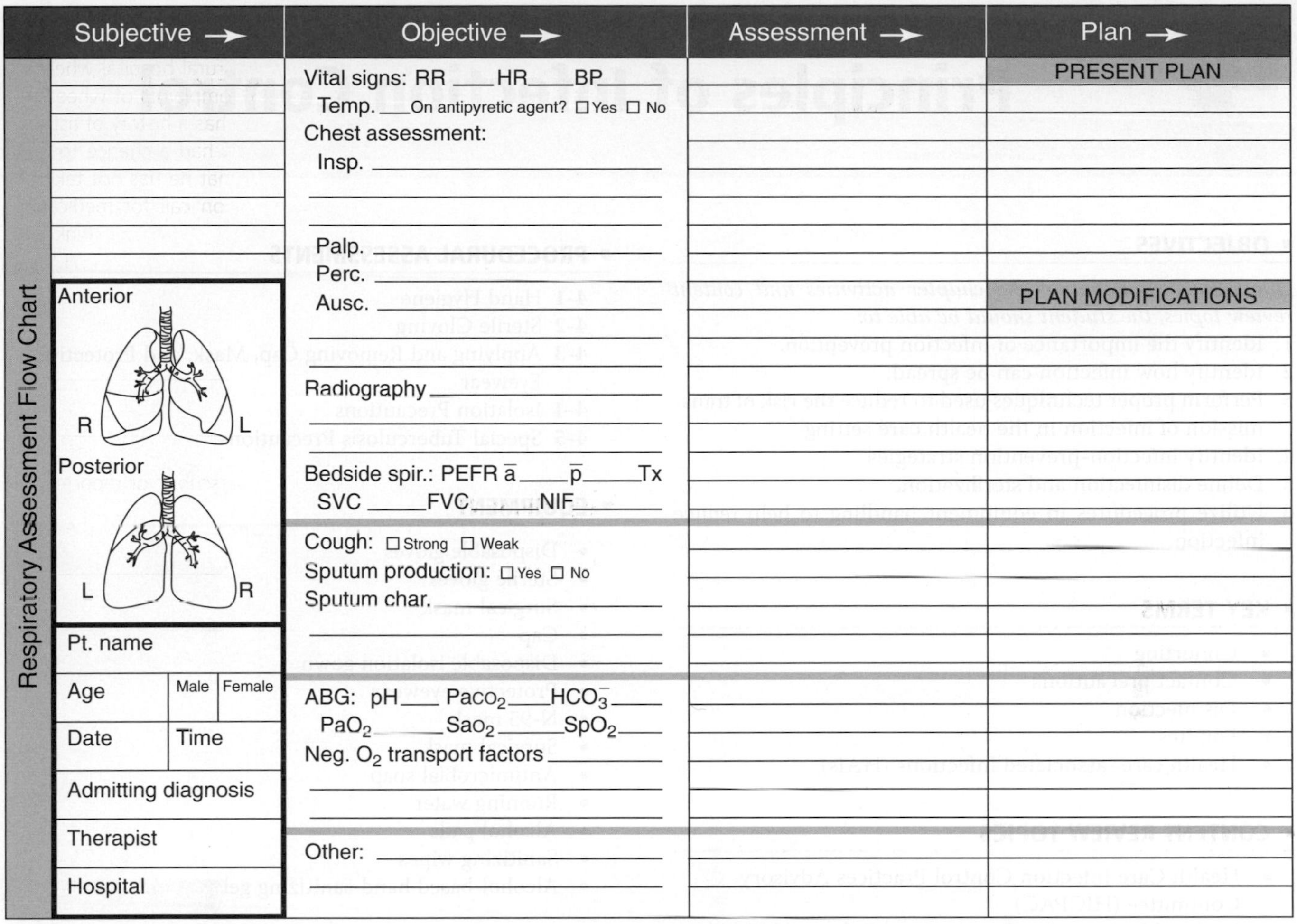

Subjective →	Objective →	Assessment →	Plan →
Anterior R L Posterior L R Pt. name Age — Male/Female Date — Time Admitting diagnosis Therapist Hospital	Vital signs: RR ____ HR ____ BP ____ Temp. ____ On antipyretic agent? ☐ Yes ☐ No Chest assessment: Insp. _____ Palp. _____ Perc. _____ Ausc. _____ Radiography _____ Bedside spir.: PEFR ā ____ p̄ ____ Tx SVC ____ FVC ____ NIF ____ Cough: ☐ Strong ☐ Weak Sputum production: ☐ Yes ☐ No Sputum char. _____ ABG: pH ____ $Paco_2$ ____ HCO_3^- ____ PaO_2 ____ Sao_2 ____ SpO_2 ____ Neg. O_2 transport factors _____ Other: _____		PRESENT PLAN PLAN MODIFICATIONS

Respiratory Assessment Flow Chart (vertical label at left)

Figure 3-5 Respiratory care progress note.

CASE STUDY 3-3

You are a student RT cleared by your instructor to assess a patient with a tracheostomy tube. You are checking the patient's chart and notice that no tracheostomy care has be performed on the patient for about 24 hours. As you approach the patient's room, a nurse stops you. She says, "This patient has been very combative and disruptive for the last 24 hours. I have not been able to take a break all morning because of him. He is finally sleeping. You cannot go in there." As you peek into the patient's room, you notice the pulse oximeter is reading 87%.

1. How would you respond to the nurse's request?

_____

_____

Principles of Infection Control

▪ OBJECTIVES

Upon the completion of the chapter activities and content review topics, the student should be able to:

1. Identify the importance of infection prevention.
2. Identify how infection can be spread.
3. Perform proper techniques used to reduce the risk of transmission of infection in the health care setting.
4. Identify infection-prevention strategies.
5. Define disinfection and sterilization.
6. Utilize procedures in equipment handling to help reduce infection.

▪ KEY TERMS

- Cohorting
- Contact precautions
- Disinfection
- Fomites
- Health care–associated infections (HAIs)

▪ CONTENT REVIEW TOPICS

- Health Care Infection Control Practices Advisory Committee (HICPAC)
- National Institute for Occupational Safety and Health (NIOSH)
- Occupational Safety and Health Administration (OSHA)
- Sterilization

▪ PROCEDURAL ASSESSMENTS

4-1 Hand Hygiene
4-2 Sterile Gloving
4-3 Applying and Removing Cap, Mask, and Protective Eyewear
4-4 Isolation Precautions
4-5 Special Tuberculosis Precautions

▪ EQUIPMENT

- Disposable gloves
- Sterile gloves
- Surgical mask
- Cap
- Disposable isolation gown
- Protective eyewear
- N-95 mask
- Surgical mask
- Antimicrobial soap
- Running water
- Alcohol pads
- Sanitizing wipes
- Alcohol-based hand-sanitizing gel

With respiratory therapists on the frontline treating all types of respiratory conditions and managing many aspects of a patient's care, it is imperative that their knowledge regarding infection control and prevention procedures be accurate and their adherence to those procedures unvarying. It has been reported that approximately 1.7 million cases of health care-associated infections (HAIs) occurred in the United States in 2002 alone.

To facilitate reduction of these infections, respiratory therapists (RTs) must participate in transmission reduction education and practice prevention control strategies to not only protect their patients but also defend themselves against infection. As an RT, you will play an important role in the prevention of these infections. Box 4-1 lists the infection prevention strategies that you should follow. This chapter will focus on understanding how infection is spread and what techniques are used to help prevent its spread.

≫ SKILL CHECK LISTS

4-1 Hand Hygiene

Proper hand hygiene is imperative. The practice of hand hygiene should start in the laboratory setting and carry over into the clinical world.

> **Reality Check** If it's wet and not yours... don't touch it without gloves.

> **Reality Check** Alcohol hand sanitizer will not kill *Clostridium difficile* spores. Three to four applications of an alcohol-based gel followed by hand washing with antimicrobial soap should be done.

BOX 4-1 Infection Preventions Strategies
for the Respiratory Therapist

BOX 4-1 Infection Preventions Strategies
for the Respiratory Therapist

- Creating a safe culture
  - Provides best practices for infection prevention by ensuring that the bedside caregiver has the appropriate time, equipment, and training to provide the best possible care
- Decreasing host susceptibility
  - Vaccination for health care personnel
  - Prevention bundles (i.e., ventilator-assisted pneumonia [VAP] bundles)
- Eliminating the source of pathogens
  - General sanitation measures
  - Specialized equipment processing
- Interrupting transmission
- Following standard precautions
  - Personal protective equipment
- Always practicing proper hand hygiene
  - Hand washing with antimicrobial soap and water for 15 seconds
  - Use of alcohol-based products
- Using gloves
- Using mouth, nose, eye, and face protection
  - Mucus membranes are vulnerable to pathogens
- Using gowns, aprons, and protective apparel
- Using respiratory protection
  - Use of N-95 mask
- Adhering to transmission-based precautions
  - Contact precautions
  - Droplet precautions
  - Airborne infection isolation
- Careful patient placement
  - Cohorting
- Careful transport of infected patients
  - Limiting transport of patients with contagious disease
  - When patients have to be transported, they need to wear appropriate barrier protection
- Proper disinfection and sterilization of equipment

Hand hygiene should be performed before and after every patient contact. The following is the step-by-step process for proper hand hygiene.

Implementation

1. Inspect forearms, hands, and fingers for cuts, abrasions, or breaks in skin.
   a. Apply dressing, if needed.
2. Inspect nails for length and condition.
   a. Cut nails if longer than $\frac{1}{4}$ inch.
   b. Remove artificial nails.
3. Remove jewelry and watch, or push watch and clothing above wrist area.
4. Perform hand antisepsis using an instant alcohol waterless antiseptic product:
   a. Dispense a proper amount of the product on the palm of the hand.

   b. Rub hands together, covering all surfaces of the hands and fingers with the antiseptic product.
   c. Rub hands together until the antiseptic product is dry.
   d. Allow hands to completely dry before applying gloves.
5. Perform hand hygiene with antimicrobial soap and warm water (Figure 4-1):
   a. Stand at the sink without touching the sink with hands, body, or clothing.
   b. Turn on water; avoid splashing.
   c. Regulate the flow and temperature of water.
   d. Wet hands and wrists with water.
   e. Apply antimicrobial soap to the palm of the hand.
   f. Lather hands by applying friction to skin surfaces for no less than 15 seconds.
   g. Interlace fingers and rub palms and backs of hands using a circular motion.
   h. Clean under fingernails.
   i. Rinse thoroughly, keeping hands below elbow level.
   j. Dry hands thoroughly, drying from fingers up to wrist and forearms.
   k. Turn off the faucet with a paper towel or pedal to avoid contamination.
   l. Discard paper towel(s) properly.
   m. Apply lotion, if needed.
   n. Allow hands to completely dry before applying gloves.
6. Avoid opening doors or touching objects with clean hands.

Evaluation of Procedure

1. Inspect the surfaces of hands and fingers.
2. Identify any unexpected outcomes.

4-2 Sterile Gloving

Certain procedures such as sterile suctioning of a tracheostomy tube require you to apply sterile gloves while performing the procedure. This skill takes practice. While in the lab setting, never in the clinical setting, you can reuse the sterile gloves to master the technique and thus not waste sterile gloves. The following is the step-by-step process for sterile gloving techniques.

Procedural Preparation

1. Review the patient's chart.
2. Examine the condition of the packaging and expiration date of gloves.
3. Determine if the patient has any latex allergy.
4. Select the proper-size gloves.

Implementation

1. Glove application (Figure 4-2):
   a. Perform proper hand hygiene.
   b. Place the package on a stable, waist-level surface.
   c. Remove the outer wrapper.
   d. Open the inner wrapper, and keep the gloves on the wrapper's inside surface.

e. With your nondominant hand, grasp the inside edge of the cuff of the glove for your dominant hand.

f. Pull the glove over your dominant hand with thumb and fingers into the proper finger spaces.

g. With your dominant hand gloved, slip fingers under the cuff of the second glove.

h. Pull the glove over your nondominant hand without contaminating the gloved dominant hand.

i. Interlock the fingers of the gloved hands to ensure proper fit.

2. Glove removal and disposal:

a. Grab the outside of one cuff with the other gloved hand, without touching the wrist.

b. Pull the glove off, turning it inside out and placing it in the palm of the gloved hand.

c. Slide the fingers of the ungloved hand underneath the cuff of the gloved hand, and pull the remaining glove inside out and over the other glove.

d. Dispose gloves in proper container.

3. Performs proper hand hygiene.

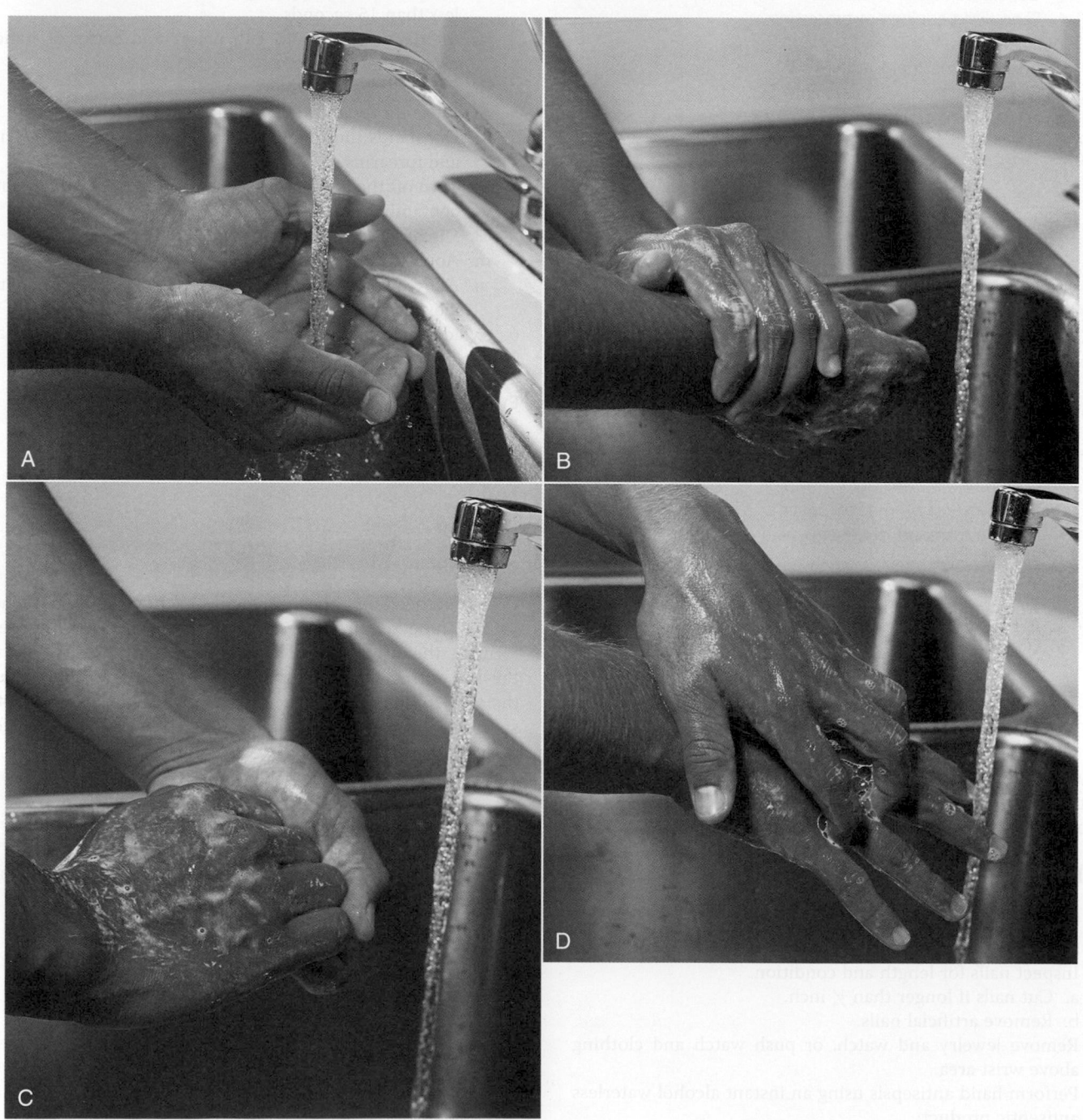

Figure 4-1 Steps for hand washing. **A,** Wet hands. **B,** Wash around wrist and forearm. **C,** Scrub palm of hand. **D,** Wash between digits on back of hand.

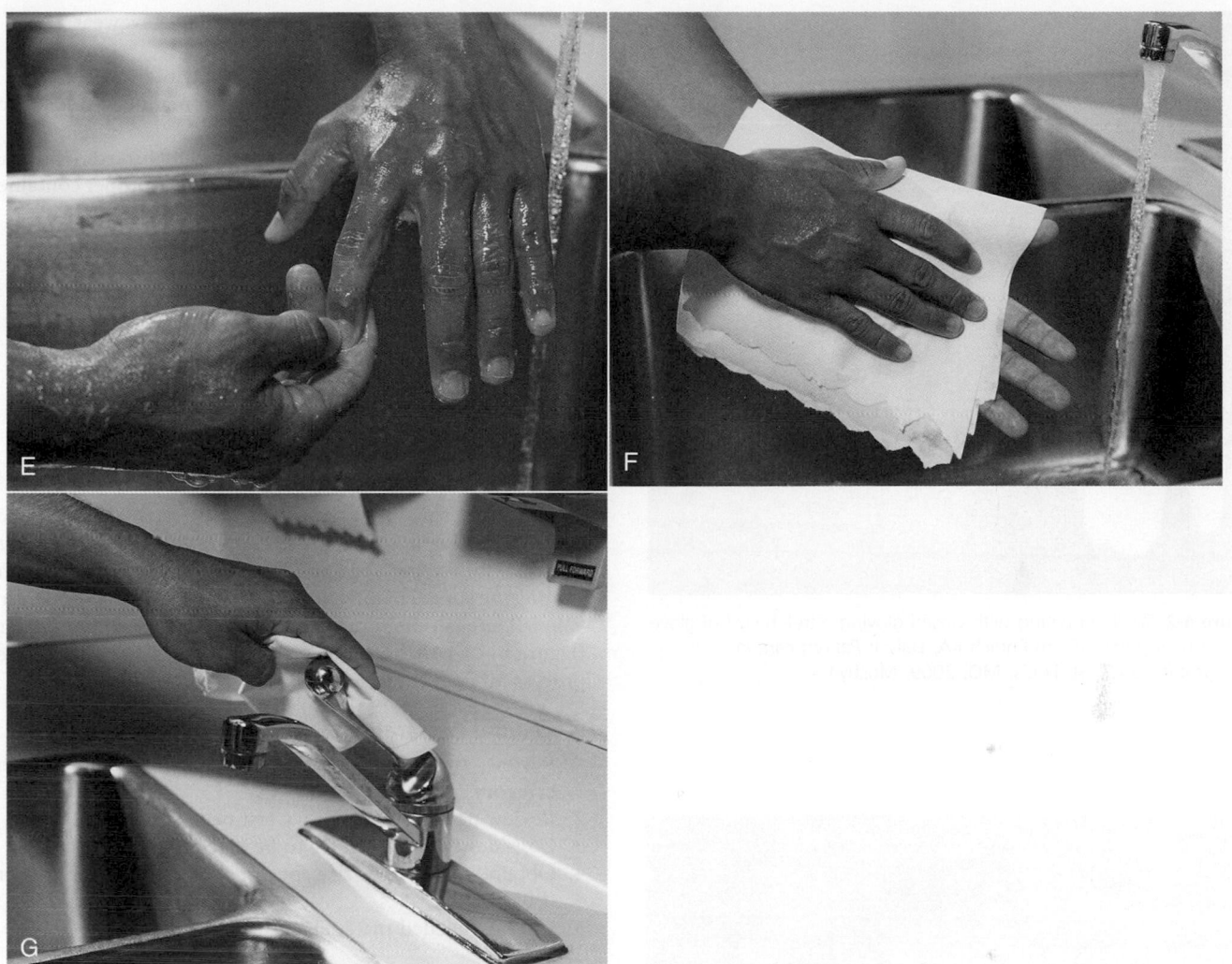

Figure 4-1 cont'd   **E,** Wash around cuticle. **F,** Dry hands with clean towel. **G,** Use paper towel to turn off faucet. (From Kacmarek RM, Stoller JK, Heuer AJ: *Egan's fundamentals of respiratory care*, ed 10 , St. Louis, MO, 2013, Mosby.)

Evaluation of Procedure

1. Identify any unexpected outcomes.

Documentation and Reporting

1. Report any exposure, according to agency protocols.

4-3 Applying and Removing Cap, Mask, and Protective Eyewear

The patients you take care of may be immunocompromised, contagious with transmittable diseases, or both. You must be knowledgeable about how to keep yourself safe and not be afraid of "catching" something. The following is the step-by-step process for applying and removing the cap, mask, and protective eyewear.

Procedural Preparation

1. Review the patient's chart.
2. Determine the need to apply the cap, mask, or protective eyewear.

3. Prepare and inspect equipment.
4. Perform proper hand hygiene, and apply gloves.

Implementation

1. Apply the cap (Figure 4-3):
   a. Secure long hair back or up.
   b. Apply the cap, covering hair completely.
2. Apply the mask:
   a. Locate the top edge of the mask.
   b. Hold the mask by the top straps, with the top edge of the mask above the nose.
   c. Pull the top straps and secure, or tie, at the top of back of head.
   d. Pull the two lower straps around the neck, or tie, with mask under chin.
   e. Pinch the upper metal bar around the bridge of the nose.
3. Apply protective eyewear:
   a. Apply eyewear or goggles comfortably, and ensure that vision is unobstructed.
   b. Ensure that the fit is snug around the forehead and face.

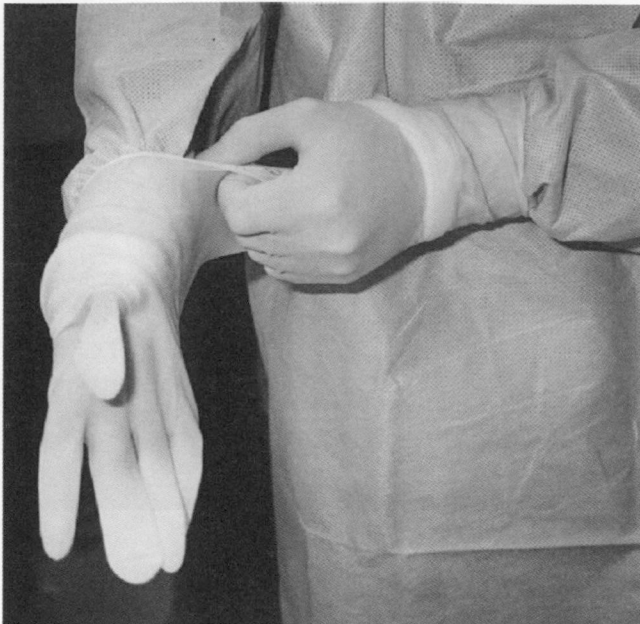

Figure 4-2 Sterile gowning with closed gloving. Stretch cuff of glove over cuff of gown. (From Ehrlich RA, Daly J: *Patient care in radiography*, ed 7, St. Louis, MO, 2009, Mosby.)

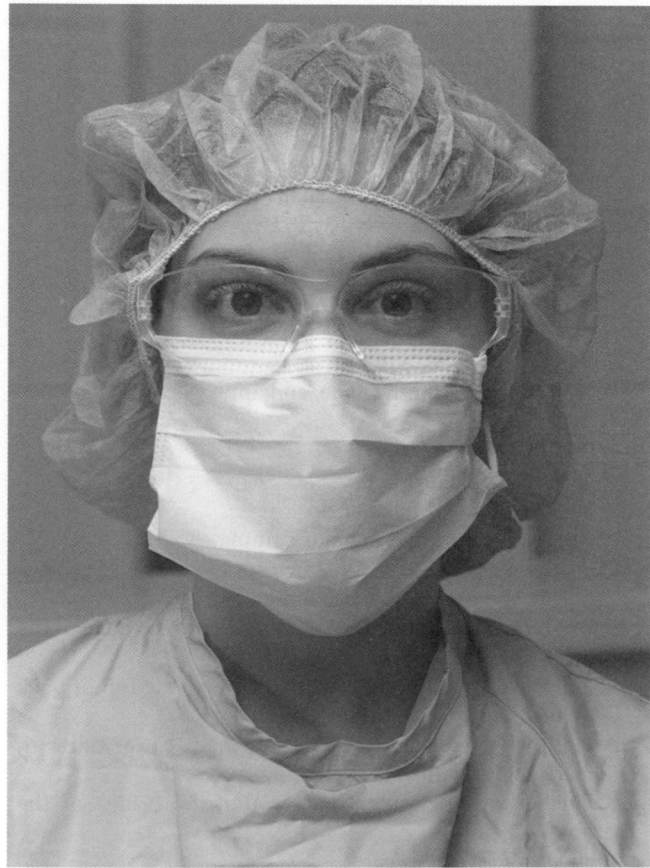

Figure 4-3 Protective cap, eyewear, and mask. (From Hupp J, Ellis E, Tucker M: *Contemporary oral and maxillofacial surgery*, ed 5, St. Louis, MO, 2008, Mosby.)

4. Dispose of the cap, mask, and protective eyewear:
   a. Remove gloves first.
   b. Remove the mask by touching only the straps or ties.
   c. Remove eyewear, and disinfect per manufacturer's specifications, if not disposable.
   d. Grasp the outer surface of the cap, and lift from the head.
   e. Discard the cap, mask, and eyewear in a proper container.
5. Perform proper hand hygiene.

Evaluation of Procedure

1. Identify any unexpected outcomes.

Documentation and Reporting

1. Report any exposure, according to agency protocols.

4-4 Isolation Precautions

Patients on isolation precautions may have diseases such as leukemia or methicillin-resistant *Staphylococcus aureus* (MRSA). Protecting your patient from further infection, preventing the spread of infection to other patients, and protecting yourself are all important aspects of isolation precautions (Figure 4-4, *A* through *C*). The following is the step-by-step process for isolation precautions.

Procedural Preparation

1. Review the patient's chart for the specific isolation category.
2. Review pertinent laboratory test needs or results.
3. Consider the type of care to be delivered to the patient.
4. Obtain the proper-size personal protective equipment (PPE).
5. Place all needed materials near work area.

Implementation

1. Perform proper hand hygiene.
2. Apply a gown:
   a. Pick up the gown by holding it at the neck.
   b. Place hands into sleeves.
   c. Push hands through the cuffs, and catch the thumb-hold, if applicable.
   d. Secure the ties at the neck, and close the gown by tying the waist ties.
3. Apply a mask and protective eyewear (see PA 4-3).
4. Apply gloves, with the edges overlying the gown cuffs.
   a. For sterile gloving, see PA 4-2.
5. Open the door with your back to enter the patient's room.
6. Explain the purpose of isolation and necessary precautions to the patient and family.
7. Remove all the isolation attire before leaving room.
   a. Remove gloves, turning them inside out.
   b. Remove the mask and protective eyewear.
   c. Remove the gown.
      i. Untie the neck and waist ties.
      ii. Pull off one sleeve by reaching inside the cuff with a finger.
      iii. Repeat for the second sleeve.
      iv. Fold the gown inside out.
8. Dispose of all isolation attire appropriately.
9. Perform proper hand hygiene before leaving the room and again outside room.

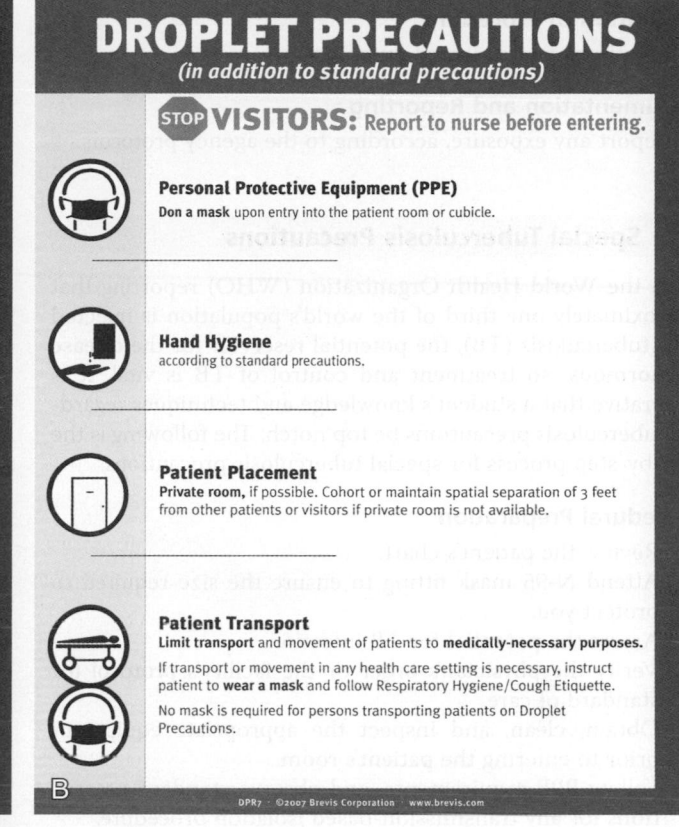

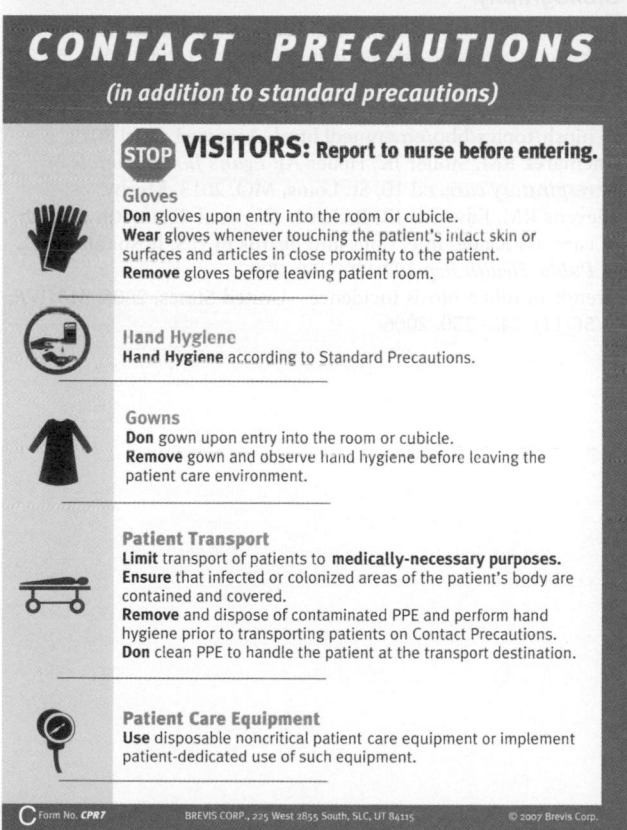

Figure 4-4 A, Contact precautions. **B,** Droplet precautions. **C,** Airborne precautions (From Brevis, Corp., Salt Lake City, UT.)

Evaluation of Procedure

1. Identify any unexpected outcomes.

Documentation and Reporting

1. Report any exposure, according to the agency protocols.

4-5 Special Tuberculosis Precautions

With the World Health Organization (WHO) reporting that approximately one third of the world's population is infected with tuberculosis (TB), the potential reservoir for the disease is enormous, so treatment and control of TB is vital. It is imperative that a student's knowledge and techniques regarding tuberculosis precautions be top notch. The following is the step-by-step process for special tuberculosis precautions.

Procedural Preparation

1. Review the patient's chart.
2. Attend N-95 mask fitting to ensure the size required to protect you.
3. Assess the potential for TB infection.
4. Verify the physician's order or the facility's protocol for standard of care.
5. Obtain, clean, and inspect the appropriate equipment prior to entering the patient's room.
6. Follow PPE requirements, and observe standard precautions for any transmission-based isolation procedure.
7. Identify the patient using two patient identifiers.
8. Introduce yourself to the patient and to the family.
9. Explain the procedure to the patient and to the family, and acknowledge the patient's understanding.
10. Perform proper hand hygiene, and put on gloves, mask, and protective eyewear, as appropriate for the procedure.

Implementation

1. Apply the N-95 mask, and check fit.
2. Enter negative pressure room, and close the door.
3. Explain the purpose of TB isolation to the patient and family.
4. Instruct the patient to always cover the mouth with a tissue when coughing and to wear a disposable surgical mask when leaving the room.
5. Provide scheduled patient care.
6. Close the door when leaving the room.
7. Remove the N-95 mask.
   a. If disposable, discard the mask in the proper receptacle.
   b. If reusable, place the mask in a labeled bag for storage, and avoid damaging the mask.
8. Perform proper hand hygiene.

Evaluation of Procedure

1. Assess the patient's laboratory data for acid-fast bacillus (AFB) smear or purified protein derivative (PPD) placement:
   a. AFB cultures are used to diagnose active *Mycobacterium tuberculosis* infections. RTs typically obtain a sputum sample for testing. A negative AFB smear means that no infection is present, and a positive AFB smear indicates a probable mycobacterial infection.
   b. The PPD skin test is a method used to diagnose TB.
2. Ask the patient or family to identify how TB may have been contracted by the patient.
3. Identify any unexpected outcomes.

Documentation and Reporting

1. Report any abnormal findings to the appropriate health care provider.

Bibliography

Centers for Disease Control and Prevention: *Guideline for hand hygiene in health-care settings*, October 25, 2002 / Vol. 51 / No. RR-16.

Center for Disease Control and Prevention: http://www.cdc.gov/niosh/topics/bbp/emergnedl.html. Accessed April 2012.

Kacmarek RM, Stoller JK, Heuer AJ: *Egan's fundamentals of respiratory care*, ed 10, St. Louis, MO, 2013, Mosby.

Klevens RM, Edwards JR, Richards CL, et al: Estimating health care-associated infections and deaths in U.S. hospitals, 2002. *Public Health Rep* 122:160–166, 2007.

Trends in tuberculosis incidence—United States, 2006. *MMWR*, 56(11), 245–250, 2006.

1. Have two different students observe you properly washing your hands with antimicrobial soap and water. Have them time you and evaluate your process to ensure that you washed them for at least 15 seconds. Have them sign below.

    Lab partner's signature: _____

    Lab partner's signature: _____

2. Repeat lab activity #1 using antiseptic product instead of antimicrobial soap and water.

    Lab partner's signature: _____

    Lab partner's signature: _____

3. Obtain a cap, a mask, and protective eyewear. Properly apply and remove the protective equipment while another student observes you and ensures that you followed all procedures correctly. Have the lab partner sign below.

    Lab partner's signature: _____

4. Why should you wear protective eyewear?

    _____

5. List a clinical situation where protective eyewear is necessary.

    _____

6. Demonstrate to your lab partner proper procedural technique used during sterile gloving. Have your partner evaluate your technique. Once you have successfully completed the procedure, have this student sign below.

    Lab partner's signature: _____

7. What is a clinical situation where sterile gloving is needed?

    _____

8. Fill in the table below with definitions for equipment processing.

Term	Definition
Cleaning	
Disinfection (general term)	
Disinfection Low-level	
Disinfection Intermediate-level	
Disinfection High-level	
Sterilization	

9. What are fomites?

Self-Assessment Questions

1. What elements must be present for transmission of infection within the health care setting?

   1. A susceptible host
   2. A source of pathogens
   3. A resistant form of a pathogen
   4. A route of transmission

   A. 2 and 3
   B. 1 and 4
   C. 1, 2, and 3
   D. 1, 2, and 4

2. The term used to describe people serving as their own source of infection is:
   A. Nosocomial infection
   B. Autogenous infection
   C. Indirect contact transmission
   D. Direct contact transmission

3. The most common route of pathogen transmission in the hospital setting is:
   A. Vector-borne transmission
   B. Droplet transmission
   C. Direct contact transmission
   D. Indirect contact transmission

4. Which of the following are considered PPE?
   A. Gloves
   B. Gowns
   C. Eye protection
   D. All of the above

5. When should gloves be changed?

   1. Between patient contacts every time
   2. Only when contaminated by blood
   3. After any direct contact with infectious material
   4. If they are torn

   A. 2 and 3 only
   B. 1 and 4 only
   C. 1, 3, and 4 only
   D. 1, 2, and 4 only

6. What disease would warrant the use of a NOISH-approved N-95 mask?
   A. Tuberculosis
   B. *Clostridium difficile* infection
   C. Oral candidiasis
   D. None of the above

7. Hand hygiene includes hand washing with antiseptic-containing soap and water for at least:
   A. 15 seconds
   B. 30 seconds
   C. 45 seconds
   D. 60 seconds

8. The practice of grouping patients with the same infection together to confine care geographically and prevent transmission to other patients is called:
   A. Isolation precautions
   B. Droplet precautions
   C. Contact precautions
   D. Cohorting

9. In-use respiratory care equipment that can spread pathogens include all of the following:

   1. Small volume nebulizers
   2. Large volume nebulizers
   3. Ventilator circuits
   4. Suction equipment

   A. 1 and 2 only
   B. 1 and 3 only
   C. 1, 2, and 3 only
   D. 1, 2, 3, and 4

10. What are common pathogens that can be transmitted via a needlestick injury?
    A. *C. difficile* and human immunodeficiency virus (HIV)
    B. Hepatitis C and HIV
    C. Methicillin-resistant *Staphylococcus Aureus* (MRSA) and vancomycin resistant enterococcus (VRE)
    D. HIV and VRE

›› CASE STUDY 4-1

Mr. Sheag is a 39-year-male patient currently hospitalized for increasing shortness of breath (SOB) with a possibility of tuberculosis. He is positive for HIV and MRSA and has a history of hypertension. He requires an arterial blood gas (ABG) sample.

1. What type of room should this patient be in?

_____

_____

_____

2. What type of transmission-based precautions should be taken with this patient?

_____

_____

_____

3. What personal protective equipment would you wear when entering his room?

_____

4. You have just finished obtaining an ABG sample from a patient. Discuss the proper way for disposing of the needle.

_____

_____

5. What should you do if you should stick yourself with a needle that had been used on this patient? (*HINT:* Go to the Centers for Disease Control and Prevention [CDC] website [www.CDC.gov] to find the most current information.)

_____

_____

_____

›› CASE STUDY 4-2

Ms. Gloria is a 67-year-old female patient with a tracheostomy tube. She receives humidification via a tracheostomy collar and a large-volume nebulizer.

1. What steps can you take to minimize infection her nebulizer may cause?

_____

_____

_____

2. What techniques should be practiced when suctioning her tracheostomy tube?

_____

_____

3. If this patient should have to be mechanically ventilated, list 10 procedures that should be followed to minimize her risk of infection.

_____

_____

_____

_____

_____

_____

_____

Patient Assessment

▪ OBJECTIVES

Upon the completion of the chapter activities and content review topics, the student should be able to:

1. Perform an assessment of the patient with respiratory problems.
2. Take a patient's medical history.
3. Measure vital signs, including:
   a. Respiratory rate
   b. Pulse rate
   c. Examination of the thorax and lungs:
      i. Inspection
      ii. Palpation
      iii. Percussion of the chest
      iv. Auscultation of the lungs
   d. Blood pressure
   e. Temperature
4. Perform pulse oximetry.
5. Document and report information in the patient chart.

▪ KEY TERMS

- Adventitious lung sounds
- Differential diagnosis
- Pertinent negatives
- Pertinent positives
- Pulsus alternans
- Pulsus paradoxus
- Respiratory frequency
- Vesicular lung sounds

▪ CONTENT REVIEW TOPICS

- Advance directive
- Differential diagnosis
- Exacerbation
- I:E ratio
- Glasgow Coma Scale (GCS)
- Modified Borg scale
- SOAP progress note
- Therapist-driven protocols

▪ PROCEDURAL ASSESSMENTS

5-1 Taking a Medical History
5-2 Taking Vital Signs: Pulse Rate, Respiratory Rate, Examination of Thorax and Lungs
5-3 Performing Pulse Oximetry
5-4 Taking Vital Signs: Blood Pressure and Temperature

▪ EQUIPMENT

- Blood pressure cuff
- Stethoscope
- Pulse oximeter
- Gloves
- Hand hygiene products
- Alcohol pads
- Lung sound DVD or other media

The profession of respiratory care is advancing before our very eyes. The modern-day respiratory therapist has greatly evolved from the "oxygen orderlies" of days past. The respiratory therapist of today plays an integral role in the management of patients, from admission to discharge to home care. Therapist-driven protocols allow for autonomy within a specific scope of practice but require strong assessment skills by the respiratory therapist (RT) for safety and function.

To effectively perform this role, the therapist's skills of medical history taking and physical examination must be exceptional. Because the pulmonary system has such an overwhelming effect on numerous body systems, great attention must be paid to the respiratory therapists' patient assessment and reassessment skills to ensure that proper modalities are being provided to the patient.

→ **Reality Check** You must be a "proactive learner" throughout your career as a student and definitely as you begin practicing as a licensed respiratory care practitioner. What this means is that when you come across a disease process, medication, therapy, and so on that you do not know about, have never heard about, or just do not understand fully, try to find out what it is! Use *Respiratory Care* and other peer-reviewed journals to keep up to date with all clinical advancements that can impact patient care.

This chapter will cover medical history taking along with skills focused on the physical assessment of a patient. As a respiratory care student, your assessment skills and medical history taking ability will need to be honed. You must practice, practice, and then practice again. Talk to your patients about their specific pulmonary disease process and how it affects them. These interactions will facilitate your further understanding of how cardiac, renal, infectious, and so many other disease processes overlap with the pulmonary system and will influence the management of your patient's respiratory care plan.

>> SKILL CHECK LISTS

5-1 Taking a Medical History

Along with the physical examination and assessment of a patient, the patient's medical history plays a fundamental role in the accurate diagnosis and appropriate treatment of the patient with respiratory disease. Thorough evaluation of the patient's chart prior to entering the room is the initial step. Box 5-1 provides information that you should obtain during the complete health history. Negative responses to questions are called pertinent negatives, whereas positive responses are called pertinent positives. For example, if the patient complains of hemoptysis but has no recent weight loss, "hemoptysis" would be a pertinent positive and "no recent weight loss" would be a pertinent negative. These types of questions help the examiner formulate a differential diagnosis, which is the determination of which of two or more diseases with similar symptoms is the one the patient has. This is accomplished by

a systematic comparing and contrasting of the clinical findings. Careful observation should be made as soon as the examiner sees the patient. How you "expect" the patient to look should be compared with how the patient "actually" looks at the time of the examination. The following is the step-by-step process for obtaining the medical history of a patient.

> ✳ **Tip** The medical history taking should begin in the patient's social space (4–12 feet) and progress into their personal space (2–4 feet).

Procedural Preparation

Note that the following eight steps are basic preparation steps that should be observed before any patient interaction.
1. Review the patient's chart.
2. Verify the physician's order or the facility's protocol for standard of care.
3. Obtain, clean, and inspect the appropriate equipment prior to entering patient's room.
4. Follow personal protective equipment (PPE) requirements, and observe standard precautions for any transmission-based isolation procedure.
5. Identify the patient using two patient identifiers.
6. Introduce yourself to the patient and to the family.

BOX 5-1	Outline of a Complete Health History

- Demographic data (obtained from admission interview):
  - Name
  - Address
  - Age
  - Birth date
  - Place of birth
  - Race
  - Nationality
  - Marital status
  - Religion
  - Occupation
  - Source of referral
- Date and source of history and estimate of the reliability of the historian
- Brief description of the patient's condition at the time the history or patient profile was taken
- Chief complaint and reason for seeking treatment
- History of present illness: chronological description of each symptom:
  - Onset: Time, type, source, setting
  - Frequency and duration
  - Location and radiation of pain
  - Severity (quantity)
  - Quality (character)
  - Aggravating and alleviating factors
  - Associated manifestations
- Past medical history:
  - Childhood diseases, hospitalizations, surgeries, injuries, accidents, and major illnesses

- Allergies
- Medications
- Family History:
  - Familial disease history
  - Marital history
  - Family relationship
- Social and environmental history:
  - Education
  - Military experience
  - Occupational history
  - Religious and social activities
  - Alcohol and cigarette consumption
  - Living arrangements
  - Hobbies and recreation
  - Satisfaction with and stresses of life situation, finances, and relationships
  - Recent travel or other event that might affect health
- Review of systems:
  - Respiratory:
    - Cough
    - Hemoptysis
    - Sputum (amount/consistency)
    - Chest pain
    - Shortness of breath
    - Hoarseness or changes in voice
    - Dizziness or fainting
    - Fever or chills
    - Peripheral edema
- Patient's printed name and signature

From Kacmarek RM, Stoller JK, Heuer, AJ: *Egan's fundamentals of respiratory care*, ed 10, St. Louis, MO, 2013, Mosby.

✳ **Tip** Upon entering a patient's room, the therapist should introduce herself or himself, state the purpose of the visit, and always refer to the patient respectfully using his or her last name.

7. Explain the procedure to the patient and to the family, and acknowledge the patient's understanding.
8. Perform proper hand hygiene, and put on gloves, mask, and protective eyewear, as appropriate for the procedure.

Implementation

1. In the social space, provide a brief introduction of yourself and your role to the patient.
2. Assess the patient's level of consciousness (orientation to person, place, and time).
3. Identify the patient respectfully using titles (e.g., Mr., Mrs., Ms.) and his or her last name.
4. Assess for factors influencing communication (e.g., language barriers, hearing impairment, anxiety, etc.).
5. Use appropriate nonverbal behaviors and active listening skills while conducting the patient interview.
6. Ensure patient privacy during the interview (e.g., close the door, pull the curtain, ask visitors to leave during assessments, etc.)
7. Structure the interview in an orderly manner (see Box 5-1):
   a. Chief complaint of the patient
   b. History of present illness
   c. Past medical history
   d. Family history
   e. Social and environmental histories
   f. Review of systems

→ **Reality Check** "Retired" is not acceptable as the answer for a patient's occupational history. Many retired patients may have worked decades in occupations that could have put them at risk for numerous pulmonary complications.

✳ **Tip** Smoking history is often recorded in:
pack-years = packs per day × years smoked

8. Ensure patient comfort before leaving the room.
9. Remove all supplies from patient's room, and clean the area, as needed.
10. Remove PPE, and perform proper hand hygiene prior to leaving the patient's room.

Evaluation of Procedure

1. Establish a baseline, or compare with previous measurements.
2. Develop appropriate respiratory care plan based on assessment data.
3. Review the chart for the presence of an advance directive.
4. Identify any unexpected outcomes.

Documentation and Reporting

1. Record your findings in the patient's chart.
2. Report any abnormal findings to the appropriate health care provider.

5-2 Taking Vital Signs

Pulse Rate

In most patients, the rate, rhythm, and strength (quality) of the pulse are evaluated using the radial artery site. Location of this site is also important because it is the most commonly accessed point for arterial blood gas (ABG) draws. Figure 5-1 illustrates the locations of the most common pulse points. A rate of 60 to 100 is considered normal for an adult person at rest. Pulmonary problems often manifest as an alteration of a patient's pulse rate. Tachycardia is a heart rate above 100 beats per minute (beats/min), whereas bradycardia is less that 60 beats/min. Table 5-1 lists some common pulse descriptions with potential causes. The following is the step-by-step process for assessing the pulse rate of a patient.

→ **Reality Check** When assessing a patient, establishing that patient's "normal" vital signs is important when trying to obtain a baseline for that patient. An athletic and fit patient may have a bradycardic heart rate which is "normal" for them.

Procedural Preparation

1. Review the patient's chart.
2. Verify the physician's order or the facility's protocol for standard of care.
3. Obtain, clean, and inspect the appropriate equipment prior to entering the patient's room.

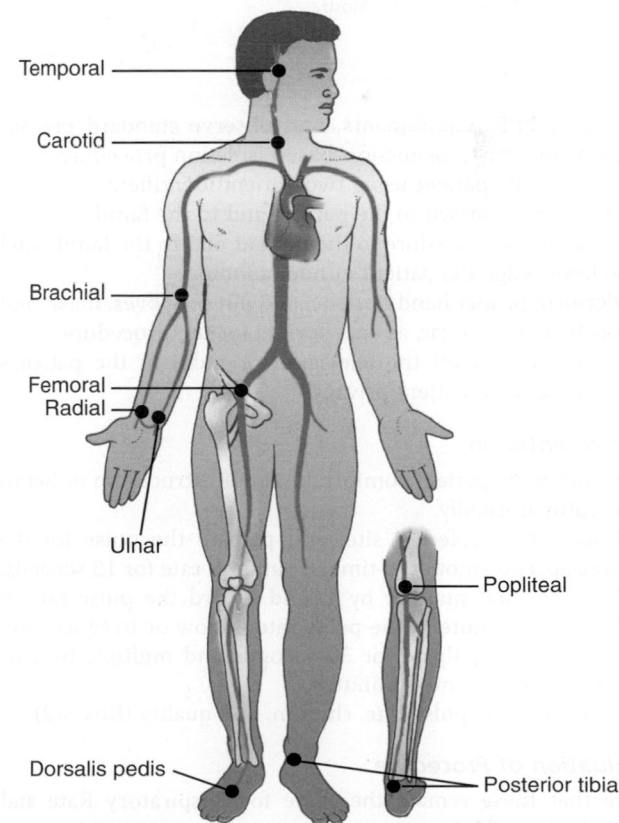

Figure 5-1 Pulse points. (From Ignatavicius D: *Medical surgical nursing*, ed 6, St. Louis, MO, 2009, Saunders.)

TABLE 5-1 Pulse Descriptions with Common Causes

Pulse Description	Common Causes
Bradycardia: rate below 60	Hypothermia, certain cardiac arrhythmias, traumatic brain injuries
Tachycardia: rate above 100	Exercise, fear, anxiety, hypotension, anemia, fever, reduced arterial blood oxygen levels, certain medications
Pulsus paradoxus: a >10 mm Hg decrease in pulse pressure with each inspiratory effort	Acute obstructive pulmonary disease, asthma exacerbation
Pulsus alternans: alternating between strong and weak heartbeats	Left-sided heart disease

---

BOX 5-2   Evaluation of Key Characteristics of the Pulse

- Is the pulse rate normal, high, or low?
- Is the rhythm regular, consistently irregular, or irregularly irregular?
- Are there any changes in the strength of the pulse in relation to respiration? Are there changes in strength from one beat to another?
- Are there any other abnormalities such as palpable vibrations (thrills or bruits)?

From Kacmarek RM, Stoller JK, Heuer, AJ: *Egan's fundamentals of respiratory care*, ed 10, St. Louis, MO, 2013, Mosby.

4. Follow PPE requirements, and observe standard precautions for any transmission-based isolation procedure.
5. Identify the patient using two patient identifiers.
6. Introduce yourself to the patient and to the family.
7. Explain the procedure to the patient and to the family, and acknowledge the patient's understanding.
8. Perform proper hand hygiene, and put on gloves, mask, and protective eyewear, as appropriate for the procedure.
9. Mute or turn off the television or radio in the patient's room. Ensure patient privacy.

Implementation

1. Position the patient comfortably, and instruct him or her to breathe normally.
2. Locate the preferred site, and palpate the pulse for the appropriate amount of time. Count the rate for 15 seconds. Multiply that number by 4, and record the pulse rate in beats per minute. If the pulse rate is slow or irregular, you may have to palpate for 30 seconds and multiple by 2 or palpate for an entire minute.
   a. Determine pulse rate, rhythm, and quality (Box 5-2).

Evaluation of Procedure

Note that these remain the same for Respiratory Rate and Auscultation of Lungs.
1. Establish a baseline of vital signs assessed, or compare with previous measurements.

2. Note any oxygen therapy needs or if changes in current therapy are indicated.
3. Identify any unexpected outcomes to the appropriate health care provider.

Documentation and Reporting

1. Describe and record the rhythm and quality of the pulse rate.

Respiratory Rate

A patient's respiratory rate (RR) can tell you a tremendous amount about his or her pulmonary status. Normal respiratory rates for an adult person at rest are 12 to 18 breaths per minute (breaths/min). Rates above normal are referred to as *tachypnea* and may be caused by hypoxemia, fever, or anxiety. Rates below normal are called *bradypnea* and may be caused by hypothermia, as a side effect of narcotic analgesics, by myocardial infarction, or by a drug overdose.

> → **Reality Check** You may not always have a thermometer, blood pressure cuff, or pulse oximeter when examining your patient and administering therapy...but, you should *always* take the respiratory rate, heart rate, and auscultate the lungs of *every* patient you see.

Procedural Preparation

1. Review the patient's chart.
2. Verify the physician's order or the facility's protocol for standard of care.
3. Obtain, clean, and inspect the appropriate equipment prior to entering the patient's room.
4. Follow PPE requirements, and observe standard precautions for any transmission-based isolation procedure.
5. Identify the patient using two patient identifiers.
6. Introduce yourself to the patient and to the family.
7. Explain the procedure to the patient and to the family, and acknowledge the patient's understanding.
8. Perform proper hand hygiene, and put on gloves, mask, and protective eyewear, as appropriate for the procedure.

Implementation

1. Place fingers on the patient's radial artery as if you were obtaining a pulse rate (PR). While doing this, you should actually be obtaining a respiratory rate, also called the respiratory frequency. Count an inspiration and the following expiration as one cycle. Using a watch with a second hand, count the number of cycles in a 15-second period. Multiply that number by 4, and record the respiratory rate in breaths per minute.
2. If you are having a difficult time visualizing the chest rise, ask the patient for permission to rest your hand on his or her abdomen or shoulder. Feel the rise of the chest during a cycle, and count the respiratory rate.

Evaluation of Procedure

1. Establish a baseline of vital signs assessed, or compare with previous measurements.
2. Note any oxygen therapy needs or if changes in current therapy are indicated.

3. Identify any unexpected outcomes to the appropriate health care provider.

Documentation and Reporting

1. Describe and record the rhythm and quality of pulse, respiratory rate, and any auscultation findings in the patient's chart.
2. Record oxygen therapy needs or if changes in current therapy are indicated.
3. Report any abnormal findings to the appropriate health care provider

Examination of the Thorax and Lungs

Proper examination of the thorax and lungs is an essential skill a respiratory care student and practitioner must acquire. Often pulmonary problems may be revealed through examination of the patient's thorax and lungs while the chest x-ray order is still pending or has yet to be ordered. The following is the step-by-step process for the examination of the thorax and lungs of a patient.

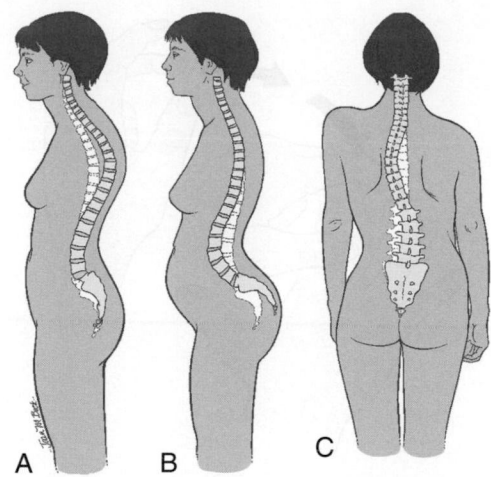

Figure 5-2 Lordosis, kyphosis, and scoliosis. (From Sanders MJ: *Mosby's paramedic textbook*, ed 3, St. Louis, MO, 2007, Mosby.)

> ✳ **Tip** To accurately assess a patient's thorax and lungs, you must expose their chest to a reasonable degree. Expose a patient's chest only as much as needed during the examination. Enlist your patient's help to move the breast, if necessary. Always explain what you are doing and why before you begin your examination. Cover the patient up as quickly as possible.

Inspection

Visual inspection of a patient's thorax plays a role in your physical assessment. An increased anteroposterior diameter, called a *barrel chest*, may be associated with emphysema. *Pectus carinatum* is the abnormal protrusion of the sternum, sometimes referred to as "pigeon-chest," whereas *pectus excavatum* is the posterior displacement of the lower aspect of the sternum, which gives the chest a "dug out" appearance. *Kyphosis* is the anteroposterior curvature that causes the patient to bend forward, and *scoliosis* is the lateral curvature of the spine. *Kyphoscoliosis* is a combination of kyphosis and scoliosis. All such deformities alter lung volumes and cause pulmonary problems. Figure 5-2 illustrates three different abnormalities.

1. Inspect the chest visually, noting the thoracic configuration and assessing for abnormalities such as increased anteroposterior diameter, pectus carinatum, pectus excavatum, kyphosis, scoliosis, and kyphoscoliosis.
2. Assess the breathing pattern and effort. Note any signs of increased work of breathing such as retractions, accessory muscle use, tracheal tugging, and the inspiration-to-expiration (I:E) ratio.

Palpation

Palpation plays a minor role in the examination of the normal thorax because the lungs are covered by the ribs and therefore cannot be directly palpated. One of the situations in which palpation may be helpful is tactile fremitus. Normal lung transmits a palpable vibration through the chest wall. This is referred to as *fremitus*. You can detect it by placing your hands firmly against either side of the chest while the patient says "ninety-nine." However, fremitus is often a very subtle finding.

1. Assess for tactile fremitus by asking the patient to repeat the word "ninety-nine" while you are palpating the thorax with the palmar aspects of your fingers. Evaluate the posterior, lateral, and anterior portions of the thorax, if possible.
2. Assess for chest wall symmetry during inhalation anteriorly by placing your hands over the anterolateral chest with your thumbs extended along the costal margin toward the xiphoid process or posteriorly by placing your hands over the posterolateral chest with your thumbs meeting at the T8 level of the patient's vertebra.
3. Have the patient exhale completely, secure your fingertips against the sides of the patient's chest, and extend your thumbs toward the middle, until the tips of the thumbs touch each other.
4. Instruct the patient to take a deep breath. Note the distance the tip of each thumb moves away from the midline.
5. Assess for air leaks by palpating the skin and subcutaneous tissue, feeling for fine air bubbles.

Percussion of the Chest

Percussion of the chest utilizes the idea that thumping on the surface of an air-filled structure such as the normal lung will produce a resonant note. If the same process is repeated over a fluid-filled or tissue-filled lung, the sound that will be generated will be relatively duller. If the normal, air-filled tissue has been displaced by fluid, as in pleural effusion, percussion will generate a dampened tone. Processes that lead to air trapping in the lung or pleural space will, however, produce a hyperresonant note on percussion. Figures 5-3, 5-4, and 5-5 illustrate percussion techniques.

1. Place your nondominant hand on your patient's chest.
2. Tap the end of the middle finger of your dominant hand quickly on the distal joint of the finger you have positioned on the chest wall.
3. Percuss the lung fields systematically and consecutively, comparing one side with the other side. Do not percuss over bony structures or over the breasts of female patients.

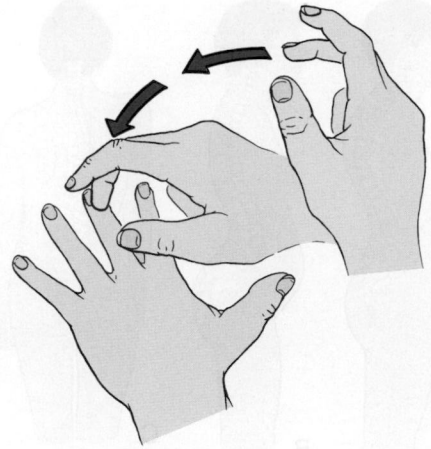

Figure 5-3 Chest percussion technique. (From Des Jardines T, Burton GG: *Clinical manifestations and assessment of respiratory disease*, ed 6, 2011, St. Louis, MO, Mosby.)

TABLE 5-2   Adventitious Lung Sounds

Sound	Mechanism	Possible Causes
Wheezes	Airflow through obstructed airways	Asthma, congestive heart failure, bronchitis
Stridor	Air flow through a partially obstructed upper airway	Croup, epiglottitis, postextubation complications
Crackles		
Inspiratory and Expiratory	Air flow moving secretion	Respiratory infection, bronchitis
Early inspiratory	Sudden opening of proximal bronchi	Bronchitis, emphysema, Asthma
Late inspiratory	Sudden opening of peripheral airways	Atelectasis, pneumonia, pulmonary edema, fibrosis

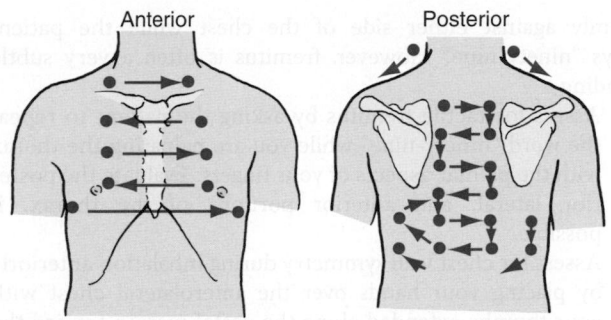

Figure 5-4 Path of systemic percussion to include all important areas. (From Des Jardines T, Burton GG: *Clinical manifestations and assessment of respiratory disease*, ed 6, 2011, St. Louis, MO, Mosby.)

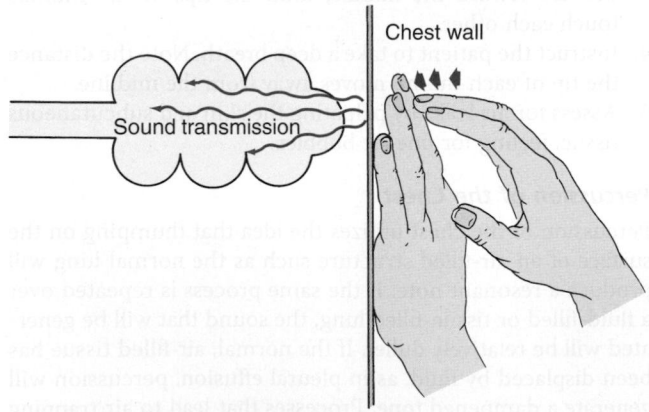

Figure 5-5 Chest percussion of a normal lung. (From Des Jardines T, Burton GG: *Clinical manifestations and assessment of respiratory disease*, ed 6, 2011, St. Louis, MO, Mosby.).

Auscultation of Lungs

Vesicular lung sounds, or normal lung sounds, are low in pitch with a soft intensity and should be heard during auscultation of the peripheral lung areas. Bronchovesicular sounds are moderate in pitch and intensity and are auscultated around

the upper portion of the sternum, between the scapulas. Tracheal breath sounds are high-pitched and loud. They are heard during auscultation over the trachea. Figure 5-6 illustrates the proper sequence for auscultating the patient's lungs during physical examination. Abnormal lung sounds, also called adventitious lung sounds, assist the practitioner in determining the patient's pulmonary difficulty. Examples of adventitious lung sounds are given in Table 5-2.

1. Use the diaphragm portion of the stethoscope to assess lung sounds. If possible, apply the diaphragm directly against the patient's chest wall. Clothing, hospital gowns, or body hair may distort lung sounds.
2. Have the patient sit upright (if possible) in a relaxed manner. The patient should be instructed to take deeper than normal tidal volume breaths through an open mouth.

> ✳ **Tip** Having the patient take deeper than normal breaths obligates them to move larger volumes of air with each breath, making lung sounds easier to hear.

3. Begin auscultation in the lung bases, compare the sounds side to side, and work upward to the apexes.
4. Record the lung sounds, making note of the location and portion of the respiratory cycle in which any adventitious lung sounds were auscultated (see Table 5-2).

5-3 Performing Pulse Oximetry

Pulse oximetry is the noninvasive measurement of a patient's SpO_2. Pulse oximetry readings are usually compared with invasive hemoximetry within ± 3% to 5%. Healthy adults should have an SpO_2 measurement of 93% to 100%. Anything below this range is considered *hypoxia*. If the patient's SpO_2 is less than 80%, it is not considered accurate. The following is the step-by-step process for performing pulse oximetry.

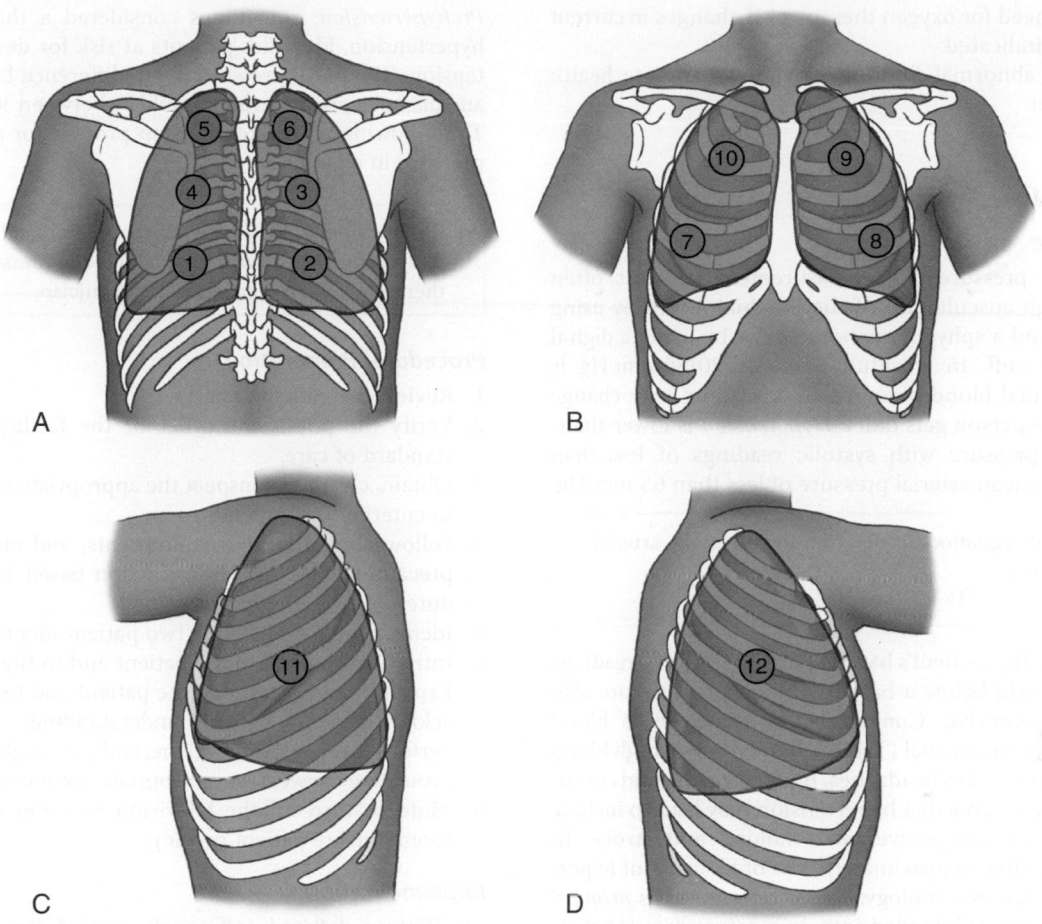

Figure 5-6 Sequencing for auscultation technique. **A,** Posterior. **B,** Anterior. **C,** Left lateral. **D,** Right lateral. (From Wilkins RL, Dexter JR, Heuer AJ: *Clinical assessment in respiratory care*, ed 6, St. Louis, MO, 2010, Mosby.)

→ **Reality Check** Severe and rapid desaturation, hypotension, hypothermia, abnormal hemoglobin, and low perfusion may cause inaccuracy in SpO₂ readings. You must be able to assess oxygenation at the bedside on the basis of the patient's clinical presentation and vital signs if the pulse oximeter fails to work.

Procedural Preparation

1. Review the patient's chart.
2. Verify the physician's order or the facility's protocol for standard of care.
3. Obtain, clean, and inspect the appropriate equipment prior to entering the patient's room.
4. Follow PPE requirements, and observe standard precautions for any transmission-based isolation procedure.
5. Identify the patient using two patient identifiers.
6. Introduce yourself to the patient and to the family.
7. Explain the procedure to the patient and to the family, and acknowledge the patient's understanding.
8. Perform proper hand hygiene, and put on gloves, mask, and protective eyewear, as appropriate for the procedure.

Implementation

1. Position the patient comfortably, and instruct him or her to breathe normally.
2. Determine the most appropriate site to attach the probe.
3. Turn on the pulse oximeter.
4. Clean the selected site with an alcohol pad.
5. Attach the probe to the selected site and secure it.
6. Observe the pulse waveform or intensity display, and correlate it with the radial pulse rate.
7. Set the alarm, and monitor skin integrity, if oximetry is continuous.

Evaluation of Procedure

1. Establish a pulse oximetry baseline, or compare with previous measurements.
2. Note any use of oxygen therapy.
3. Identify any unexpected outcomes.
4. Correlate your findings with the ABG measurement.

Documentation and Reporting

1. Record pulse oximetry, pulse rate, and patient's current oxygen use and amount, if applicable.
2. Record whether pulse oximetry is continuous or intermittent.

3. Record the need for oxygen therapy or if changes in current therapy are indicated.
4. Report any abnormal findings to the appropriate health care provider.

5-4 Taking Vital Signs

Blood Pressure

Arterial blood pressure (BP) measurement is most often attained through auscultation of the brachial artery by using a stethoscope and a sphygmomanometer or by using a digital blood pressure cuff. In an adult person, 120/80 mm Hg is considered normal blood pressure. This reading may change over time as the person gets older. *Hypotension* is lower-than-normal blood pressure with systolic readings of less than 90 mm Hg or a mean arterial pressure of less than 65 mm Hg.

> **✳ Tip** This is the equation for determining the mean arterial pressure (MAP)
>
> $$[2 \times D] + \text{systolic}] \div 3$$

Compared with a patient's baseline measurements, readings that are 40 mm Hg below a baseline blood pressure are also considered hypotensive. Conversely, *hypertension* is blood pressure higher than normal (Table 5-3). Persistent high blood pressure may manifest as headaches, blurred vision, and confusion. Potential problems that hypertension may lead to include renal insufficiency, congestive heart failure, and stroke. In the adult population, approximately 90% of all cases of hypertension are of unknown etiology. This is referred to as *primary hypertension* and is subdivided into two categories: (1) *stage I hypertension* and (2) *stage II hypertension* (Table 5-4).

TABLE 5-3 Average Blood Pressures by Age

From	To	Average	Minimum	Maximum
15	19	117/77	105/73	120/81
20	24	120/79	108/75	132/83
25	29	121/80	109/76	133/84
30	34	121/81	110/77	134/85
35	39	123/82	111/78	135/86
40	44	125/83	112/79	137/87
45	49	127/84	115/80	138/88
50	54	129/85	116/81	142/89
55	59	131/86	118/82	144/90
60	64	134/87	121/83	147/91

From: High Blood Pressure Info.org: http://www.highbloodpressureinfo.org/normal-blood-pressure-range.html. Accessed April 3, 2012; Dao HH, Essalihi R, Bouvet C, Moreau P: Evolution and modulation of age-related medial elasto-calcinosis: impact on large artery stiffness and isolated systolic hypertension. *Cardiovasc Res* 66(2):307–317, 2005.

TABLE 5-4 Hypertension Categories and Ranges

Hypertension Category	Pressures
Prehypertension	Systolic BP 120–139 mm Hg
Stage I	Systolic BP 140–159 mm Hg or diastolic BP 90–99 mm Hg
Stage II	Systolic BP >160 mm Hg or diastolic BP >100 mm Hg

Prehypertension, sometimes considered a third category of hypertension, identifies patients at risk for developing hypertension. The pulse pressure is the difference between systolic and diastolic pressures and should be between 30 to 40 mm Hg. The following is the step-by-step process for assessing blood pressure in a patient.

> **→ Reality Check** Very often, the patient's blood pressure and temperature are taken with digital blood pressure cuffs and thermometers by a patient care technician.

Procedural Preparation

1. Review the patient's chart.
2. Verify the physician's order or the facility's protocol for standard of care.
3. Obtain, clean, and inspect the appropriate equipment prior to entering the patient's room.
4. Follow personal PPE requirements, and observe standard precautions for any transmission-based isolation procedure.
5. Identify the patient using two patient identifiers.
6. Introduce yourself to the patient and to the family.
7. Explain the procedure to the patient and to the family, and acknowledge the patient's understanding.
8. Perform proper hand hygiene, and put on gloves, mask, and protective eyewear, as appropriate for the procedure.
9. Mute or turn off the television or radio in the patient's room. Ensure patient privacy.

Implementation

1. Wrap a deflated cuff snugly around the patient's upper arm. The lower edge of the cuff should be 1 inch above the antecubital fossa.
2. While palpating the brachial artery for a pulse, inflate the cuff to approximately 30 mm Hg above the point at which the brachial pulse can no longer be felt (Figure 5-7).
3. Place the diaphragm portion of the stethoscope over the brachial artery and slowly deflate the cuff at a rate of 2 mm Hg per second while observing the manometer.
4. Note the systolic pressure. The first sound heard is the systolic pressure.
5. Note the diastolic pressure. The point at which the sounds disappear is the diastolic pressure.
6. Remove the cuff in a timely manner.
7. Return the volume of the television or radio to the previous level.
8. Ensure patient comfort and safety.
9. Remove the supplies from the patient's room, and clean the area, as needed
10. Remove PPE, and perform proper hand hygiene prior to leaving the room.

Evaluation of Procedure

1. Establish a baseline of vital signs assessed, or compare with previous measurements.
2. Note any use of oxygen therapy.
3. Identify any unexpected outcomes.

Documentation and Reporting

1. Record the blood pressure in mm Hg in the patient's chart.

2. Record oxygen therapy needs or if changes in current therapy are indicated.
3. Report any abnormal findings to the appropriate health care provider.

Temperature

Although it is seldom the responsibility of the RT to obtain a patient's temperature, you must know how body temperature can affect the respiratory system. Normal body temperature may vary, depending on the site where it is measured. Table 5-5 lists the sites where temperature can be measured with the correlating normal values. Normal rectal temperatures are 37.1°C to 38.1°C. Temperatures above this range are referred to as *hyperthermia* and those below this range are *hypothermia*. Fever in a patient will increase the rate of metabolism, raising cellular oxygen demand and increasing the production of carbon dioxide. The following is the step-by-step process for assessing the temperature of a patient.

TABLE 5-5 Normal Temperature Ranges

Site	Fahrenheit	Celsius
Oral	97.0°–99.5°	36.5°–37.5°
Axillary	96.7°–98.5°	35.9°–36.9°
Rectal	98.7°–100.5°	37.1°–38.1°
Ear	38.7°–100.5°	37.1°–38.1°

Modified from Heuer AJ, Scanlan CL: *Wilkins' clinical assessment in respiratory care*, ed 7, St. Louis, MO, 2014, Mosby.

Procedural Preparation

1. Review the patient's chart.
2. Verify the physician's order or the facility's protocol for standard of care.
3. Obtain, clean, and inspect the appropriate equipment prior to entering the patient's room.
4. Follow PPE requirements, and observe standard precautions for any transmission-based isolation procedure.
5. Identify the patient using two patient identifiers.
6. Introduce yourself to the patient and to the family.
7. Explain the procedure to the patient and to the family, and acknowledge the patient's understanding.
8. Perform proper hand hygiene, and put on gloves, mask, and protective eyewear, as appropriate for the procedure.
9. Mute or turn off the television or radio in the patient's room. Ensure patient privacy.

Implementation

1. Position the patient comfortably, and instruct him or her to breathe normally.
2. Determine the most appropriate site to obtain temperature.
3. Place a disposable sheath on thermometer probe. Turn the device on, and press **START**.
4. Take the temperature. When the thermometer indicates completion of reading (often beeps), remove it from the measuring site; dispose of the sheath; clean, if needed.
5. Record the temperature and the site where it was taken.

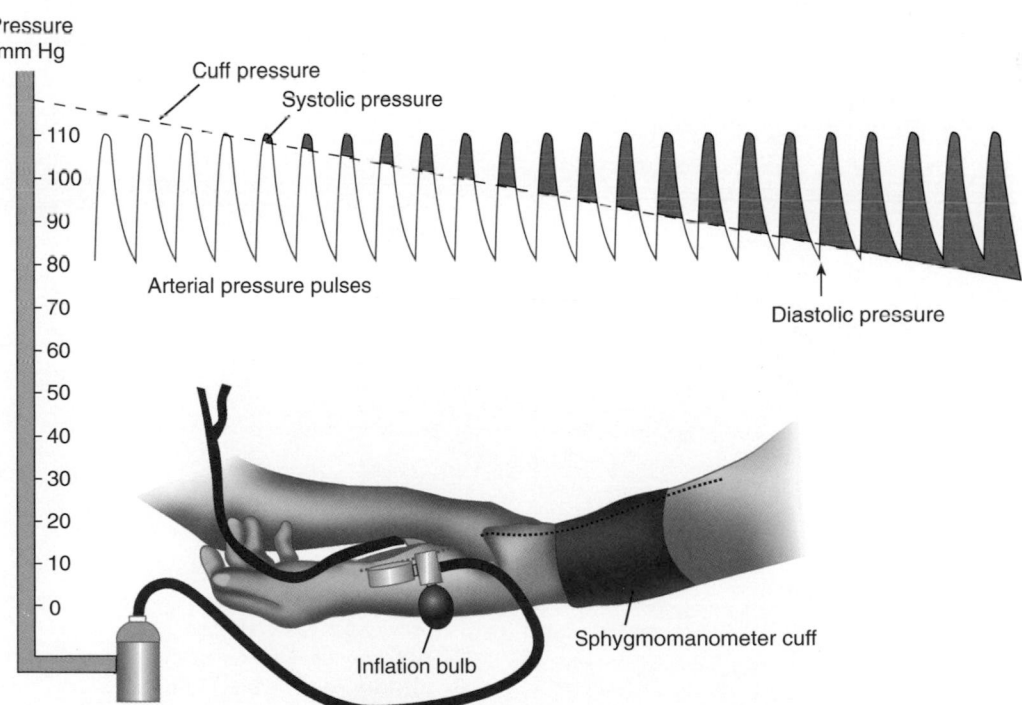

Figure 5-7 Auscultation method for measuring arterial blood pressure, using a sphygmomanometer and a stethoscope. (From Kacmarek RM, Stoller JK, Heuer AJ: *Egan's fundamentals of respiratory care*, ed 10, St. Louis, MO, 2013, Mosby.)

> **✳ Tip** This is the formula to convert Fahrenheit to Celsius, and vice versa:
>
> $$°F = \left(°C \times \frac{9}{5}\right) + 32$$
>
> $$°C = (°F - 32) \times \frac{5}{9}$$

Documentation and Reporting

1. Record the temperature in either degrees Celsius or Fahrenheit.

Bibliography

Des Jardins T, Burton GG: *Clinical manifestation and assessment of respiratory diseases*, ed 6, St. Louis, MO, 2009, Mosby.

Heuer AJ, Scanlan CL: *Wilkins' clinical assessment in respiratory care*, ed 7, St. Louis, MO, 2014, Mosby.

Ignatavicius D: *Medical surgical nursing*, ed 6, St. Louis, MO, 2009, Saunders.

Kacmarek RM, Stoller JK, Heuer AJ: *Egan's fundamentals of respiratory care*, ed 10, St. Louis, MO, 2013, Mosby.

Lab Activities

Taking a Medical History

1. Organize the following information into one of the appropriate categories in the chart (Table 5-6).

- a. Onset, time, and type of pain
- b. Patient's name and address
- c. Reason patient is seeking treatment
- d. Education
- e. Occupational history
- f. Alcohol and cigarette use
- g. Living arrangements

- h. Medications
- i. Allergies
- j. Childhood diseases
- k. Marital history
- l. Recent travel
- m. Hobbies and recreation
- n. Aggravation and alleviating factors of chief complaint

TABLE 5-6 Taking a Medical History

Demographic Data	Chief Complaint	History of Present Illness	Past Medical History	Family History	Social and Environmental History

2. Using a lab partner as your patient, perform medical history taking and physical assessment. Record the information in the patient chart provided. Be certain to use all of the procedural assessments discussed in this chapter to ensure a complete physical examination (Figure 5-8).

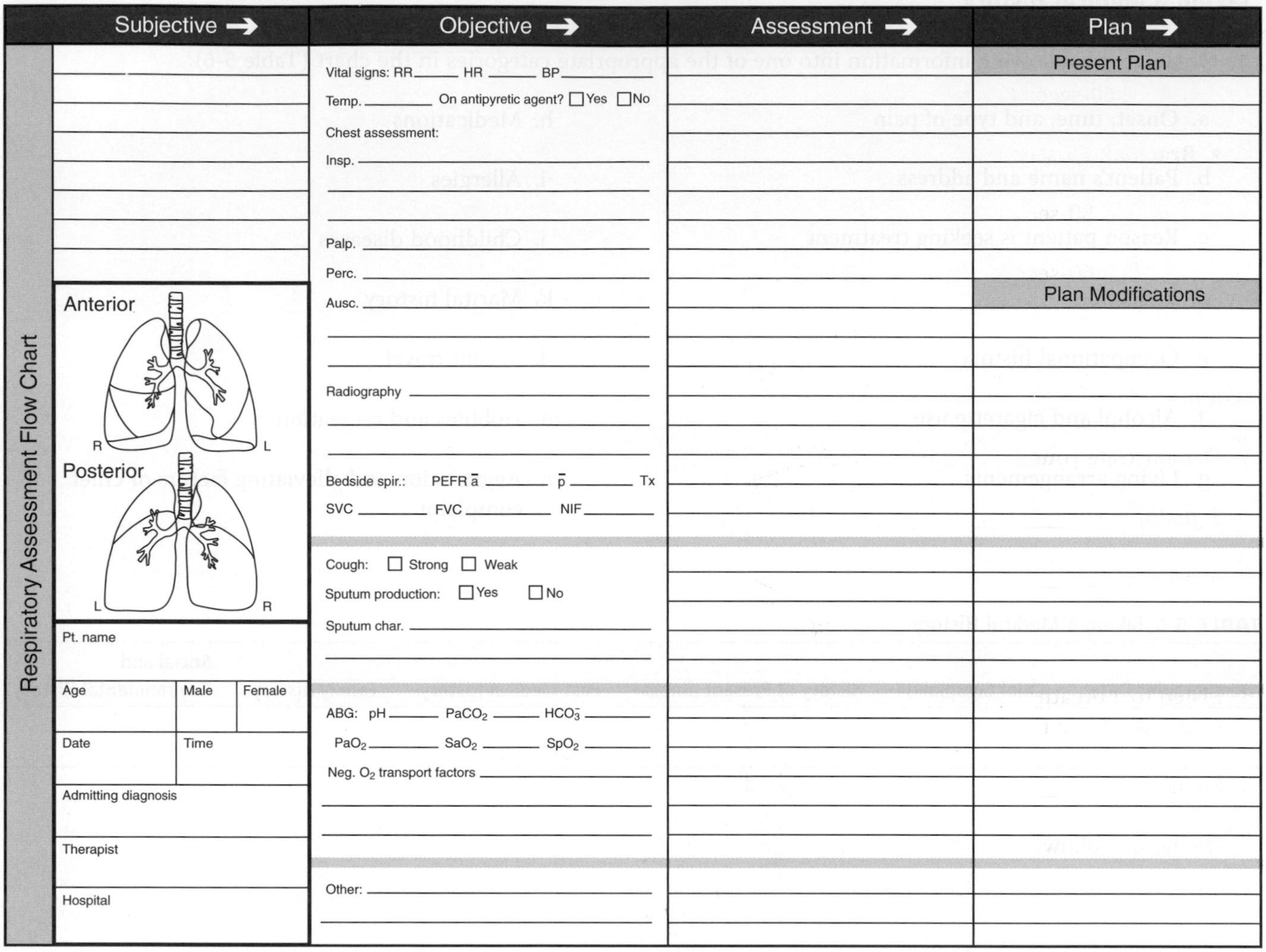

Subjective →	Objective →	Assessment →	Plan →
	Vital signs: RR____ HR ____ BP____		Present Plan
	Temp. ____ On antipyretic agent? ☐Yes ☐No		
	Chest assessment:		
	Insp. ____		
	Palp. ____		
	Perc. ____		
	Ausc. ____		Plan Modifications
	Radiography ____		
	Bedside spir.: PEFR $\bar{a}$ ____ $\bar{p}$ ____ Tx		
	SVC ____ FVC ____ NIF ____		
	Cough: ☐ Strong ☐ Weak		
	Sputum production: ☐Yes ☐No		
	Sputum char. ____		
	ABG: pH ____ $PaCO_2$ ____ HCO_3^- ____		
	PaO_2____ SaO_2 ____ SpO_2 ____		
	Neg. O_2 transport factors ____		
	Other: ____		

Respiratory Assessment Flow Chart

Anterior — R — L
Posterior — L — R

Pt. name
Age | Male | Female
Date | Time
Admitting diagnosis
Therapist
Hospital

Figure 5-8 SOAP form. (From Des Jardines T, Burton GG: *Clinical manifestations and assessment of respiratory disease*, ed 6, 2011, St. Louis, MO, Mosby.)

Locating Pulse Points and Measuring Pulse Rates

3. Identify the following pulse points on yourself using Figure 5-1 for guidance:

- Carotid
- Ulnar
- Femoral
- Temporal

- Posterior tibial
- Dorsalis pedis
- Popliteal

4. Using your lab partner, locate and measure his or her radial and brachial pulse rate using the 15-second, 30-second, and 60-second measurements. Then compare the findings.

- **Radial:** 15-seconds = _____ × 4 = _____ beats per minute

  30-seconds = _____ × 2 = _____ beats per minute

  60-seconds = _____ beats per minute

- **Brachial:** 15-seconds = _____ × 4 = _____ beats per minute

  30-seconds = _____ × 2 = _____ beats per minute

  60-seconds = _____ beats per minute

Examination of the Thorax and Lungs

5. Demonstrate your auscultation technique on three different students. Obtain their signatures.

   Signature:_____

   Signature:_____

   Signature:_____

6. Listen to a breath sound DVD, or go online to listen to different types of adventitious lung sounds with a fellow classmate. Have the partner sign off that this assignment has been completed.

   Signature:_____

7. Define the following ventilatory patterns. Give an example of a clinical condition in which each could occur.

   a. Tachypnea:_____

   b. Cheyne-Stokes:_____

   c. Bradypnea:_____

   d. Kussmaul:_____

   e. Biot:_____

   f. Apnea:_____

   g. Hyperpnea:_____

   h. Eupnea:_____

8. List the four basic parts of the stethoscope.

   _____

9. Using your lab partner, identify the following imaginary lines on his or her chest wall (Figures 5-9, 5-10, and 5-11). Obtain his or her signature in the table below for each item.

Imaginary Line	Signature
Midclavicular line	
Midsternal line	
Anterior axillary line	
Midaxillary line	
Posterior axillary line	
Left scapular line	
Midspinal line	
Right scapular line	

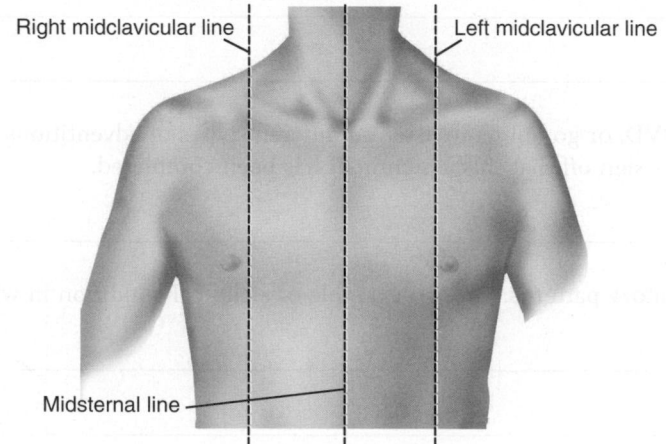

Figure 5-9 Imaginary lines on the anterior chest wall. (From Kacmarek RM, Stoller JK, Heuer AJ: *Egan's fundamentals of respiratory care*, ed 10, St. Louis, MO, 2013, Mosby.)

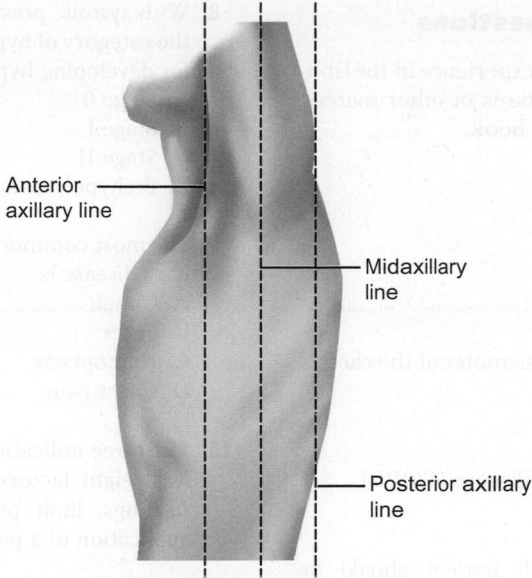

Figure 5-10 Imaginary lines on the lateral chest wall. (From Kacmarek RM, Stoller JK, Heuer AJ: *Egan's fundamentals of respiratory care*, ed 10, St. Louis, MO, 2013, Mosby.)

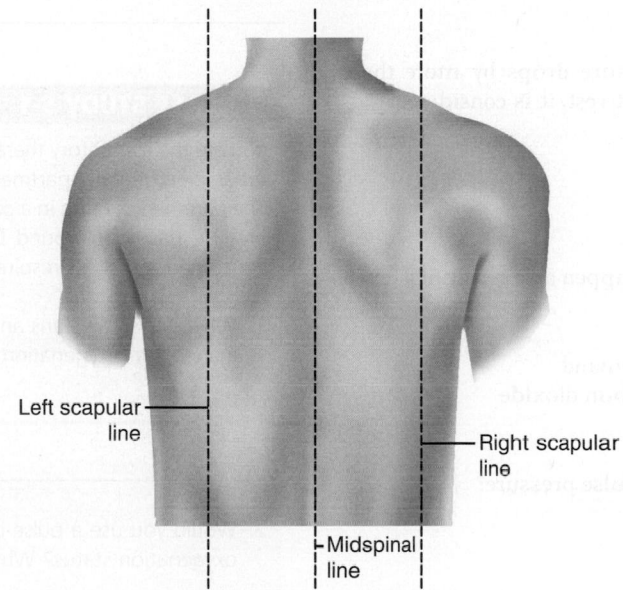

Figure 5-11 Imaginary lines on a posterior chest wall. (From Kacmarek RM, Stoller JK, Heuer AJ: *Egan's fundamentals of respiratory care*, ed 10, St. Louis, MO, 2013, Mosby.)

Blood Pressure Measurement

10. Assess the blood pressure on three different students. Obtain their signatures.

Signature:_____

Signature:_____

Signature:_____

Self-Assessment Questions

The following questions may need your experience in the laboratory or information gleaned from lectures or other sources. Answers can be found at the end of the book.

1. Fever is most often the result of:
   A. Brain tumor
   B. Infection
   C. Anxiety
   D. Exercise

2. An increase in the anteroposterior diameter of the chest is often associated with:
   A. Asthma
   B. Congestive heart failure
   C. Chronic obstructive pulmonary disease (COPD)
   D. Tuberculosis

3. A pulse rate of 135 in an adult patient should be considered:
   A. Bradycardia
   B. Tachycardia
   C. Hyperpnea
   D. Tachypnea

4. When the systolic blood pressure drops by more than 10 mm Hg during inhalations at rest, it is considered:
   A. Pulsus paradoxus
   B. Auscultatory gap
   C. Korotkoff sounds
   D. Pulsus alternans

5. Which of the following could happen as a result of a fever in your patient?
   A. Tachypnea
   B. Increased cellular oxygen demand
   C. Increased production of carbon dioxide
   D. All of the above

6. What is the normal range for pulse pressure?
   A. 30–40 mm Hg
   B. 40–50 mm Hg
   C. 50–60 mm Hg
   D. 60–80 mm Hg

7. What is the normal respiratory rate for an adult person at rest?
   A. 5–10 breaths/min
   B. 7–12 breaths/min
   C. 12–20 breaths/min
   D. 18–24 breaths/min

8. With systolic pressures ranging from 120 to 139 mm Hg, the category of hypertension that identifies patients at risk for developing hypertension is:
   A. Stage 0
   B. Stage I
   C. Stage II
   D. Prehypertension

9. The most common symptom seen in patients with pulmonary disease is:
   A. Cough
   B. Fever
   C. Hemoptysis
   D. Chest pain

10. List three indications for using pulse oximetry; and list at least eight factors, agents, or situations that may affect readings, limit precision, or limit the performance or application of a pulse oximeter.

_____

_____

_____

▶▶ CASE STUDY 5-1

You are the respiratory therapist (RT) on the night shift in a busy urban emergency department (ED) of a level-one trauma center. The paramedics bring in a patient who was pulled from a house fire. He has soot around both nares but no burns. You are concerned about his respiratory status.

1. What are some signs and symptoms that indicate inadequate oxygenation this patient may display?

_____

_____

2. Would you use a pulse oximeter to measure your patient's oxygenation status? Why, or why not?

_____

_____

3. How should you determine this patient's oxygenation status?

_____

_____

Electrocardiogram Interpretation

▪ OBJECTIVES

Upon the completion of the chapter activities and content review topics, the student should be able to:
1. Describe the purpose of the electrocardiogram (ECG).
2. Obtain a 12-lead electrocardiogram.
3. Describe the anatomic locations of standard lead placement.
4. Identify the numeric values assigned to the ECG paper.
5. Identify the various abnormal electrocardiographic recordings.

▪ KEY TERMS

- Augment
- Bipolar leads
- Depolarization
- Electrodes
- Precordial leads
- Repolarization
- Unipolar leads

▪ CONTENT REVIEW TOPICS

- Advanced cardiac life support (ACLS)
- Automaticity
- Telemetry unit

▪ PROCEDURAL ASSESSMENTS

6-1 Obtaining a 12-Lead ECG
6-2 Interpreting an ECG

▪ EQUIPMENT

- ECG machine
- Self-sticking electrodes for 4 limb leads and 6 chest leads

I n numerous medical facilities, it is the respiratory therapists (RTs) who are responsible for obtaining ECGs for evaluation of cardiac arrhythmias. The ability to recognize life-threatening arrhythmias while obtaining a patient's ECG and while monitoring a patient in the intensive care unit (ICU) is a necessary skill for RTs. The ECG is a vital piece of the comprehensive care plan of a patient with a respiratory complaint, as cardiac events may initially present as shortness of breath (SOB). Whether the ECG is used diagnostically or as a monitoring tool, obtaining and interpreting it must be a part of an RT's skill set.

> → **Reality Check** The ECG measures the electrical activity of the heart, not the mechanical activity. So, you must treat the patient, not the ECG rhythm.

In the ICU, monitoring a single lead, usually lead II, is the standard. The lead is displayed on the monitor with other diagnostic parameters. Many of the respiratory care treatments we perform, for example, the delivery of aerosolized adrenergic bronchodilators and suctioning a patient's airway, may directly affect the heart. Therefore, the ability to continuously monitor a patient's heart rate and rhythm is crucial. If a complete assessment of the heart's electrical activity is needed in the patient complaining of chest pain that may be cardiac in origin, a 12-lead ECG will be ordered. Other complaints that may elicit the need for a 12-lead ECG are listed in Box 6-1. Through the use of 10 specifically placed electrodes, a 12-lead ECG allows for 12 different views of the heart's electrical activity.

> ✳ **Tip** Think of the lungs as hands that cradle the heart. This visualization with help you understand the involvement of the cardiovascular system in respiratory care.

ECG interpretation takes practice, but it can enable you to become a well-rounded therapist who can successfully function in many areas of the hospital and other medical settings. This chapter covers the basic principles regarding heart rates, durations, and amplitudes may be determined from ECG recordings and methods to obtain a 12-lead ECG for interpretation.

≫ SKILL CHECK LISTS

6-1 Obtaining a 12-Lead Electrocardiogram

Obtaining an ECG is a noninvasive procedure that can be quickly performed in the emergent setting. To obtain a 12-lead ECG, electrodes are placed in locations on the arms, legs, and chest of the patient. An electrode is a device that contains a conductive material. Electrodes are applied to the patient at specific locations to view the heart's electrical activity. Figure 6-1 illustrates the view that the limb leads produce.

The limb leads consist of four electrodes placed on the extremities giving you six views of the heart. These views are denoted as leads I, II, III, aV_R, aV_L, and aV_F. Leads I, II, and III make up the standard limb leads and are considered bipolar leads. That is, their measurement of electrical activity happens in two different directions. Figure 6-2 illustrates the views

- Chest pain
- Shortness of breath
- Dyspnea with palpitations
- Weakness
- Lethargy
- Syncope

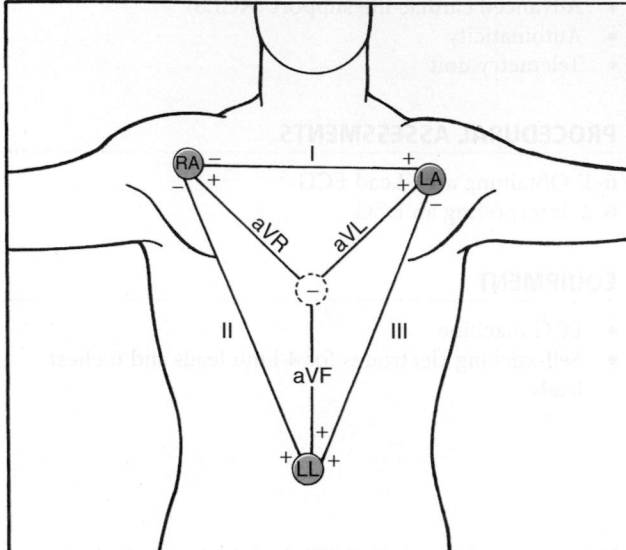

Figure 6-1 View of the standard limb leads and augmented leads. (From Aehlert B: *ECGs made easy*, ed 4, St. Louis, MO, 2009, Mosby.)

obtained by leads I, II, and III. The augmented limb leads are unipolar. Electrical potential produced by the augmented leads is relatively small, so the ECG machine magnifies, or augments, the amplitude of the electrical potentials.

> → **Reality Check** Typically, when the ECG is being used as a monitoring tool, lead II will be utilized.

The chest leads, referred to as precordial leads, are denoted V_1, V_2, V_3, V_4, V_5, and V_6. Unlike the limb leads, these leads are unipolar. That is, their measurement of electrical activity happens in only one direction. Lead placement is important. ECGs could be misinterpreted because of improper lead placement. Figure 6-3 illustrates proper chest lead placement.

Procedural Preparation

Note that the following eight steps are basic preparation steps that should be observed before any patient interaction.
1. Review the patient's chart.
2. Verify the physician's order or the facility's protocol for standard of care.
3. Obtain, clean, and inspect the appropriate equipment prior to entering the patient's room.
4. Follow personal protective equipment (PPE) requirements, and observe standard precautions for any transmission-based isolation procedure.

5. Identify the patient using two patient identifiers.
6. Introduce yourself to the patient and to the family.
7. Explain the procedure to the patient and to the family, and acknowledge the patient's understanding.
8. Perform proper hand hygiene, and put on gloves, mask, and protective eyewear, as appropriate for the procedure.

Implementation

1. Position the patient in the semi-Fowler position, and instruct him or her to breathe normally.
2. Provide privacy.
3. Clean and prepare the patient's skin, as needed.
4. Apply self-sticking electrodes, and attach leads to the chest and the extremities.
   a. For the four limb leads: Place one on each wrist (RA, on right wrist or LA, on left wrist) and one on each ankle (RL, ground electrode on right ankle or LL, on left ankle).

> → **Reality Check** They are called *limb leads* and should be placed on the extremities, not on the upper chest and abdomen of the patient.

   b. For the six chest leads: Follow this order beginning with V_1: fourth intercostal space to the right of the sternum; V_2: fourth intercostal space to the left of the sternum; V_4: fifth intercostal space at the midclavicular line; V_3: directly between leads V_2 and V_4; V_5: level with V_4 at the left anterior axillary line; V_6: level with V_5 at the left midaxillary line (directly under the midpoint of the armpit).
5. Turn on the ECG machine, and enter the patient's demographic information.
6. Obtain a tracing.
7. Inspect the printout for clarity, and repeat, if necessary.
8. Disconnect the leads, clean the skin, and reposition the patient.
9. Discard any disposable equipment.
10. Remove the supplies from the patient's room, and clean the area, as needed.
11. Remove PPE, and perform proper hand hygiene prior to leaving the patient's room.

Evaluation of Procedure

1. Establish a baseline, or compare with previous measurements.

Documentation and Reporting

1. Attach the ECG tracing to the patient's chart.
2. Report about or deliver the ECG tracing to the appropriate health care provider.
3. Report any abnormal findings immediately to the appropriate health care provider.

6-2 Interpreting an Electrocardiogram

Being systematic in your evaluation of an ECG strip helps ensure that interpretation is accurate and that no subtleties are overlooked. To properly interpret an ECG, you must first understand the graph paper the ECG is printed on. The

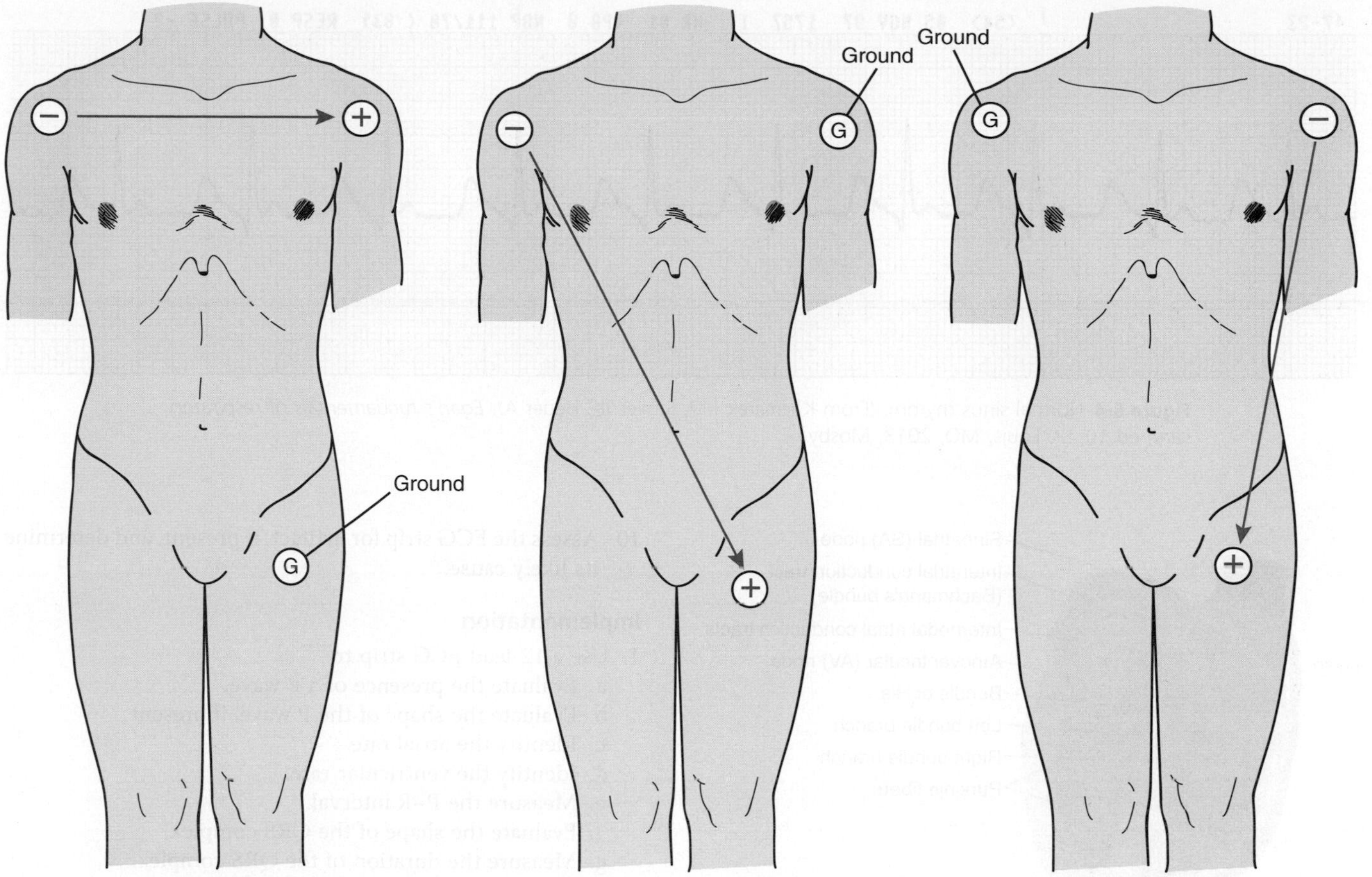

Figure 6-2 Electrode placement on the patient's limbs for lead I, lead II, and lead III. (From Aehlert B: *ECGs made easy*, ed 4, St. Louis, MO, 2009, Mosby.)

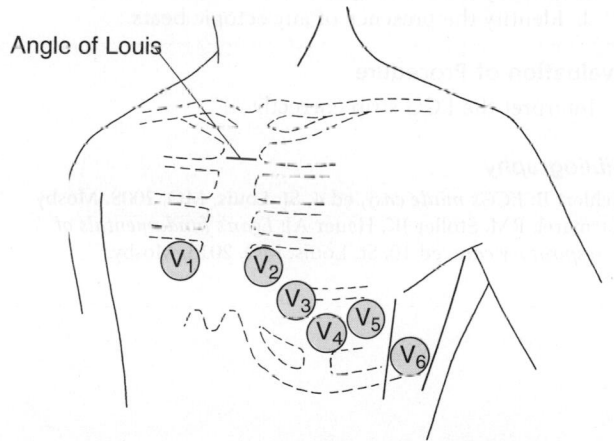

Figure 6-3 Proper precordial lead placement. (From Heuer AJ, Scanlan C: *Wilkins' clinical assessment in respiratory care*, ed 7, St. Louis, MO, 2014, Mosby.)

horizontal axis of the ECG paper corresponds to time, and as a rule, it typically records at a speed of 25 millimeters per second (mm/s). The graph paper consists of small and large boxes. The small boxes are 1 mm wide and 1 mm high, and the large boxes consist of five times five small boxes. The large boxes have darker lines around them.

Voltage, measured in millivolts (mV), also called *amplitude*, which is measured in millimeters (mm), is represented on the vertical axis of the paper. Voltage may be a positive or negative value. You cannot diagnose an ECG finding as abnormal, if you do not know what a normal finding looks like. Figure 6-4 is an ECG tracing of a normal sinus rhythm, and Figure 6-5 illustrates the normal conducting system of the human heart.

If you look at an ECG as electricity measured over time, understanding of abnormalities may be a bit easier. The following is the step-by-step process for the "Implementation" portion of the procedural assessment for interpreting an electrocardiogram.

> → **Reality Check** Sometimes "way too fast" or "way too slow" is all the interpretation you will need to realize your patient is in trouble.

Procedural Preparation

1. Review the patient's chart.
2. Verify the physician's order or the facility's protocol for standard of care.
3. Obtain, clean, and inspect the appropriate equipment prior to entering the patient's room.
4. Follow PPE requirements, and observe standard precautions for any transmission-based isolation procedure.
5. Identify the patient using two patient identifiers.
6. Introduce yourself to the patient and to the family.

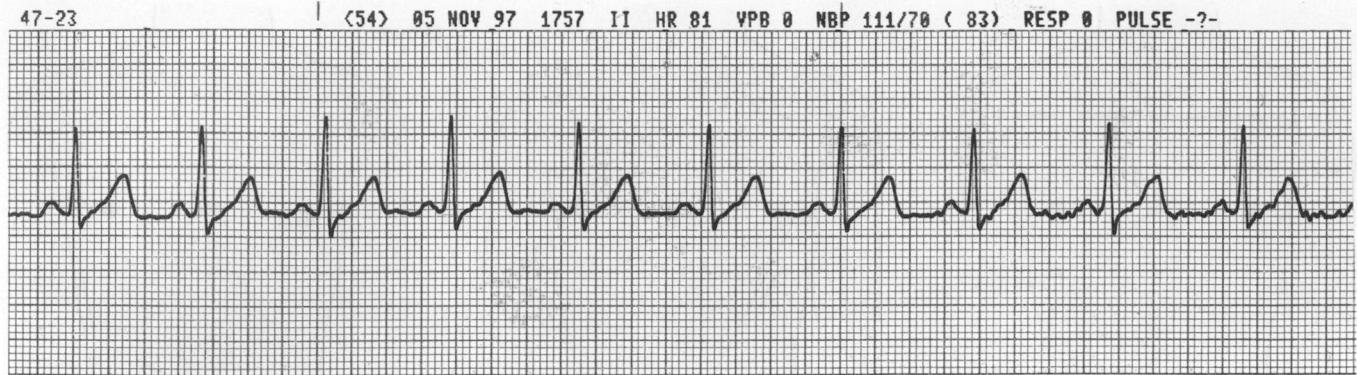

47-23   (54) 05 NOV 97 1757 II HR 81 VPB 0 NBP 111/70 (83) RESP 0 PULSE -?-

Figure 6-4 Normal sinus rhythm. (From Kacmarek RM, Stoller JK, Heuer AJ: *Egan's fundamentals of respiratory care*, ed 10, St. Louis, MO, 2013, Mosby.)

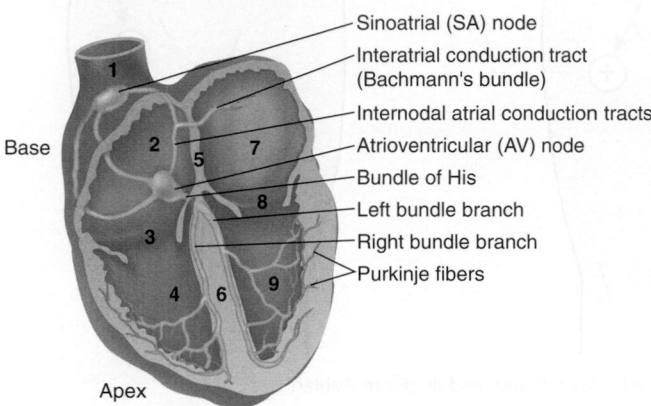

Base

- Sinoatrial (SA) node
- Interatrial conduction tract (Bachmann's bundle)
- Internodal atrial conduction tracts
- Atrioventricular (AV) node
- Bundle of His
- Left bundle branch
- Right bundle branch
- Purkinje fibers

Apex

1. Superior vena cava
2. Right atrium
3. Tricuspid valve
4. Right ventricle
5. Interatrial septum
6. Interventricular septum
7. Left atrium
8. Mitral valve
9. Left ventricle

Figure 6-5 Conducting system of the human heart. (From Kacmarek RM, Stoller JK, Heuer AJ: *Egan's fundamentals of respiratory care*, ed 10, St. Louis, MO, 2013, Mosby.)

7. Explain the procedure to the patient and to the family, and acknowledge the patient's understanding.
8. Perform proper hand hygiene, and put on gloves, mask, and protective eyewear, as appropriate for the procedure.
9. Obtain a 12-lead ECG strip for interpretation.

10. Assess the ECG strip for artifact, if present, and determine its likely cause.

Implementation

1. Use a 12-lead ECG strip to:
   a. Evaluate the presence of a P wave.
   b. Evaluate the shape of the P wave, if present.
   c. Identify the atrial rate.
   d. Identify the ventricular rate.
   e. Measure the P–R interval.
   f. Evaluate the shape of the QRS complex.
   g. Measure the duration of the QRS complex.
   h. Evaluate the shape of the T wave.
   i. Evaluate the ST segment.
   j. Measure the R–R interval.
   k. Identify the mean QRS axis.
   l. Identify the presence of any ectopic beats.

Evaluation of Procedure

1. Interpret the ECG strip correctly.

Bibliography

Aehlert B: *ECGs made easy*, ed 4, St. Louis, MO, 2008, Mosby.
Kacmarek RM, Stoller JK, Heuer AJ: *Egan's fundamentals of respiratory care*, ed 10, St. Louis, MO, 2013, Mosby.

1. Label the time intervals and box heights on the ECG graph paper in Figure 6-6 below.

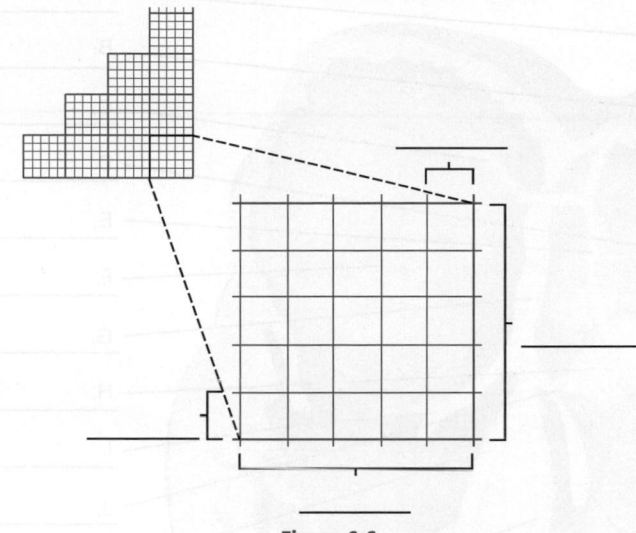

Figure 6-6

2. Label Figure 6-7 *A-J*, then answer the following questions *a* through *d*.

a. Which of the letters corresponds to ventricular depolarization?

b. Which of the letters is the Q wave?

c. Which of the letters corresponds with the P–R interval?

d. Which of the letters corresponds to atrial depolarization?

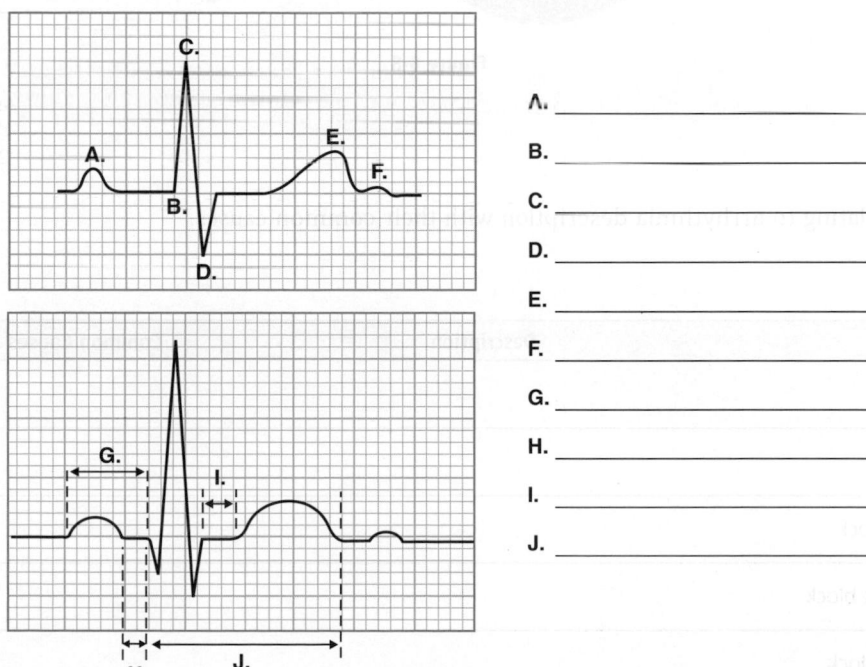

A. _____

B. _____

C. _____

D. _____

E. _____

F. _____

G. _____

H. _____

I. _____

J. _____

Figure 6-7

3. Label Figure 6-8.

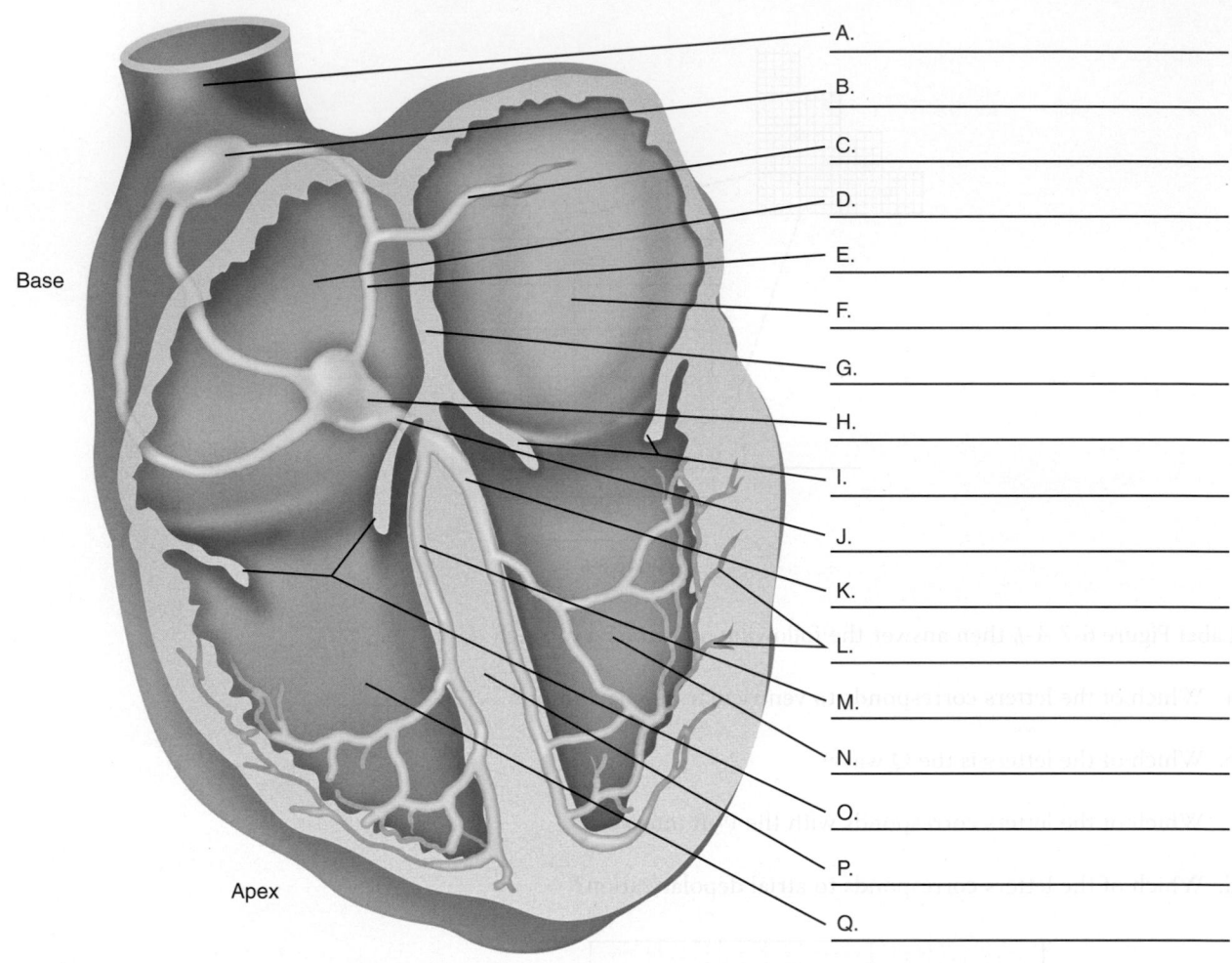

Base

Apex

A. _____

B. _____

C. _____

D. _____

E. _____

F. _____

G. _____

H. _____

I. _____

J. _____

K. _____

L. _____

M. _____

N. _____

O. _____

P. _____

Q. _____

Figure 6-8

4. Fill in Table 6-1 relating to arrhythmia description with their common causes.

TABLE 6-1

Arrhythmias	Description	Common Causes
Sinus tachycardia		
Sinus bradycardia		
First-degree heart block		
Second-degree heart block		
Third-degree heart block		

Arrhythmias	Description	Common Causes
Atrial flutter		
Atrial fibrillation		
Ventricular tachycardia		
Ventricular fibrillation		
Pulseless electrical activity (PEA)		
Asystole		

5. Fill in Table 6-2 relating to the waves, intervals, complexes, and segments used in interpreting an ECG with normal values and corresponding events.

TABLE 6-2

What You Are Evaluating	How to Evaluate	Normal Value	Corresponding Event in the Heart
P wave			
P–R interval			
QRS complex			
T wave			
ST segment			
R–R interval			
QRS axis			

6. Fill in Table 6-3 relating to rate determination.

TABLE 6-3

Rate	Method Used to Determine Rate
Atrial rate	
Ventricular rate	

7. Obtain a 12-lead ECG machine. Work in pairs; one student will be the patient *(note that it is preferred that you use a male student as the patient),* and the other student will be connecting the 12-lead electrodes. Perform the following tasks:

a. Have the patient lie on a hospital bed, and attach a 12-lead ECG. Print out a 12-lead strip. Then print out at least a 6-second strip of lead II, and answer the following questions:

   i. What is the atrial rate?_____

   ii. What is the ventricular rate?_____

   iii. Are P waves present? If so, are they all similar in shape? Is a QRS complex present after every P wave?

   _____

   iv. What is the P–R interval?_____

   v. Is a QRS complex present?_____

   vi. What is the duration of the QRS complex?_____

   vii. Is a T wave present? _____If so, is it upright? _____

   viii. Is the ST segment flat, elevated, or depressed?_____

   ix. Is the rhythm regular?_____

   x. What is your interpretation of the rhythm?_____

b. Now, move the electrodes of V_1 and V_2 about three inches apart. Print out a 12-lead strip, and compare it with the correct 12-lead strip from the previous ECG. What differences do you notice? Re-adjust the electrodes to proper placement when done.

   _____

c. Replace an electrode for one of the upper limb leads without securing it completely to the skin, and run a 12-lead ECG strip. What do you notice? Re-adjust the electrode to proper placement when done.

   _____

d. Switch the left and right upper limb leads, and run a 12-lead ECG strip. What do you notice? Re-adjust the electrodes to proper placement when done.

   _____

e. With the patient correctly attached to the ECG machine, set it in monitor mode to display lead II. Wheel the patient around the halls, or have the patient move around in the bed. What do you notice?

   _____

8. Using Figure 6-9 answer the following questions:

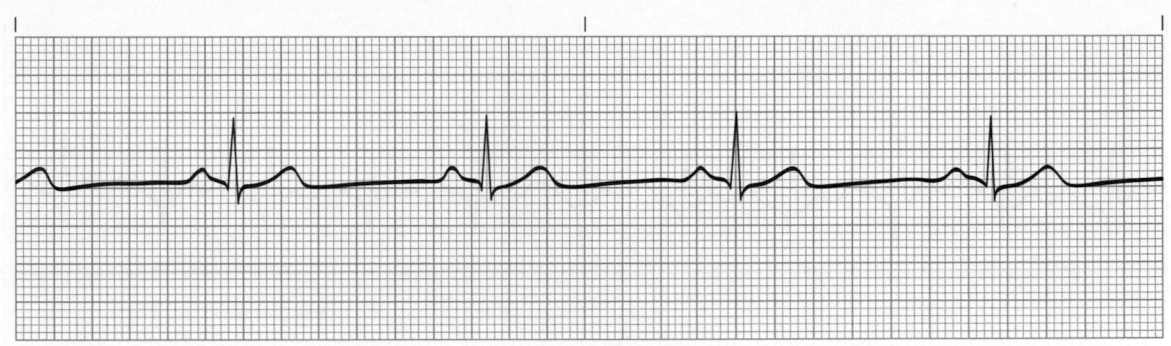

Figure 6-9

a. What is the atrial rate?

_____

b. What is the ventricular rate?

_____

c. Are P waves present? If so, are they all similar in shape? Is a QRS complex present after every P wave?

_____

d. What is the P–R interval?

_____

e. Is a QRS complex present? If so, what is its duration?

_____

f. Is a T wave present? If so, is it upright?

_____

g. Is the ST segment flat, elevated, or depressed?

_____

h. Is the rhythm regular?

_____

i. What is your interpretation of the rhythm?

_____

j. What are some common causes of this rhythm?

_____

9. Using Figure 6-10 to answer the following questions:

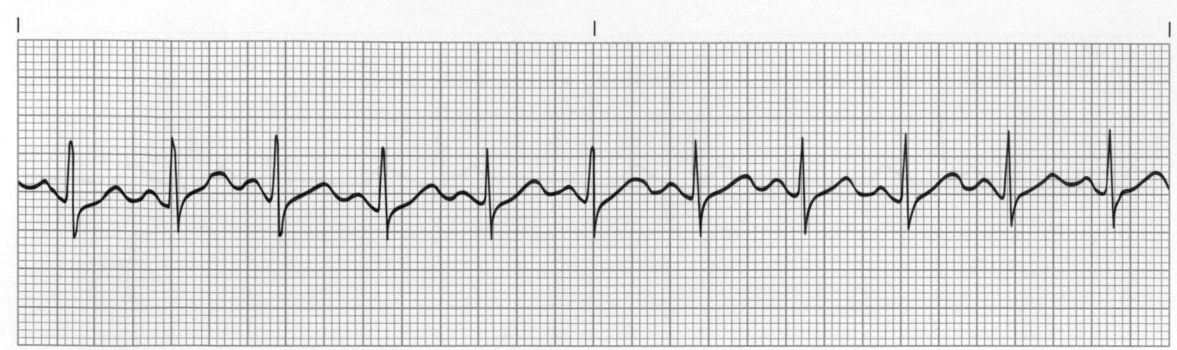

Figure 6-10

a. What is the atrial rate?

_____

b. What is the ventricular rate?

_____

c. Are P waves present? If so, are they all similar in shape? Is a QRS complex present after every P wave?

_____

d. What is the P–R interval?

_____

e. Is a QRS complex present? If so, what is its duration?

_____

f. Is a T wave present? If so, is it upright?

_____

g. Is the ST segment flat, elevated, or depressed?

_____

h. Is the rhythm regular?

_____

i. What is your interpretation of the rhythm?

_____

j. What are some common causes of this rhythm?

_____

10. Using Figure 6-11 to answer the following questions:

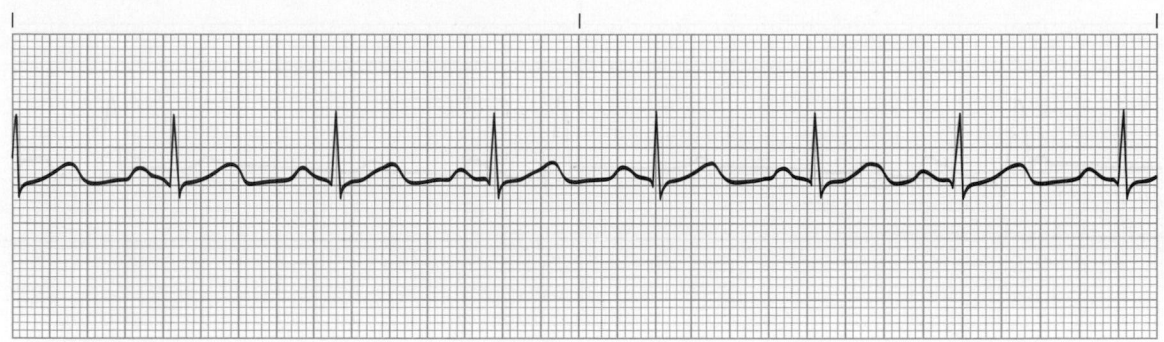

Figure 6-11 From Kacmarck RM, Stoller JK and Heuer AJ: Egan's fundamentals of respiratory care, ed 10, St. Louis, MO, 2013, Elsevier.

a. What is the atrial rate?

_____

b. What is the ventricular rate?

_____

c. Are P waves present? If so, are they all similar in shape? Is a QRS complex present after every P wave?

_____

d. What is the P–R interval?

_____

e. Is a QRS complex present? If so, what is its duration?

_____

f. Is a T wave present? If so, is it upright?

_____

g. Is the ST segment flat, elevated, or depressed?

_____

h. Is the rhythm regular?

_____

i. What is your interpretation of the rhythm?

_____

11. Using Figure 6-12 answer the following questions:

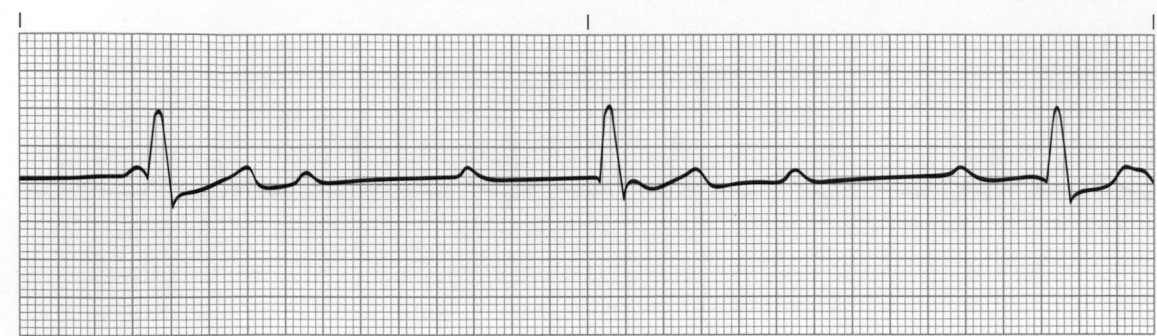

Figure 6-12

a. What is the atrial rate?

_____

b. What is the ventricular rate?

_____

c. Are P waves present? If so, are they all similar in shape? Is a QRS complex present after every P wave?

_____

d. What is the P–R interval?

_____

e. Is a QRS complex present? If so, what is its duration?

_____

f. Is a T wave present? If so, is it upright?

_____

g. Is the ST segment flat, elevated, or depressed?

_____

h. Is the rhythm regular?

_____

i. What is your interpretation of the rhythm?

_____

j. What are some common causes of this rhythm?

_____

12. Using Figure 6-13 answer the following questions:

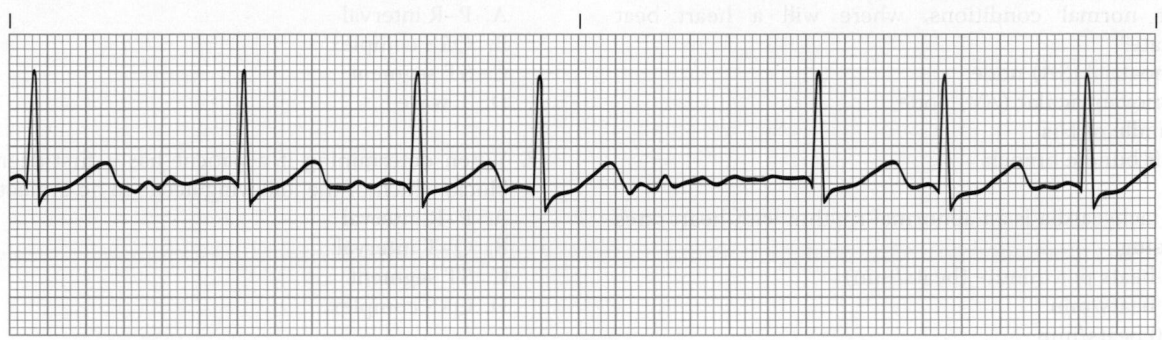

Figure 6-13

a. What is the atrial rate?

_____

b. What is the ventricular rate?

_____

c. Are P waves present? If so, are they all similar in shape? Is a QRS complex present after every P wave?

_____

d. What is the P–R interval?

_____

e. Is a QRS complex present? If so, what is its duration?

_____

f. Is a T wave present? If so, is it upright?

_____

g. Is the ST segment flat, elevated, or depressed?

_____

h. Is the rhythm regular?

_____

i. What is your interpretation of the rhythm?

_____

j. What are some common causes of this rhythm?

_____

Self-Assessment Questions

1. Under normal conditions, where will a heart beat originate?
   A. Sinoatrial (SA) node
   B. Atrioventricular (AV) node
   C. Bundle of His
   D. Left bundle branch

2. Sinus tachycardia is an abnormal rhythm with heart rates exceeding:
   A. 60 beats per minute (beats/min)
   B. 80 beats/min
   C. 100 beats/min
   D. 120 beats/min

3. How many seconds are indicated by each small box on the ECG paper?
   A. 0.02
   B. 0.04
   C. 0.08
   D. 0.10

4. The horizontal axis of the ECG paper corresponds with time, and as a rule, it typically records at a speed of:
   A. 25 millimeters per second (mm/s)
   B. 25 mm/0.04 s
   C. 20 mm/s
   D. 20 mm/0.04 s

5. In which of the following situations would a 12-lead typically be ordered?

   1. Syncope in a 78-year-old male patient
   2. Cough with chest pain in a 3-year-old patient
   3. Sudden onset of shortness of breath in a 25-year-old patient with a heart transplant
   4. Wheezing and shortness of breath in a 12-year-old patient with asthma

   A. 1 and 4 only
   B. 1 and 3 only
   C. 1, 2, and 3 only
   D. 1, 2, 3, and 4

6. Depolarization of the ventricles is represented on an ECG as the:
   A. P–R interval
   B. QRS complex
   C. ST segment
   D. T wave

7. When determining if a patient has a first-degree heart block, which of the following needs to be evaluated?
   A. P–R interval
   B. Q–T interval
   C. ST segment
   D. QRS complex

8. The rapid return of a cell to the polarized position in which the electrical imbalance across the membrane is reestablished is called:
   A. Depolarization
   B. Repolarization
   C. Hyperpolarization
   D. Hypopolarization

9. A negative QRS complex in lead I is consistent with right-axis deviation and is often caused by:
   A. Congestive heart failure
   B. Asthma
   C. Cor pulmonale
   D. Chronic obstructive pulmonary disease (COPD)

10. For which of the following arrhythmias would you apply shock to the heart immediately?
    A. PEA
    B. Asystole
    C. Atrial fibrillation
    D. Ventricular fibrillation

CASE STUDY 6-1

While suctioning a patient's tracheostomy tube, you observe the ECG tracing as shown in Figure 6-14. The patient is currently on a tracheostomy ("trach") collar with an FIO₂ (fraction of inspired oxygen) of 0.28.

1. What arrhythmia are you seeing?

_____

_____

2. What are some common causes of the disturbance?

_____

_____

_____

3. What should you do to correct the problem?

_____

_____

_____

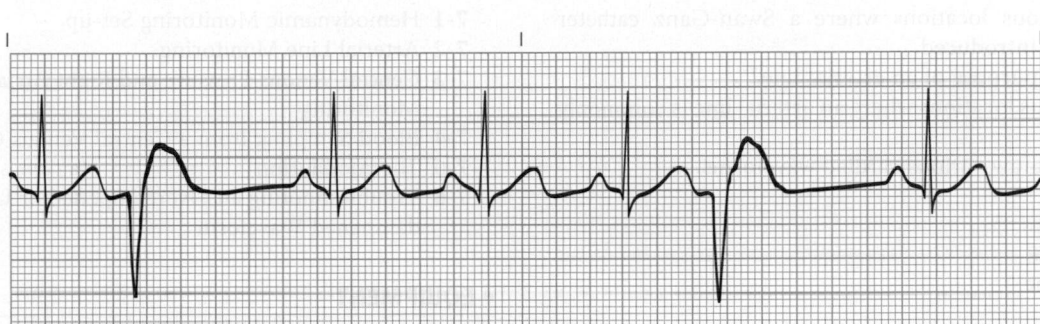

Figure 6-14

Hemodynamic Monitoring

Jonathan R. Marino

▪ OBJECTIVES

Upon the completion of the chapter activities and content review topics, the student should be able to:

1. Identify and assemble a hemodynamic monitoring set-up.
2. Describe the function of each component of a hemodynamic monitoring set-up.
3. Identify and explain the purpose of each component of a Swan-Ganz catheter.
4. List the various locations where a Swan-Ganz catheter is commonly introduced.
5. Describe the purpose of an arterial line.
6. List the various locations where an arterial line is commonly introduced.
7. Identify and draw various cardiac waveforms.

▪ KEY TERMS

- Arterial line
- Artifact
- End-diastolic volume (EDV)
- Injectate
- Isovolumetric
- Lumen
- Thermodilution
- Swan-Ganz catheter (pulmonary artery catheter)

▪ CONTENT REVIEW TOPICS

- Cardiac anatomy and physiology
- Pulmonary anatomy and physiology
- Patient assessment
- Sterile gloving

▪ PROCEDURAL ASSESSMENTS

7-1 Hemodynamic Monitoring Set-up
7-2 Arterial Line Monitoring
7-3 Central Venous Pressure and Right Atrial Pressure Monitoring
7-4 Blood Sampling from a Central Venous Catheter
7-5 Thermodilution
7-6 Troubleshooting an Overdampened or Underdampened Waveform

▪ EQUIPMENT

- PAC or A-line catheter
- Three-way stopcock
- Rigid-pressure tubing
- Pressure transducer
- 500-mL normal saline solution bag as the flush system
- Pressure bag
- Transducer cable
- Monitor

As a respiratory therapist (RT), hemodynamic monitoring and analysis are important when working with critically ill patients. Knowledge about monitoring, interpreting, and analyzing the information provided by various hemodynamic catheters and transducers will help you understand how your patient's cardiac function and fluid balance relates to his or her pulmonary system. This information helps guide your choices and decision making with regard to their care plan. Moreover, hemodynamic monitoring will allow you to implement therapies that may improve your patient's health status.

> ✳ **Tip** The word "hemodynamic" is made up of the word parts *hemo-*, which refers to "blood," and *-dynamic*, which refers to motion or movement. The opposite of *dynamic* is *static*, which means "*stationary.*"

Hemodynamic monitoring refers to the observation of blood pressure, blood volume, and cardiac output (CO; or cardiac flow), as well as cardiac preload and afterload, and systemic and pulmonary vascular resistance in real time (Box 7-1). Special indwelling catheters such as the Swan-Ganz catheter are inserted into a specific artery or vein by a trained physician

or RT. A Swan-Ganz catheter is a useful device for measuring dynamic pressures in the heart, the vena cava, and the pulmonary artery. The catheter is typically introduced through the internal jugular vein, the subclavian vein, or the femoral vein. The position of the catheter determines which pressure the monitor will display.

Modern-day catheters have many passages called lumens. Some catheters have up to six lumens; the catheter pictured in Figure 7-1 is a quadruple lumen catheter equipped with an inflatable balloon at the tip and a monitor connector to transmit data from the thermistor to the monitor. The lumen opening that is the closest to the various ports is called the *proximal lumen*. Similarly, the lumen opening that is farthest from the ports is called the *distal lumen*. The third lumen is dedicated for medication or fluid administration by injection. This catheter, in the proper position, is capable of measuring dynamic blood pressure in the vena cava, the right atrium, the right ventricle, or the pulmonary artery. If the balloon at the tip is properly inflated, an indirect measurement of the left atrial pressure is obtained. The catheters are attached to pressure transducers, which send data to a monitor for visual observation. From this data, a pressure-time graphic is visualized, and mean pressures are calculated and displayed on the monitor. This chapter will focus on the monitoring and analysis of hemodynamic data that are relevant to the field of respiratory care.

BOX 7-1   Characteristics of a Reliable Monitoring System

- The system should be as simple as possible. Extra stopcocks and manifolds decrease the fidelity of the monitoring system and increase the risk of fluid leak, microbial line contamination, and air bubble collection.
- The bores of monitoring catheters should be no smaller than 18 gauge or 7 French. Small bores result in overdampening.
- All connecting tubing should be of low compliance (stiff) and no longer than 3 to 4 feet. Low-compliance tubing is identified on packaging as "monitoring tubing."
- Tubing connectors should be tight. Use Luer-Lok connections, and inspect frequently for fluid leaks.
- The catheter and connection tubing must be patent. Use a continuous-flush device for cardiovascular pressure monitoring, and inspect frequently to see that the pressure bag is inflated to 300 mm Hg. Routinely "fast-flush" the monitoring systems of patients with hypercoagulability.
- The system must be free of air bubbles or clots. Even pinpoint-sized air bubbles decrease the fidelity of monitoring systems.
- Keep the connecting tubing away from areas of patient movement. Jostling of tubing results in an externally induced whip artifact.

From Darovic GO: *Handbook of hemodynamic monitoring*, ed 2, St. Louis, MO, 2003, Saunders.

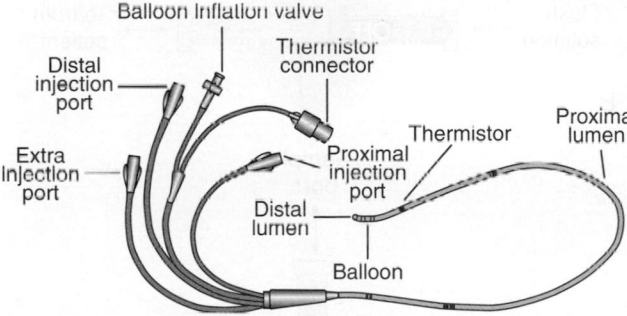

Figure 7-1   Example of a Swan-Ganz catheter. (From Cairo JM: *Pilbeam's mechanical ventilation*, ed 5, St. Louis, MO, 2013, Mosby.)

›› SKILLS CHECK LIST

7-1 Hemodynamic Monitoring Set-up

Correct set-up of equipment is the first step in the monitoring process. Figure 7-2 shows a schematic of a hemodynamic monitoring set-up. The functions of these components of the set-up are listed in Box 7-2. The following is the step-by-step process for hemodynamic monitoring set-up:

Procedural Preparation

1. Review the patient's chart.
2. Verify the physician's order or the facility's protocol for standard of care.

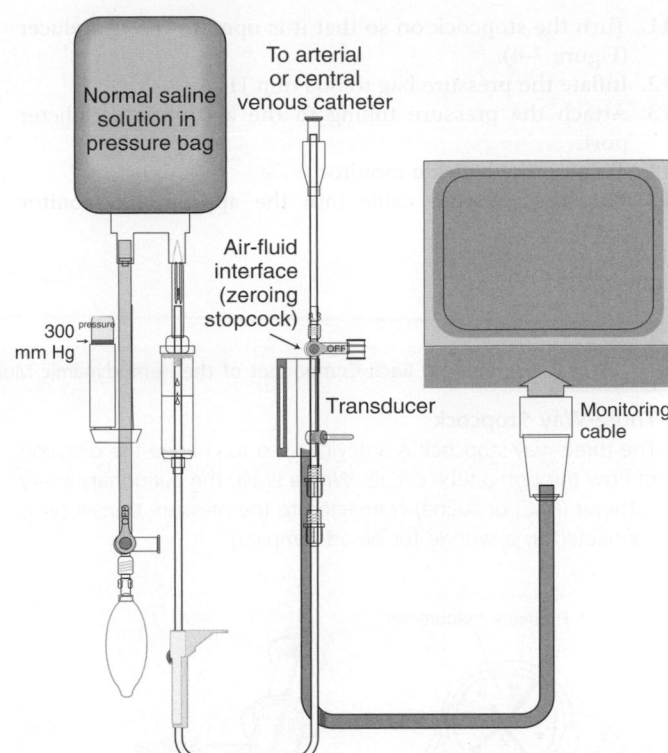

Figure 7-2   Single-pressure transducer system. (Drawing by Paul W. Schiffmacher, Thomas Jefferson University, Philadelphia, PA, copyright, 2004)

3. Obtain, clean, and inspect the appropriate equipment prior to entering the patient's room.
4. Follow the personal protective equipment (PPE) requirements, and observe the standard precautions for any transmission-based isolation procedure.
5. Identify the patient using two patient identifiers.
6. Introduce yourself to the patient and to the family.
7. Explain the procedure to the patient and to the family, and acknowledge the patient's understanding.
8. Perform proper hand hygiene, and put on gloves, mask, and protective eyewear, as appropriate for the procedure.

Implementation

1. Place the patient in the supine position, with the head of the bed no higher than 45 degrees.
2. Open the prepackaged pressure transducer kit.
3. Tighten all the connections.
4. Attach the transducer clamp to the intravenous (IV) pole, and place the transducer inline with the patient's phlebostatic axis.
5. Open the bag of heparinized saline, and insert it into the pressure bag.
6. Spike the bag, and hang the bag from the IV pole.
7. Turn the stopcock off to the patient, and attach the pressure tubing to the transducer stopcock (Figure 7-3).
8. Open the roller clamp, and prime the drip chamber.
9. Flush the tubing, and attach it to the pressure transducer.
10. Turn the stopcock off to the patient, and flush through the transducer.

11. Turn the stopcock on so that it is open to the transducer (Figure 7-4).
12. Inflate the pressure bag to 300 mm Hg.
13. Attach the pressure tubing to the appropriate catheter port.
14. Turn on the bedside monitor.
15. Plug the pressure cable into the appropriate monitor port.

16. Turn on the chosen parameter (pulmonary artery [PA], right atrial [RA], arterial).
17. Set the appropriate scale.
18. Level the transducer and set to zero (Figure 7-5).
19. Remove the supplies from the patient's room, and clean area, as needed.
20. Remove the PPE, and perform proper hand hygiene prior to leaving the patient's room.

BOX 7-2   Function of Each Component of the Hemodynamic Monitor Set-up

Three-Way Stopcock

The three-way stopcock is a device used to change the direction of flow through a tube circuit. With a twist, the pulmonary artery catheter (PAC; or A-line) connected to the pressure transducer is connected to a syringe for blood sampling.

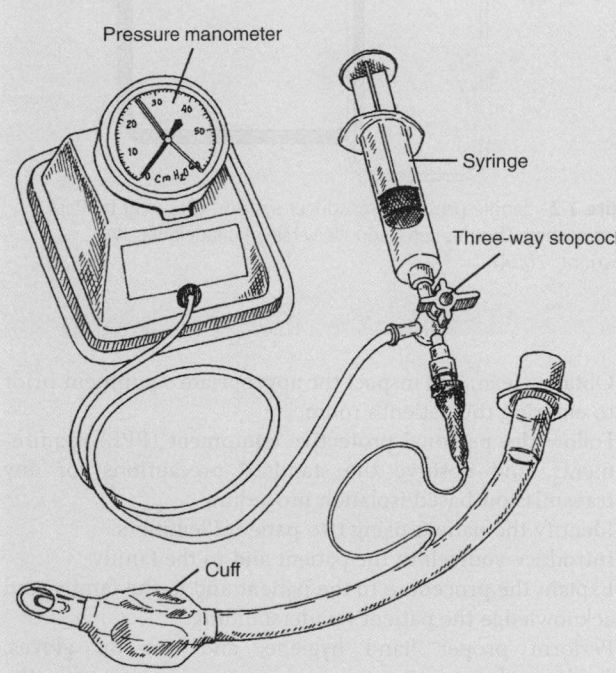

Pressure manometer
Syringe
Three-way stopcock
Cuff

Cuff measuring device made from pressure manometer, three-way stopcock, and 10-mL syringe. (From Sills JR: *The comprehensive respiratory therapist exam review entry and advanced levels*, ed 5, 2010, St. Louis, MO, Mosby.)

Another reason to turn the stopcock is to calibrate or "zero," the system to barometric pressure. Readings from the pressure transducer are relative to barometric pressure; therefore, it is essential that the system be properly calibrated.

Pressure Transducer

These devices convert the pressure impulse of the blood from within the vein or the artery into an electrical signal. The electrical signal is then sent to the monitor.

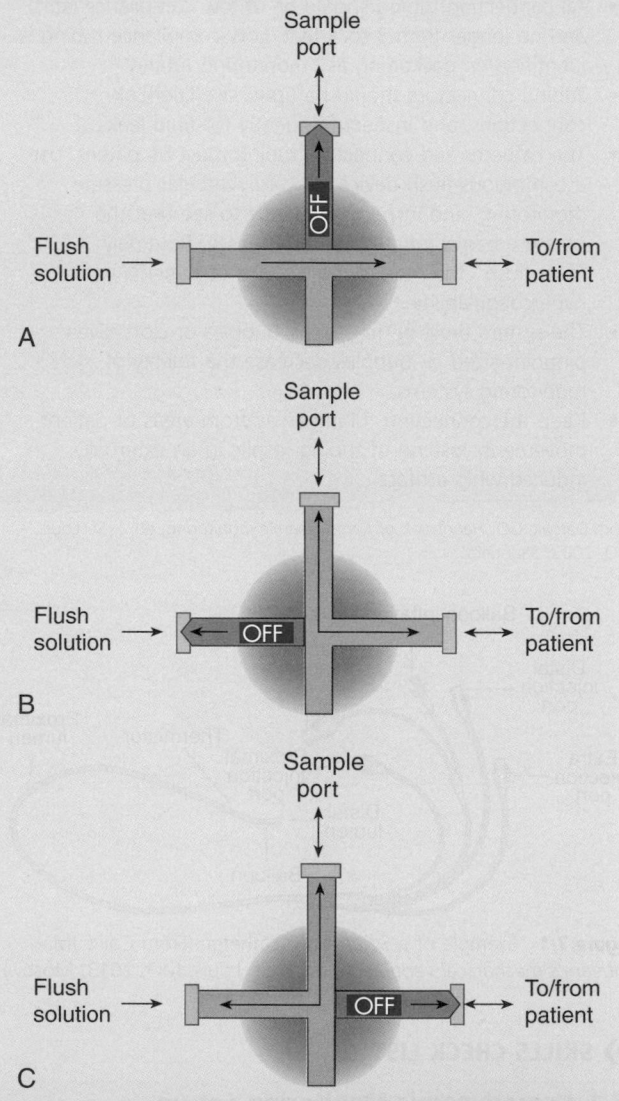

A three-way stopcock for use in an arterial line system. **A,** The normal operating position of the stopcock that allows fluid to flow to the patient (and the blood pressure to be monitored if assembled for continuous blood pressure monitoring). **B,** The stopcock position that allows blood to be withdrawn from the patient through the sample port. The flush solution port is closed. **C,** The stopcock position for flush solution to go to the sample port to clear out any blood. When the stopcock is turned to a 45-degree angle between any two ports, all of the ports are closed. (From Kacmarek RM, Stoller JK, Heuer AJ: *Egan's fundamentals of respiratory care*, ed 10, St. Louis, 2013, Mosby.)

| BOX 7-2 | Function of Each Component of the Hemodynamic Monitor Set-up—cont'd |

Rigid-Pressure Tubing

This type of tubing is used to preserve pressure or prevent the loss of pressure between the patient's vein or artery and the pressure transducer. Think of it as a basketball; if the basketball is fully inflated (rigid), it is easy to dribble or bounce, and if it is not fully inflated (soft), it is very difficult to bounce. The rigid tubing provides an easy surface for the pressure to be transmitted to the transducer.

500-mL Heparinized Saline with Pressure Bag

The 500-mL bag of heparinized saline is inserted into a pressure bag, which is inflated to, and maintained at, a pressure of

300 mm Hg. The purpose of this flush system is to keep the line clear of any blood that might backflow through the catheter. It is important to keep the catheter clear of blood because stagnant blood may form clots.

Monitor

The monitor receives the electrical signal from the pressure transducer and converts it to a pressure-time graphic so that various pressures can be visualized. Using this data, the monitor will calculate the mean, or average, pressure at a given location.

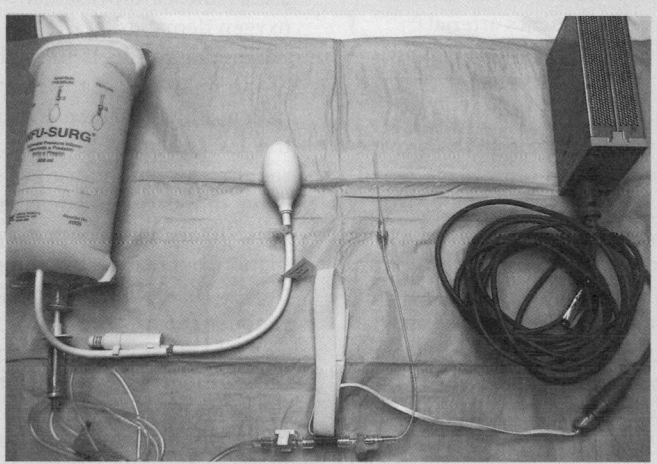

Pressure transducer fluid monitoring set. A pressurized saline (heparinized solution may be substituted) is connected to an intravascular line and arterial catheter, which is then fixed to a three-way stopcock. The fluid wave is directly monitored by the electromechanical transducer, which records pressure cycles and displays multiple hemodynamic values. (From Roberts J, Hedges J: *Clinical procedures in emergency medicine*, ed 5, St. Louis, MO, 2009, Saunders.)

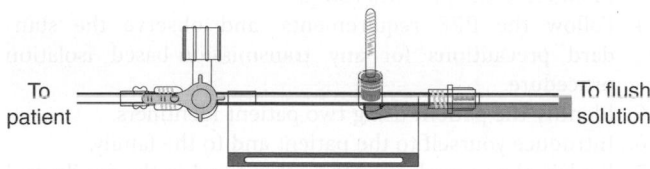

Figure 7-3 Stopcock is off to the patient. (Drawing by Paul W. Schiffmacher, Thomas Jefferson University, Philadelphia, PA, copyright, 2004)

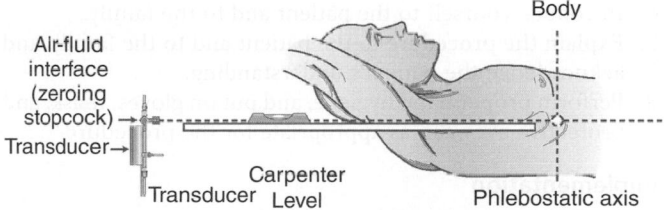

Figure 7-5 Air–fluid interface (zeroing stopcock) is leveled with the phlebostatic axis by using a carpenter level. (Drawing by Paul W. Schiffmacher, Thomas Jefferson University, Philadelphia, PA, copyright, 2004)

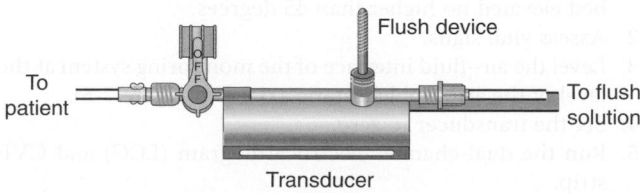

Figure 7-4 Stopcock is open to the transducer. (Drawing by Paul W. Schiffmacher, Thomas Jefferson University, Philadelphia, PA, copyright, 2004)

Evaluation of Procedure

1. Establish a baseline, or compare with previous measurements.
2. Develop the appropriate respiratory plan based on assessment data.
3. Identify any unexpected outcomes.
4. Correlate your findings with noninvasive data, if applicable.

Documentation and Reporting

1. Record your findings in the patient's chart.
2. Report any abnormal findings to the appropriate health care provider.

7-2 Arterial Line Monitoring

An arterial line is a single-lumen catheter commonly used in critical care when frequent arterial blood samples are anticipated and to monitor arterial blood pressure dynamically.

> → **Reality Check** Monitoring blood pressure with an arterial line provides the ability to observe the patient's arterial blood pressure in real time.

With proper calibration, invasive monitoring systems provide more accurate techniques compared with noninvasive monitoring techniques.

Like an arterial blood gas (ABG) puncture, introduction of an arterial line is commonly done in the radial artery or, less commonly, in the brachial, femoral, or dorsalis pedis artery. Medication is not introduced through an arterial line because serious tissue damage could result. The following is the step-by-step process for arterial line monitoring.

Procedural Preparation

1. Review the patient's chart.
2. Verify the physician's order or the facility's protocol for standard of care.
3. Obtain, clean, and inspect the appropriate equipment prior to entering the patient's room.
4. Follow the personal PPE requirements, and observe the standard precautions for any transmission-based isolation procedure.
5. Identify the patient using two patient identifiers.
6. Introduce yourself to the patient and to the family.
7. Explain the procedure to the patient and to the family, and acknowledge the patient's understanding.
8. Perform proper hand hygiene, and put on gloves, mask, and protective eyewear, as appropriate for the procedure.

Implementation

1. Position the patient in a comfortable position.
2. Assess vital signs.
3. Visually inspect the catheter.
4. Assess the arterial catheter insertion site and the involved extremity for postinsertion complications.
5. Set the transducer to zero.
6. Obtain the tracing.
7. Assess the waveform.
8. Remove the supplies from the patient's room, and clean the area, as needed.
9. Remove PPE, and perform proper hand hygiene prior to leaving the patient's room.

Evaluation of Procedure

1. Establish a baseline, or compare with previous measurements.

2. Attach the tracing to the patient's chart, if applicable.
3. Identify any unexpected outcomes.

Documentation and Reporting

1. Record your findings in the patient's chart.
2. Report any abnormal findings to the appropriate health care provider.

7-3 Central Venous Pressure and Right Atrial Pressure Monitoring

The main purpose of monitoring central venous pressure (CVP) and right atrial pressure in the critically ill patient is to assess the cardiovascular system and its response to tissue oxygen demands.

The CVP reflects the right atrial pressure and the function of the right side of the heart and provides an insight into the patient's fluid balance. Monitoring the CVP is appropriate for the assessment of cardiac function in acutely ill patients who require close monitoring of fluid balance as well as in patients being monitored for their response to certain cardiac medications. In acutely ill patients who are receiving mechanical ventilation, increased intrathoracic pressures may require that the CVP be kept at a higher-than-normal level to maintain venous return.

Right atrial pressure monitoring is not only appropriate for the assessment of cardiac function and fluid balance, but it also provides information about right ventricular functionality and may help diagnose pulmonary hypertension. The following is the step-by-step process for CVP and right atrial pressure monitoring.

Procedural Preparation

1. Review the patient's chart.
2. Verify the physician's order or the facility's protocol for standard of care.
3. Obtain, clean, and inspect the appropriate equipment prior to entering the patient's room.
4. Follow the PPE requirements, and observe the standard precautions for any transmission-based isolation procedure.
5. Identify the patient using two patient identifiers.
6. Introduce yourself to the patient and to the family.
7. Explain the procedure to the patient and to the family, and acknowledge the patient's understanding.
8. Perform proper hand hygiene, and put on gloves, mask, and protective eyewear, as appropriate for the procedure.

Implementation

1. Place the patient in the supine position, with the head of the bed elevated no higher than 45 degrees.
2. Assess vital signs.
3. Level the air–fluid interface of the monitoring system at the level of the atria (phlebostatic axis) (see Figure 7-5).
4. Set the transducer to zero.
5. Run the dual-channel electrocardiogram (ECG) and CVP strip.
6. Measure the pressures at the end of expiration.
7. Reassess vital signs.
8. Remove the supplies from the patient's room, and clean the area, as needed.

9. Remove PPE, and perform proper hand hygiene prior to leaving the patient's room.

Evaluation of Procedure

1. Establish a baseline, or compare with previous measurements.
2. Develop an appropriate respiratory plan based on assessment data.
3. Identify any unexpected outcomes.

Documentation and Reporting

1. Record your findings in the patient's chart.
2. Report any abnormal findings to the appropriate health care provider.

7-4 Blood Sampling from a Central Venous Catheter

In addition to monitoring pressures, central venous catheters may be used to sample venous blood from patients who require frequent blood draws, and mixed venous samples may be acquired from the PA for purposes of analyzing oxygen consumption. Although blood may be sampled from a central venous catheter, it should not be inserted for the sole purpose of collecting blood samples. The following is the step-by-step process for blood sampling from a central venous catheter.

Procedural Preparation

1. Review the patient's chart.
2. Verify the physician's order or the facility's protocol for standard of care.
3. Obtain, and inspect the appropriate equipment prior to entering the patient's room.
4. Follow PPE requirements, and observe the standard precautions for any transmission-based isolation procedure.
5. Identify the patient using two patient identifiers.
6. Introduce yourself to the patient and to the family.
7. Explain the procedure to the patient and to the family, and acknowledge the patient's understanding.
8. Perform proper hand hygiene, and put on gloves, mask, and protective eyewear, as appropriate for the procedure.

Implementation

1. Place the patient in a comfortable position.
2. Assess vital signs.
3. Inspect the catheter for leaks or air bubbles.
4. Clean the needleless cap at the top of the stopcock with alcohol or other antiseptic solution.
5. Attach the needleless blood sampling device to the capped stopcock of the monitoring system.
6. Suspend the right atrial pressure or central venous pressure monitoring alarm.
7. Turn the stopcock off to the monitoring system, and flush the system.
8. Insert a blood specimen tube into the blood sampling device.
9. Remove the discarded blood specimen tube, and dispose of it appropriately.

a. Newer systems do not require you to dispose of blood. Blood is withdrawn by utilizing a syringe at the transducer. After the sample is obtained, this blood is returned to the patient through a needleless system, and the system is flushed.
10. Insert the blood specimen tube into the blood sampling device to obtain a specimen.
11. Detach the blood sampling device from the capped stopcock, and dispose of it appropriately.
12. Cleanse the needleless cap at the top of the stopcock with alcohol or other antiseptic solution.
13. Attach a 10-mL syringe filled with sterile normal saline solution to the needleless capped stopcock.
14. Gently flush the normal saline solution into the needleless cap.
15. Turn the stopcock off to the blood sampling device.
16. Fast-flush the remaining blood in the central venous catheter back into the patient until the line runs clear.
17. Observe the monitor for return of the right atrial pressure or central venous pressure waveform.
18. Turn the alarms on.
19. Label the specimen.
20. Dispose of the used supplies in an appropriate container.
21. Send the specimen for analysis.
22. Remove the supplies from the patient's room, and clean the area, as needed.
23. Remove the PPE, and perform proper hand hygiene prior to leaving the patient's room.

Evaluation of Procedure

1. Establish a baseline, or compare with previous measurements.
2. Develop an appropriate respiratory plan based on assessment data.
3. Identify any unexpected outcomes.

Documentation and Reporting

1. Record your findings in the patient's chart.
2. Report any abnormal findings to the appropriate health care provider.

7-5 Thermodilution

Blood volume and CO may also be measured by using a technique called thermodilution. Thermodilution is done by positioning the proximal lumen in the right atrium of the heart and then introducing an injectate with a known volume and temperature into the proximal injection port. An injectate is simply material that is injected; in this case, it is 5% dextrose in water (D_5W). As the heart pumps blood and the introduced fluid to the PA, the thermistor detects the change in temperature. The data are then converted to CO using mathematic formulas. Once various pressures are obtained and CO is computed, the average systemic and pulmonary vascular resistance is calculated with ease. The following is the step-by-step process for performing thermodilution:

Procedural Preparation

1. Review the patient's chart.
2. Verify the physician's order or the facility's protocol for standard of care.

3. Obtain, and inspect the appropriate equipment prior to entering the patient's room.
4. Follow the PPE requirements, and observe the standard precautions for any transmission-based isolation procedure.
5. Identify the patient using two patient identifiers.
6. Introduce yourself to the patient and to the family.
7. Explain the procedure to the patient and to the family, and acknowledge the patient's understanding.
8. Perform proper hand hygiene, and put on gloves, mask, and protective eyewear, as appropriate for the procedure.

Implementation

1. Place the patient in the supine position, with the head of the bed no higher than 20 degrees.
2. Select cold or room-temperature injectate.
3. Select the injectate bolus amount, typically 10 mL.
4. Connect the CO cable to the PA catheter.
5. Select the computation constant.
6. Connect and turn on the CO computer.
7. Record the temperature of the injectate.
8. Verify the position of the PA catheter by assessing the RA and PA waveforms.
9. Observe the patient's cardiac rate and rhythm.
10. Aseptically connect the IV tubing to the injectate solution.
11. Hang the IV injectate solution on an IV pole, and prime the tubing.
12. Remove the sterile cap from the proximal lumen of the PA catheter.
13. Connect the injectable tubing to the proximal lumen of the PA catheter via a three-way stopcock.
14. Connect the injectate syringe to the three-way stopcock.
15. Connect the inline temperature probe.
16. If using cold injectate, set up the cold injectate system.
17. Turn the stopcock so that it is open to the injectate solution (closed to the patient), and withdraw 10 mL of the injectate solution into the syringe.
18. Turn the stopcock so that it is closed to the injectate solution and open to the patient.
19. Activate the CO computer.
20. Observe for steady baseline temperature on the monitor screen.
21. Observe the patient's respiratory pattern.
22. Begin administering the injectate at end expiration to decrease variance in CO measurements caused by the respiratory cycle.
23. Administer the injectate rapidly and smoothly in 4 seconds or less.
24. Assess the CO curve and value on the monitor screen.
25. Repeat steps 17 through 24 up to three times for cold injectate and up to five times for room-temperature injectate.
26. Determine the mean CO measurement.
27. Return the proximal stopcock at the RA lumen to the original position.
28. Continue infusions delivered through the introducer or other central lines.
29. Observe the PA and RA waveforms on the monitor.
30. Appropriately dispose of used supplies.

31. Remove the PPE, and perform proper hand hygiene prior to leaving the patient's room.

Evaluation of Procedure

1. Establish a baseline, or compare with previous measurements.
2. Develop an appropriate respiratory plan based on assessment data.
3. Identify any unexpected outcomes.

Documentation and Reporting

1. Record your findings in the patient's chart.
2. Report any abnormal findings to the appropriate health care provider.

7-6 Troubleshooting an Overdampened or Underdampened Waveform

If a waveform is dampened or suppressed, the data shown are inaccurate for your patient. Inaccurate data may lead to inappropriate decisions being made or red flags going unnoticed. A waveform may be overdampened or underdampened.

With overdampened waveforms, waveforms are more rounded than normal, the dicrotic notch vanishes, and the systolic peak does not reach its true peak. Overdampened waveforms may result in a falsely low systolic pressure and falsely high diastolic pressure. This may be a result of energy losses caused by rigid pressure tubing being absent from the system, larger air bubbles, blood clots in the system, loose connections, or kinked tubing or catheter. If the wrong type of tubing is in the system, remove the existing tubing, and replace it with rigid tubing. If the problem persists, ensure that the connections are secure, that the tubing is not kinked, and that the tubing is free of air bubbles or clots. If the catheter is found to be kinked, a physician will have to be consulted to adjust the catheter position.

Underdampened waveforms may result in a falsely high systolic pressure and a falsely low diastolic pressure or artifact may be present. Artifact may be described as "noise," or additional signals presenting themselves on the waveform. If underdampening is present, the tubing may be too long and should be shortened, if possible. Often, tubing extensions are present or extra components (stopcocks etc.) are inline and should be removed. The transducer may be defective as well, in which case it should be replaced.

The following is the step-by-step process for troubleshooting an overdampened or underdampened waveform:

Procedural Preparation

1. Review the patient's chart.
2. Verify the physician's order or the facility's protocol for standard of care.
3. Obtain, and inspect the appropriate equipment prior to entering the patient's room.
4. Follow the PPE requirements, and observe the standard precautions for any transmission-based isolation procedure.
5. Identify the patient using two patient identifiers.
6. Introduce yourself to the patient and to the family.
7. Explain the procedure to the patient and to the family, and acknowledge the patient's understanding.

8. Perform proper hand hygiene, and put on gloves, mask, and protective eyewear, as appropriate for the procedure.

Implementation

1. Identify the problem waveform.

Overdampened Waveform

   a. Check the patient for hypotension.
   b. Perform a dynamic response test.
   c. Ensure that the flush bag has fluid and a maintained pressure of 300 mm Hg.
   d. Check the positioning of the arterial line.
   e. Check the system for air bubbles.
   f. Check the tubing system for disconnections or leaks.
   g. Check for appropriate rigid tubing.
   h. Aspirate before flushing, if applicable.
   i. Flush the line clear.

Underdampened Waveform

   a. Perform a dynamic response test.
   b. Check the system for air bubbles.
   c. Check the length of the pressurized tubing system.
2. Reassess vital signs.
3. Remove the supplies from the patient's room, and clean the area, as needed.

4. Remove PPE, and perform proper hand hygiene prior to leaving the patient's room.

Evaluation of Procedure

1. Establish a baseline, or compare with previous measurements.
2. Reevaluate blood pressure, if needed.
   a. Overdampened waveform
   b. Underdampened waveform
3. Identify any unexpected outcomes.

Documentation and Reporting

1. Record your findings in the patient's chart.
2. Report any abnormal findings to the appropriate health care provider.

Bibliography

American Association of Colleges of Nursing: *Procedure manual for critical care*, ed 6, St. Louis, MO, 2010, Saunders.

Darovic GO: *Handbook of hemodynamic monitoring*, ed 2, St. Louis, MO, 2004, Saunders.

Kacmarek RM, Stoller JK, Heuer AJ: *Egan's fundamentals of respiratory care*, ed 10, St. Louis, MO, 2013, Mosby.

Klabunde RE: *Cardiovascular physiology concepts*, ed 2, Philadelphia, PA, 2012, Lippincott Williams & Wilkins.

1. Describe the function of each component of a hemodynamic monitoring set-up.

   a. Three-way stopcock

   _____

   b. Pressure transducer

   _____

   c. Rigid-pressure tubing

   _____

   d. 500-mL normal saline with pressure bag

   _____

   e. Monitor

   _____

2. Which locations are common sites to introduce a Swan-Ganz catheter?

   _____

3. What are the two indications for placement of an arterial line?

   _____

4. Explain in your own words why the dicrotic notch becomes visible on a pulmonary artery pressure-time waveform.

   _____

5. What are the five indications for the insertion of a Swan-Ganz catheter?

   _____

   _____

   _____

6. What is a cardiac cycle?

   _____

7. If an arterial line blood pressure waveform is overdampened, how do you correct the overdampening?

   _____

8. Identify the labeled parts of the Swan-Ganz catheter.

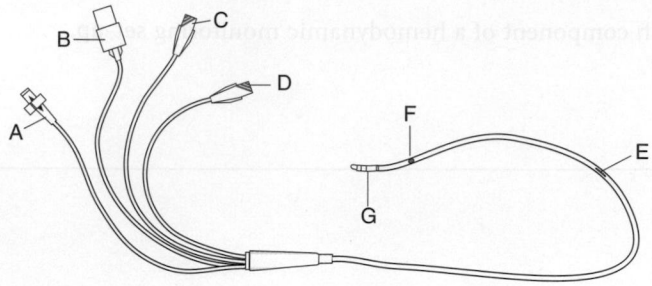

9. Draw each of the following:

a. Right atrial waveform

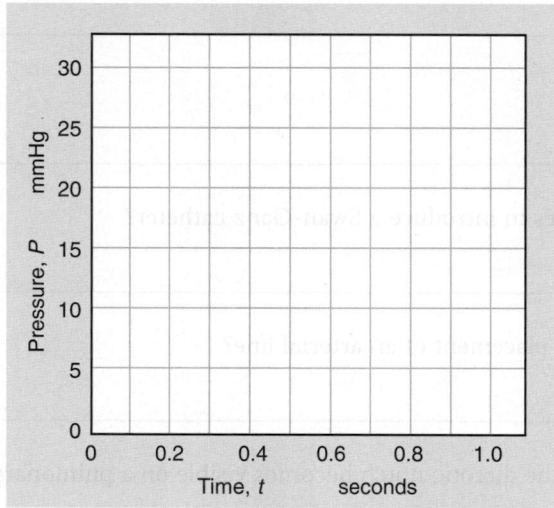

b. Right ventricular waveform

c. Pulmonary artery waveform

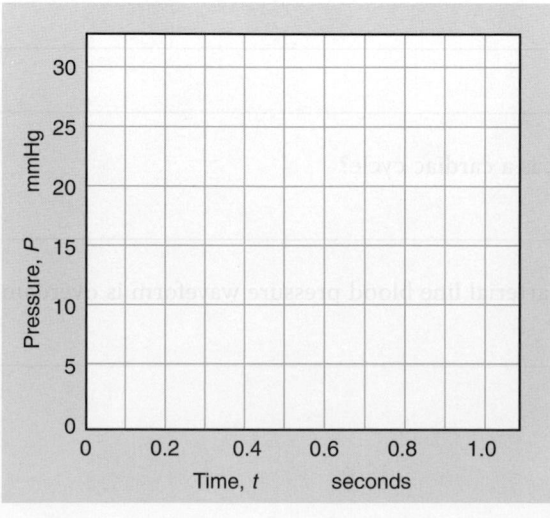

Self-Assessment Questions

1. What is the function of a pressure transducer?
   A. It transfers the pressure from the line into the monitor.
   B. It acts as a conduit for saline from the pressure bag.
   C. It is a blood pressure–regulating device.
   D. It converts a blood pressure into an electrical signal.

2. Why is rigid-pressure tubing important?
   A. It reduces the amount of pressure loss through the tubing.
   B. It ensures the tubing will not kink.
   C. It causes overdampening.
   D. It makes drawing blood samples easier to perform.

3. If a Swan-Ganz catheter is properly inserted into the pulmonary artery, under normal conditions, which waveform can you expect to see on the monitor?

A.

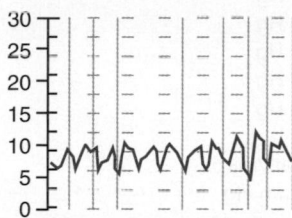

B.

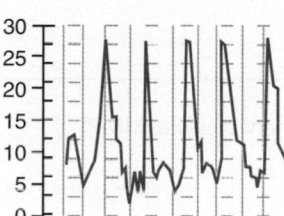

C.

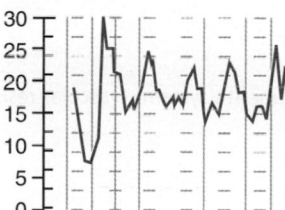

D.

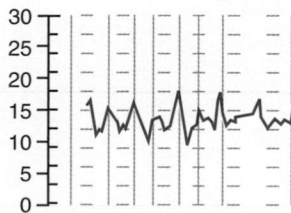

(A. - D. Redrawn from Abbott Critical Care Systems, Mountain View, CA)

4. Calculate the pulmonary vascular resistance for the following data:

CO	7.5 L/min
CVP	10 mm Hg
PAWP	22 mm Hg
PA	44/28 mm Hg
RA	9 mm Hg

   A. 149 dynes second cm^{-5}
   B. 121 dynes second cm^{-5}
   C. 207 dynes second cm^{-5}
   D. 235 dynes second cm^{-5}

5. For the answer above, this patient's pulmonary vascular resistance is:
   A. Low
   B. Normal
   C. High
   D. Not enough information is available.

6. Calculate the pulmonary vascular resistance for the following data:

CO	3.5L/min
CVP	18 mm Hg
PAWP	25 mm Hg
BP	155/120 mm Hg

   A. 1,683 dynes second cm^{-5}
   B. 2,364 dynes second cm^{-5}
   C. 2,598 dynes second cm^{-5}
   D. 2,819 dynes second cm^{-5}

7. For the answer above, this patient's pulmonary vascular resistance is:
   A. Low
   B. Normal
   C. High
   D. Not enough information is available.

8. The use of mechanical ventilation causes intrathoracic pressure to increase. This increase makes it important that the patient's central venous pressure remain _____.
   A. Slightly low
   B. Within normal limits
   C. Slightly high
   D. Not enough information is available.

9. A Swan-Ganz catheter may be placed for the sole purpose of obtaining blood samples.
   A. Yes, this is common practice.
   B. Only if an arterial line is unavailable.
   C. Only if the patient is a difficult stick.
   D. Never for the sole purpose of obtaining blood samples.

10. The hemodynamic data below are recorded for a patient who is being mechanically ventilated.

CO	6.2 L/min
PAP	52/31 mm Hg
PCWP	14 mm Hg
CVP	12 mm Hg

These data are most consistent with:

A. Hypovolemia
B. Pulmonary hypertension
C. Nonelevated ST myocardial infarction
D. Right ventricular failure

» CASE STUDY 7-1

A 48-year-old patient was brought to the emergency department (ED) via emergency medical services (EMS) earlier today with chest pain, shortness of breath, peripheral cyanosis, diminished breath sounds, and moderate diaphoresis. The patient coded in the emergency room, was resuscitated, and intubated. An arterial line was placed, and the patient was transferred to the intensive care unit (ICU). A Swan-Ganz catheter was inserted and the data revealed:

PAP (pulmonary artery pressure)	55/25 mm Hg
PCWP (pulmonary capillary wedge pressure)	22 mm Hg
CVP (central venous pressure)	10 mm Hg
PvO$_2$ (mixed venous oxygen tension)	20 mm Hg
PaO$_2$ (partial pressure of oxygen)	75 mm Hg
PaCO$_2$ (partial pressure of carbon dioxide)	65 mm Hg
HCO$_{3-}$ (bicarbonate ion)	28 mm Hg
pH	7.25
Heart rate	138 beats/min
Dynamic blood pressure	80/40 mm Hg
FiO$_2$ (fraction of inspired oxygen)	0.60

1. Interpret the patient's blood gas at this time.

_____

2. Calculate this patient's mean systemic artery pressure (MSAP) and mean pulmonary artery pressure (MPAP).

   a. MSAP: _____

   b. MPAP: _____

3. Are these mean pressures within elevated, decreased, or normal limits?

4. Through thermodilution, the patient's CO was found to be 3.2 L/min. Calculate this patient's systemic vascular resistance (SVR) and pulmonary vascular resistance (PVR).

   a. SVR: _____

   b. PVR: _____

5. Are these resistance values within elevated, decreased, or normal limits?

_____

6. On the basis of your answers, what is a probable diagnosis for this patient?

_____

7. Would you anticipate this patient's ejection fraction to be within normal limits? If not, do you expect it to be elevated or decreased? Why?

_____

Analysis and Monitoring of Gas Exchange

Jonathan R. Marino

▪ OBJECTIVES

Upon the completion of the chapter activities and content review topics, the student should be able to:

1. Perform the modified Allen's test.
2. Perform an arterial puncture.
3. Perform an arterial line insertion.
4. Obtain a capillary blood sample.
5. Obtain an arterial blood sample from an arterial line.
6. Place and maintain a transcutaneous blood gas probe.
7. Connect an end-tidal carbon dioxide monitor.
8. Interpret arterial blood gas data.

▪ KEY TERMS

- Arterial blood gas
- Acidemia
- Acidosis
- Alkalemia
- Alkalosis
- Capnography
- Capnometry
- Contagion
- Gradient
- Hypoxemia
- Invasive
- Allen's test
- Noninvasive
- Point-of-care testing

▪ CONTENT REVIEW TOPICS

- Arterial blood gas (ABG) interpretation
- Neonatal arterial blood gas values
- Adult arterial blood gas values

▪ PROCEDURAL ASSESSMENTS

8-1 Performing a Modified Allen's Test
8-2 Performing an Arterial Puncture
8-3 Placing a Radial Arterial line
8-4 Blood Sampling from an Indwelling Arterial Catheter
8-5 Capillary Blood Sampling
8-6 Monitoring Transcutaneous Blood Gas
8-7 Monitoring End-Tidal Carbon Dioxide

▪ EQUIPMENT

- Standard personal protective equipment (gloves, safety goggles)
- 2-inch by 2-inch sterile gauze
- Alcohol prep pads
- Blood gas puncture arm
- Indwelling catheter syringe tip
- Needle-capping device
- Patient or sample label
- Preheparinized blood gas syringe (1–3 mL)
- Sample indwelling catheter setup
- Sharps container
- Short-bevel 20-gauge to 22-gauge needle with a clear hub
- Tape
- Towels

B oth invasive and noninvasive diagnostic tests may be used to assess and monitor a patient's gas exchange status.

> → **Reality Check** Having knowledge of how well your patient is oxygenating and ventilating puts you in a position to recognize what to do, or not to do, for your patients.

If your patient does not have adequate gas exchange, he or she is at risk of becoming hypoxemic, hypercapnic, or hypocapnic, and this may lead to acidemia or alkalemia. The focus of this

chapter is to explore various procedures and techniques of clinically analyzing and monitoring gas exchange.

❯❯ SKILL CHECK LISTS

8-1 Performing a Modified Allen's Test

The modified Allen's test is performed prior to radial artery puncture to ensure that adequate collateral circulation is present through the ulnar artery to the hand in the event that the radial artery is damaged during an arterial puncture procedure (Figure 8-1). Radial artery puncture should not be

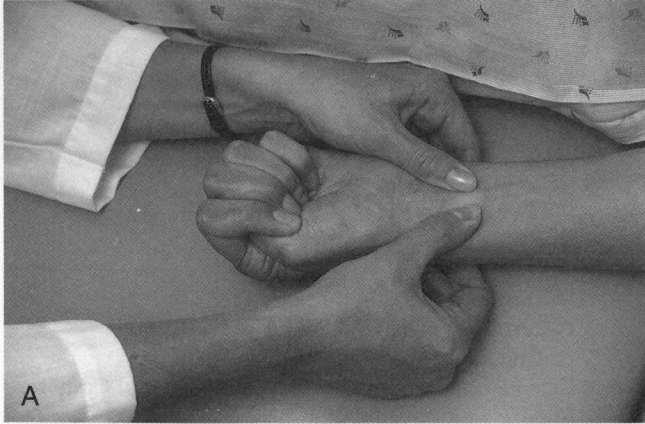

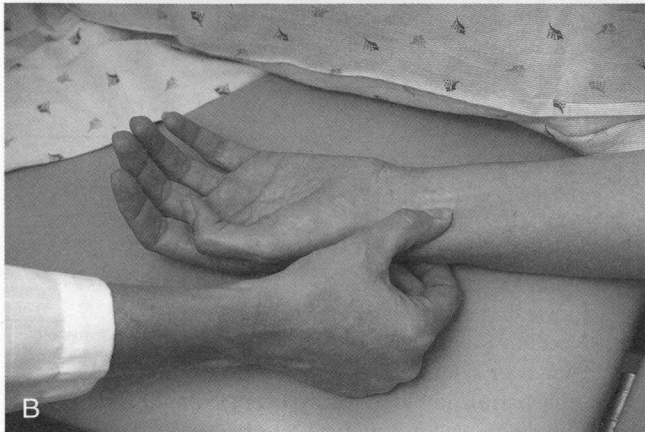

Figure 8-1 A modified Allen's test assesses circulation for the hand. (From Pagana K: *Mosby's manual of diagnostic and laboratory testing*, ed 2, St. Louis, MO, 2010, Mosby.)

performed when the modified Allen's test results are negative. The following is the step-by-step process for performing a modified Allen's test.

Procedural Preparation

1. Review the patient's chart.
2. Verify the physician's order or the facility's protocol for standard of care.
3. Obtain, clean, and inspect the appropriate equipment prior to entering the patient's room.
4. Follow the PPE requirements, and observe the standard precautions for any transmission-based isolation procedure.
5. Identify the patient using two patient identifiers.
6. Introduce yourself to the patient and to the family.
7. Explain the procedure to the patient and to the family, and acknowledge the patient's understanding.
8. Perform proper hand hygiene, and put on gloves, mask, and protective eyewear, as appropriate for the procedure.

Implementation

1. Place the patient in a comfortable position, and instruct him or her to breathe normally.
2. Assess vital signs.
3. Instruct the patient to form a tight fist or raise the arm above the heart level for several seconds.

4. Apply direct pressure to the radial and ulnar arteries, thus obstructing arterial blood flow to the hand while the patient opens and closes the fist rapidly several times.
5. Instruct the patient to open the hand or keep the arm above the heart level with the radial artery compressed.
6. Examine the palmar surface for an erythematous blush or pallor within 6 seconds:
   a. An erythematous blush indicates ulnar artery patency and is interpreted as a positive Allen's test result. Radial arterial puncture may be performed at this site.
   b. Pallor indicates occlusion of the ulnar artery and is interpreted as a negative Allen's test result. Radial arterial puncture should not be done.
7. Remove the supplies from the patient's room, and clean the area, as needed.
8. Remove PPE, and perform proper hand hygiene prior to leaving the patient's room.

Evaluation of Procedure

1. Establish a baseline, or compare with previous measurements.
2. Identify any unexpected outcomes.
3. Evaluate alternative sites for arterial puncture if the Allen's test result is negative.

Documentation and Reporting

1. Record your findings in the patient's chart.
2. Report any abnormal findings to the appropriate health care provider.

8-2 Performing an Arterial Puncture

Arterial sampling is indicated when a patient's oxygenation, ventilation, or acid–base status, as well as the blood's oxygen carrying capacity, need to be evaluated. It may also be utilized as a tool to evaluate a patient's response to therapeutic intervention, diagnostic evaluation, or to monitor the severity and progression of a disease process.

Blood may be sampled by performing an arterial puncture. The radial, brachial, and dorsalis pedis arteries are common sites for arterial puncture. The femoral artery may be used but usually requires a special order from a physician. Figure 8-2 illustrates common arteries used for puncture.

> **✳ Tip** Lesions and sites distal to or through a surgical shunt should also be avoided.

As with any invasive procedure, you need to be aware of certain hazards and complications. When inserting a needle into a patient's artery, a chance of introducing a contagion at the sampling site or of introducing a contagion to the sampler by accidental needle stick exists. Trauma, occlusion, or spasm of the artery may also occur. Other possible complications include air or clotted blood emboli, hematoma, or hemorrhage at the trauma site; vasovagal response; and pain. Images of arterial puncture of the radial artery are provided in Figure 8-3. The following is the step-by-step process for arterial puncture.

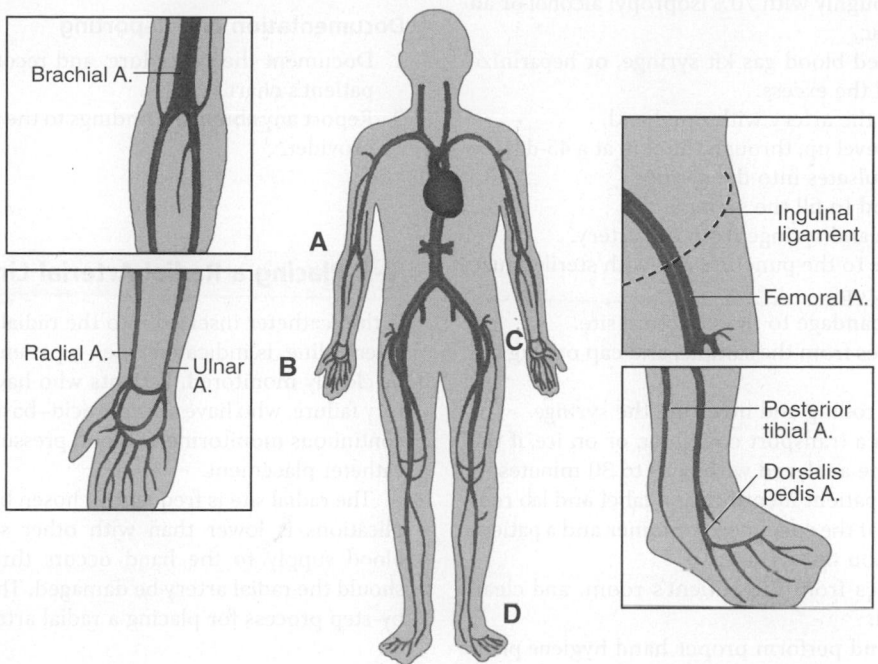

Figure 8-2 Arteries used for arterial puncture. **A,** Brachial artery. **B,** Radial artery. **C,** Femoral artery. **D,** Dorsalis pedis. The radial artery is the preferred site. (From Kacmarek RM, Stoller JK, Heuer AJ: *Egan's fundamentals of respiratory care*, ed 10, St. Louis, MO, 2013, Mosby.)

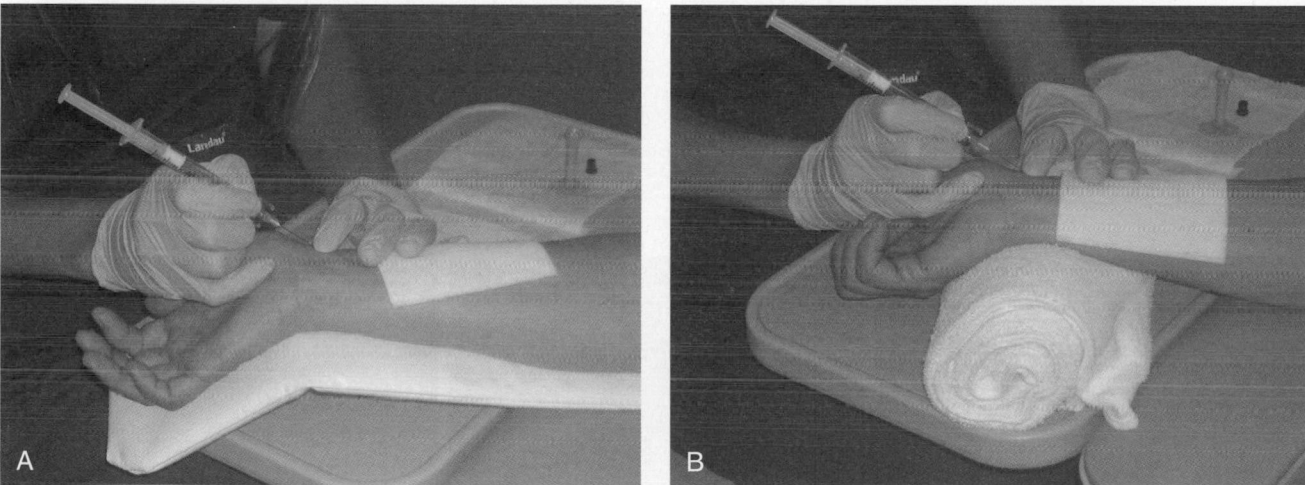

Figure 8-3 A, Arterial puncture with arm board. **B,** Arterial puncture with towel. (From Mottram C: *Ruppel's manual of pulmonary function testing*, ed 10, St. Louis, MO, 2013, Mosby.)

Procedural Preparation

1. Review the patient's chart.
2. Verify the physician's order or the facility's protocol for standard of care.
3. Obtain, clean, and inspect the appropriate equipment prior to entering the patient's room.
4. Follow the PPE requirements, and observe the standard precautions for any transmission-based isolation procedure.
5. Identify the patient using two patient identifiers.
6. Introduce yourself to the patient and to the family.
7. Explain the procedure to the patient and to the family, and acknowledge the patient's understanding.

8. Perform proper hand hygiene, and put on gloves, mask, and protective eyewear, as appropriate for the procedure.

Implementation

1. Position the patient by extending the patient's wrist approximately 30 degrees, and instruct him or her to breathe normally.
2. Assess vital signs, and estimate the oxygen concentration or fraction of inspired oxygen (FIO_2) that the patient is receiving.
3. Perform an Allen's test, if radial artery puncture is used (See PA 8-1).

4. Clean the site thoroughly with 70% isopropyl alcohol or an equivalent antiseptic.
5. Use a preheparinized blood gas kit syringe, or heparinize a syringe and expel the excess.
6. Palpate and secure the artery with one hand,
7. Insert the needle, bevel up, through the skin at a 45-degree angle until blood pulsates into the syringe.
8. Allow 1 mL of blood to fill the syringe.
9. Remove the needle and syringe from the artery.
10. Apply firm pressure to the puncture site with sterile gauze until the bleeding stops.
11. Apply dressing or bandage to the puncture site.
12. Expel any air bubbles from the sample, and cap or plug the syringe.
13. Mix the sample by rolling and inverting the syringe.
14. Place the sample in a transport container, or on ice, if the specimen will not be analyzed within 10 to 30 minutes.
15. Attach the correct patient identification label and lab requisition to the side of the specimen container and a patient identification label on the syringe.
16. Remove the supplies from the patient's room, and clean the area, as needed.
17. Remove the PPE, and perform proper hand hygiene prior to leaving the patient's room.

Evaluation of Procedure

1. Establish a baseline, or compare with previous measurements.
2. Develop an appropriate respiratory care plan based on assessment data.
3. Note any use of oxygen therapy.
4. Check the puncture site after 20 minutes for hematoma and adequacy of distal circulation.
5. Identify any unexpected outcomes.
6. Correlate findings with SpO_2, if available.

Documentation and Reporting

1. Document the procedure, and record your findings in the patient's chart.
2. Report any abnormal findings to the appropriate health care provider.

8-3 Placing a Radial Arterial Line

A thin catheter inserted into the radial artery, that is, a radial arterial line, is indicated when a patient's blood gases need to be closely monitored. Patients who have experienced respiratory failure, who have a severe acid–base disorder, or who need continuous monitoring of blood pressure benefit from arterial catheter placement.

The radial site is frequently chosen because the risk of complications is lower than with other sites because collateral blood supply to the hand occurs through the ulnar artery should the radial artery be damaged. The following is the step-by-step process for placing a radial arterial line (Figure 8-4).

Procedural Preparation

1. Review the patient's chart.
2. Verify the physician's order or the facility's protocol for standard of care.
3. Obtain, clean, and inspect the appropriate equipment prior to entering the patient's room.
4. Follow the PPE requirements, and observe the standard precautions for any transmission-based isolation procedure.
5. Identify the patient using two patient identifiers.
6. Introduce yourself to the patient and to the family.

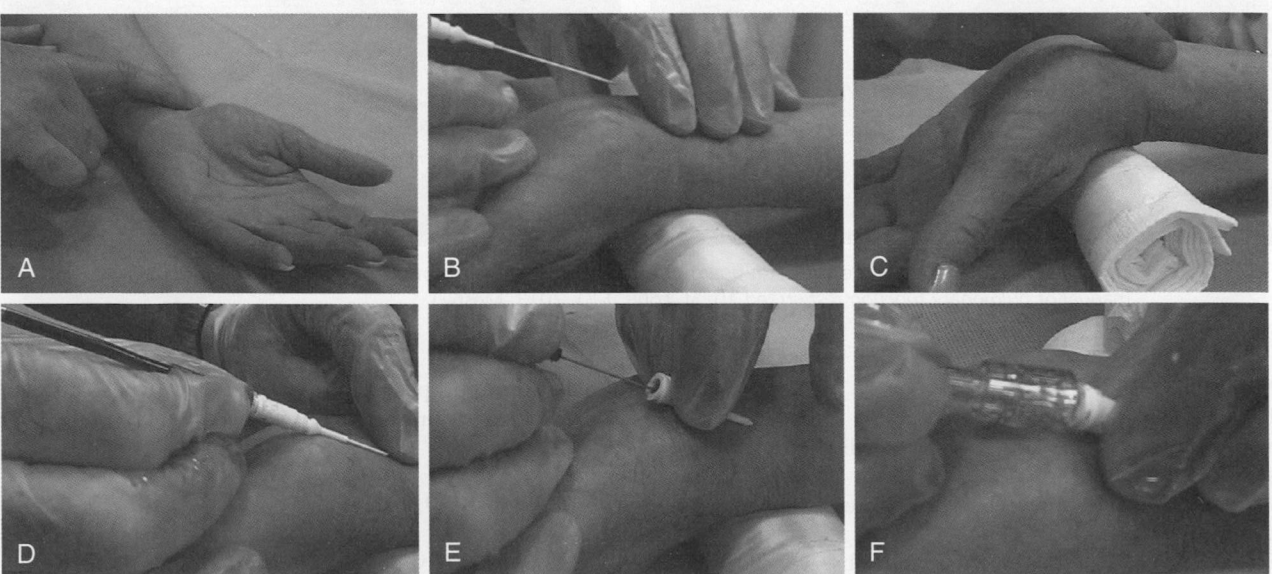

Figure 8-4 Radial arterial line placement. **A,** To approach the radial artery, you need to go over the thenar eminence. **B,** Extending the wrist allows a straight shot to the radial artery. **C,** Approach at a shallow angle to get the needle in, and slide up a little more to get the catheter in as well. **D,** Make sure the blood keeps flowing as you advance. **E,** Slide the catheter in, and hold down above the line so that blood does not squirt out. **F,** Use of the Luer-Lok is recommended to avoid disconnecting the line. (From Jeremias A, Brown D: *Cardiac intensive care*, ed 2, St. Louis, MO, 2010, Saunders.)

7. Explain the procedure to the patient and to the family, and acknowledge the patient's understanding.
8. Perform proper hand hygiene, and put on gloves, mask, and protective eyewear, as appropriate for the procedure.

Implementation

1. Place the patient in a comfortable position that gives adequate access to the placement site, and instruct him or her to breathe normally.
2. Assess vital signs.
3. Perform an Allen's test (See PA 8-1).
4. Position the patient's wrist and hand, and dorsiflex the wrist over a towel pad or padded bedside table.
5. Put on sterile gloves and protective eyewear.
6. Prepare the entry site with betadine, chlorhexidine, or other skin cleanser.
7. Apply sterile drape at the entry site.
8. Identify the radial artery.
9. Stabilize the artery by pulling the skin taut.
10. Using sterile technique, insert the arterial needle into the skin just distal to the palpated arterial site at a 30- to 60-degree angle
11. Advance the needle into the artery until pulsatile bright red blood enters the column.
12. Advance the guidewire.
13. Advance plastic catheter over the guidewire.
14. Connect to the pressure tubing and the transducer.
15. Level and set the transducer to zero, and verify the arterial waveform.
16. Clean the area of any blood; allow the site to dry.
17. Apply Benzoin to the cleansed area, and allow the site to dry and become tacky.
18. Secure the arterial line with tape or Steri-strips, and cover with a Tegaderm dressing.
19. Secure the tubing to prevent it from being pulled.
20. Remove the supplies from the patient's room, and clean the area, as needed.
21. Remove PPE, and perform proper hand hygiene prior to leaving the patient's room.

Evaluation of Procedure

1. Establish a baseline, or compare with previous measurements.
2. Develop an appropriate respiratory care plan based on assessment data.
3. Identify any unexpected outcomes.

Documentation and Reporting

1. Record your findings in the patient's chart.
2. Report any abnormal findings to the appropriate health care provider.

8-4 Blood Sampling from an Indwelling Arterial Catheter

In the intensive care unit (ICU) setting, for patients requiring mechanical ventilation for treatment of respiratory failure or severe acid–base disturbances, frequent arterial blood sampling is typically required as part of their respiratory care plan. Rather than repeated arterial punctures, an arterial catheter is placed to facilitate the recurrent arterial blood sampling.

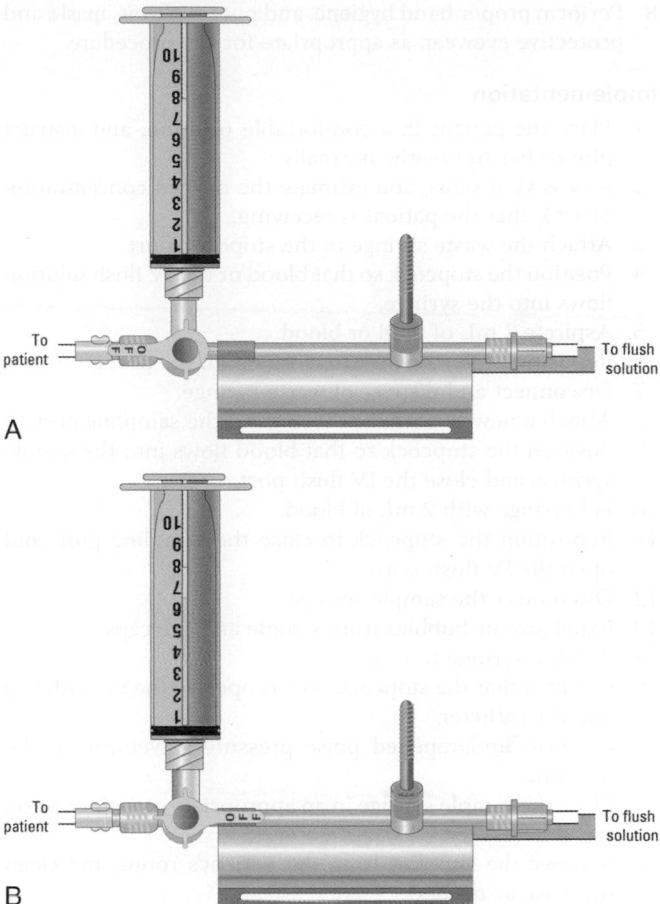

Figure 8-5 A, A syringe attached to the port of the three-way stopcock. The stopcock is turned "off" to the patient. **B,** A syringe attached to the top of the three-way stopcock. The stopcock is turned "off" to the flush solution. (Drawing by Paul WS, Thomas Jefferson University Hospital, Philadelphia, PA, copyright, 2004.)

Drawing blood from an arterial line is a convenient way to acquire an arterial blood sample and reduces the pain and discomfort a patient experiences from repetitive needle sticks. Another benefit of drawing blood from an indwelling catheter is that it reduces the possibility of pathogens being introduced through numerous puncture sites. Images of this process are provided in Figure 8-5. The following is the step-by-step process for blood sampling from an indwelling arterial catheter.

Procedural Preparation

1. Review the patient's chart.
2. Verify the physician's order or the facility's protocol for standard of care.
3. Obtain, clean, and inspect the appropriate equipment prior to entering the patient's room.
4. Follow the PPE requirements, and observe the standard precautions for any transmission-based isolation procedure.
5. Identify the patient using two patient identifiers.
6. Introduce yourself to the patient and to the family.
7. Explain the procedure to the patient and to the family, and acknowledge the patient's understanding.

8. Perform proper hand hygiene, and put on gloves, mask, and protective eyewear, as appropriate for the procedure.

Implementation

1. Place the patient in a comfortable position, and instruct him or her to breathe normally.
2. Assess vital signs, and estimate the oxygen concentration or FIO_2 that the patient is receiving.
3. Attach the waste syringe to the stopcock port.
4. Position the stopcock so that blood or the IV flush solution flows into the syringe.
5. Aspirate 2 mL of fluid or blood.
6. Reposition the stopcock to close off all the ports.
7. Disconnect and dispose of waste syringe.
8. Attach a new heparinized syringe to the sampling port.
9. Position the stopcock so that blood flows into the sample syringe, and close the IV flush port.
10. Fill syringe with 2 mL of blood.
11. Reposition the stopcock to close the sampling port, and open the IV flush port.
12. Disconnect the sample syringe.
13. Expel any air bubbles from sample and the caps.
14. Roll the syringe to mix.
15. Confirm that the stopcock port is open to the IV flush bag and the catheter.
16. Confirm undampened pulse pressure waveform on the monitor.
17. Place the sample syringe in an appropriate container, or on ice, if necessary.
18. Remove the supplies from the patient's room, and clean the area, as needed.
19. Remove PPE, and perform proper hand hygiene prior to leaving the patient's room.

Evaluation of Procedure

1. Establish a baseline, or compare with previous measurements.
2. Develop an appropriate respiratory care plan based on assessment data.

3. Make changes to the FIO_2, if indicated.
4. Identify any unexpected outcomes.
5. Correlate your findings with the noninvasive measurements, if applicable.

Documentation and Reporting

1. Record your findings in the patient's chart.
2. Report any abnormal findings to the appropriate health care provider.

8-5 Capillary Blood Sampling

Although arterial samples are preferred, capillary blood gases are often used to analyze ventilation and acid–base balance in infants and children experiencing respiratory failure. To obtain a valid sample, capillary puncture sites are warmed to facilitate capillary dilation and increased blood flow to the area. PO_2 values may be used for trending purposes but have no value in the estimation and interpretation of arterial oxygenation. The following is the step-by-step process for capillary blood gas sampling (Figure 8-6).

Implementation

1. Place the patient in a comfortable position, and select the site.
2. Assess vital signs, and estimate the oxygen concentration or FIO_2 that the patient is receiving.
3. Warm the site to 42°C for 10 minutes by using a compress, heat lamp, or commercial hot pack.
4. Clean the skin with an antiseptic solution.
5. Puncture the skin with a lancet.
6. Wipe away the first drop of blood, and observe free flow.
7. Fill the sample tube from the middle of the blood drop until the tube is completely full.
8. Place the metal flea in the capillary tube, and seal the tube ends.
9. Tape sterile cotton or a bandage over the puncture wound.

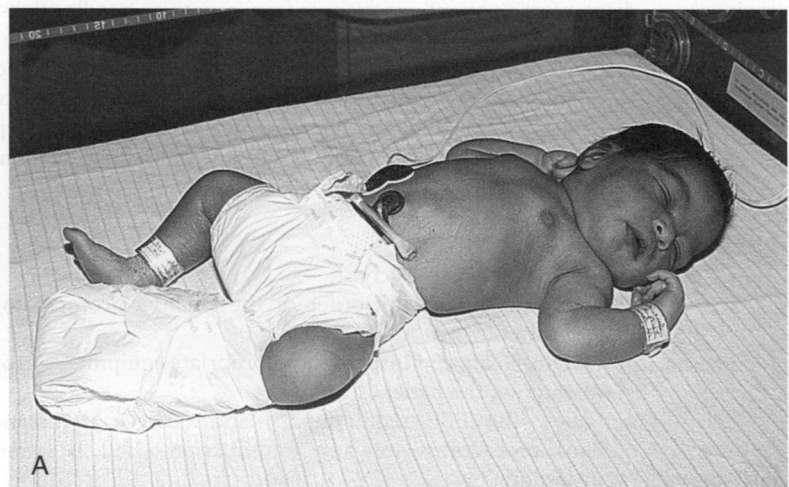
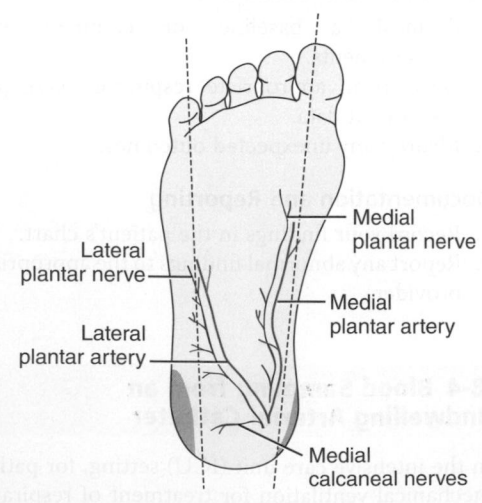

Figure 8-6 Heel stick. **A,** Newborn with foot wrapped for warmth to increase blood flow to extremity before heel stick. **B,** Heel stick sites (*shaded areas*) on infant's foot for obtaining samples of capillary blood. (**A,** Courtesy of Marjorie Pyle, RNC, Lifecircle, Costa Mesa, CA. **A** and **B,** From Perry S, Hockenberry M, Lowdermilk D, Wilson D: *Maternal child nursing care*, ed 4, St. Louis, MO, 2010, Mosby.)

10. Mix the sample by moving the magnet back and forth along the capillary tube.
11. Chill the sample immediately, or analyze it within 10 to 15 minutes, if left at room temperature.
12. Remove the supplies from the patient's room, and clean the area, as needed.
13. Remove PPE, and perform proper hand hygiene prior to leaving the patient's room.

Evaluation of Procedure

1. Establish a baseline, or compare with previous measurements.
2. Develop an appropriate respiratory care plan based on assessment data.
3. Note any use of oxygen therapy.
4. Identify any unexpected outcomes.

Documentation and Reporting

1. Record your findings in the patient's chart.
2. Report any abnormal findings to the appropriate health care provider.

8-6 Monitoring Transcutaneous Blood Gas

Transcutaneous blood gas monitoring is a noninvasive way to monitor a patient's blood gas. The monitor itself is a small probe that can read oxygen and carbon dioxide levels through the skin (Figure 8-7). This method is appropriate for continuous or extended monitoring or when direct arterial blood measurement is not available or accessible. Transcutaneous monitoring is also an effective diagnostic tool for assessment of functional cardiac shunts. The following is the step-by-step process for transcutaneous blood gas monitoring.

Procedural Preparation

1. Review the patient's chart.
2. Verify the physician's order or the facility's protocol for standard of care.
3. Obtain, clean, and inspect the appropriate equipment prior to entering the patient's room.

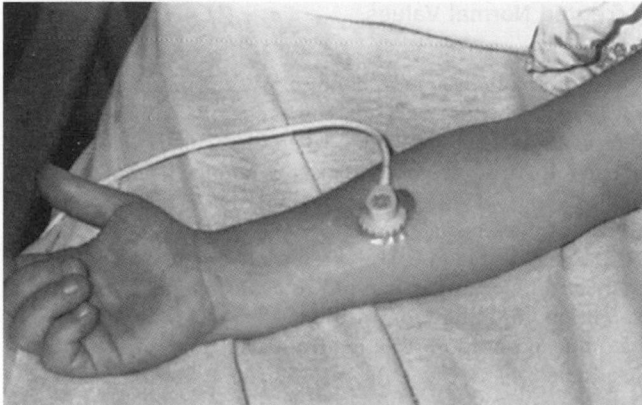

Figure 8-7 Transcutaneous oxygen monitor electrode placed on a child's arm. (From Walsh B, Czervinski M, DiBlasi R: *Perinatal and pediatric respiratory care*, ed 3, St. Louis, MO, 2010, Saunders.)

4. Follow the PPE requirements, and observe the standard precautions for any transmission-based isolation procedure.
5. Identify the patient using two patient identifiers.
6. Introduce yourself to the patient and to the family.
7. Explain the procedure to the patient and to the family, and acknowledge the patient's understanding.
8. Perform proper hand hygiene, and put on gloves, mask, and protective eyewear, as appropriate for the procedure.

Implementation

1. Place the patient in a comfortable position.
2. Place the monitor at the bedside, and turn it on, as specified by the manufacturer.
3. Assess vital signs, and estimate the oxygen concentration or FiO_2 that the patient is receiving.
4. Select the monitoring site.
5. Prepare the sensor.
6. Select the appropriate probe temperature, as specified by the manufacturer.
7. Prepare the monitoring site.
8. Attach the probe to the patient.
9. Allow for stabilization time.
10. Set the alarm.
11. Remove the supplies from the patient's room, and clean the area, as needed.
12. Remove the PPE, and perform proper hand hygiene prior to leaving the patient's room.

Evaluation of Procedure

1. Establish a baseline, or compare with previous measurements.
2. Develop an appropriate respiratory care plan based on assessment data.
3. Correlate with ABG measurements, if applicable.
4. Identify any unexpected outcomes.
5. Establish the change time of the probe site, and document it.
6. Monitor the probe site for complications.

Documentation and Reporting

1. Record your findings in the patient's chart.
2. Report any abnormal findings to the appropriate health care provider.

8-7 Monitoring End-Tidal Carbon Dioxide

ABG interpretation provides information about your patient's ventilatory status, but CO_2 can be measured by capnometry as well. Capnometry is the measurement of CO_2 in a volume of gas, usually by using methods of infrared absorption or mass spectrometry. In a critical care setting, a capnometer is placed on the ventilator circuit closest to the patient airway.

> **✱ Tip** The two types of capnometers are *mainstream* and *sidestream* capnometers.

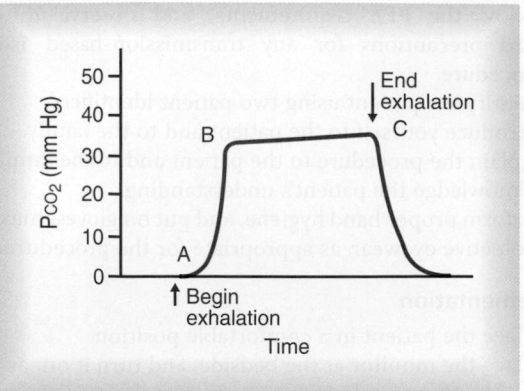

Figure 8-8 Normal single-breath capnograph tracing. (From Kacmarek RM, Stoller JK, Heuer AJ: *Egan's fundamentals of respiratory care*, ed 10, St. Louis, MO, 2013, Mosby.)

The capnometer sends the information to the monitor and displays the information as an end-tidal carbon dioxide tension (P_{ETCO_2})-time waveform or capnogram. P_{ETCO_2} is an end-tidal gas, that is, the gas sampled at the end of the exhalation. It usually averages 3 to 5 mm Hg less than the $PaCO_2$ obtained through ABG sampling. Figure 8-8 illustrates a normal single breath capnograph tracing. The following is the step-by-step process for end-tidal CO_2 monitoring.

Procedural Preparation

1. Review the patient's chart.
2. Verify the physician's order or the facility's protocol for standard of care.
3. Obtain, clean, and inspect the appropriate equipment prior to entering the patient's room.
4. Follow the PPE requirements, and observe the standard precautions for any transmission-based isolation procedure.
5. Identify the patient using two patient identifiers.
6. Introduce yourself to the patient and to the family.
7. Explain the procedure to the patient and to the family, and acknowledge the patient's understanding.
8. Perform proper hand hygiene, and put on gloves, mask, and protective eyewear, as appropriate for the procedure.

Implementation

1. Assess vital signs, and estimate the oxygen concentration or FiO_2 that the patient is receiving.
2. Connect the monitor to the electrical outlet.
3. Calibrate the monitor to the known CO_2 level.
4. Connect the monitor to the patient's airway:
   a. Directly to the airway for a mainstream monitor
   b. Using an adapter for a sidestream monitor
5. Reassess vital signs.
6. Remove the supplies from the patient's room, and clean the area, as needed.
7. Remove the PPE, and perform proper hand hygiene prior to leaving the patient's room.

Evaluation of Procedure

1. Establish a baseline, or compare with previous measurements.

TABLE 8-1   Normal Arterial Blood Gas Components

ACID–BASE COMPONENT	
pH	7.35–7.45
$PaCO_2$	35–45 mm Hg
HCO_3^-	22–26 mEq/L
BE	±2 mEq/L
OXYGENATION COMPONENT	
PaO_2	80–100 mm Hg
SaO_2	95%–100%

2. Correlate your findings with an arterial $PaCO_2$ measurement.
3. Develop an appropriate respiratory care plan based on assessment data.
4. Identify any unexpected outcomes.

Documentation and Reporting

1. Record your findings in the patient's chart.
2. Report any abnormal findings to the appropriate health care provider.

Components of Arterial Blood Gases

Interpretation of arterial blood provides a diagnostic snapshot of lung–blood gas exchange and the acid–base status of blood. When used in conjunction with CO-oximetry, the analysis provides valuable information about blood's ability to transport oxygen from the lungs to the tissues.

Once the sample is obtained, the analysis is performed by a blood gas analyzer. Common blood gas analyzers *measure* pH, $PaCO_2$, and PaO_2, and *calculate* HCO_3^-, SaO_2, and BE. An analyzer capable of CO-oximetry also measures concentrations of oxyHb, deoxyHb, or reduced Hb, COHb, and MetHb as a percentage of the total hemoglobin concentration.

If you know the patient's hemoglobin level, PaO_2, and SaO_2, you will be able to calculate the total amount of oxygen in the systemic arteries, or the *arterial oxygen content* (CaO_2).

Accepted Normal Values

pH

Under normal physiologic conditions, the body is able to keep the blood pH within a very narrow range—7.38 to 7.42. Clinical intervention is recommended when the pH falls below 7.35 or above 7.45. In other words, pH values ranging from 7.35 to 7.38 and 7.42 to 7.45 are abnormal but not critical enough to warrant intervention.

Decreased blood pH is referred to as *acidemia*, and increased blood pH is referred to as *alkalemia*. A pathologic condition resulting from acidemia is called *acidosis*, and a pathologic condition resulting from alkalemia is called *alkalosis* (Table 8-1).

$PaCO_2$

$PaCO_2$ is the acidic component of the pH. Many studies have characterized the normal value for $PaCO_2$. They have stated that the normal levels for men and women differ slightly but that values from 30 to 46 mm Hg cover the entire population. Clinically, however, the accepted normal range is 35 to 45 mm Hg (see Table 8-1).

HCO_3^-

The alkaline or buffer component of the pH is HCO_3^-, which is calculated using the Henderson-Hasselbalch equation. This equation describes the relationship between pH, HCO_3^-, and CO_2, where the ionization constant, pKc, is 6.1 (Table 8-1).

$$pH = pKc + log\frac{[HCO_3^-]}{[CO_2]}$$

CO_2 concentration can be converted from $PaCO_2$ mm Hg by multiplying it by the conversion factor: 0.03 mEq/L/mm Hg. Thus,

$$pH = 6.1 + log\frac{[HCO_3]}{0.03 \cdot PaCO_2}$$

Using basic algebra, HCO_3^- can be calculated by rearranging the preceding equation into the following form:

$$[HCO_3^-] = 0.03 \cdot PaCO_2 \cdot 10^{(pH-6.1)}$$

If the median normal value for pH and $PaCO_2$ are inserted into this equation,

$$[HCO_3^-] = 0.03\frac{mEq/L}{mmHg} \cdot 40\,mmHg \cdot 10^{(7.40-6.1)}$$

we can find the median value for HCO_3^-, which is 24 mEq/L. The accepted clinical normal value for HCO_3^- ranges from 22 to 26 mEq/L.

Base Excess

Another point of view in measuring the alkaline component of the pH is *base excess* (BE). BE is the concentration of strong acid (mEq/L), which has to be added or taken from blood at 37°C to return the pH to 7.40 (see Table 8-1).

The accepted normal value for BE is ±2. If BE is more than 2, BE is present, and strong acid would have to be added to bring the pH to 7.40; similarly, if BE is less than −2, strong acid would have to be removed to bring the pH to 7.40. A BE that is negative is also called *base deficit*.

Blood gas machines calculate BE from the Van Slyke equation, which was derived experimentally in 1978 by Dr. Ole Siggaard-Andersen.

$$[HCO_3^-] - 24.4 = -\frac{(2.3\,Hb + 7.7) \cdot (pH - 7.40) + BE}{(1 - 0.023\,Hb)}$$

Rearranged to solve for BE,

$$BE = (1 - 0.023\,Hb) \cdot ([HCO_3^-] - 24.4 + (2.3\,Hb + 7.7)$$
$$\cdot (pH - 7.40))$$

Blood gas machines that are capable of analyzing CO-oximetry use the measured hemoglobin level for this calculation; however, machines that are not capable of analyzing

CO-oximetry approximate BE by substituting a normal value for hemoglobin, for example, 9.309 mmol/L (1 g/dL equals approximately 0.6206 mmol/L; therefore, 15 g/dL = 9.309 mmol/L). In this case, the Van Slyke equation reduces to:

$$BE = 0.786\,([HCO_3^-] - 24.4 + 29.11(pH - 7.40))$$

PaO_2

The amount of oxygen dissolved in arterial plasma is measured as a PaO_2. A dissolved oxygen level below the clinical normal level is called *hypoxemia* and that above the accepted normal level is called *hyperoxemia*. The measure of PaO_2 is a tool used to assess tissue hypoxia (see Table 8-1).

Normal PaO_2 values vary with age, body position, and elevation above sea level. In older patients, for example, a study has shown a mean variation in PaO_2 of approximately 6 mm Hg in the sitting position versus the supine position in a sample of 46 healthy older patients.

For clinical purposes, PaO_2 is classified as follows:
Over 100 mm Hg = hyperoxemia
80–100 mm Hg = normal oxygenation
60–79 mm Hg = mild hypoxemia
40–69 mm Hg = moderate hypoxemia
<40 mm Hg = severe hypoxemia

SaO_2

The amount of oxygen bound to arterial hemoglobin is measured as a percentage (SaO_2). A hemoglobin molecule is capable of binding four oxygen molecules. If each of the four sites has an oxygen molecule bound to it, it is 100% saturated. If three of the four sites have an oxygen molecule bound to it, it is 75% saturated. The average of all of the hemoglobin that has oxygen bound to it in a given sample is the SaO_2 (see Table 8-1).

For clinical purposes, SaO_2 is classified as follows:
95–100% = normal oxygenation
90–94% = mild hypoxemia
75–89% = moderate hypoxemia
<75% = severe hypoxemia

Blood Gas Interpretation

Interpreting blood gas is an easy four-step process. The first three steps assess the patient's acid–base status. The last step assesses the patient's oxygenation status.

Categorization of pH

Is the pH within normal range, and if not, what condition is present?

Recall that for clinical purposes, normal blood pH is between 7.35 and 7.45. Decreased blood pH is referred to as *acidemia*, and increased blood pH is referred to as *alkalemia*. A pathologic condition resulting from acidemia is called *acidosis* and a pathologic condition resulting from alkalemia is called *alkalosis*.

pH	Condition
<7.35	Acidosis
7.35–7.45	Normal
>7.45	Alkalosis

Assessment of Respiratory or Metabolic Origin

What is causing the imbalance of pH?

Recall that for clinical purposes, CO_2 levels between 35 and 45 mm Hg and bicarbonate levels between 22 and 26 mEq/L are considered normal.

If CO_2 levels decrease below 35, it is contributing to alkalosis; if it goes above 45, it is creating excess acid and is contributing to acidosis.

If bicarbonate levels are below 22, it is not as able to buffer acids as it should and therefore is contributing to acidosis; if it is above 26, it is overbuffering the acids and thus contributing to alkalosis.

CO_2	Contribution
<35	Alkalosis
35–45	Normal
>45	Acidosis

Bicarbonate	Contribution
<22	Acidosis
22–26	Normal
>26	Alkalosis

The origin of the pH disorder is CO_2 (respiratory in nature), bicarbonate (metabolic in nature), or both. The contribution that matches the pH condition is the origin of the disorder. For example, if the pH condition is acidosis, the CO_2 contribution is acidosis, and the bicarbonate contribution is alkalosis; then, because the CO_2 contribution matches the pH condition, the CO_2 is the origin of the disorder.

Assessment for Compensation

Does a compensatory response exist, and if so, what is it, and is it adequate?

When a pH disorder is present, the body will make an effort to balance the pH or compensate for the imbalance, and if the disorder is respiratory in nature, the body will attempt to compensate metabolically, and vice versa.

The way to determine a compensatory response is to note the respiratory or metabolic factor that is *not* contributing to the pH disorder. In the example in step 2, the contributing factor is respiratory; in this step, we look at the metabolic factor. If the metabolic factor is normal, no compensation is present, and it is considered an acute disorder. If the metabolic factor is contributing to compensation, the bicarbonate contribution will be alkalosis.

Is the compensation adequate? To determine this, we have to look back at the pH. If the pH is abnormal, it is considered partially compensated. If the pH is within normal limits, it is considered fully compensated.

Categorization of Oxygenation

Recall the PaO_2 classification given on p. 145. View the patient's PaO_2 value, and assign the appropriate classification.

Bibliography

Sorbini CA, Grassi V, Solinas E, Muiesan G: Arterial oxygen tension in relation to age in health subjects, *Resp Int J Thorac Med* 25(1):3-13, 1968.

Dantzker DR: Ventilation-perfusion inequality in lung disease, *Chest* 91(5):749-754, 1987.

Wagner PD, Dantzker DR, Dueck R, et al: Ventilation-perfusion inequality in chronic obstructive pulmonary disease, *J Clin Invest* 59:203-216, 1977.

Cruz JC, Hartley LH, Vogel JA: Effect of altitude relocations upon $AaDO_2$ at rest and during exercise, *J Appl Physiol* 39(3):469-474, 1975.

Hardie JA, Vollmer WM, Buist AS, et al: Reference values for arterial blood gases in the elderly, *Chest* 125(6):2053-2060, 2004.

Walsh B, Czervinski M, DiBlasi R: *Perinatal and pediatric respiratory care*, ed 3, St. Louis, MO, 2010, Saunders.

Kacmarek RM, Stoller JK, Heuer AJ: *Egan's fundamentals of respiratory care*, ed 10, St. Louis, MO, 2013, Mosby.

Minty BP, Nunn JF: Regional quality control survey of blood gas analysis, *Ann Clin Biochem* 14(5):245-253, 1977.

Pinnock C, Lin T, Smith T: *Fundamentals of anaesthesia*, ed 2, Cambridge, U.K., 2003, Cambridge University Press.

McPherson RA, Pincus MR: *Henry's clinical diagnosis and management by laboratory methods*, ed 22, St. Louis, MO, 2012, Saunders.

Siggard-Anderson O: The van Slyke equation, *Scand J Clin Lab Invest Suppl* 146:15-20, 1977.

1. List three indications for obtaining an arterial blood gas sample.

a. _____

b. _____

c. _____

2. List 10 precautions and possible complications involved with sampling for arterial blood gas analysis.

_____

_____

_____

_____

_____

3. List 10 clinical indications for arterial blood gas analysis.

_____

_____

_____

_____

_____

4. List five indications for capillary blood gas sampling in neonatal and pediatric patients.

a. _____

b. _____

c. _____

d. _____

e. _____

5. What is the age contraindication for capillary blood gas sampling?

_____

6. List two indications for transcutaneous blood gas monitoring for neonatal and pediatric patients.

a. _____

b. _____

7. List eight indications for capnometry during mechanical ventilation.

_____

_____

_____

_____

_____

8. What are some causes of sudden high P_{ETCO_2} levels?

a. _____

b. _____

c. _____

9. What are some causes of sudden low P_{ETCO_2} levels?

a. _____

b. _____

c. _____

d. _____

e. _____

f. _____

g. _____

10. Using three different students in your lab, perform a modified Allen's test. Be sure to explain the procedure to each of them. Obtain their signatures.

Signature:_____

Signature:_____

Signature:_____

11. Locate and palpate the common sites below for arterial blood gas sampling on yourself. Check them off once you have located them.

Radial:_____

Brachial:_____

Femoral:_____

Dorsalis pedis:_____

12. With a lab partner, use an arterial puncture arm to perform three radial and three brachial artery punctures. Obtain your partner's signatures upon successful puncture.

Radial:_____

Radial:_____

Radial:_____

Brachial:_____

Brachial:_____

Brachial:_____

13. Using your lab partner as your patient, locate and palpate his or her radial pulse. Trace the radial pulse up the forearm to the brachial artery. Obtain his or her signature.

Signature:_____

14. With a partner, obtain a sample from a practice indwelling catheter successfully three different times. Obtain his or her signatures.

Signature:_____

Signature:_____

Signature:_____

15. Set up a sidestream or mainstream end-tidal CO_2 monitor. Have your instructor sign off once you correctly set it up.

Signature:_____

16. Define the following, and give a clinical situation where each would occur:

a. Respiratory acidosis

_____

_____

b. Respiratory alkalosis

_____

_____

c. Metabolic acidosis

_____

_____

d. Metabolic alkalosis

_____

_____

Self-Assessment Questions

1. After changing the FIO_2 delivered to a patient with healthy lungs, how much time should pass before performing arterial blood gas sampling?
   A. 5–10 minutes
   B. 10–20 minutes
   C. 20–30 minutes
   D. 30–45 minutes

2. After changing the FIO_2 delivered to a patient with chronic obstructive pulmonary disease (COPD), how much time should pass before performing arterial blood gas sampling?
   A. 5–10 minutes
   B. 10–20 minutes
   C. 20–30 minutes
   D. 30–45 minutes

3. Which of the following affect the accuracy or precision of pulse oximeter readings?

   1. Presence of $Hbco$
   2. Presence of HbF
   3. Elevated bilirubin levels
   4. Magnetic resonance imaging

   A. 1 and 2
   B. 1 and 3
   C. 1 and 4
   D. 2 and 3

4. The modified Allen's test is a procedure that:
   A. Locates the position of the radial artery.
   B. Confirms collateral circulation to the hand.
   C. Confirms the correct location of the puncture site.
   D. Aids the practitioner in visualizing the radial artery.

5. Air bubbles in a blood gas sample can cause:

   1. Increased oxygen tension
   2. Decreased oxygen tension
   3. Increased carbon dioxide tension
   4. Decreased carbon dioxide tension

   A. 1 and 3
   B. 1 and 4
   C. 2 and 3
   D. 2 and 4

6. As the gradient between $Paco_2$ and $Petco_2$ increases, what can you assume has happened to dead space volume in relation to tidal volume?
   A. Dead space volume has increased.
   B. Dead space volume has decreased.
   C. Dead space volume has remained the same.
   D. Dead space volume requires a tidal volume to be assessed.

7. What potential hazard do end-tidal CO_2 monitors pose to the patient?
   A. May contribute to necrosis and endotracheal fistula
   B. May cause burns to the upper airway
   C. May decrease the concentration of oxygen reaching the patient
   D. May create leaks or act as an obstruction

8. Which is best able to measure hemoglobin saturation?
   A. Pulse-oximeter
   B. Clark electrode in a blood gas analyzer
   C. Transcutaneous oxygen monitor
   D. CO-oximeter

9. What is the purpose of heating the puncture site prior to a capillary puncture?
   A. Warmer blood allows the PO_2 to better correlate with PaO_2.
   B. Capillary blood at the typical puncture sites is located closer to the surface of the skin. Warming increases the blood temperature so that it is closer to core temperature, and this eliminates the need for temperature correction during analysis.
   C. It distracts the patient from the anxiety associated with the pain of the coming puncture. Anxiety increases ventilation and will skew the results.
   D. It arterializes the capillary bed because heating an area increases perfusion to that area.

10. Which arterial sample site is the most hazardous to sample from?
    A. Radial
    B. Brachial
    C. Femoral
    D. Dorsalis pedis

>> **CASE STUDY 8-1**

A patient is in respiratory distress on a non-rebreather mask with an estimated FiO_2 of 0.80. The doctor orders arterial blood gas assessment. Arterial puncture is performed according to hospital policy. You show the sample to the doctor because of its dark color. The doctor orders CO-oximetry analysis to be performed as well. The blood gas reveals:

pH	7.437
$Paco_2$	36.7
Pao_2	153
HCO_3^-	24.3
Sao_2	99.2
Hb	9.3 g/dL
O_2Hb-ox	80.1%
MetHb-ox	19.1% (critical)
COHb-ox	0.0%

1. Given barometric pressure of 760 mm Hg, what is the patient's A-aDO$_2$ (alveolar–arterial oxygen difference)?

_____

_____

2. What does this A-aDO$_2$ indicate?

_____

_____

3. Given the hemoglobin results, what is the effective arterial oxygen content?

_____

_____

Pulmonary Function Testing

Toni L. Rodriguez

▪ OBJECTIVES

Upon the completion of the chapter activities and content review topics, the student should be able to:

1. Identify lung volumes and capacities.
2. Identify general types of instruments that measure gas volume and flow.
3. Perform calibration of volume displacement and flow-sensing spirometers.
4. Perform simple spirometry.
5. Perform a forced vital capacity.
6. Interpret pulmonary function test results.

▪ KEY TERMS

- Expiratory reserve volume (ERV)
- Forced vital capacity (FVC)
- Forced expiratory flow between 25% and 75% ($FEF_{25\%-75\%}$)
- Forced expired volume in 1 second (FEV_1)
- Forced expired volume in 1 second-to-vital capacity ratio (FEV_1/FVC)
- Functional residual capacity (FRC)
- Inspiratory capacity (IC)
- Inspiratory reserve volume (IRV)
- Obstructive pulmonary disease
- Restrictive pulmonary disease
- Residual volume (RV)
- Slow vital capacity (SVC)
- Tidal volume (V_T)
- Total lung capacity (TLC)
- Vital capacity (VC)

▪ CONTENT REVIEW TOPICS

- American Thoracic Society (ATS)
- Spirometry calibration
- Mechanical quality control

▪ PROCEDURAL ASSESSMENTS

9-1 Performing Simple Spirometry
9-2 Performing Forced Vital Capacity Maneuver
9-3 Performing Flow-Volume Curves

▪ EQUIPMENT

- Barometer
- Calibration syringe
- Disposable mouth pieces
- Manometer
- Respirometer
- Scale with height measurement
- Spirometer
- Spirometer hoses
- Thermometer
- Wastebasket

Pulmonary function tests (PFTs) are used to evaluate lung volumes and capacities, rates of flow, and gas exchange. Indications for PFTs include the need to identify and quantify changes in pulmonary function; evaluate need and quantify therapeutic effectiveness; perform epidemiologic surveillance for pulmonary disease; assess patients for risk of postoperative pulmonary complications; and determine pulmonary disability. Diagnosis of pulmonary diseases commonly requires PFTs, and respiratory therapists (RTs) usually administer the variety of tests involved. Categories of these tests are given in Box 9-1.

Basic diagnostic and therapeutic questions for pulmonary function testing are provided in Box 9-2. Pulmonary function tests do not diagnose specific diseases but, rather, classify patterns of impairment to include obstructive and restrictive impairments. These two types of impairments may occur together and are referred to as *mixed impairment* (Box 9-3). RTs need to be familiar with PFTs because these tests reveal quantitative data about a patient's pulmonary pathology. A diagrammatic representation of lung volumes and capacities is given in Figure 9-1.

The primary measuring instruments used in performing PFTs include spirometers, which measure gas volume, and pneumotachometers, which measure gas flow. Simple PFTs may be performed at the bedside or in the patient's home. But more detailed and complex physiologic assessments need to be performed in a pulmonary function laboratory. Basic precautions for infection control during assessment are important and are outlined in Box 9-4. Most spirometers in laboratories use computer generated graphics. Testing formats include screenings, bedside testing, and complete pulmonary function survey. Criteria for acceptability for some common tests are summarized in Table 9-1. Reversibility of airway obstruction is determined by performing spirometry before and after the administration of bronchodilators. The formula used to calculate improvement is given in Box 9-5 and pretest instructions

---

BOX 9-1 Categories of Pulmonary Function Tests

Airway Function
1. Simple spirometry
   a. VC, ERV, IC
2. Forced vital capacity maneuver
   a. FVC, FEV_1, FEF, PEF
      (1) Pre–bronchodilator and post–bronchodilator challenges
      (2) Pre–bronchodilator and post–bronchodilator challenges
   b. MEFV curves $\dot{V}_{max}$
      (1) Pre–bronchodilator and post–bronchodilator challenges
      (2) Pre–bronchodilator and post–bronchodilator challenges
3. Maximal voluntary ventilation (MVV)
4. Maximal inspiratory/expiratory pressures (MIP/MEP)
5. Airway resistance (Raw) and compliance (C_1)

Lung Volumes and Ventilation
1. FRC
   a. Open-circuit (N_2 washout)
   b. Closed-circuit/rebreathing (Helium [He] dilution)
   c. Thoracic gas volume (VTG)

2. TLC, RV, RV/TLC ratio
3. Minute ventilation, alveolar ventilation, and dead space
4. Distribution of ventilation
   a. Multiple-breath N_2
   b. Helium equilibration
   c. Single-breath techniques

Carbon Monoxide Diffusion Capacity (DLCO) Tests
1. Single-breath (breath holding)
2. Steady state
3. Other techniques

Blood Gases and Gas Exchange Tests
1. Blood gas analysis and blood oximetry
   a. Shunt studies
2. Pulse oximetry
3. Capnography

Cardiopulmonary Exercise Tests
1. Simple noninvasive tests
2. Tests with exhaled gas analyses
3. Tests with blood gas analyses

Metabolic Measurements
1. Resting energy expenditure (REE)
2. Substrate utilization

From Mottram C: *Ruppel's manual of pulmonary function testing*, ed 10, St. Louis, MO, 2013, Mosby.

BOX 9-2 Questions for Clinical Pulmonary Function Testing

Diagnostic
- Is lung disease present?
- What type of lung impairment is present?
- What is the degree of lung impairment?
- Is more than one type of lung impartment present?
- Can multiple lung diseases be separated?

Therapeutic
- Is therapy indicated?
- What treatments are most effective?
- To what degree is the disease reversible?
- Can treatments be evaluated?
- Is rehabilitation feasible?

BOX 9-3 Examples of Obstructive and Restrictive Diseases

Obstructive
- Chronic obstructive pulmonary disease (COPD); emphysema and chronic bronchitis
- Asthma
- Bronchiectasis
- Cystic fibrosis

Restrictive
- Interstitial lung diseases
- Diseases of the chest wall and pleura
- Neuromuscular disorders
- Congestive heart failure (CHF)
- Obesity
- Lung resection

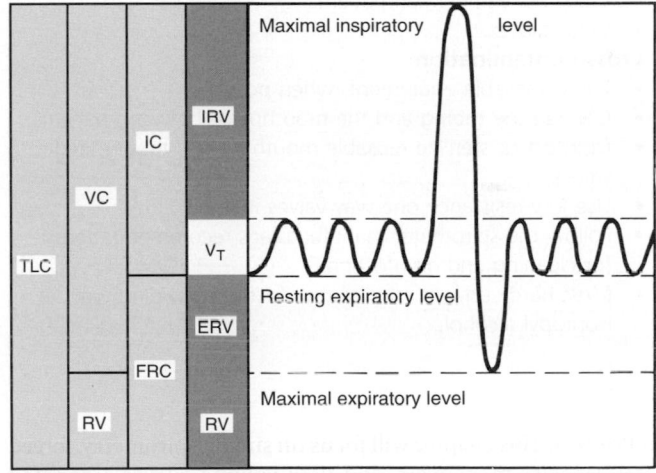

Figure 9-1 Diagrammatic representation of lung volumes and capacities based on a simple spirogram. Relationships between the subdivisions and relative sizes as compared with TLC are shown (*shaded areas*). Resting expiratory level is used as a starting point for FRC determinations because it remains more stable than other identifiable points during repeated measurements. *ERV*, expiratory reserve volume; *FRC*, functional residual capacity; *IC*, inspiratory capacity; *IRV*, inspiratory reserve volume; *RV*, residual volume; *TLC*, total lung capacity; *VC*, vital capacity; *VT*, tidal volume. (From Mottram C: *Ruppel's manual of pulmonary function testing*, ed 10, St. Louis, MO, 2013, Mosby.)

TABLE 9-1 Criteria for Acceptability

Vital Capacity (VC)	Forced Vital Capacity (FVC)	Flow-Volume (F-V) Loop
• End-expiratory volume varies by less than 100 mL for three preceding breaths • Volume plateau is observed at maximal inspiration and expiration • Two acceptable VC maneuvers should be obtained; volumes within 150 mL	• Maximal effort: no cough, or glottis closure during the first second; no leaks or obstructions of the mouthpiece • Good start-of-test; back-extrapolated volume less than 5% of FVC or 150 mL, whichever is greater • Tracing shows 6 seconds of exhalation or an obvious plateau; no early termination or cutoff; or subject cannot or should not continue to exhale • Three acceptable spirograms obtained; two largest FVC values within 150 mL; two largest forced expired volume in 1 second (FEV_1) values within 150 mL • Report the highest FVC and highest FEV_1, even if they come from separate maneuvers; The FEV_1/FVC ration is derived from these values	• Rapid rise from maximal inspiration to peak expiratory flow (PEF) • Maximal effort until flow returns to zero baseline; no glottis closure or abrupt end of flow • Maximal inspiratory effort with return of volume to point of maximal inspiration • At least three acceptable loops recorded; superimposed or side-by-side loops should be repeatable, unless bronchospasm occurs • Report the F-V loop from the single best test maneuver

---

BOX 9-4   Hygiene and Infection Control

Hand Washing
- Wash hands immediately after direct contact with contaminated mouthpieces, tubing, valves, and equipment surfaces.
- Wash hands between patients.
- Wear gloves.

Cross-Contamination
- Use disposable equipment, when possible.
- Change the tubing and the mouthpiece between patients.
- Disinfect or sterilize reusable mouth pieces, tubing, and valves.
- Use low-resistance one-way valves in line.
- Follow the spirometer manufacturer's recommendations for cleaning and disinfecting.
- Most hard surfaces may be disinfected by wiping with isopropyl alcohol.

BOX 9-5   Formula to Calculate Pulmonary Function Improvement

$$\% \text{ improvement} = \frac{Post - Pre}{Pre} \times 100$$

"Pre" is the pulmonary function variable before using a bronchodilator, and "Post" is the pulmonary function variable after using a bronchodilator. The calculation is used to determine how much the pulmonary function variable improved after taking a bronchodilator challenge.

BOX 9-6   Pulmonary Function Testing Pretest Instructions

- Do not smoke 1 hour prior to the test.
- Do not consume alcoholic beverages 4 hours before the test.
- Do not take caffeine 4 hours before the test.
- Avoid eating a large meal 2 hours before the test.
- Do not use bronchodilators 4 to 6 hours before the test, if tolerated.
- Refrain from heavy exercise a minimum of 30 minutes before the test.
- Reschedule the test if you have symptoms of a cold or flu.
- Notify the testing center if special accommodations are needed.

in Box 9-6. This chapter will focus on simple spirometry, forced vital capacity maneuvers, and flow-volume curves associated with airway function testing.

›› SKILL CHECK LISTS

9-1 Performing Simple Spirometry

Vital capacity (VC), also referred to as slow vital capacity (SVC), is a basic index of pulmonary function and measures the largest volume of air that can be expired after a maximal inspiratory effort. It gives valuable information about the strength of the respiratory muscles and other aspects of pulmonary function. Subdivisions of VC include IC and ERV. IC is about 75% of VC with the ERV measuring about 25% of VC. If VC is reduced, further testing is indicated. The following is the step-by-step process for performing simple spirometry.

Procedural Preparation
1. Review the patient's chart.
2. Verify the physician's order or the facility's protocol for standard of care.
3. Obtain, clean, and inspect the appropriate equipment prior to entering the patient's room.
4. Follow personal protective equipment (PPE) requirements, and observe standard precautions for any transmission-based isolation procedure.
5. Identify the patient using two patient identifiers.

6. Introduce yourself to the patient and to the family.
7. Explain the procedure to the patient and to the family, and acknowledge the patient's understanding.
8. Perform proper hand hygiene, and put on gloves, mask, and protective eyewear, as appropriate for the procedure.

Implementation

1. Place the patient in a comfortable position, in the sitting or high-Fowler position.
2. Assess vital signs.
3. Provide instructions, and demonstrate the tests to the patient before administering them.
4. Position the nose clips, if applicable.
5. Position the mouthpiece resting on top of patient's tongue.
6. Instruct the patient to gently bite down with the teeth and seal the lips firmly around the mouthpiece.
7. Place the spirometer hose or flow sensor in the patient's hand, and instruct him or her to breathe quietly for several breaths.
8. For VC:
   a. Instruct the patient to inspire maximally and then exhale completely.
   b. Instruct the patient to perform the maneuver slowly and completely.
9. For IC:
   a. Instruct the patient to breathe normally for three or four breaths.
   b. Instruct the patient to inhale maximally.
10. For ERV:
    a. Instruct the patient to breathe normally for three or four breaths.
    b. Instruct the patient to exhale maximally.
11. Ensure that the patient performs procedure until acceptability and repeatability criteria are achieved.
12. Remove the supplies from patient's room, and clean the area, as needed.
13. Remove the PPE, and perform proper hand hygiene prior to leaving the patient's room.

Evaluation of Procedure

1. Establish a baseline, or compare with previous measurements.
2. Assess the patient during the test to identify any distress or physical complications.
3. Interpret the results.
4. Develop an appropriate respiratory care plan based on assessment data.
5. Identify any unexpected outcomes.

Documentation and Reporting

1. Record your findings in the patient's chart as a percent of the predicted body temperature pressure saturated (BTPS).
2. Report any abnormal findings to the appropriate health care provider.

9-2 Performing Forced Vital Capacity Maneuver

Pulmonary function tests are used to determine the type of pulmonary impairment the patient is suffering from and, if present, its severity. Obstructive disease typically affects the

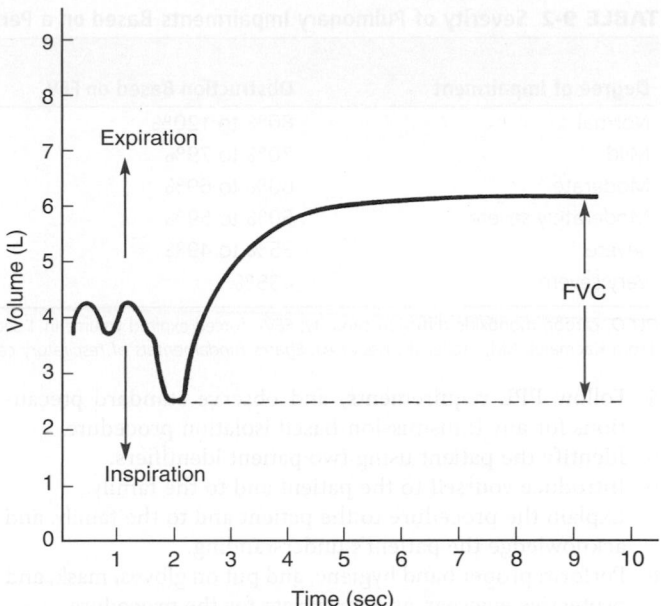

Figure 9-2 This is a typical spirogram tracing that plots volume against time as the patient exhales forcefully. In this tracing, expiration causes an upward deflection; in some systems, the tracing is inverted. The patient inspires to the maximal inspiratory level (*dashed line*), at which point lung volume is close to total lung capacity (TLC). The patient then expires as forcefully and rapidly as possible to the maximal expiratory level, at which point the lungs contain residual volume (RV) only. (From Mottram C: *Ruppel's manual of pulmonary function testing*, ed 10, St. Louis, MO, 2013, Mosby.)

airways of the patient, and breathing is difficult during expiration. Flow rates are useful measurements for obstructive diseases. Comparatively, restrictive disease typically affects the lung parenchyma, and inhalation is the difficult phase of breathing. Tests that involve measurements of volumes and capacities are useful. One of the most commonly performed tests is the FVC maneuver. A typical spirogram plotting volume against time as the patient forcefully exhales can be seen in Figure 9-2. This test is extremely effort dependent and usually requires the RT administering the test to coach the patient throughout the procedure. To determine the presence or the severity of a patient's pulmonary impairment, a comparison of the patient's predicted and measured values are used. The following equation is used to compare:

$$\% \text{ Predicted} = \frac{\text{Measured value}}{\text{Predicted normal value}} \times 100$$

FVC is used to measure FEV_T values by timing the FVC maneuver at specific time intervals. Table 9-2 describes the severity of pulmonary impairment based on a percentage of the predicted normal values. The following is the step-by-step process for performing a forced vital capacity maneuver.

Procedural Preparation

1. Review the patient's chart.
2. Verify the physician's order or the facility's protocol for standard of care.
3. Obtain, clean, and inspect the appropriate equipment prior to entering the patient's room.

TABLE 9-2 Severity of Pulmonary Impairments Based on a Percentage of Predicted Normal Values

Degree of Impairment	Obstruction Based on FEV₁	Restriction or Obstruction Based on TLC, FRC, RV	Gas Exchange Based on DLCO
Normal	80% to 120%	80% to 120%	80% to 120%
Mild	70% to 79%	70% to 79% or 121% to 130%	61% to 79%
Moderate	60% to 69%	60% to 69% or 131% to 140%	40% to 60%
Moderately severe	50% to 59%	50% to 59% or 141% to 150%	
Severe	35% to 49%	35% to 49% or 151% to 165%	<40%
Very severe	<35%	Very severe <35% or >165%	

DLCO, carbon monoxide diffusion capacity; FEV₁, forced expired volume in 1 second; FRC, functional residual capacity; RV, residual volume; TLC, total lung capacity. (From Kacmarek RM, Stoller JK, Heuer AJ: *Egan's fundamentals of respiratory care*, ed 10, St. Louis, MO, 2013, Mosby.)

4. Follow PPE requirements, and observe standard precautions for any transmission-based isolation procedure.
5. Identify the patient using two patient identifiers.
6. Introduce yourself to the patient and to the family.
7. Explain the procedure to the patient and to the family, and acknowledge the patient's understanding.
8. Perform proper hand hygiene, and put on gloves, mask, and protective eyewear, as appropriate for the procedure.

Implementation

1. Place the patient in a comfortable position, in the sitting or high-Fowler position or sitting upright with feet flat on the floor.
2. Assess vital signs:
   a. Ask the patient to loosen any tight clothing.
   b. Ask about the presence and fit of dentures.
3. Provide instructions, and demonstrate the tests to the patient before administering them.
4. Position nose clips.
5. Position the mouthpiece to rest on top of the patient's tongue.
6. Instruct the patient to gently bite down with the teeth and seal the lips firmly around the mouthpiece.
7. Place the spirometer hose or flow sensor in the patient's hand, and instruct him or her to breathe quietly for several breaths.
8. Instruct the patient to take a maximal inspiration and then to expel the air out forcefully.
9. Encourage the patient to continue to blow.
10. Ensure that the patient performs procedure until acceptability and repeatability criteria are achieved.
11. Remove the supplies from the patient's room, and clean the area, as needed.
12. Remove the PPE, and perform proper hand hygiene prior to leaving the patient's room.

Evaluation of Procedure

1. Establish a baseline, or compare with previous measurements.
2. Assess the patient during the test to identify any distress or physical complications.
3. Interpret the results.
4. Develop an appropriate respiratory care plan based on assessment data.
5. Identify any unexpected outcomes.

Documentation and Reporting

1. Record your findings in the patient's chart as a percent of the predicted BTPS.

2. Report any abnormal findings to the appropriate health care provider.

9-3 Performing Flow-Volume Curves

→ **Reality Check** You may not work in a pulmonary function lab, but understanding the information provided from various types of PFTs is vital to understanding the overall pulmonary function of your patients.

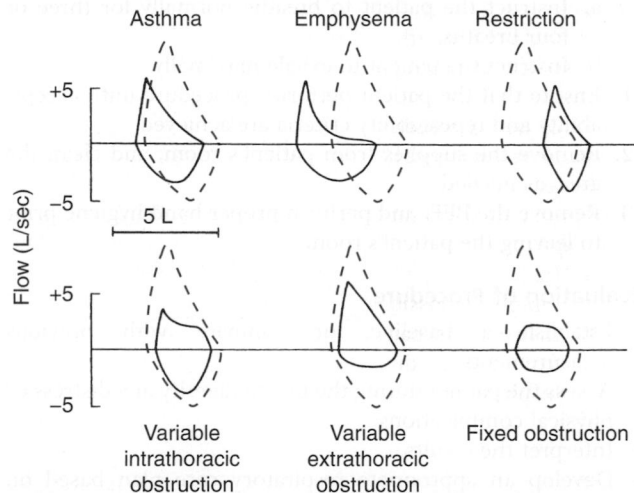

Figure 9-3 Six abnormal flow-volume loop pattern curves are shown plotting flow in liters per second (L/s) against the FVC on an absolute volume scale, with the expected curve shown as dashed lines. In patients who have asthma and emphysema, the expiratory curve is characteristically concave. The TLC and RV points are consistent with hyperinflation, air trapping, or both. In patients with lung or chest wall restriction, the shape of the loop is preserved but FVC is decreased. TLC and RV are displaced toward lower lung volume. The bottom three examples depict types of large airway obstruction. Variable intrathoracic obstruction shows reduced flows on expiration ("what's in is out") despite near-normal flows on inspiration. Variable extrathoracic obstruction shows an opposite pattern. Inspiratory flow is reduced, whereas expiratory flow is relatively normal ("what's out is in"). Fixed large airway obstruction is characterized by equally reduced inspiratory and expiratory flows. (From Mottram C: Ruppel's *Manual of Pulmonary Function Testing*, ed 10, St. Louis, MO, 2012, Mosby)

Flow-volume loops are the expiratory and inspiratory flow-volume curves plotted together. Graphically displaying both the maximal forced expiratory and inspiratory air flow together may help classify a patient's impairment as obstructive, restrictive, or mixed. Abnormal flow-volume loop patterns are given in Figure 9-3. The following is the step-by-step process for performing flow-volume curves.

Procedural Preparation

1. Review the patient's chart.
2. Verify the physician's order or the facility's protocol for standard of care.
3. Obtain, clean, and inspect the appropriate equipment prior to entering the patient's room.
4. Follow PPE requirements, and observe standard precautions for any transmission-based isolation procedure.
5. Identify the patient using two patient identifiers.
6. Introduce yourself to the patient and to the family.
7. Explain the procedure to the patient and to the family, and acknowledge the patient's understanding.
8. Perform proper hand hygiene, and put on gloves, mask, and protective eyewear, as appropriate for the procedure.

Implementation

1. Place the patient in the sitting or high-Fowler position or sitting upright with feet flat on the floor.
2. Assess vital signs.
3. Provide instructions, and demonstrate the tests to the patient before administering them.
4. Position nose clips.
5. Position the mouthpiece to rest on top of patient's tongue.
6. Instruct patient to gently bite down with the teeth and seal the lips firmly around the mouthpiece.
7. Place the spirometer hose or flow sensor in the patient's hand, and instruct him or her to breathe quietly for several breaths.
8. For maximal expiratory flow-volume (MEFV) and maximal inspiratory flow volume (MIFV):
   a. Instruct the patient to inspire fully and then exhale as rapidly as possible.
   b. Instruct the patient to inspire as rapidly as possible from the maximal expiratory level back to maximal inspiration.

9. Ensure that the patient performs the procedure until acceptability and repeatability criteria are achieved.
10. Remove the supplies from the patient's room, and clean the area, as needed.
11. Remove the PPE, and perform proper hand hygiene prior to leaving the patient's room.

Evaluation of Procedure

1. Establish a baseline, or compare with previous measurements.
2. Assess the patient during the test to identify any distress or physical complications.
3. Interpret the results.
4. Develop an appropriate respiratory care plan based on assessment data.
5. Identify any unexpected outcomes.

Documentation and Reporting

1. Record your findings in the patient's chart as a percent of the predicted BTPS.
2. Report any abnormal findings to the appropriate health care provider.

Bibliography

American College of Occupational and Environmental Medicine: Spirometry in the occupational health setting 2011 Update, *JOEM* 53:569-584, 2011.

American Thoracic Society/European Respiratory Society: General considerations for lung function testing, *Eur Resp J* 26:153-161, 2005.

American Thoracic Society/European Respiratory Society: Standardization of spirometry, *Eur Resp J* 26:319–338, 2005.

Centers for Disease Control and Prevention: *National Institute for Occupational Safety and Health spirometry training guide*, Morgantown, West Virginia, 2003, CDC.

Hankinson JL, Odencranz JR, Fedan KB: Spirometric reference values from a sample of the general population, *Am J Resp Med* 159:179-187, 1999.

Kacmarek RM, Stoller JK, Heuer AJ: *Egan's fundamentals of respiratory care*, ed 10, St. Louis, MO, 2012, Mosby.

Mottram C: *Ruppel's of pulmonary function testing*, ed 10, St. Louis, MO, 2012, Mosby.

1. List at least five indications for spirometry.

_____

_____

2. List at least five relative contraindications for spirometry.

_____

_____

3. Working with a lab partner, practice interviewing him or her, and fill in the following chart:

PULMONARY HISTORY

1. Age_____ Sex _____ Standing height _____
   Weight _____ Race_____

2. Current diagnosis or reason for test:

   _____

3. Family history: Did anyone in your immediate family (mother, father, brother or sister) ever have the following?
   - Tuberculosis **Y / N**
   - Emphysema **Y / N**
   - Chronic bronchitis **Y / N**
   - Asthma **Y / N**
   - Hay fever or allergies **Y / N**
   - Lung cancer **Y / N**
   - Other lung disorders **Y / N**

4. Personal history: Have you ever had, or been told that you had, the following?
   - Tuberculosis **Y / N**
   - Emphysema **Y / N**
   - Chronic bronchitis **Y / N**
   - Asthma **Y / N**
   - Recurrent lung infections **Y / N**
   - Pneumonia or pleurisy **Y / N**
   - Hay fever or allergies **Y / N**
   - Chest injury **Y / N** (if yes, what kind?) _____

   _____

   - Chest surgery **Y / N** (if yes, what kind?) _____

   _____

5. Occupational/environmental exposure:
   - What is, or was, your occupation? _____

   _____

   - Have you ever been exposed to gases, dusts or fumes that caused breathing problems? If so, what were they?_____

   _____

- Do you have hobbies or other activities that cause breathing problems? If so, what are they? _____

   _____

6. Smoking habits: Have you ever smoked the following?
   - Cigarettes (how many packs per day?)_____
   - Cigars (how many per day?)_____
   - Pipe (how many bowls per day?)_____
     How long?_____ years
   - Do you still smoke? **Y / N**   If no, how long ago did you stop? _____ years.
   - Do you live with a smoker? **Y / N**

7. Cough
   - On most days, do you have a cough? **Y / N**
   - How long have you had this cough? _____
   - Is the cough productive or nonproductive? _____

8. Dyspnea: Do you get short of breath at the following times?
   - At rest? **Y / N**
   - On exertion? **Y / N**   If yes, what causes it? _____

   _____

9. Current medications (for heart, lung, blood pressure, other)

Medication	Last taken

Figure 9-4

4. Label the following figure:

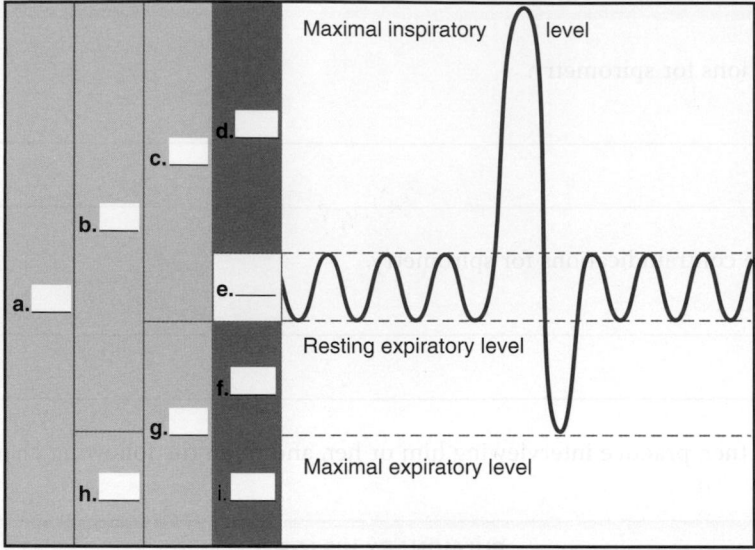

Figure 9-5 (Modified from Mottram C: *Ruppel's manual of pulmonary function testing*, ed 10, St. Louis, MO, 2013, Mosby.)

5. Match the following abnormal flow-volume loop patterns with the correct description:

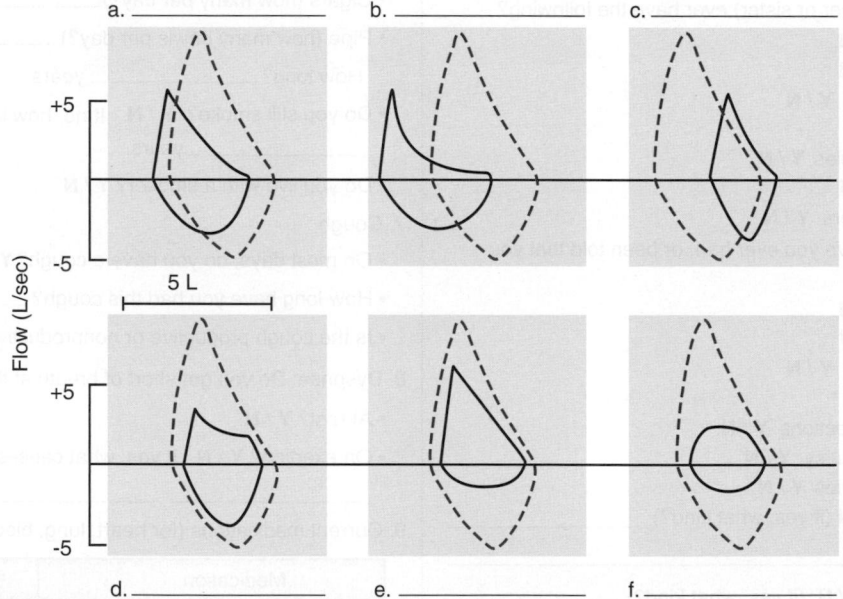

Figure 9-6 (Modified from Mottram C: *Ruppel's manual of pulmonary function testing*, ed 10, St. Louis, MO, 2013, Mosby.)

- Restriction
- Variable intrathoracic obstruction
- Asthma

- Fixed obstruction
- Emphysema
- Variable extrathoracic obstruction

Use the figures provided to answer the following questions:

6. Determine the FVC by measuring the highest point on the tracing plateau.

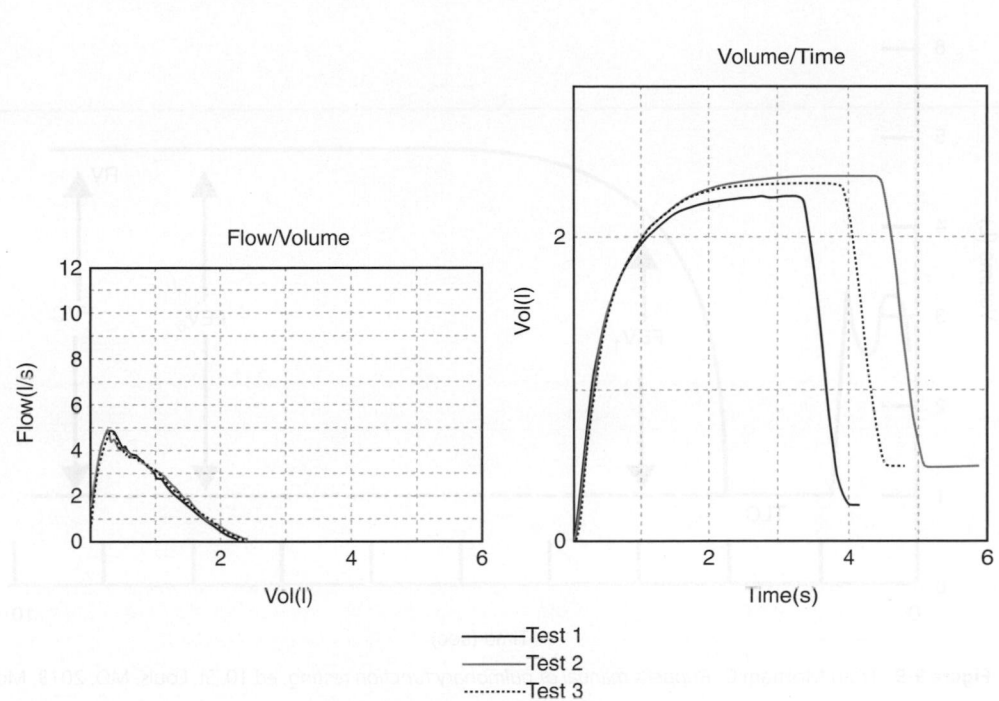

Figure 9-7 (From Mottram C: *Ruppel's manual of pulmonary function testing*, ed 10, St. Louis, MO, 2013, Mosby.)

7. Draw a back-extrapolation line on the volume–time curve by aligning a straight edge on the steepest part of the curve to identify time zero. The point where the back-extrapolation line crosses the time line becomes time zero.

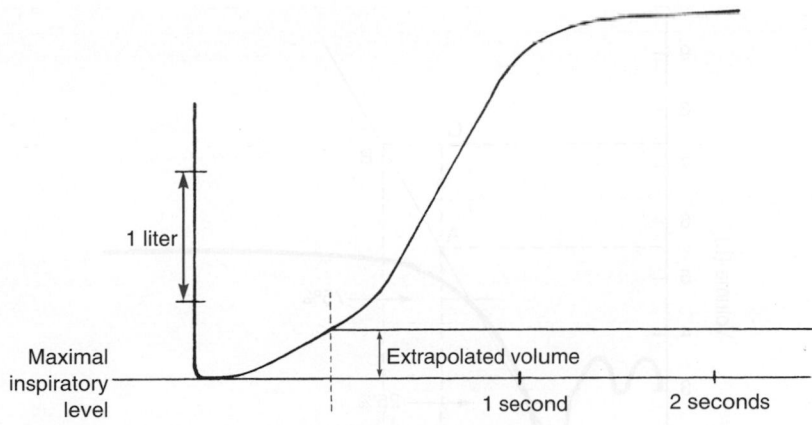

Figure 9-8 (From Mottram C: *Ruppel's manual of pulmonary function testing*, ed 10, St. Louis, MO, 2013, Mosby.)

✳**Tip** The extrapolated volume from back-extrapolation must be less than 5% or 150 mL of FVC for a tracing to be considered valid.

8. Determine the FEV_1 by measuring one second over from time zero, and measure up the identified 1-second line to read the volume. Also, determine the FEV_6. FEV_1 _____ FEV_6 _____

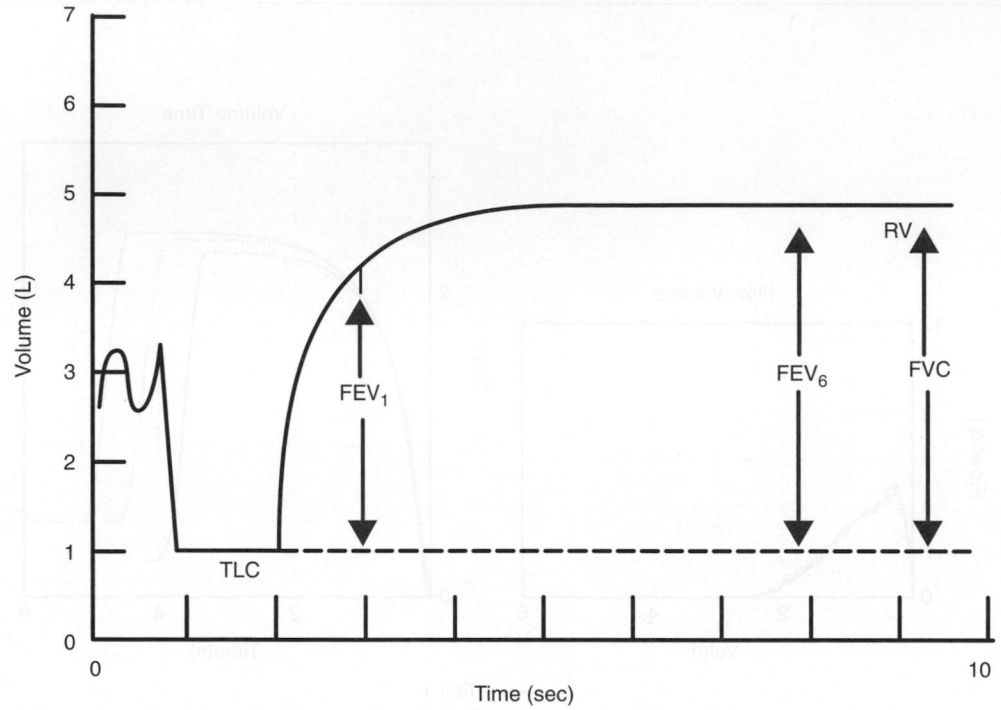

Figure 9-9 (From Mottram C: *Ruppel's manual of pulmonary function testing*, ed 10, St. Louis, MO, 2013, Mosby.)

a.   Divide the FEV_1 by the FVC, and multiply the result by 100 to determine the FEV_1:FVC ratio as a percent.

_____

9. Use Figure 9-10 to answer the questions below.

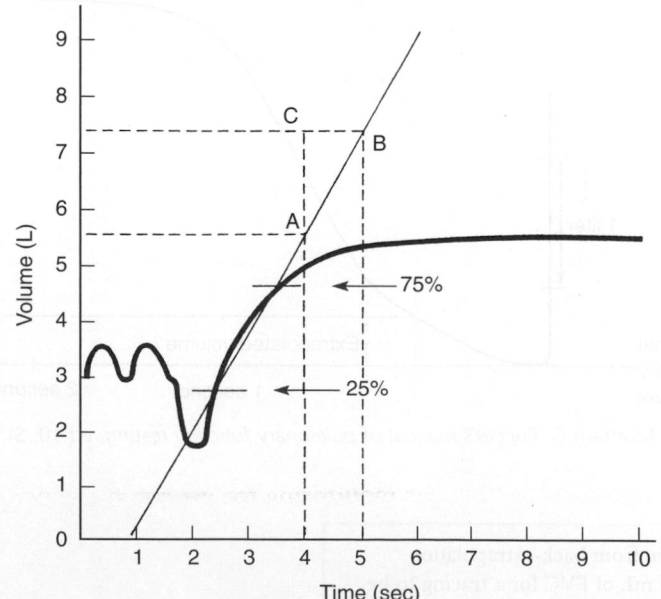

Figure 9-10 (From Mottram C: *Ruppel's manual of pulmonary function testing*, ed 10, St. Louis, MO, 2013, Mosby.)

a. Calculate 25% of the FVC : _____; mark the volume as a point on the volume–time curve.

b. Calculate 75% of the FVC : _____; mark the volume as a point on the volume–time curve.

c. On Figure 9-10, label any two points that are 1-second apart. Use this to determine FEV_1 _____

d. Calculate the FEV_1/FVC ratio: _____

e. Measure the volume at each point identified in step d. The difference between these two volumes is the $FEF_{25-75\%}$ in liters per second.

   i. FVC _____

   ii. FEV_1 _____

   iii. FEV1:FVC Ratio _____

   iv. $FEF_{25-75\%}$ _____

10. Use the flow-volume loop to calculate the following:

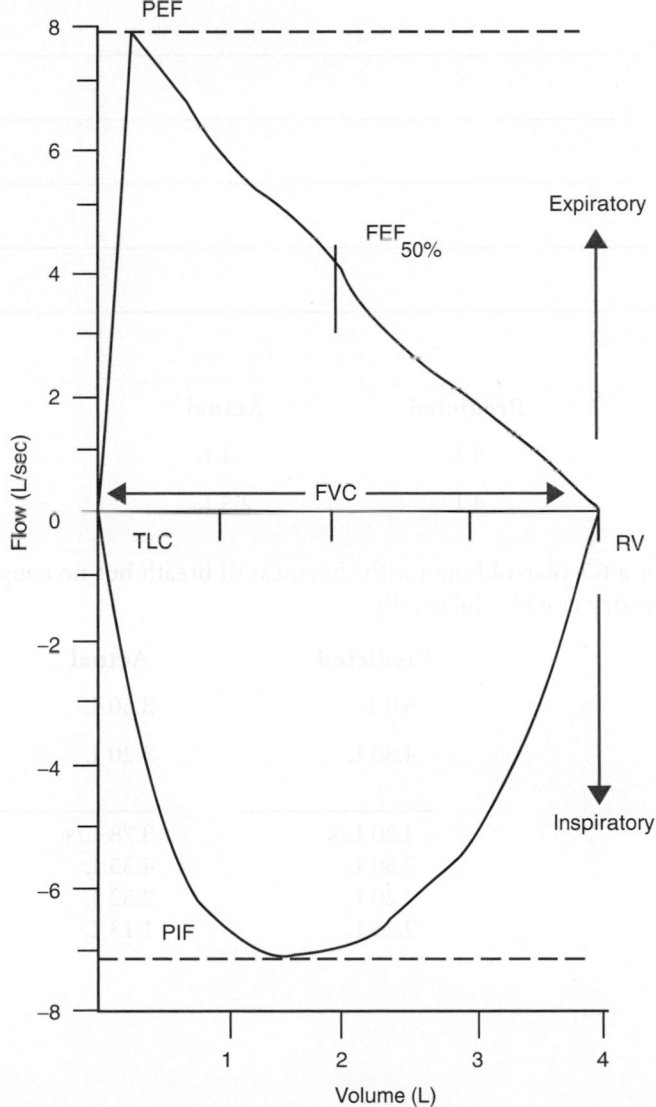

Figure 9-11 (From Mottram C: *Ruppel's manual of pulmonary function testing*, ed 10, St. Louis, MO, 2013, Mosby.)

a. Determine the FVC by measuring the volume across the center of the loop. _____

b. Determine the peak expiratory flow (PEFR) by measuring the flow at the highest point on the expiratory curve.

_____

c. Determine the peak inspiratory flow (PIFR) by measuring the flow at the highest point on the inspiratory curve.

_____

d. Calculate 25% of the FVC value. Mark this volume as a point on the FVC line. Extend this point up to the expiratory curve, and record the flow rate as $FEF_{25\%}$. _____

e. Calculate 50% of the FVC value. Mark this volume as a point on the FVC line. Extend this point up to the expiratory curve, and record the flow rate and record the flow rate as $FEF_{50\%}$. _____

f. Calculate 75% of the FVC value. Mark this volume as a point on the FVC line. Extend this point up to the expiratory curve, and record the flow rate as the $FEF_{75\%}$. _____

11. Answer the following questions about lung capacities:

a. $IRV + V_T + ERV + RV = $ _____

b. $FRC - ERV = $ _____

c. $TLC - VC = $ _____

d. $VT + IRV = $ _____

e. $ERV + RV = $ _____

12. Fill in the following chart:

	Predicted	Actual	Percent Predicted
FVC liters (L)	5 L	4 L	_____
FEV_1 (L)	4 L	2.5 L	_____

13. Fill in the following chart for a 65-year-old man with shortness of breath but no cough or wheezing. His examination is significant for dry crackles bilaterally:

	Predicted	Actual	Percent Predicted
FVC liters (L)	6.0 L	3.60 L	_____
FEV_1 (L)	4.80 L	3.20 L	_____
$\%FEV_1/FVC$	_____	_____	N/A
$FEF_{25\%-75\%}$ L/s	4.20 L/s	3.78 L/s	
TLC (L)	7.50 L	4.35 L	
FRC (L)	4.20 L	2.52 L	
RV (L)	2.25 L	1.13 L	

Self-Assessment Questions

1. Maximal inspiratory pressure primarily measures:
   A. Inspiratory muscle strength
   B. Inspiratory muscle duration
   C. Functional residual capacity
   D. Inspiratory capacity

2. Which of the following are examples of volume-displacement type spirometers?

   1. Dry rolling-seal
   2. Bellows
   3. Pneumotachs
   4. Turbine

   A. 1 and 2 only
   B. 1 and 3 only
   C. 1, 2, and 4 only
   D. 1, 2, 3, and 4

3. A volume-displacement spirometer is being calibration-checked with a 3 L calibration syringe. Which of the following test results would be considered acceptable?
   A. 2.80 L
   B. 2.98 L
   C. 3.15 L
   D. 3.20 L

4. Pretest instructions for pulmonary function studies include:

   1. No alcohol ingestion 4 hours before the test
   2. No caffeine 4 hours before the test
   3. No smoking 1 hour before the test
   4. Avoid eating a large meal 4 hours before the test

   A. 3 only
   B. 1 and 3 only
   C. 1, 2, and 3 only
   D. 1, 2, 3, and 4

5. The number of acceptable spirograms that should be obtained during testing is:
   A. Two
   B. Three
   C. Five
   D. Eight

6. Pulmonary function testing provides the basis for the classification of two major disease categories. Which of the following are these?
   A. Pulmonary and cardiac
   B. Obstructive and restrictive
   C. Reversible and irreversible
   D. Temporary and chronic

7. The acceptable limit for back-extrapolated volume as a percent of FVC is less than:
   A. 2% or 0.50 L of the FVC, whichever is greater
   B. 3% or 0.10 L of the FVC, whichever is greater
   C. 5% or 0.150 L of the FVC, whichever is greater
   D. 6% or 0.200 L of FVC, whichever is greater

8. The volume of gas inspired per the amount of inspiratory effort is termed:
   A. Resistance
   B. Compliance
   C. Tidal volume
   D. Inspiratory capacity

9. An indication for spirometry is:
   A. Unstable cardiovascular status
   B. Pneumothorax
   C. Recent eye surgery
   D. Change in lung function over time

10. Total lung capacity may be calculated by:
    A. $IRV + VC$
    B. $IC + V_T + FRC$
    C. $FRC + IC$
    D. $VC + V_T$

CASE STUDY 9-1

Miss Kova is a 30-year-old female in good health and runs about two miles every day. When she sprints during her runs, she experiences shortness of breath. She has a history of seasonal allergies. She does not smoke. Her pulmonary function testing values are as follows:

	Pre-drug	Predicted	% Predicted	Post-drug	% Predicted	% Change
FVC liters (L)	6.0	5.9	101%	5.8	98%	−3
FEV₁ (L)	4.4	4.5	97%	5.1	113%	16
% FEV₁/FVC	73	76	N/A	87	N/A	
FEF₂₅%–₇₅% liters per second (L/s)	3.6	4.8	75%	4.6	98	27

1. What is your interpretation of the pre–bronchodilator spirometry?

_____

_____

2. Did she exhibit a response to the bronchodilator? _____

3. What is the cause of the patient's symptoms?

_____

_____

4. What types of medications would you recommend?

_____

_____

Chest Radiography Interpretation

▪ OBJECTIVES

Upon the completion of the chapter activities and content review topics, the student should be able to:

1. Demonstrate a systematic review of a chest radiograph.
2. Evaluate the normal anatomic structures seen on a chest radiograph.
3. Describe common radiographic abnormalities.
4. Perform radiograph interpretation of a radiograph.

▪ KEY TERMS

- Air bronchograms
- Cephalization
- Infiltrates
- Kerley B lines
- Picture archive communication system (PACS)
- Radiolucent
- Radiopaque
- Subcutaneous emphysema

▪ CONTENT REVIEW TOPICS

- Cardiopulmonary pathology
- Computed tomography
- Computed tomographic angiography
- Magnetic resonance imaging
- Ultrasonography

▪ PROCEDURAL ASSESSMENTS

10-1 Interpreting Chest Radiographs

▪ EQUIPMENT

- Digital imaging files of chest radiographs
- Radiographs showing multiple views of chest
- Radiograph view box

As a respiratory therapy student, you develop and improve assessment skills by examining every patient you come in contact with. This same rigor should be applied to becoming proficient in interpreting a chest radiograph. Students are not expected to be experts in interpreting a chest radiograph. But, normal chest radiographic findings along with common abnormalities associated with pulmonary pathologies should be recognizable. Figure 10-1 illustrates normal chest radiographic findings.

> → **Reality Check** Remember, you are looking at a two-dimensional representation of a three-dimensional patient.

Although no single perfect way to interpret a radiograph exists, you must find your own technique and stick to it. Consistency with your approach to the interpretation of radiographs will help to ensure that you will not be tempted to focus on just the obvious and fail to notice a subtle detail that will be essential to a patient's diagnosis and treatment. Although it is the physician who orders a radiograph, the respiratory therapist (RT) is frequently the health care team member who conducts patient assessment on the mechanically ventilated patient and notices a need for a radiograph. Indications for obtaining a chest radiograph are given in Box 10-1.

> ✳ **Tip** When viewing digital radiographs, you may need to change your position or the computer screen's position to see certain features. If you are not directly in front of the screen, some things are not as readily apparent.

In the majority of hospitals, radiographs are viewed using an imaging system such as the picture archive communication system (PACS). These systems make it possible to capture, disseminate, and store radiographs in a digital format that is viewable on computer screens around the hospital. Reviewing a digital imaging system of radiographs, some with a radiologist's explanation, will help you improve your interpretation skills.

This chapter summarizes a basic technique for interpreting chest radiographs.

≫ SKILL CHECK LIST

10-1 Interpreting Chest Radiographs

Interpreting a chest radiograph should begin in the same way for all patients. Initially, you should check patient details such as name and date of birth to ensure that you are looking at the right radiograph for the right patient. The date the radiograph was taken should also be noted.

> ✳ **Tip** Start by understanding a normal radiograph and becoming proficient in interpreting all the anatomic structures. Then move on to the abnormalities seen on chest radiographs of the patient with pulmonary problems.

Looking for markers and noting the patient's positioning during the radiograph are also important. Also, check the adequacy of inspiration by noting the number of ribs. Eight to ten

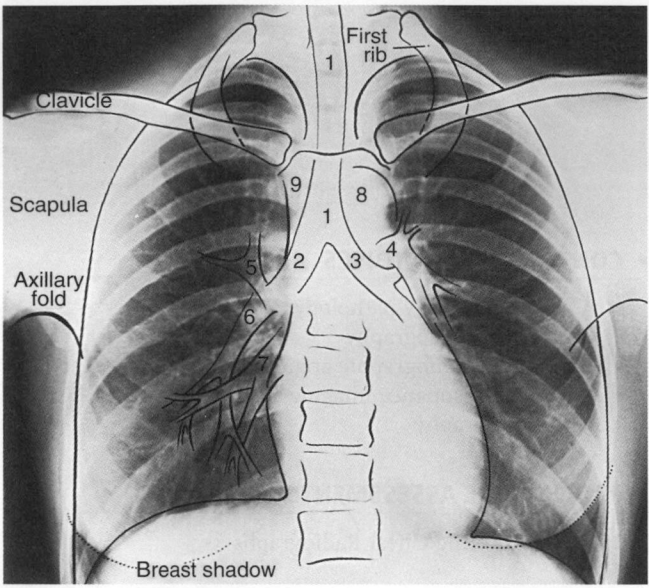

Figure 10-1 Posteroanterior (PA) projection of normal chest radiograph showing the trachea (1), right main bronchus (2), left main bronchus (3), left pulmonary artery (4), right upper lobe pulmonary artery (5), right interlobar artery (6), right lower and middle lobe veins (7), aortic knob (8), and superior vena cava (9). (From Heuer AJ, Scanlan CL: *Clinical assessment for respiratory care*, ed 7, St. Louis, MO, 2014, Mosby.)

pairs of ribs should be seen posteriorly to consider a chest radiograph adequate in terms of inspiration.

When evaluating the quality of the radiograph and the exposure, remember that overexposed radiographs look darker and underexposed radiographs look whiter than normal. To evaluate penetration you should look for intervertebral bodies. If penetration is sufficient, you should see the intervertebral disk spaces through the shadow of the heart with the blood vessels of the peripheral lung regions visible. On underpenetrated radiographs, you will not be able to differentiate the vertebral bodies and spaces. Conversely, an overpenetrated radiograph will not display the peripheral blood vessels, leaving the lung parenchyma black. Adjusting the contrast may overcome some, but not all, of the problems associated with improper penetration. The following is an extended version of the step-by-step process for interpreting a chest radiograph.

> → **Reality Check** Become familiar with the features offered in the viewing of radiographs. Each radiographic package may have different features. The zoom feature is helpful for looking for air bronchograms and Kerley B lines. The inversion feature is useful for looking at fluid verses atelectasis, and the wheel on the mouse makes scrolling through a computed tomography (CT) scan very helpful.

BOX 10-1	Common Clinical Indications for Obtaining a Chest Radiograph

Symptoms
- New or unexplained dyspnea
- Cough, sputum, and fever
- Chest pain
- Hemoptysis

Medical History
- Recent history of chest trauma
- History of aspiration of foreign body
- History of tuberculosis
- History of chronic obstructive pulmonary disease (COPD)
- Significant smoking history
- History of pulmonary fibrosis
- Employment history consistent with inhalation of certain dusts

Physical Examination
- Crackles or wheezes on auscultation
- Sudden drop in blood pressure during mechanical ventilation
- Unilateral decrease in breath sounds
- Extensive use of accessory muscles
- Respiratory rate >30 breaths/min at rest
- Loud P_2 sound
- Pedal edema
- Cardiac murmurs
- Signs of trauma

Arterial Blood Gas Levels
- Severe hypoxemia
- Acute hypercapnia

Pulmonary Function Tests
- Evidence of air trapping (e.g., increase in residual volume or functional residual capacity)
- Reduction in expiratory flows or lung volumes
- Reduced diffusing capacity of lung for carbon monoxide

Postprocedure Factors
- Intubation
- Central venous pressure line or pulmonary artery catheter placement
- Nasogastric tube placement
- Chest tube placement
- Thoracentesis
- Pericardiocentesis
- Bronchoscopy with transbronchial biopsy
- Percutaneous needle biopsy of the lung
- Abdominal or thoracic surgery

Other
- Sudden increase in peak airway pressure (with volume-targeted ventilation) during mechanical ventilation
- After cardiopulmonary resuscitation
- Routine for mechanically ventilated patients
- Routine screening for infectious disease

From Heuer AJ, Scanlan CL: *Clinical assessment for respiratory care*, ed 7, St. Louis, MO, 2014, Mosby.

Procedural Preparation

1. Review the patient's chart.

Implementation

1. Confirm the patient's name and the date the chest radiograph was taken.
2. Identify the type of radiograph:
   a. Posteroanterior radiograph (PA)
   b. Anteroposterior radiograph (AP)
3. Look for markers, and note the position of the patient:
   a. Left and right
   b. PA
   c. AP
   d. Supine, upright, lateral, decubitus
   e. Patient rotation
4. Evaluate the quality of the radiograph:
   a. Overexposed
   b. Underexposed
   c. Intervertebral bodies
5. Evaluate the airway:
   a. Ensure that the trachea is visible and in midline.
   b. Ensure that the trachea gets pushed away from abnormality such as a pleural effusion or tension pneumothorax.
   c. Ensure that the trachea gets pulled towards abnormality such as atelectasis.
   d. Ensure that the trachea normally narrows at the vocal cords.
   e. Identify the carina.
   f. Follow view out to both main-stem bronchi.
6. Evaluate the cardiac silhouette:
   a. Look at size of the heart, and estimate the cardiothoracic ratio (width of heart to the thoracic is normally less than 1:2).
   b. Check whether the silhouette is appropriate or blunted.
   c. If a thin rim of air is present around the heart, think of pneumomediastinum.
   d. Check the aorta.
7. Evaluate the bones:
   a. Fractures
   b. Deformities
8. Evaluate the hemidiaphragms and lung edges:
   a. Note the position.
   b. Are they elevated?
   c. Are they flattened?
   d. Costophrenic angle (*Note*: Effusions cause blunting.)
   e. Right hemidiaphragm (*Note*: Should be higher than the left.)
   f. If much higher, think of effusion, lobar collapse, and diaphragmatic paralysis.
   g. If you cannot see parts of the diaphragm, consider infiltrate or effusion.
9. Evaluate the lung fields:
   a. Are they symmetrical?
   b. Note any opacities.
   c. Check for infiltrates, evaluate their location, and identify the pattern of infiltration.
   d. Keep in mind that the right middle lobe should be adjacent to the heart.
   e. The lingula should be adjacent to the left side of the heart.
   f. Look for lobar collapse.
   g. Look for air bronchograms and Kerley B lines.
   h. Pay attention to the apices.
   i. Check for granulomas, tumors, and pneumothorax.
10. Evaluate the hilum:
    a. Check the position and size bilaterally.
    b. Most hilar shadows represent the right and left pulmonary arteries (the left one should be more superior than the right one).
11. Evaluate soft tissue:
    a. Subcutaneous emphysema
12. Evaluate for the presence of instrumentation:
    a. Artificial airway
    b. Chest tubes
    c. Intravenous (IV) lines
    d. Electrocardiography (ECG) leads
    e. Surgical drains
    f. Pacemaker
    g. Surgical wires and pins
    h. Nasogastric tube

Evaluation of Procedure

1. Establish a baseline, or compare with previous measurements.
2. Trend data, if multiple radiographs are available.
3. Develop an appropriate respiratory care plan based on assessment data.
4. Interpret from general data to specific data.

Documentation and Reporting

1. Report any abnormal findings to the appropriate health care provider.

Bibliography

Eisenberg R, Johnson N: *Comprehensive radiographic pathology*, ed 5, St. Louis, MO, 2011, Mosby.

Heuer AJ, Scanlan CL: *Clinical assessment for respiratory care*, ed 7, St. Louis, MO, 2014, Mosby.

Kacmarek RM, Stoller JK, Heuer AJ: *Egan's fundamentals of respiratory care*, ed 10, St Louis, MO, 2013, Mosby.

1. Define the following terms:

a. Radiolucent

_____

b. Radiopaque

_____

c. Air bronchograms

_____

d. Infiltrates

_____

e. Kerley B lines

_____

f. Cephalization

_____

g. Subcutaneous emphysema

_____

h. Bleb

_____

i. Consolidation

_____

2. Label the images below:

a. Figure 10-2

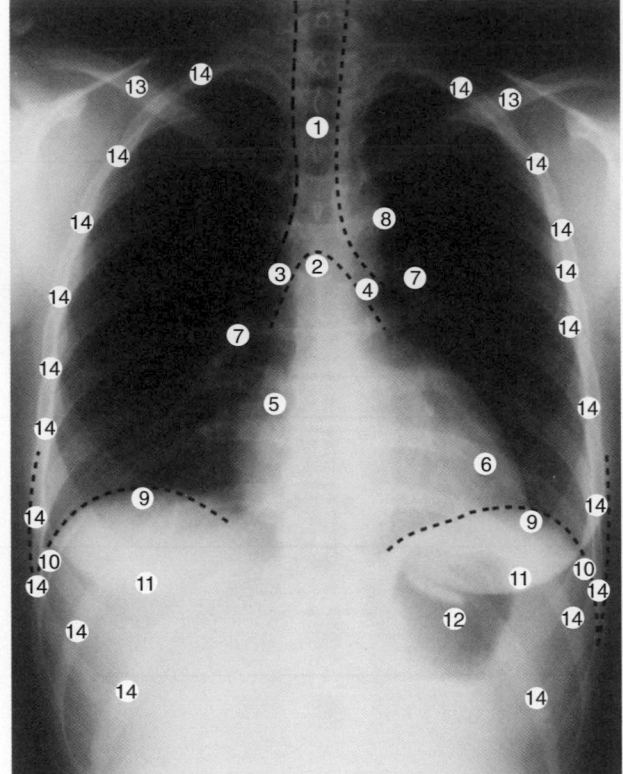

Figure 10-2 (From DesJardins T, Burton GG: *Clinical manifestations and assessment of respiratory disease,* ed 6, 2011, St. Louis, MO, Mosby.)

1. _____

2. _____

3. _____

4. _____

5. _____

6. _____

7. _____

8. _____

9. _____

10. _____

11. _____

12. _____

13. _____

14. _____

b. Figure 10-3

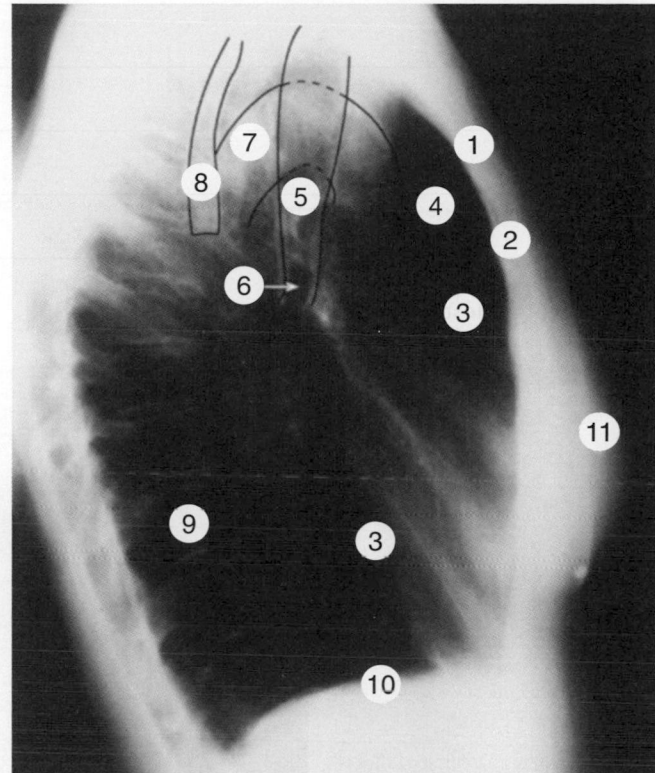

Figure 10-3 (From DesJardins T, Burton GG: *Clinical manifestations and assessment of respiratory disease*, ed 6, 2011, St. Louis, MO, Mosby.)

1. _____
2. _____
3. _____
4. _____
5. _____
6. _____
7. _____
8. _____
9. _____
10. _____
11. _____

3. List the five technical factors that should be routinely assessed when reading a chest radiograph:

a. _____

b. _____

c. _____

d. _____

e. _____

4. Use Figure 10-4 to answer the following questions:

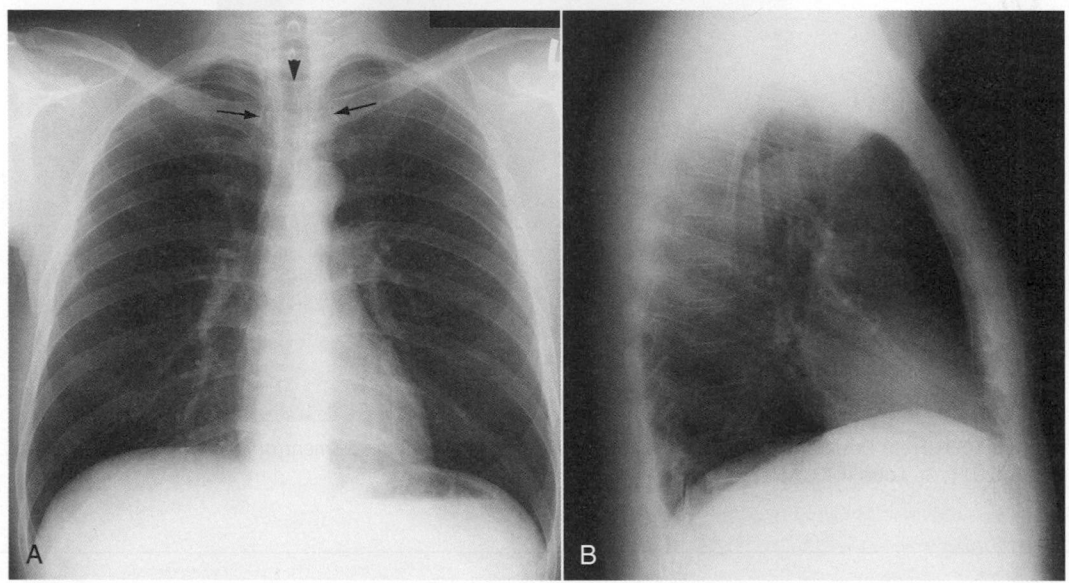

Figure 10-4 (From Kacmarek RM, Stoller JK, Heuer AJ: *Egan's fundamentals of respiratory care*, ed 10, St. Louis, MO, 2013, Mosby.)

a. Which image is a PA radiograph?_____

b. Is the patient positioned appropriately? _____

c. Label the right and left clavicles.

d. Is the quality of the radiograph acceptable for interpretation?_____

e. Is the trachea in midline?_____

f. Label the trachea.

g. Are any fractured bones visible?_____

h. Is the heart of normal size?_____

i. Label the heart.

j. Are the hemidiaphragms normal?_____

k. Label the right and left hemidiaphragms.

l. The right hemidiaphragms are usually a bit higher than the left. Why?_____

m. Are the costophrenic angles sharp?_____

n. How many ribs do you see?_____

o. Are any pulmonary masses present?_____

p. Are any soft tissue abnormalities present?_____

q. Is an artificial airway present?_____

r. What is your interpretation of this film?_____

5. Use Figure 10-5 to answer the following questions:

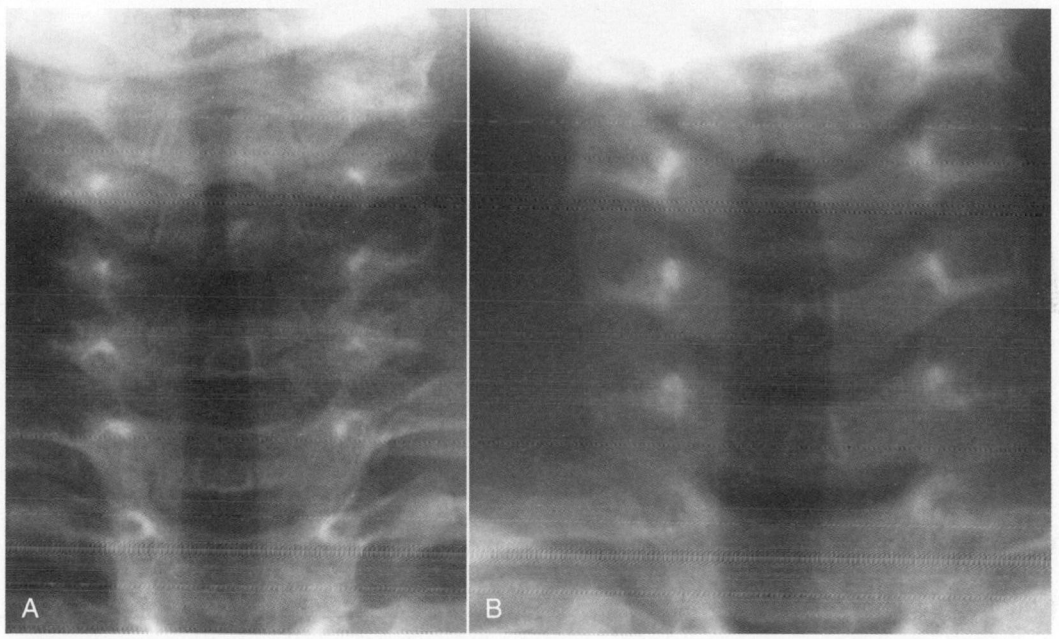

Figure 10-5 (From Eisenberg R, Johnson N: *Comprehensive radiographic pathology*, ed 5, St. Louis, MO, 2011, Mosby.)

a. Is the trachea visible and in midline in Figure 10-5, *A*?_____

b. Is the trachea visible and in midline in Figure 10-5, *B*?_____

c. In which figure is an abnormality seen?_____

Use Figure 10-5, *B*, to answer the following questions:

d. What pathology is commonly associated with this radiographic finding?_____

e. What treatment could you deliver to this patient as a respiratory therapist?_____

f. In an adult patient, what is the narrowest part of the trachea?_____

g. In an infant patient, what is the narrowest part of the trachea?_____

6. Use Figure 10-6 to answer the following questions:

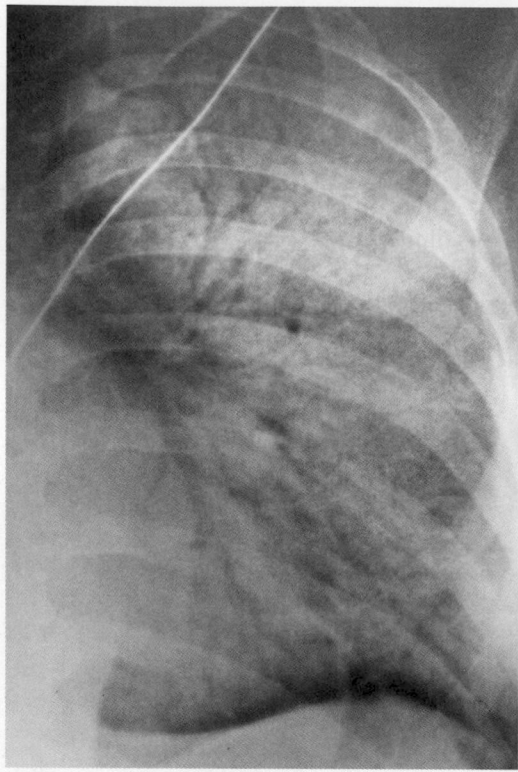

Figure 10-6 (From Eisenberg R, Johnson N: *Comprehensive radiographic pathology*, ed 5, St. Louis, MO, 2011, Mosby.)

a. How many ribs do you see?_____

b. What radiographic abnormality do you see?_____

c. Label the abnormality.

d. What process causes this radiographic appearance?_____

e. What abnormalities may you see in this patient's complete blood cell count?_____

7. Use Figure 10-7 to answer the following questions:

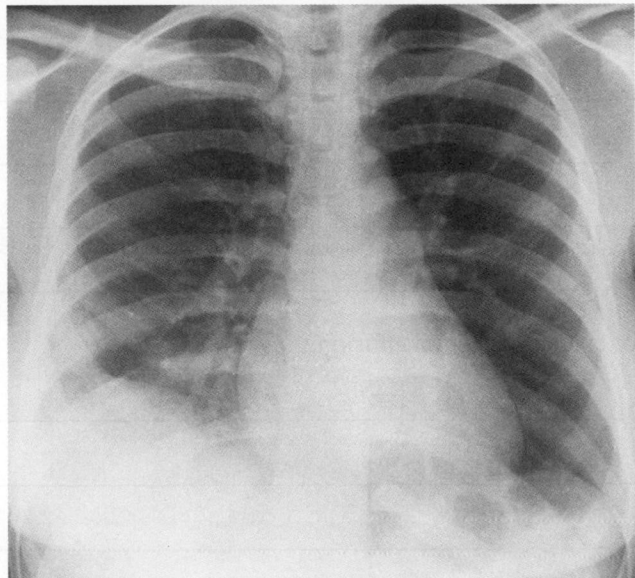

Figure 10-7 (From Eisenberg R, Johnson N: *Comprehensive radiographic pathology*, ed 5, St. Louis, MO, 2011, Mosby.)

a. What type of projection is this radiograph? _____

b. Is the patient positioned appropriately? _____

c. Label the right and left clavicles.

d. Is the quality of the radiograph acceptable for interpretation? _____

e. Is the trachea in midline? _____

f. Label the trachea.

g. Are any fractured bones visible? _____

h. Is the heart of normal size? _____

i. Label the heart.

j. Are both hemidiaphragms visible? _____

k. Are the costophrenic angles sharp? _____

l. How many ribs do you see? _____

m. Are any pulmonary masses present?_____

n. Are any soft tissue abnormalities present?_____

o. Is an artificial airway present?_____

p. What is your interpretation of this radiograph?_____

q. For further evaluation of the pathology that causes this radiographic abnormality, what type of radiograph can be ordered?_____

8. a. List the common causes of transudative pleural effusion:

1. _____

2. _____

3. _____

4. _____

5. _____

b. List the common causes of exudative pleural effusion:

1. _____

2. _____

3. _____

4. _____

5. _____

6. _____

9. Use Figure 10-8 to answer the following questions:

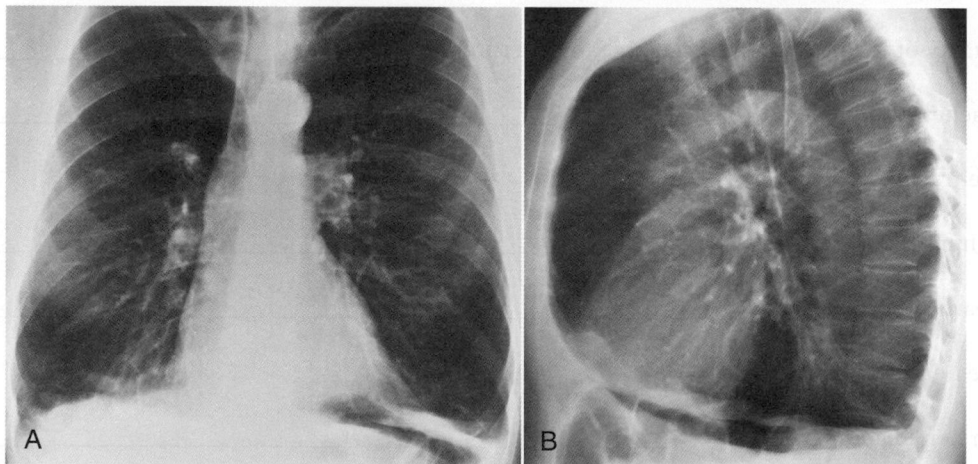

Figure 10-8 (From Eisenberg R, Johnson N: *Comprehensive radiographic pathology*, ed 5, St. Louis, MO, 2011, Mosby.)

a. What types of projections are these radiographs? _____

b. Describe the hemidiaphragms. _____

c. Does the image in Figure 10-8, *B*, demonstrate a normal anteroposterior (AP) diameter? _____

d. Do these images demonstrate underinflation, normal inflation, or hyperinflation of the lungs? _____

e. What is your interpretation of this radiograph? _____

f. Exacerbation of what pulmonary pathology are these types of images associated with? _____

10. Use Figure 10-9 to answer the following questions:

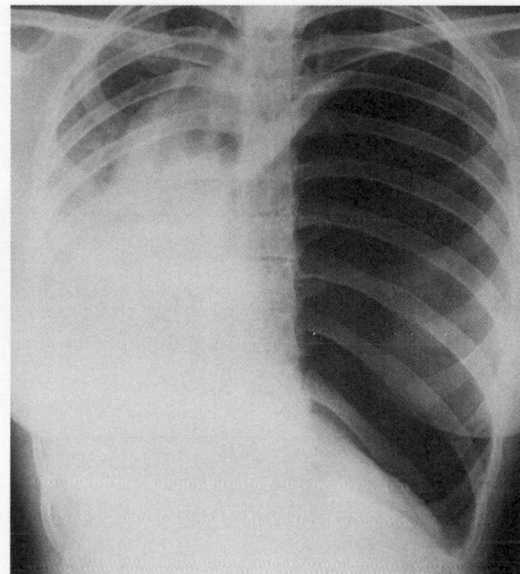

Figure 10-9 (From Eisenberg R, Johnson N: *Comprehensive radiographic pathology*, ed 5, St. Louis, MO, 2011, Mosby.)

a. Which type of projection is this radiograph? _____

b. Is the patient positioned appropriately? _____

c. Label the right and left clavicles.

d. Is the quality of the radiograph acceptable for interpretation? _____

e. Is the trachea in midline? _____

f. Label the trachea.

g. Are any fractured bones visible? _____

h. Is the heart of normal size? _____

i. Are the hemidiaphragms normal? _____

j. Are the costophrenic angles sharp? _____

k. How many ribs do you see? _____

l. Are any soft tissue abnormalities present? _____

m. What is your interpretation of this radiograph? _____

n. What is the treatment for this pathology? _____

11. Use Figure 10-10 to answer the following questions:

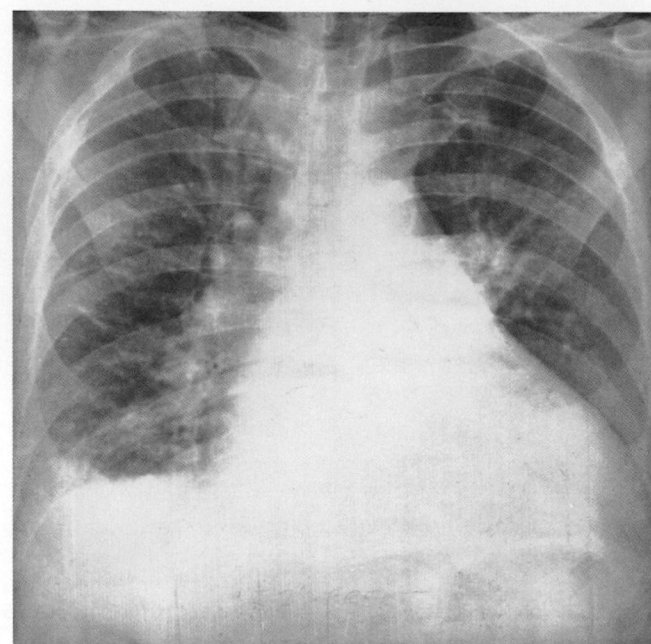

Figure 10-10 Heuer AJ, Scanlan C: *Clinical assessment in respiratory care*, ed 6, St. Louis, MO, 2014, Mosby.)

a. Which type of projection is this radiograph? _____

b. Is the patient positioned appropriately? _____

c. Label the right and left clavicles.

d. Is the quality of the radiograph acceptable for interpretation? _____

e. Is the trachea in midline? _____

f. Label the trachea.

g. Are any fractured bones visible? _____

h. Is the heart of normal size? _____

i. Are the hemidiaphragms normal? _____

j. Are the costophrenic angles sharp? _____

k. How many ribs do you see? _____

l. Are any soft tissue abnormalities present? _____

m. What is your interpretation of this radiograph? _____

n. What is the treatment for this pathology? _____

Self-Assessment Questions

1. In what situation would you suggest obtaining a chest radiograph?

   1. Sudden onset of dyspnea
   2. Plateau pressures changing from 32 cmH_2O to 22 cmH_2O
   3. PaO_2 changing from 98 mm Hg to 42 mm Hg in 30 minutes
   4. Pulmonary artery catheter placement

   A. 1 and 2 only
   B. 2 only
   C. 1, 2, and 3 only
   D. 1, 3, and 4 only

2. Following a normal physical examination of your 26-year-old male patient, you pull up his chest radiograph and observe that the heart is located on the right side of the radiograph. What is the most likely cause?
   A. Dextrocardia
   B. Mislabeling of the radiograph
   C. The patient has a pneumothorax, which is pushing his heart to the right side of his chest
   D. Situs inversus

3. Hyperinflation with flattened hemidiaphragms is a common radiographic finding in:
   A. Exacerbation of asthma
   B. Acute pulmonary edema
   C. Pulmonary embolism
   D. Bacterial pneumonia

4. Radiographic signs of cardiac decompensation include:

   1. Cardiac enlargement
   2. Pleural effusion
   3. Kerley B lines
   4. Alveolar filling

   A. 1 and 2 only
   B. 2, 3, and 4 only
   C. 1 and 4 only
   D. 1, 2, 3, and 4

5. The term *bat-wing appearance* is used to describe:
   A. COPD
   B. Acute respiratory distress syndrome (ARDS)
   C. Pulmonary edema
   D. Tuberculosis

6. Movement of air into the mediastinum is termed:
   A. Pneumothorax
   B. Pneunomediastinum
   C. Bleb
   D. Subcutaneous emphysema

7. Instrumentation visible on a chest radiograph includes:

   1. Endotracheal tubes
   2. Tracheostomy tubes
   3. Central lines
   4. Chest tubes

   A. 1 and 2 only
   B. 1 only
   C. 1, 2, and 4 only
   D. 1, 2, 3, and 4

8. A blunted costophrenic angle is commonly seen in:
   A. Pulmonary edema
   B. Pneumothorax
   C. Pleural effusion
   D. Pulmonary fibrosis

9. The most common radiographic view of an intubated patient receiving mechanical ventilation is:
   A. PA radiograph
   B. AP radiograph
   C. Lateral radiograph
   D. Lateral decubitus radiograph

10. When pleural effusion is suspected, what type of radiographic view should be ordered?
    A. PA radiograph
    B. AP radiograph
    C. Lateral radiograph
    D. Lateral decubitus radiograph

CASE STUDY 10-1

Your patient was intubated and manually ventilated in the emergency department (ED) prior to transfer to the intensive care unit (ICU). Following transfer from the gurney to the ICU bed, the patient is hooked up to the ventilator, and the high pressure alarm and low exhaled tidal volume alarms are activated. A STAT (immediate) radiograph is ordered, as pictured in Figure 10-11.

1. Identify and label the endotracheal tube.

_____

_____

2. Identify and label any instrumentation.

_____

_____

3. What is your interpretation?

_____

_____

4. How would you correct this problem?

_____

_____

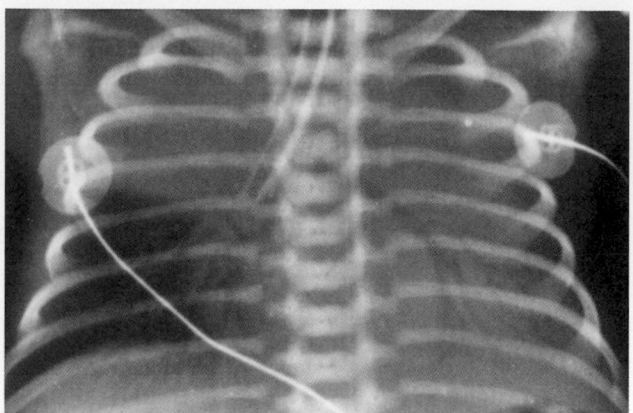

Figure 10-11 (From Eisenberg R, Johnson N: *Comprehensive radiographic pathology*, ed 5, St. Louis, MO, 2011, Mosby.)

Airway Management

▪ OBJECTIVES

Upon the completion of the chapter activities and content review topics, the student should be able to:

1. Identify normal airway anatomy.
2. Perform oropharyngeal suctioning.
3. Perform sterile open and in-line suctioning.
4. Collect a sputum sample by way of suctioning.
5. Perform insertion of an oropharyngeal airway.
6. Perform orotracheal and nasotracheal intubation on an adult patient.
7. Perform endotracheal tube care.
8. Monitor cuff pressure.
9. Perform tracheostomy care.
10. Perform changing a tracheostomy tube.
11. Perform extubation of orotracheal and nasotracheal tubes.
12. Describe the advantages and disadvantages of alternative airway devices.
13. Describe how to assist with bronchoscopy.

▪ KEY TERMS

- Bronchoscopy
- Decannulation
- Extubation
- Intubation

▪ CONTENT REVIEW TOPICS

- American Society for Testing and Materials (ASTM)
- Mallampati Classification
- Normal cough mechanism
- Spontaneous breathing trial (SBT)
- Rigid tube bronchoscopy
- Tracheal stenosis
- Tracheomalacia

▪ PROCEDURAL ASSESSMENTS

11-1 Oropharyngeal Suctioning
11-2 Endotracheal Tube Suctioning
11-3 Nasotracheal Suctioning
11-4 Collecting Sputum Samples by Suctioning
11-5 Inserting an Oropharyngeal Airway
11-6 Oral Endotracheal Intubation
11-7 Nasotracheal Intubation
11-8 Inserting Alternative Airway Devices
11-9 Endotracheal Tube Care
11-10 Monitoring Cuff Pressures
11-11 Tracheostomy and Stoma Care
11-12 Changing a Tracheostomy Tube
11-13 Orotracheal or Nasotracheal Extubation
11-14 Assisting with Bronchoscopy

▪ EQUIPMENT

- Airway management mannequin and silicone spray
- Bag valve mask
- Bronchoscopy equipment-optional
- Calibrated, adjustable regulator
- Cuff pressure monitoring device
- Disposable gloves
- Endotracheal tubes
- Human patient simulator (optional)
- In-line suction device
- Laryngoscope handle with different blades
- Lukens trap or sterile sputum trap
- Mask
- Oropharyngeal airways
- Oxygen source with connections
- Protective eye-wear
- Sterile gloves
- Sterile water or normal saline and cup
- Stethoscope
- Suction catheters
- Tape
- Tracheostomy tubes
- Unit-dose saline vials
- Vacuum source
- Water-soluble lubricant
- Yankauer suction device

M anagement of a patient's airway in various scenarios is the responsibility of the respiratory therapist (RT). These scenarios include inserting and maintaining artificial airways, bronchial hygiene, and assisting physicians in special procedures involving the airway.

Any deficiencies in airway management may have grave consequences for patients. Care must be taken at every point of a patient's airway care. Figure 11-1 shows normal airway anatomy. An RT's expertise and knowledge relating to its structures and functions are essential for top-quality airway care.

This chapter will cover numerous skills an RT needs to perform airway clearance techniques, insert and maintain artificial airways, and assist in procedures related to the airway.

⟫ SKILL CHECK LISTS

11-1 Oropharyngeal Suctioning

Any type of retained airway secretions may impose an increased work of breathing for a patient and cause a myriad

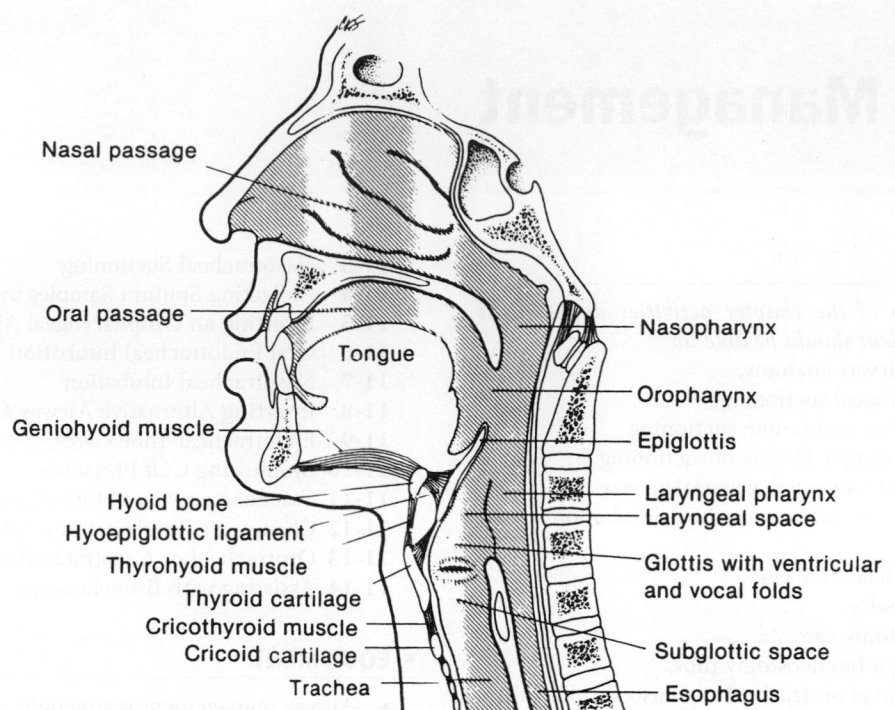

Figure 11-1 Normal airway anatomy. (From Benumof, JL (ed): Clinical procedures in anesthesia and intensive care, Philadelphia, 1992, pp 89-114, JB Lippincott)

BOX 11-1   Oral Care

- Brush the patient's teeth with a brush or a foam swab to remove dental plaque.
- Use toothpaste.
- Have the patient rinse, or wipe the patient's mouth clean.
- Use a water-soluble moisturizer to assist in the maintenance of healthy lips and gums at least once every 2 hours.
- Avoid lemon glycerin swabs.
- Assess the oral cavity.

---

of pulmonary complications. Upper airway suctioning is called *oropharyngeal suctioning*. It may be performed on all types of patients with a variety of artificial airway and includes oral care. Box 11-1 describes the key points of oral care.

> **Reality Check** Oral care in the clinical setting may be either a respiratory technician's responsibility or a nurse's responsibility.

Oropharyngeal suctioning is also performed as part of oral hygiene, aspiration precautions, prior to endotracheal intubation, and part of other respiratory procedures.

A type of suction device, called a *Yankauer suction device*, can be seen in Figure 11-2. The following is the step-by-step process for oropharyngeal suctioning of a patient's airway.

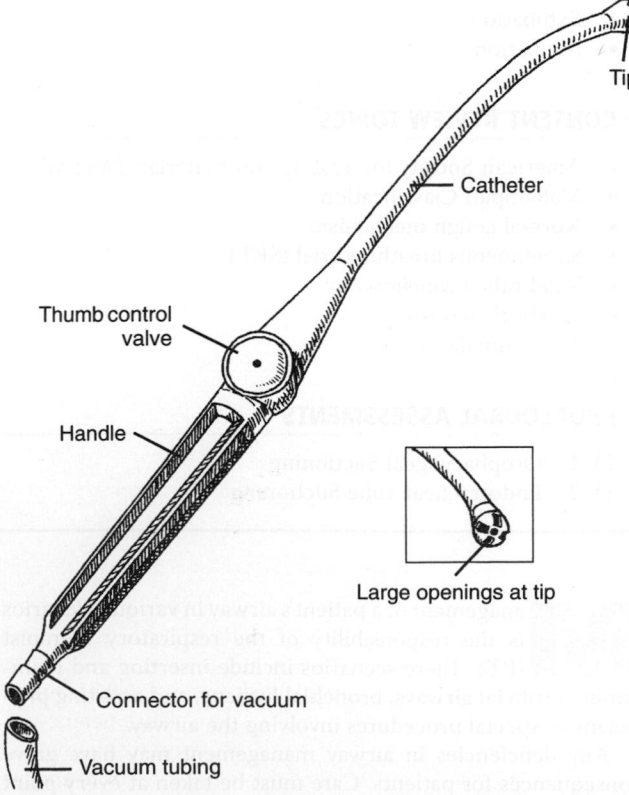

Figure 11-2 Yankauer suction device. (From Sills JR: *The comprehensive respiratory therapist exam review*, ed 5, St. Louis, MO, 2010, Mosby.)

Procedural Preparation

1. Review the patient's chart.
2. Verify the physician's order or the facility's protocol for standard of care.
3. Obtain, clean, and inspect the appropriate equipment prior to entering the patient's room.
4. Follow personal protective equipment (PPE) requirements, and observe standard precautions for any transmission-based isolation procedure.
5. Identify the patient using two patient identifiers.
6. Introduce yourself to the patient and to the family.
7. Explain the procedure to the patient and to the family, and acknowledge the patient's understanding.
8. Perform proper hand hygiene, and put on gloves, mask, and protective eyewear, as appropriate for the procedure.

Implementation

1. Place the patient in a comfortable position, and instruct him or her to breathe normally.
2. Assess vital signs and symptoms of upper airway obstruction requiring oropharyngeal suctioning.
3. Connect the tubing, and turn on suction device.
4. Remove the oxygen mask, if present.
5. Insert the rigid tonsillar device, the Yankauer, or the catheter into patient's mouth.
6. Cover, if needed, the thumb-control valve, and suction the patient's mouth.
7. Rinse the catheter, and turn off the suction device.
8. Wipe the patient's face, if needed.
9. If removed, replace patient's oxygen mask.
10. Remove the supplies from the patient's room, and clean the area, as needed.
11. Remove PPE, and perform proper hand hygiene prior to leaving the patient's room.

Evaluation of Procedure

1. Establish a baseline, or compare with respiratory assessment before and after suctioning.
2. Repeat suctioning, if needed.
3. Reposition the patient.
4. Identify any unexpected outcomes.

Documentation and Reporting

1. Record your findings in the patient's chart.
2. Report any abnormal findings to the appropriate health care provider.

11-2 Endotracheal Tube Suctioning

With a bypassed upper airway, the patient's normal cough mechanism and secretion management abilities are compromised. It is the responsibility of the RT to ensure patency of a patient's airway. Suctioning is part of required maintenance of an artificial airway so that adequate ventilation and gas exchange can take place. Additionally, the RT should be aware of the complications associated with suctioning. Box 11-2 lists the complications that can be seen with this procedure.

> **BOX 11-2 Complications Associated with Suctioning**
>
> - Cardiac dysrhythmias
> - Hypertension
> - Hypotension
> - Atelectasis
> - Hypoxia or hypoxemia
> - Excessive coughing
> - Trauma
> - Discomfort and pain
> - Nosocomial infection
> - Nasal irritation (for nasal suctioning)
> - Mucosal hemorrhage

> **BOX 11-3 Indications for the Use of the Closed Suctioning Technique**
>
> Mechanically ventilated patients, especially neonates and patients with:
> - PEEP ≥10 cm H_2O
> - Mean airway pressure ≥20 cm H_2O
> - Inspiratory time ≥1.5 seconds
> - F_iO_2 ≥0.60
> - Frequent suctioning (≥6 times/day)
> - Hemodynamic instability associated with ventilator disconnection
> - Respiratory infections requiring airborne or droplet precautions
> - Inhaled agents that cannot be interrupted by ventilator disconnection (i.e., nitric oxide, helium and oxygen mixture)

From Kacmarek RM, Stoller JK, Heuer AJ: *Egan's fundamentals of respiratory care*, ed 10, St. Louis, MO, 2013, Mosby.

> **Reality Check** Do not "schedule" airway suctioning for your patient. Assess the patient, and suction only when needed.

Indications for the closed suctioning technique are provided in Box 11-3. The following is the step-by-step process for endotracheal tube suctioning.

Procedural Preparation

1. Review the patient's chart.
2. Verify the physician's order or the facility's protocol for standard of care.
3. Obtain, clean, and inspect the appropriate equipment prior to entering the patient's room.
4. Follow PPE requirements, and observe standard precautions for any transmission-based isolation procedure.
5. Identify the patient using two patient identifiers.
6. Introduce yourself to the patient and to the family.
7. Explain the procedure to the patient and to the family, and acknowledge the patient's understanding.
8. Perform proper hand hygiene, and put on gloves, mask, and protective eyewear, as appropriate for the procedure.

Implementation

1. Position the patient.
2. Assess vital signs and need for suctioning.
3. Hyperoxygenate the patient, according to institutional protocol and the patient's condition.
   a. F_IO_2 of 1.0 for 30 to 60 seconds for pediatric and adults
   b. 0.1 increase from set F_IO_2 for neonates
4. Perform closed in-line suctioning:
   a. Unlock the suction control mechanism.
   b. Pick up the suction catheter with the dominant hand, and stabilize the endotracheal airway tube with the other hand.
   c. Insert the catheter without applying suction:
      i. For deep suctioning, insert the catheter until resistance is met.
      ii. For shallow suctioning, insert catheter the length of the airway plus the adapter (recommended for infants and children).
   d. Apply suctioning while withdrawing catheter for no more than 15 seconds (5 seconds in the neonate).
   e. Completely withdraw the catheter, and rinse, if needed.
   f. To rinse, place a saline vial in-line, squeezing it while applying suction.
   g. Lock the suction control mechanism.
5. Perform sterile suctioning.
   a. Open the sterile suctioning kit.
   b. Apply the sterile glove to the dominant hand.
   c. Open the sterile water container, and fill it with sterile water for suction line irrigation.
   d. Wrap the suction catheter with the dominant hand.
   e. Insert the catheter without applying suction.
   f. Apply suction while withdrawing the catheter.
   g. Maintain sterile technique.
6. Hyperoxygenate using the same method as in Step 3.
7. Perform oral suctioning, if indicated.
8. Remove the supplies from the patient's room, and clean the area, as needed.
9. Remove PPE, and perform proper hand hygiene prior to leaving the patient's room.

> **Reality Check** Open sterile suctioning is typically used on patients with a tracheostomy tube.

Evaluation of Procedure

1. Establish a baseline, or compare with the patient's respiratory assessment before and after suctioning.
2. Repeat suctioning, if needed.
3. Reposition the patient, if needed.
4. Identify any unexpected outcomes.

Documentation and Reporting

1. Record your findings in the patient's chart.
2. Report any abnormal findings to the appropriate health care provider.

11-3 Nasotracheal Suctioning

In the patient who does not have an artificial airway, nasotracheal suctioning is used to clear maintained secretions. It may also be used to obtain a sputum sample for microbiology testing. The following is the step-by-step process for nasotracheal suctioning.

> ✳ **Tip** Always have oropharyngeal suctioning equipment and an emesis basin ready in case the patient vomits during this procedure.

Procedural Preparation

1. Review the patient's chart.
2. Verify the physician's order or the facility's protocol for standard of care.
3. Obtain, clean, and inspect the appropriate equipment prior to entering the patient's room.
4. Follow PPE requirements, and observe standard precautions for any transmission-based isolation procedure.
5. Identify the patient using two patient identifiers.
6. Introduce yourself to the patient and to the family.
7. Explain the procedure to the patient and to the family, and acknowledge the patient's understanding.
8. Perform proper hand hygiene, and put on gloves, mask, and protective eyewear, as appropriate for the procedure.

Implementation

1. Place the patient in a comfortable position, and instruct him or her to breathe normally.
2. Assess vital signs and need for suctioning.
3. Assemble and check the equipment.
4. Preoxygenate the patient, as indicated.
5. Remove the oxygen delivery device, if present.
6. Coat the distal end of the suction catheter with a water-soluble lubricant.
7. Apply a sterile glove to the dominant hand.
8. Insert the catheter gently through the nostril; direct it toward the septum and floor of the nasal cavity; twist the catheter to ease insertion.
9. Have the patient assume a "sniffing" position (Figure 11-3).
10. Advance the catheter until resistance is felt or the patient coughs.

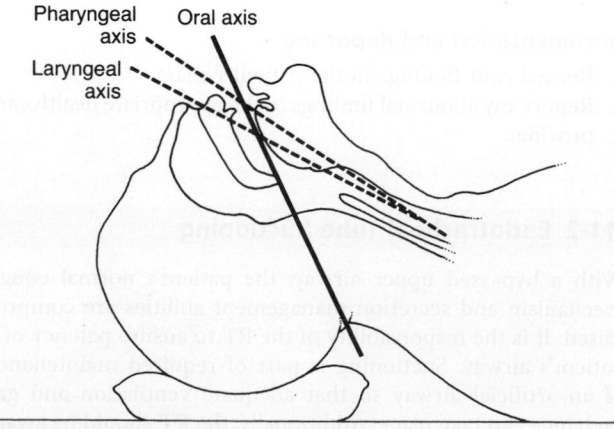

Figure 11-3 Sniffing position. (From Aehlert B: ACLS study guide, ed 4, 2011, St. Louis, MO, Mosby.)

11. Apply suction while withdrawing the catheter for no more than 15 seconds.
12. Maintain sterile technique.
13. Oxygenate according to procedure, as needed.
14. Suction the oropharynx, if needed.
15. Remove the supplies from the patient's room, and clean the area, as needed.
16. Remove PPE, and perform proper hand hygiene prior to leaving the patient's room.

Evaluation of Procedure

1. Establish a baseline, or compare with the patient's respiratory assessment before and after suctioning.
2. Repeat suctioning, if needed.
3. Reposition the patient.
4. Identify any unexpected outcomes.

Documentation and Reporting

1. Record your findings in the patient's chart.
2. Report any abnormal findings to the appropriate health care provider.

11-4 Collecting Sputum Samples by Suctioning

Identification of the pathogen, or pathogens, responsible for a patient's pulmonary infection is an important part in their treatment plan. Proper identification ensures the proper antibiotics are administered. A sterile sputum sample must be obtained using a specimen trap. Figure 11-4 provides an example of one of these containers, frequently referred to as a *Lukens trap*. The following is the step-by-step process for collecting a sputum sample by suctioning.

Procedural Preparation

1. Review the patient's chart.
2. Verify the physician's order or the facility's protocol for standard of care.
3. Obtain, clean, and inspect the appropriate equipment prior to entering the patient's room.

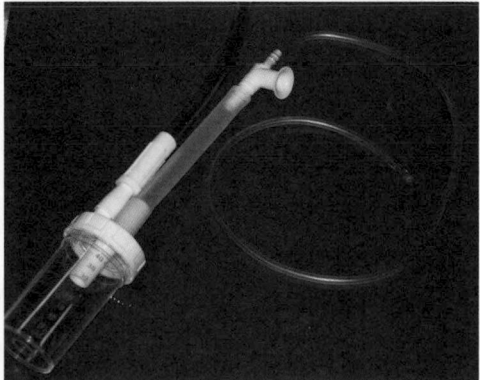

Figure 11-4 Specimen container placement between the suction catheter and wall suction source. (From Kacmarek RM, Stoller JK, Heuer AJ: *Egan's fundamentals of respiratory care*, ed 10, St. Louis, MO, 2013, Mosby.)

4. Follow PPE requirements, and observe standard precautions for any transmission-based isolation procedure.
5. Identify the patient using two patient identifiers.
6. Introduce yourself to the patient and to the family.
7. Explain the procedure to the patient and to the family, and acknowledge the patient's understanding.
8. Perform proper hand hygiene, and put on gloves, mask, and protective eyewear, as appropriate for the procedure.

Implementation

1. Place the patient in a comfortable position, and instruct him or her to breathe normally.
2. Assess vital signs.
3. Place a new catheter just before a suction sample is taken, if a closed suction system is being used.
4. Apply a sterile glove to the dominant hand.
5. Insert the specimen trap without applying suction.
6. Suction for no more than 15 seconds.
7. Collect 2 to 10 mL of sputum, and label per your facility's policy.
8. Detach the catheter from the sputum trap and cover while maintaining sterile technique.
9. Remove the supplies from the patient's room, and clean the area, as needed.
10. Remove PPE, and perform proper hand hygiene prior to leaving the patient's room.

Evaluation of Procedure

1. Establish a baseline, or compare with the patient's respiratory assessment before and after suctioning.
2. Repeat suctioning, if needed.
3. Reposition the patient.
4. Identify any unexpected outcomes.

Documentation and Reporting

1. Record your findings in the patient's chart.
2. Report any abnormal findings to the appropriate health care provider.

11-5 Inserting an Oropharyngeal Airway

Establishing and maintaining the airway of an unconscious patient is a critical part of the respiratory care plan, especially during emergency life support. The tongue could easily impede the airway, making it difficult, even impossible, for ventilation to ensue. Oropharyngeal airways (OPAs) may be used to displace the tongue and maintain the patency of a patient's airway. OPAs may also be used as a bite block for the orally intubated patient. These types of airways are illustrated in Figure 11-5. The following is the step-by-step process for inserting an oropharyngeal airway.

Procedural Preparation

1. Review the patient's chart.
2. Verify the physician's order or the facility's protocol for standard of care.
3. Obtain, clean, and inspect the appropriate equipment prior to entering the patient's room.
4. Follow PPE requirements, and observe standard precautions for any transmission-based isolation procedure.
5. Identify the patient using two patient identifiers.

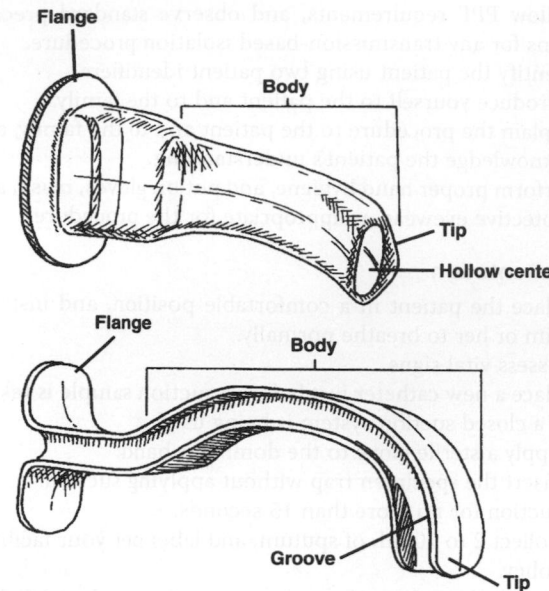

Figure 11-5 Oropharyngeal airways. (From Sills: *The comprehensive respiratory therapist exam review*, ed 5, St. Louis, MO, 2010, Mosby.)

6. Introduce yourself to the patient and to the family.
7. Explain the procedure to the patient and to the family, and acknowledge the patient's understanding.
8. Perform proper hand hygiene, and put on gloves, mask, and protective eyewear, as appropriate for the procedure.

Implementation

1. Position the patient.
2. Assess vital signs and for presence of a gag reflex.
3. Open the patient's mouth.
4. Insert the oral airway, with curved end up and to one side of the oropharynx; turn the airway over after reaching the back of the throat.
5. Suction the airway, if needed (see PA 11-1).
6. Remove the supplies from patient's room, and clean the area, as needed.
7. Remove the PPE, and perform proper hand hygiene prior to leaving the patient's room.

Evaluation of Procedure

1. Establish a baseline, or compare with the patient's respiratory assessment before and after oral airway insertion.
2. Determine the use of the airway (i.e., bite block or intermittent until endotracheal intubation is used to secure the airway) (see PA 11-6).
3. Reposition the patient, if needed.
4. Identify any unexpected outcomes.

Documentation and Reporting

1. Record your findings in the patient's chart.
2. Report any abnormal findings to the appropriate health care provider.

11-6 Oral Endotracheal Intubation

When a patient can no longer protect his or her airway, oral endotracheal intubation may be necessary.

> → **Reality Check** Before any aggressive airway management technique is performed, check the patient's code status to make sure that you are following his or her wishes.

Extensive practice in the lab with mannequins is required before you should attempt this procedure on a patient. The entire procedure of oral endotracheal intubation should take no more than 30 seconds. If an intubation attempt fails, and OPA should be placed followed by 3 to 5 minutes of manual ventilation and oxygenation. The following is the step-by-step process for oral endotracheal intubation.

Procedural Preparation

1. Review the patient's chart.
2. Verify the physician's order or the facility's protocol for standard of care.
3. Obtain, clean, and inspect the appropriate equipment prior to entering the patient's room.
4. Follow PPE requirements, and observe standard precautions for any transmission-based isolation procedure.
5. Identify the patient using two patient identifiers.
6. Introduce yourself to the patient and to the family.
7. Explain the procedure to the patient and to the family, and acknowledge the patient's understanding.
8. Perform proper hand hygiene, and put on gloves, mask, and protective eyewear, as appropriate for the procedure.

Implementation

1. Position the patient.
2. Manually ventilate and oxygenate the patient with bag-mask device, 100% oxygen, suctions if needed (see PA 11-1).
3. Insert the laryngoscope correctly:
   a. Hold the laryngoscope in the left hand.
   b. Open the patient's mouth using the right hand.
   c. Insert the laryngoscope into the right side of the mouth, and move it toward the center to displace the tongue to the left.
   d. Advance the tip of the blade along the curve of the tongue until the epiglottis is visualized.
4. Insert the endotracheal tube within 15 seconds, and inflate the cuff per your facility's policy.
5. Ventilate with a bag-mask device, and assess for proper tube placement:
   a. Visualize the tube passing through the cords.
   b. Use a CO_2 detector.
   c. Visualize the condensation in the tube.
6. Visualize equal chest rise.
7. Auscultate the epigastric region.
8. Auscultate the left and then the right lung fields.
9. Secure the tube.
10. Order a chest radiograph to confirm placement.
11. Order proper ventilator settings (see PA 22-1).
12. Remove the supplies from the patient's room, and clean the area, as needed.
13. Remove PPE, and perform proper hand hygiene prior to leaving the patient's room.

Evaluation of Procedure

1. Ensure appropriate ventilation and oxygenation.
2. Identify any unexpected outcomes.

Documentation and Reporting

1. Record your findings in the patient's chart.
2. Report any abnormal findings to the appropriate health care provider.

11-7 Nasotracheal Intubation

Although more difficult to execute compared with oral endotracheal intubation, nasotracheal intubation may be required to secure the airway in patients with maxillofacial injuries and in those undergoing oral surgery. Box 11-4 details the equipment and steps involved in the direct visualization or blind passage techniques. The following is the step-by-step process for inserting a nasotracheal airway.

Procedural Preparation

1. Review the patient's chart.
2. Verify the physician's order or the facility's protocol for standard of care.

BOX 11-4 | **Techniques for Nasotracheal Intubation with Required Equipment**

Equipment Needed
- A mixture of 0.25% phenylephrine and 3% lidocaine applied to nasal mucosa with a long cotton-tipped swab
- Suction equipment
- Manual resuscitation bag with mask
- Laryngoscope with assorted blades
- Endotracheal tubes
- Tape or commercial tube holder
- Magill forceps
- Towels
- Personal protective equipment (PPE)
- patient must be breathing

Direct Visualization Technique
- Lubricate the tube with water-soluble gel.
- Position the patient.
- To insert the tube, position the tube with the bevel toward the septum, and advance along the floor of the meatus inferiorly.
- When the top of the tube is in the patient's oropharynx, open the patient's mouth, and insert the laryngoscope.
- Visualize the glottis.
- Use the Magill forceps to grasp the tube above the cuff, and direct it between the vocal cords.
- Advance the tube, confirm placement, and stabilize the tube.
- You may use a bronchoscope to aid in the passage of the tube.

Blind Passage Technique
- Lubricate the tube with water-soluble gel.
- Place the patient in the supine or sitting position.
- To insert the tube, position the tube with the bevel toward the septum, and advance along the floor of the meatus inferiorly.
- As the tube approaches the larynx, listen through the tube for air movement.
- Successful passage of the tube is indicated by a harsh cough, followed by vocal silence.
- Confirm placement, and stabilize the tube.
- A light wand may help ensure proper placement.

---

3. Obtain, clean, and inspect the appropriate equipment prior to entering the patient's room.
4. Follow PPE requirements, and observe standard precautions for any transmission-based isolation procedure.
5. Identify the patient using two patient identifiers.
6. Introduce yourself to the patient and to the family.
7. Explain the procedure to the patient and to the family, and acknowledge the patient's understanding.
8. Perform proper hand hygiene, and put on gloves, mask, and protective eyewear, as appropriate for the procedure.

Implementation

1. Position the patient.
2. Manually ventilate and oxygenate the patient with a bag-mask device and 100% oxygen, and suction, if needed (see PA 11-1).
3. Apply the appropriate medication to the nasal mucosa.
4. Lubricate the tube with water-soluble gel.
5. Insert the tube properly by using direct visualization or blind passage technique (see Box 11-4), and inflate the cuff per your facility's policy.
6. Ventilate with a bag-mask device, and assess for proper tube placement:
   a. Visualize the tube passing through the cords.
   b. Use an end-tidal CO_2 detector.
7. Visualize equal chest rise.
8. Auscultate the epigastric region.
9. Auscultate the left and then the right lung fields.
10. Secure the tube.
11. Order a chest radiograph to confirm placement.
12. Order proper ventilator settings (see PA 22-1).
13. Remove the supplies from the patient's room, and clean the area, as needed.
14. Remove the PPE, and perform proper hand hygiene prior to leaving the patient's room.

Evaluation of Procedure

1. Ensure appropriate ventilation and oxygenation.
2. Identify any unexpected outcomes.

Documentation and Reporting

1. Record your findings in the patient's chart.
2. Report any abnormal findings to the appropriate health care provider.

11-8 Inserting Alternative Airway Devices

At times, endotracheal intubation is not possible. Alternative methods are used to temporarily secure the airway until an airway can be permanently secured. A laryngeal mask airway (LMA) and double-lumen airway are pictured in Figures 11-6 and 11-7. The following is the step-by-step process for inserting alternative airway devices.

Procedural Preparation

1. Review the patient's chart.
2. Verify the physician's order or the facility's protocol for standard of care.
3. Obtain, clean, and inspect the appropriate equipment prior to entering the patient's room.
4. Follow PPE requirements, and observe standard precautions for any transmission-based isolation procedure.

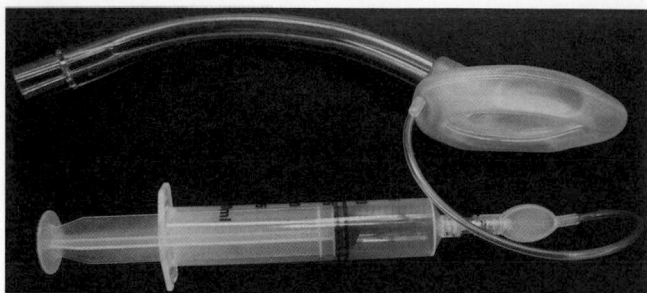

Figure 11-6 Laryngeal airway. (From Cairo J: *Mosby's respiratory care equipment*, ed 8, St. Louis, MO, 2010, Mosby.)

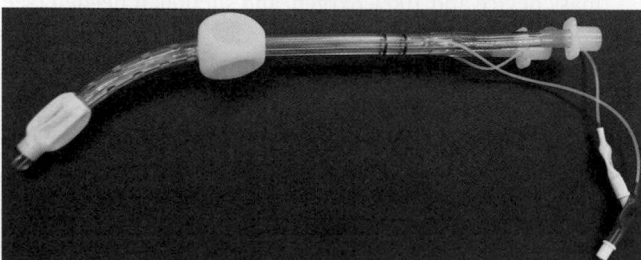

Figure 11-7 Double-lumen airway device, which is useful after failed intubation. (From Cairo J: *Mosby's respiratory care equipment*, ed 8. St. Louis, MO, 2010, Mosby.)

5. Identify the patient using two patient identifiers.
6. Introduce yourself to the patient and to the family.
7. Explain the procedure to the patient and to the family, and acknowledge the patient's understanding.
8. Perform proper hand hygiene, and put on gloves, mask, and protective eyewear, as appropriate for the procedure.

Implementation

1. Position the patient.
2. Assess vital signs.
3. Manually ventilate and oxygenate the patient with the bag-mask device and 100% oxygen.
4. Suction the airway, if needed.
5. Perform LMA placement:
   a. Lubricate the posterior surface of the mask with a water-soluble gel.
   b. Ensure that the cuff is fully deflated.
   c. Use the index finger to guide the insertion of the laryngeal mask along the palate and down into the oropharynx.
   d. Inflate the cuff to a maximum of 60 cm H_2O.
6. Perform double-lumen airway placement:
   a. Insert the airway blindly through the oropharynx into the trachea or esophagus.
   b. Inflate the distal cuff with 12 to 15 mL of air.
   c. Auscultate the chest and abdomen for breath sounds or gurgling in the epigastrium.
   d. In the case of a tracheal entry, inflate both cuffs (the proximal cuff with 85 to 100 mL of air and the distal with 15 mL of air) to prevent air from escaping through the esophagus.

7. Manually ventilate the patient.
8. Visualize equal chest rise.
9. Auscultate the epigastric region.
10. Auscultate the left and then the right lung fields.
11. Secure the tube.
12. Remove the supplies from the patient's room, and clean the area, as needed.
13. Remove PPE, and perform proper hand hygiene prior to leaving the patient's room.

Evaluation of Procedure

1. Ensure appropriate ventilation and oxygenation.
2. Identify any unexpected outcomes.
3. Use temporary airway until endotracheal intubation can be performed.

Documentation and Reporting

1. Record your findings in the patient's chart.
2. Report any abnormal findings to the appropriate health care provider.

11-9 Endotracheal Tube Care

Endotracheal tube (ETT) care helps maintain the patency of a patient's airway, along with minimizing tube movement, which helps prevent trauma and injury to the trachea. It also helps prevent accidental extubations.

Tape or commercial tube holders are two acceptable methods for securing ETTs. Care must be taken when using

> **✱ Tip** Always have emergency airway equipment and a manual resuscitation bag hooked to oxygen at hand when changing the securing device of an endotracheal tube in case the tube slips out of place.

tape because it may be loosened by saliva, vomitus, or other oral secretions.

The following is the step-by-step process for endotracheal tube care.

Procedural Preparation

1. Review the patient's chart.
2. Verify the physician's order or the facility's protocol for standard of care.
3. Obtain, clean, and inspect the appropriate equipment prior to entering the patient's room.
4. Follow PPE requirements, and observe standard precautions for any transmission-based isolation procedure.
5. Identify the patient using two patient identifiers.
6. Introduce yourself to the patient and to the family.
7. Explain the procedure to the patient and to the family, and acknowledge the patient's understanding.
8. Perform proper hand hygiene, and put on gloves, mask, and protective eyewear, as appropriate for the procedure.

Implementation

1. Place the patient in a comfortable position; observe for signs and symptoms of need to perform ETT care and oral hygiene.
2. Assess vital signs and baseline ventilation.

3. Assess ETT depth.
4. Place a towel across the patient's chest.
5. Perform oropharyngeal suctioning (see PA 11-1).
6. Remove the old tape or device from the tube and the patient's face with the dominant hand while stabilizing the ETT with the other hand.
7. Clean the adhesive from the patient's face.
8. Remove the oral airway or bite block, and place it on a towel.
9. Clean the patient's mouth and teeth on both sides of the ETT using a brush or foam swab.
10. Suction any residue.
11. Clean the patient's face.
12. Apply skin protectant.
13. Secure the ETT with tape or commercial tube-holding device.
14. Clean and reinsert the oral airway or the bite block.
15. Reassess the patient.
16. Remove the supplies from the patient's room, and clean the area, as needed.
17. Remove PPE, and perform proper hand hygiene prior to leaving the patient's room.

Evaluation of Procedure

1. Compare assessments before and after the procedure.
2. Note the depth and position of the ETT.
3. Ensure that the ETT is secure.
4. Note any skin damage or breakdown.
5. Identify any unexpected outcomes.

Documentation and Reporting

1. Record your findings in the patient's chart.
2. Report any abnormal findings to the appropriate health care provider.

11-10 Monitoring Cuff Pressures

Laryngeal and tracheal lesions are injuries associated with tracheal tubes, and every attempt must be made to minimize complications. Aspiration, extubation, and further airway compromise may be caused by inappropriate management of cuff pressures. Cuff pressures should be maintained between 20 to 30 cm H_2O. Figure 11-8 illustrates the sequelae that may develop from tracheal cuff injuries. The following is the step-by-step process for monitoring cuff pressures.

Procedural Preparation

1. Review the patient's chart.
2. Verify the physician's order or the facility's protocol for standard of care.
3. Obtain, clean, and inspect the appropriate equipment prior to entering the patient's room.
4. Follow PPE requirements, and observe standard precautions for any transmission-based isolation procedure.
5. Identify the patient using two patient identifiers.
6. Introduce yourself to the patient and to the family.
7. Explain the procedure to the patient and to the family, and acknowledge the patient's understanding.
8. Perform proper hand hygiene, and put on gloves, mask, and protective eyewear, as appropriate for the procedure.

Implementation

1. Position the patient, and locate the pilot balloon; ensure that a 10-mL syringe is available.
2. Assess vital signs.
3. Measure the cuff pressure:
   a. Obtain a three-way stopcock.
   b. Attach the three-way stopcock or cufflator to the cuff inflation valve.
   c. Read the cuff pressure (place the stopcock in the OFF position to the syringe if using a manometer).
4. Adjust cuff pressure to 20 to 30 cm H_2O.
5. Remove the three-way stopcock or cufflator from the inflation valve when measurements are completed.
6. Remove the supplies from the patient's room, and clean the area, as needed.
7. Remove PPE, and perform proper hand hygiene prior to leaving the patient's room.

Evaluation of Procedure

1. Ensure appropriate ventilation and oxygenation.
2. Identify any unexpected outcomes.

Documentation and Reporting

1. Record your findings in the patient's chart.
2. Report any abnormal findings to the appropriate health care provider.

11-11 Tracheostomy and Stoma Care

A patient's secretion production and stoma condition will determine the frequency of tracheostomy and stoma care. Daily management is usually required. Emergency inner cannula changing may be needed if a mucus plug lodges in the cannula obstructing it. Regular bedside assessments are essential for all tracheostomy patients. The following is the step-by-step process for tracheostomy and stoma care.

Procedural Preparation

1. Review the patient's chart.
2. Verify the physician's order or the facility's protocol for standard of care.
3. Obtain, clean, and inspect the appropriate equipment prior to entering the patient's room.
4. Follow PPE requirements, and observe standard precautions for any transmission-based isolation procedure.
5. Identify the patient using two patient identifiers.
6. Introduce yourself to the patient and to the family.
7. Explain the procedure to the patient and to the family, and acknowledge the patient's understanding.
8. Perform proper hand hygiene, and put on gloves, mask, and protective eyewear, as appropriate for the procedure.

Implementation

1. Place the patient in a comfortable position, and instruct him or her to breathe normally.
2. Assess vital signs.
3. Suction the patient, as needed (see PA 11-2).

Pathogenesis of Tracheal Cuff Site Injury

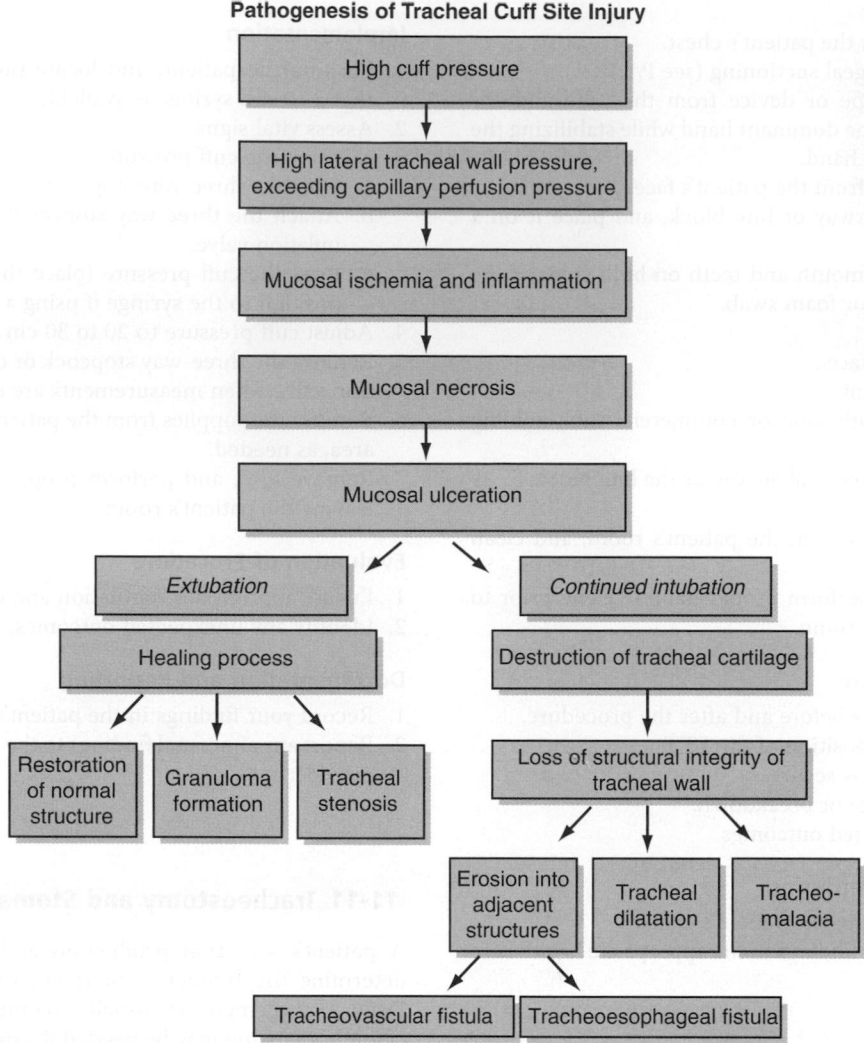

Figure 11-8 Tracheal injury may occur secondary to trauma from the cuff. (From Kacmarek RM, Stoller JK, Heuer AJ: *Egan's fundamentals of respiratory care*, ed 10, St. Louis, MO, 2013, Mosby.)

4. Remove the inner cannula, and reinsert a new cannula.
5. Remove the dressing and tracheostomy ties.
6. Clean the stoma with an appropriate cleanser and sterile water.
7. Apply new dressing and tracheostomy ties.
8. Remove the supplies from the patient's room, and clean the area, as needed.
9. Removes PPE, and performs proper hand hygiene prior to leaving the patient's room.

Evaluation of Procedure

1. Ensure the stability of the tracheostomy tube throughout the procedure.
2. Note any increase in the need for oxygen therapy throughout the procedure.
3. Return the patient to previous therapy.
4. Identify any unexpected outcomes.

Documentation and Reporting

1. Record your findings in the patient's chart.
2. Report any abnormal findings to the appropriate health care provider.

11-12 Changing a Tracheostomy Tube

When a problem with the tracheostomy tube develops or a different size tube is needed, the entire tracheostomy tube has to be changed. Figure 11-9 illustrates causes requiring a tracheostomy tube to be changed. Preparation is imperative when changing a tracheostomy tube in case it becomes difficult or impossible to reinsert it. Only a physician should change the tube size if this has to be performed before the stoma is completely healed. The following is the step-by-step process for changing a tracheostomy tube.

Procedural Preparation

1. Review the patient's chart.
2. Verify the physician's order or the facility's protocol for standard of care.
3. Obtain, clean, and inspect the appropriate equipment prior to entering the patient's room.
4. Follow PPE requirements, and observe standard precautions for any transmission-based isolation procedure.
5. Identify the patient using two patient identifiers.
6. Introduce yourself to the patient and to the family.

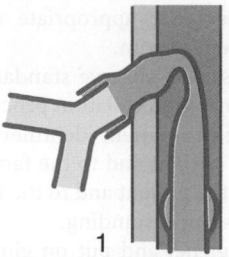 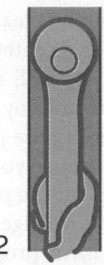 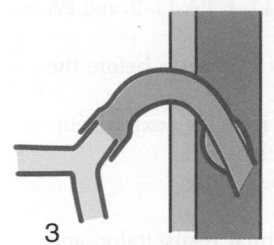 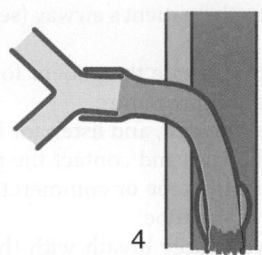

Figure 11-9 Tube obstruction may be caused by (1) kinking of the tube or the patient biting on the tube, (2) herniation of the cuff over the tube tip, (3) obstruction of the tube orifice against the tracheal wall, and (4) mucus plugging. (Modified from Sykes MK, McNichol MW, Campbell, EJM: Respiratory failure, ed 2, Wiley-Blackwell, 1976, Hoboken, NJ.)

7. Explain the procedure to the patient and to the family, and acknowledge the patient's understanding.
8. Perform proper hand hygiene, and put on gloves, mask, and protective eyewear, as appropriate for the procedure.

Implementation

1. Place the patient in a comfortable semi-Fowler position, and instruct him or her to breathe normally.
2. Assess vital signs.
3. Perform suctioning (see PA 11-2).
4. Prepare and inspect the new tracheostomy tube, and place it in a prepared sterile field.
5. Remove the inner cannula of the new tracheostomy tube, and insert the obturator into the outer cannula.
6. Attach clean ties to one side of the phalange, and check the integrity of the cuff by inflating it; then deflate it.
7. Apply sterile water-soluble lubricant to the tip of the new tracheostomy tube.
8. On the patient's current tracheostomy tube, loosen the ties and deflate the cuff, if inflated.
9. Remove any oxygen or humidity device.
10. Remove the old tracheostomy tube by pulling it out with gentle steady pressure in the same direction as you would when removing an inner cannula.
11. Put on sterile gloves.
12. Push the new tracheostomy tube into the tracheostomy site, using gentle force, while pushing back and then down until the posterior trachea is reached; then follow the posterior wall until the tube is fully inserted.
13. Remove the obturator, allow air to flow, and insert the inner cannula.
14. Attach new tracheostomy ties, inflate the cuff, and place dressing around the stoma, if necessary.
15. Reapply the oxygen or humidity device.
16. Remove the supplies from the patient's room, and clean the area, as needed.
17. Remove PPE, and perform proper hand hygiene prior to leaving the patient's room.

Evaluation of Procedure

1. Establish a baseline, or compare the patient's respiratory assessments before and after tracheostomy tube change.
2. Ensure that a spare tracheostomy tube of the same size and of the size below and a manual resuscitation bag are available at the patient's bedside.
3. Identify any unexpected outcomes.

Documentation and Reporting

1. Record your findings in the patient's chart.
2. Report any abnormal findings to the appropriate health care provider.

11-13 Orotracheal or Nasotracheal Extubation

Whether it was a temporary intubation for a surgical procedure or an intubation following a long illness, extubation should be accomplished as soon as the patient is capable of maintaining his or her own airway and gas exchange. Assessment of extubation readiness includes, but is not limited to, the patient's ability to follow directions and take a deep breath, manage secretions and have a strong cough, successful completion of a spontaneous breathing trial (SBT), and the presence of a cuff leak. SBT and extubation readiness are discussed in Chapter 25. Many facilities have protocols in place for extubation readiness.

> → **Reality Check** Some facilities extubate and immediately apply oxygen and humidity therapy.

The following is the step-by-step process for extubation of orotracheal or nasotracheal tubes.

Procedural Preparation

1. Review the patient's chart.
2. Verify the physician's order or the facility's protocol for standard of care.
3. Obtain, clean, and inspect the appropriate equipment prior to entering the patient's room.
4. Follow PPE requirements, and observe standard precautions for any transmission-based isolation procedure.
5. Identify the patient using two patient identifiers.
6. Introduce yourself to the patient and to the family.
7. Explain the procedure to the patient and to the family, and acknowledge the patient's understanding.
8. Perform proper hand hygiene, and put on gloves, mask, and protective eyewear, as appropriate for the procedure.

Implementation

1. Place the patient in a comfortable position, and instruct him or her to breathe normally.
2. Assess vital signs.

3. Suction the patient's airway (see PA 11-1, PA 11-2, and PA 11-3).
4. Hyperoxygenate the patient for 1 to 2 minutes before the extubation procedure.
5. Deflate the cuff, and listen for leaks; if no leak exists, reinflate the cuff, and contact the physician.
6. Remove the tape or commercial tube holder.
7. Remove the tube.
   a. Give a large breath with the manual resuscitator, and remove the tube at peak inspiration.
   b. Alternatively, have the patient cough and pull the tube during the expulsive expiratory phase.
8. Apply appropriate oxygen and humidity therapy; have racemic epinephrine ready.
9. Auscultate the patient; confirm that no stridor is present.
10. Remove the supplies from the patient's room, and clean the area, as needed.
11. Remove the PPE, and perform proper hand hygiene prior to leaving the patient's room.

Evaluation of Procedure

1. Ensure that no immediate complications have resulted from the extubation.
2. Note any use of oxygen or humidity therapy.
3. Identify any unexpected outcomes.

Documentation and Reporting

1. Record your findings in the patient's chart.
2. Report any abnormal findings to the appropriate health care provider.

11-14 Assisting with Bronchoscopy

Bronchoscopy is frequently performed in the intensive care unit. But it may also be performed emergently to remove objects, for visualization during procedures, and for inspection of the airway. As an RT, you must be continuously assessing the patient during a procedure for any adverse effects. Figure 11-10 shows a flexible fiberoptic bronchoscope. The following is the step-by-step process for assisting with bronchoscopy.

Procedural Preparation

1. Review the patient's chart.
2. Verify the physician's order or the facility's protocol for standard of care.

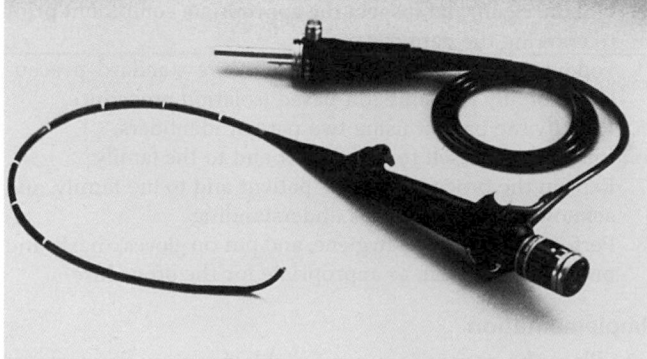

Figure 11-10 Flexible fiberoptic bronchoscope. (Courtesy of Olympus America, Inc. Center Valley, PA.)

3. Obtain, clean, and inspect the appropriate equipment prior to entering the patient's room.
4. Follow PPE requirements, and observe standard precautions for any transmission-based isolation procedure.
5. Identify the patient using two patient identifiers.
6. Introduce yourself to the patient and to the family.
7. Explain the procedure to the patient and to the family, and acknowledge the patient's understanding.
8. Perform proper hand hygiene, and put on gloves, mask, and protective eyewear, as appropriate for the procedure.
9. Assess respiratory status.
10. Determine time patient last ingested food.

Implementation

1. Assess the IV access (see PA 24-3); establish a new IV line, if required.
2. Prepare any patient-monitoring equipment.
3. Assist the patient in maintaining the required position.
4. Turn off the alarms, if the patient is currently receiving mechanical ventilation.
5. Place the suction catheter near the patient's mouth.
6. Instruct the patient not to swallow as the local anesthetic is sprayed.
7. Attach the bronchoscope to the machine to provide light.
8. Explain each step to the patient as it occurs.
9. Reassess the respiratory status continually throughout procedure.
10. Note the characteristics of the suctioned material.
11. Label all the specimens collected.
12. Wipe the patient's mouth and nose to remove any lubricant after the bronchoscope has been removed.
13. Return the alarm settings to the acceptable range if the patient is receiving mechanical ventilation.
14. Remove the supplies from the patient's room, and clean the area, as needed.
15. Clean and disinfect the bronchoscope per manufacturer specifications.
16. Remove PPE, and perform proper hand hygiene prior to leaving the patient's room.

Evaluation of Procedure

1. Observe sputum production.
2. Develop an appropriate respiratory care plan based on assessment data.
3. Note any use of oxygen therapy or ventilatory changes, if applicable.
4. Note the monitoring devices used during the procedure.
5. Identify any unexpected outcomes.
6. Correlate your findings with other lab findings.

Documentation and Reporting

1. Record your findings in the patient's chart.
2. Report any abnormal findings to the appropriate health care provider.

Bibliography

Heuer AJ, Scanlan CL: *Wilkins' clinical assessment in respiratory care*, ed 7, St. Louis, MO, 2014, Mosby.

Kacmarek, RM, Stoller JK, Heuer AJ: *Egan's fundamentals of respiratory care*, ed 10, St. Louis, MO, 2013, Mosby.

1. Obtain a flexible suction catheter, a Yankauer, and an in-line suction catheter from your lab instructor. Set them up and test each one to make sure that they are working properly. Indicate the clinical situations where each would be appropriate.

   a. Flexible suction catheter:

   _____

   b. Yankauer:

   _____

   c. In-line suction catheter:

   _____

2. Fill in the following table information regarding the advantages and disadvantages of different tracheal airway routes:

Route	Advantages	Disadvantages
Oral intubation		
Nasal intubation		
Tracheostomy		

3. Using the following step-by-step outline, practice oral endotracheal intubation with a mannequin in the lab. Perform the procedure three times successfully, and have your lab partner sign below.

   a. Place the mannequin in the "sniffing" position by placing a folded towel under the mannequin's neck.

   b. Hyperoxygenate using a manual resuscitation bag and mask.

   c. Holding the laryngoscope in your left hand, insert the blade of the laryngoscope to the right of the mannequin's tongue and gradually move the blade to the center of the mouth, pushing the tongue to the left.

   d. Slowly advance the blade, and locate the epiglottis.

e. Displace the epiglottis properly, depending on the blade you are using:

    i. With the curved blade (MacIntosh), the epiglottis is displaced indirectly by advancing the tip of the blade into the vallecula and lifting the blade up and forward.

    ii. With the straight blade (Miller), the epiglottis is displaced directly by advancing the tip of the blade over its posterior surface and lifting forward.

> **✳ Tip** Avoid bending your wrist or rocking the blade against the patient's teeth.

f. Lifting the laryngoscope at a 45-degree angle exposes the cords.

g. The tube should not obstruct your view of the vocal cords.

h. Pass the tube through the vocal cords until the cuff disappears into the trachea.

i. Remove the stylet, and advance the tube until the cuff is 3 to 4 cm beyond the vocal cords (19–21 cm at the teeth in females, 21–23 cm at the teeth in males).

j. Inflate the cuff, and oxygenate and ventilate.

k. Assess the tube position.

Signature: _____

Signature: _____

Signature: _____

4. After completing the steps in lab activity #3, secure the ETT with tape and note the depth of the ETT. Now, change the tape and resecure the tube by using a commercial tube holder. Have your lab partner sign below to confirm use of proper technique.

Signature: _____

5. Define the terms, and answer the question below:

a. Tracheomalacia

_____

b. Tracheal stenosis

_____

c. How can they be prevented?

_____

6. Using a human patient simulator, or a mannequin, practice measuring cuff pressures with your lab partner. Perform the procedure three times successfully, and have your lab partner sign below. Be sure not to completely deflate the cuff.

Signature: _____

Signature: _____

Signature: _____

7. Practice setting up a new tracheostomy tube from scratch. This should include setting up and attaching new tracheostomy ties or Velcro tracheostomy tube holder. Using a mannequin, demonstrate the proper technique of changing the entire tracheostomy tube to your instructor. Have the instructor sign below.

Instructor's signature: _____

8. List the four causes of tube obstructions.

a. _____

b. _____

c. _____

d. _____

9. What are some hazards and complications involved in the removal of an ETT?

_____

10. Decannulation is the removal of a tracheostomy tube. List the three ways decannulation may be accomplished.

a. _____

b. _____

c. _____

11. Fill in the following table information regarding the advantages and disadvantages of alternatives to endotracheal intubation for maintaining upper airway patency.

Airway	Advantages	Disadvantages
Oral or nasal airway		
Double-lumen airway		
Laryngeal mask airway		

12. List the nine hazards and complications involved in bronchoscopy assisting.

a. _____

b. _____

c. _____

d. _____

e. _____

f. _____

g. _____

h. _____

i. _____

Self-Assessment Questions

1. How often should you perform endotracheal tube suctioning on a patient?
   A. Every 2 hours
   B. After any ventilator adjustment
   C. When assessment indicates the need
   D. Before the physician assesses the patient

2. Following a motor vehicle collision, a patient's airway is severely compromised by a multiple maxillary fracture. What procedure would you suggest for airway maintenance that may be required for about 24 to 36 hours?
   A. Oral endotracheal intubation
   B. Laryngeal mask airway
   C. Oropharyngeal airway
   D. Nasotracheal intubation

3. You are a member of the rapid response team with the responsibility for stocking the airway kit. What oral endotracheal intubation equipment should be in the kit?
   A. Obturator, stylet, numerous tracheostomy tube sizes, manual resuscitation device
   B. Suction equipment, oxygen apparatus, two laryngoscopes and assorted blades, five tubes, syringe, stylet
   C. A variety of oxygen masks
   D. Suction equipment, oxygen apparatus, manual resuscitation device

4. How long should an endotracheal intubation attempt take?
   A. No more than 30 seconds
   B. No more than 1 minute
   C. No more than 2 minutes
   D. As long as it takes to secure the patient's airway

5. Following a spinal cord injury, it is thought that a patient will need continuous mechanical ventilation for approximately 4 to 5 months. What procedure would you suggest for airway maintenance for this particular patient?
   A. Oral endotracheal intubation
   B. Laryngeal mask airway
   C. Tracheostomy tube placement
   D. Nasotracheal intubation

6. Following endotracheal extubation, a nurse calls you because your patient has stridor that is audible even without a stethoscope. What is your next step?
   A. Have her administer a nasal cannula at 2 L/min
   B. Obtain racemic epinephrine for delivery via small volume nebulizer with mask
   C. Reintubate the patient
   D. Apply heated humidification

7. When troubleshooting airway emergencies, what situations may occur?
   1. Tube obstruction
   2. Cuff leak
   3. Accidental extubation
   4. Wrong tube size insertion

   A. 1 and 3 only
   B. 1, 2, and 3 only
   C. 1 and 4 only
   D. 3 and 4 only

8. Indications for using closed suctioning include:
   1. $F_IO_2 \geq 0.60$
   2. PEEP ≥ 10 cm H_2O
   3. Once daily suctioning needed
   4. Patient on droplet precautions

   A. 1 and 3 only
   B. 1 and 2 only
   C. 1, 2, and 4 only
   D. 1, 2, 3, and 4

9. Contraindications for nasotracheal intubation include:
   1. Occluded nasal passages
   2. Visible secretions in the airway
   3. Epiglottitis
   4. Bronchospasm

   A. 1 only
   B. 2 and 3 only
   C. 1, 3, and 4 only
   D. 1, 2, 3, and 4

10. When managing airway emergencies, clinical monitoring tools should include:
    1. Patient's level of consciousness
    2. Symmetry of chest movement
    3. Ease of ventilation
    4. Presence and character of breath sounds

    A. 1 only
    B. 2 and 3 only
    C. 1, 2, and 3 only
    D. 1, 2, 3, and 4

CASE STUDY 11-1

You have a patient who is orally intubated and receiving mechanical ventilation in the intensive care unit. The patient has deep mucous plugs that cannot be removed with deep suctioning of the endotracheal tube.

1. What procedure would you recommend to the physician?

_____

_____

2. What equipment would you need for this procedure?

_____

_____

3. What patient support and monitoring equipment would you need for this procedure?

_____

_____

4. Would you need to administer any medications?

_____

_____

5. You are attempting endotracheal intubation of the patient with a MacIntosh blade on the laryngoscope, and you cannot see the vocal cords or the epiglottis. What troubleshooting techniques can you use?

_____

_____

Emergency Life Support

▪ OBJECTIVES

Upon the completion of the chapter activities and content review topics, the student should be able to:
1. Manage effectively all aspects of a code.
2. Perform cardiopulmonary resuscitation (CPR) on adults, children, and infants.
3. Provide manual ventilation with a bag-mask device.
4. Describe the steps to use an automated external defibrillator (AED).
5. Describe ways of restoring ventilation.
6. Perform placement of a nasopharyngeal airway.
7. Identify complications that may result from CPR.
8. Describe common advanced life support algorithms.

▪ KEY TERMS

- Defibrillation
- Synchronized cardioversion
- Trismus
- Bag-mask device

▪ CONTENT REVIEW TOPICS

- Advanced cardiac life support (ACLS) algorithms
- American Heart Association (AHA)
- Basic life support (BLS)
- Biphasic defibrillation
- Monophasic defibrillation

▪ PROCEDURAL ASSESSMENTS

12-1 Code Management
12-2 Manual Ventilation With A Bag-Mask Device
12-3 Using An Automated External Defibrillator
12-4 Inserting A Nasopharyngeal Airway

▪ EQUIPMENT

- AED with mannequin for defibrillation (optional)
- CPR mannequins for neonates, infants, and adults
- Disposable gloves
- Mannequin
- Manual resuscitation mask
- Mask
- Nasopharyngeal airways (various sizes)
- Protective eyewear
- Water-soluble gel

Respiratory therapists (RTs) are involved in many aspects of patient care that may entail the need for emergency life support. Whether in an intensive care unit (ICU) or an emergency department (ED) or flying as a part of a medical transports team, RTs find themselves as key players in a patient's care during a medical emergency.

BLS is initiated to restore ventilation and circulation to patients with occluded airways, respiratory arrest, cardiac arrest, or both. BLS skills are only adequate until ACLS equipment with capable personnel becomes available. Both BLS and ACLS are offered in many respiratory care programs as part of the curriculum. If not, you should inquire about where these courses are offered so that you can achieve your BLS and ACLS certifications.

This chapter covers the basics of code management, manual ventilation, and use of an AED. ACLS algorithms, including pharmacology, are also covered.

❯❯ SKILL CHECK LISTS

12-1 Code Management

With RTs involved in airway management, especially in the emergent setting, being at the head of the bed often lends itself to managing the code. In the hospital setting, help is usually readily available. However, the RT must be familiar with the skills and practices of both one- and two-rescuer CPR for adults, children, and infants. Table 12-1 lays out the steps involved in CPR. The following is the step-by-step process for code management.

> ✳ **Tip** BLS and ACLS are often requirements for employment. Pediatric advanced life support (PALS) and neonatal resuscitation program (NRP) are also formal courses you can attend. These are helpful if you plan on practicing in the neonatal and pediatric populations.

> → **Reality Check** You must be very familiar with your facility's policies involving "code blue" or "calling a code."

TABLE 12-1 Steps for Cardiopulmonary Resuscitation in the Adult, Child, and Infant

Procedure	Adult	Child	Infant
COMPRESSIONS			
Where to check pulse (Limit pulse check to <10 seconds)	Carotid artery	Carotid or femoral artery	Brachial artery
Hand placement	Heel of one hand on sternum in center of chest, between nipples. Second hand on top of first with hands overlapped and parallel	Lower half of sternum with heel of one hand or with two hands (for larger children) Do not compress over xiphoid	Sternum with two fingers placed just below nipple line in center of chest
Compression-to-ventilation ratio	One or two rescuers: 30:2	One rescuer: 30:2 Two rescuers: 15:2	One rescuer: 30:2 Two rescuers: 15:2
Cycles of compression and ventilation	5	5	5
Depth of compressions (push in hard and fast, allow chest to fully recoil)	2	At least one third the anteroposterior diameter of chest or 2 inches (5 cm)	At least one third anteroposterior diameter of chest 1.5 inches (4 cm)
Compression rate	100/min	100/min	100/min
BREATHING			
Obstructive procedure	*Responsive:* If mild, allow the victim to clear the airway by coughing. If severe, repeat abdominal thrusts until the foreign body is expelled, or the choking victim becomes unresponsive. Consider chest thrusts if the abdominal thrusts are not effective, or if the rescuer is unable to encircle the victim's abdomen, or if the victim is in the late stages of pregnancy. *Unresponsive:* Carefully move the patient to the ground, immediately activate the EMS, and then begin CPR, but look into the mouth before giving breaths. If a foreign body is seen, it should be removed. Follow ventilation with chest compressions.	Same as for adult	*Responsive:* If mild, allow the infant to clear the airway by coughing. If the infant is unable to make a sound (severe obstruction), deliver five back blows (slaps) followed by chest thrusts repeatedly until the object is expelled, or the infant becomes unresponsive. Abdominal thrusts should not be done on infants because they may damage the largely unprotected liver. *Unresponsive:* Activate the EMS and then begin CPR, but look into the mouth before giving breaths. If a foreign body is seen, it should be removed. Follow ventilation with chest compressions.
RESCUE BREATHING			
(Palpable pulse, but no spontaneous breaths, or inadequate breathing)	10–12/min, 1 breath every 5–6 seconds	12–20/min, 1 breath every 3–5 sec, if palpable pulse ≥60/min	20/min, 1 breath every 3 sec, if palpable pulse ≥60/min

From Kacmarek RM, Stoller JK, Heuer AJ: *Egan's fundamentals of respiratory care*, ed 10, St. Louis, MO, 2013, Mosby.

Procedural Preparation

1. Follow PPE requirements and perform proper hand hygiene, and put on gloves, mask, and protective eyewear, as appropriate for the procedure.
2. Establish unresponsiveness in the patient.
3. Initiate code notification procedures based on your facility's protocol for standard of care.

Implementation

1. Restore circulation:
   a. Determine pulselessness.
   b. Perform chest compressions.
2. Restore the airway:
   a. Inspect for any neck or facial trauma.
   b. Perform either the head-tilt or the chin-lift method or the jaw thrust maneuver to open the airway.
   c. Perform oropharyngeal suctioning, if needed (see PA 11-1).
   d. Insert the oropharyngeal airway (see PA 11-5).
3. Restore breathing:
   a. Perform appropriate method for artificial ventilation (see PA 11-8).
4. Perform defibrillation:
   a. Apply and use the AED (see PA 12-3).
5. Remove the supplies from the patient's room, and clean the area, as needed.
6. Remove PPE and perform proper hand hygiene prior to leaving the patient's room.

Evaluation of Procedure

1. Reassess the patient throughout the code management.
2. Observe for any spontaneous return of respirations or pulse.

> **✳ Tip** Never delay compressions!

3. Develop an appropriate respiratory care plan based on assessment data.
4. Identify the causes of sudden cardiac or respiratory arrest.
5. Identify any unexpected outcomes.

Documentation and Reporting

1. Record the location of respiratory or cardiopulmonary arrest.
2. Record your findings in the patient's chart.
3. Record the arrest situation, per your facility's protocol.

12-2 Manual Ventilation with a Bag-Mask Device

Management of a patient's airway is typically the responsibility of the RT. Manual ventilation with a bag-mask device is necessary during airway emergencies, CPR, as well as transport of the mechanically ventilated patient (Figure 12-1).

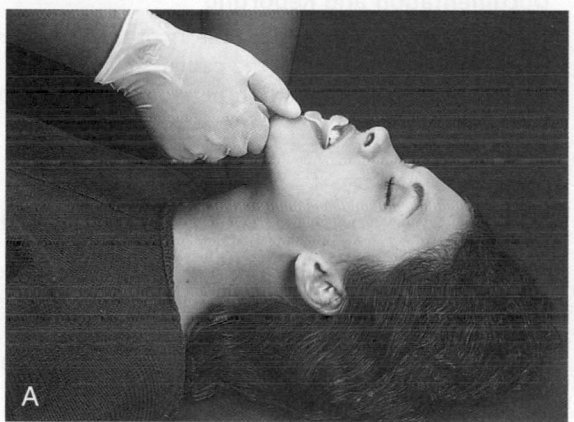
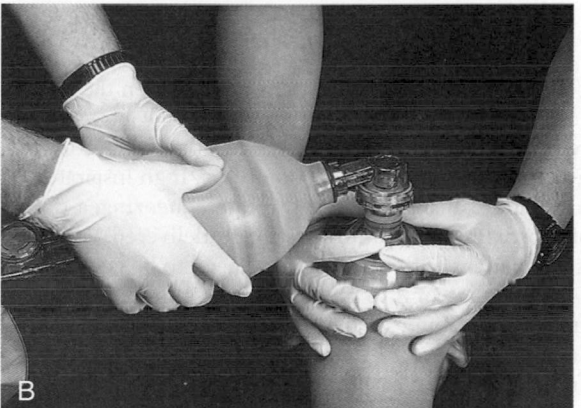
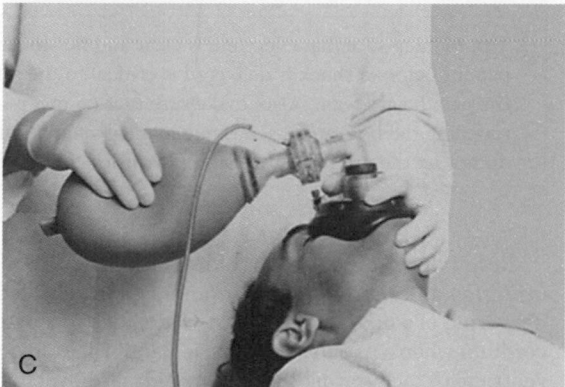

Figure 12-1 A, The flange of the oral airway should rest on the patient's lips. **B,** Ventilating using the bag-mask device. **C,** Bag-mask device without an oral airway. (**A & B,** From Aehlert B: *ACLS study guide*, ed 4, St. Louis, MO, 2012, Mosby. **C,** From Malamed S: *Sedation*, ed 5, St. Louis, MO, 2010, Mosby.)

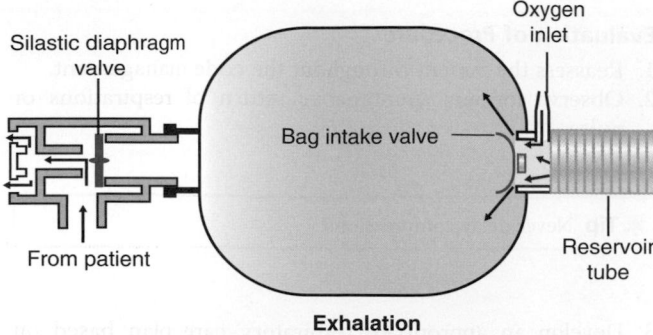

Exhalation

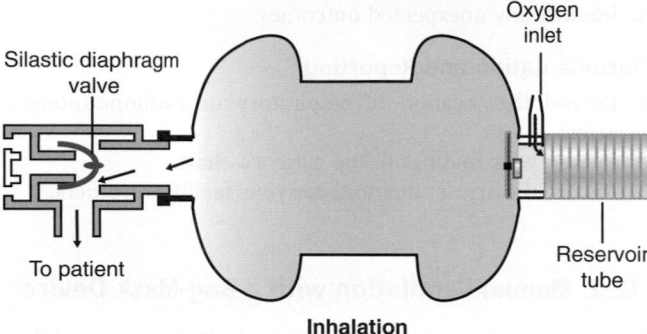

Inhalation

Figure 12-2 Components of a bag-mask device. (From Kacmarek RM, Stoller JK, Heuer AJ: *Egan's fundamentals of respiratory care*, ed 10, St. Louis, MO, 2013, Mosby.)

A bag-mask device is used most effectively when the RT is standing at the head of the bed. The components of a bag-mask device are provided in Figure 12-2. The full-bag volume of an adult bag-mask device is usually 2000 or less. If an inspiratory time of 1 second can be obtained through squeezing, a tidal volume of approximately 500 mL is typically delivered. Ventilation rates in a patient with cardiac arrest need to be controlled and kept in the range of 8 to 10 breaths per minute (breaths/min). Large tidal volumes ranging from greater than 6 to 7 mL/kg and rates above 12 breaths/min have been shown to be harmful to patients in cardiopulmonary arrest. The following is the step-by-step process for manually ventilating a patient with a bag-mask device.

> → **Reality Check** You should never perform mouth-to-mouth on a patient in the hospital setting. Always use a barrier device.

Procedural Preparation

1. Review the patient's chart.
2. Verify the physician's order or the facility's protocol for standard of care.
3. Obtain, clean, and inspect the appropriate equipment prior to entering the patient's room.
4. Follow PPE requirements, and observe standard precautions for any transmission-based isolation procedure.

5. Identify the patient using two patient identifiers.
6. Introduce yourself to the patient and to the family.
7. Explain the procedure to the patient and to the family, and acknowledge the patient's understanding.
8. Perform proper hand hygiene, and put on gloves, mask, and protective eyewear, as appropriate for the procedure.

Implementation

1. Position the patient.
2. Clear the airway of secretions, vomitus, and foreign objects (see PA 11-1).
3. Insert an oropharyngeal airway (see PA 11-5).
4. Connect the device to an oxygen source, and set the flowmeter to 15 liters per minute (L/min).
5. Place the mask on the patient's face; make a tight seal, or apply a manual resuscitator to the artificial airway device.
6. Compress the bag to ventilate at an appropriate volume and rate based on the patient's age and size.
7. Assess the adequacy of ventilation.
8. Remove the supplies from the patient's room, and clean the area, as needed.
9. Remove PPE, and perform proper hand hygiene prior to leaving the patient's room.

Evaluation of Procedure

1. Reassess the patient for adequate ventilation; reposition to open the airway, as necessary.
2. Develop an appropriate care plan based on assessment data.
3. Identify any unexpected outcomes.

Documentation and Reporting

1. Record the location of respiratory or cardiac arrest.
2. Record your findings in the patient's chart.
3. Record the arrest situation per your facility's protocol for standard of care.

12-3 Using an Automated External Defibrillator

With numerous personnel trained in ACLS available in code situations in the hospital setting, AEDs are not always needed. Conversely, in skilled nursing facilities and low-acuity facilities, AEDs are part of the code management situation, and the RT should be familiar with their use.

> ✳ **Tip** Making sure that everyone is clear and not touching the patient before a shock is delivered is critical to the safety of the health care team. Also, make sure that no one is touching the bed, and discontinue manual ventilation (but do not let the weight of the bag-mask dislodge the airway).

Respiratory therapists should not confuse the terms *defibrillation* and *synchronized cardioversion*. Defibrillation is the delivering of a direct electrical countershock to a patient's precordium when a patient is in ventricular fibrillation or pulseless ventricular tachycardia. Synchronized cardioversion, on the other hand, is used in ACLS algorithms to deliver a countershock synchronized with the heart's electrical activity and is frequently initiated at lower joule settings.

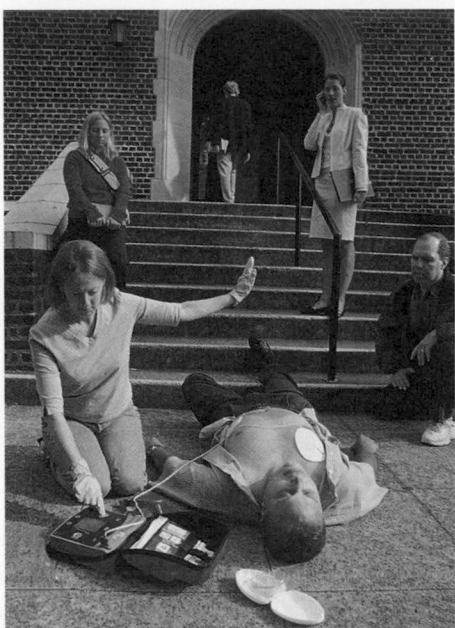

Figure 12-3 Automated external defibrillator (AED) with pads attached. (From Perry P, Potter P: *Clinical nursing skills and techniques*, ed 7, St. Louis, MO, 2010, Mosby.)

The American Heart Association (AHA) recommends the use of an AED on children over the age of one who are in cardiac arrest. The AED has different pads for use in pediatric and adult patients. An AED with adult pads is shown in Figure 12-3. Once turned on, some AEDs even give audible prompts to the rescuer such as "analyzing" and "shock advised." The rescuer must never delay chest compressions for the AED to analyze a rhythm. The following is the step-by-step process for using an AED.

Procedural Preparation

1. Ensure that an AED is available and functions properly.
2. Perform proper hand hygiene, and put on gloves, mask, and protective eyewear, as appropriate for the procedure.
3. Establish unresponsiveness.
4. Initiate code notification procedures based on your facility's protocol for standard of care.
5. Start CPR until the AED arrives.

Implementation

1. Place the AED near the patient's head.
2. Turn on the power.
3. Attach the pads per device instructions.
4. Clear the rescuers away from the patient.
5. Allow the AED time to analyze the rhythm.
6. Deliver a shock, as indicated by the AED.
7. Continue chest compressions for 2 minutes.
8. Allow the AED to resume analysis of the rhythm.
9. Repeat steps 5 through 8 until return of spontaneous circulation (ROSC) or the physician pronounces death.
10. Remove the supplies from the patient's room, and clean the area, as needed.
11. Remove PPE, and perform proper hand hygiene prior to leaving the patient's room.

Evaluation of Procedure

1. Observe for any ROSC.
2. Never delay chest compressions.
3. Develop an appropriate respiratory care plan based on assessment data.
4. Identify the causes of sudden cardiac arrest.
5. Identify any unexpected outcomes.

Documentation and Reporting

1. Record the location of respiratory or cardiopulmonary arrest, time and number of AED shocks, medications given, procedures performed, cardiac rhythm, and use of CPR.
2. Record your findings in the patient's chart.
3. Record the arrest situation per your facility's protocol.

12-4 Inserting a Nasopharyngeal Airway

Circumstances such as seizure activity or trismus, the involuntary contraction of the jaw muscles, may limit your ability to insert an oral airway in the emergency setting. In adults, the option of placing a nasopharyngeal airway may help stabilize the airway during manual resuscitation. Nasopharyngeal airways may also facilitate nasotracheal suctioning (see Chapter 11).

Proper sizing of a nasopharyngeal airway is accomplished by measuring from earlobe to nose tip. Sizes usually range from 26 French (Fr) to 32 Fr. Use should be limited to the adult patient, since the nasal passages in infants and children are very small. Figure 12-4 illustrates some common nasopharyngeal airways and how to measure for use. The following is the step-by-step process for nasopharyngeal insertion.

Procedural Preparation

1. Review the patient's chart.
2. Verify the physician's order or the facility's protocol for standard of care.
3. Obtain, clean, and inspect the appropriate equipment prior to entering the patient's room.
4. Follow PPE requirements, and observe standard precautions for any transmission-based isolation procedure.
5. Identify the patient using two patient identifiers.
6. Introduce yourself to the patient and to the family.
7. Explain the procedure to the patient and to the family, and acknowledge the patient's understanding.
8. Perform proper hand hygiene, and put on gloves, mask, and protective eyewear, as appropriate for the procedure.

Implementation

1. Position the patient's head, tilting it slightly backward.
2. Lubricate the nasopharyngeal airway with water-soluble gel.
3. Position the airway perpendicular to the frontal plane of the patient's face.
4. Advance the airway slowly through the inferior meatus, with the beveled edge facing the septum.
5. Visualize and confirm placement using a tongue depressor.
6. Suction airway, if needed (see PA 11-1).
7. Remove the supplies from the patient's room, and clean the area, as needed.

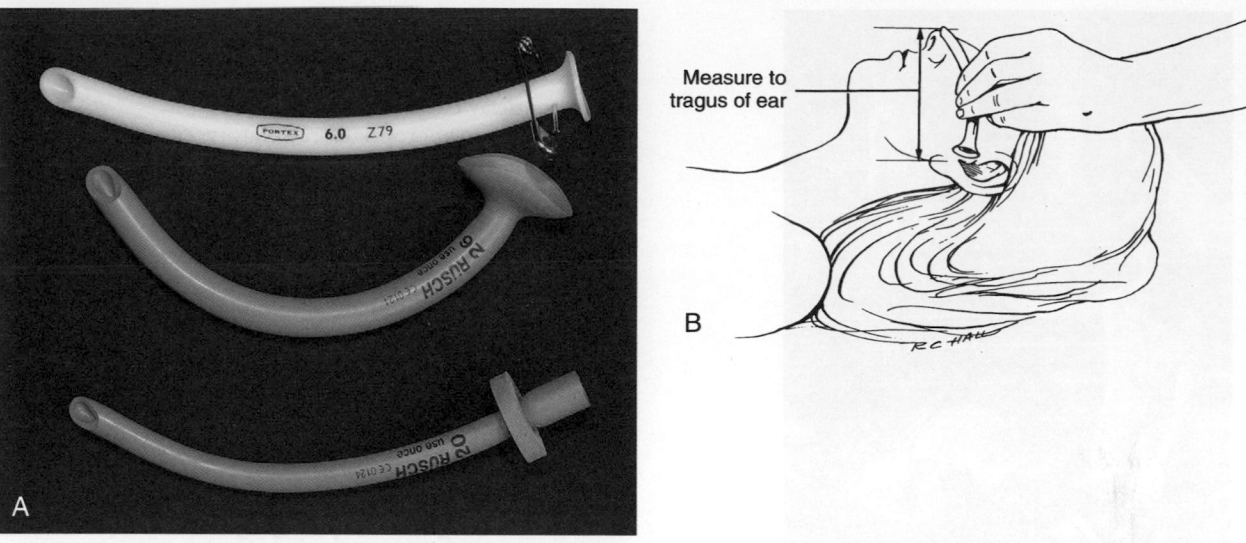

Figure 12-4 **A,** Nasopharyngeal airways. **B,** Proper measurement of the nasopharyngeal airway. (A, From Malamed S: *Medical emergencies in the dental office*, ed 6, St. Louis, MO, 2008, Mosby. B, From Eubanks DH, Bone RC: *Comprehensive respiratory care*, ed 2, St. Louis, MO, 1990, Mosby.)

8. Remove PPE, and perform proper hand hygiene prior to leaving the patient's room.

Evaluation of Procedure

1. Establish a baseline, or compare with the patient's respiratory assessment before and after airway insertion.
2. Determine the use of an airway for nasotracheal suctioning intermittently or until endotracheal intubation is used to secure airway (see PA 11-6).
3. Reposition the patient.
4. Identify any unexpected outcomes.

Documentation and Reporting

1. Record your findings in the patient's chart.
2. Report any abnormal findings to the appropriate health care provider.

Bibliography

Kacmarek RM, Stoller JK, Heuer AJ: *Egan's fundamentals of respiratory care*, ed 10, St. Louis, MO, 2013, Mosby.

1. Review the current CPR guidelines for the adult, child, and infant. Using mannequins, demonstrate one- and two-rescuer guidelines for each. Have your lab partner sign on the lines below after he or she has observed you perform each demonstration.

   Adult: 1 rescuer/Signature_____

   Adult: 2 rescuers/Signature_____

   Child: 1 rescuer/Signature_____

   Child: 2 rescuers/Signature_____

   Infant: 1 rescuer/Signature_____

   Infant: 2 rescuers/Signature_____

2. Fill in the following chart information regarding the steps of CPR in adults, children, and infants:

	ADULT	CHILD	INFANT
Compressions			
Where to check pulse (limit to <10 seconds)			
Hand placement			
Compression-to-ventilation ratio			
Cycles of compressions			
Depth of compressions			
Compression rate			
Breathing			
Obstructive procedure			
Rescue Breathing			
Palpable pulse, no spontaneous breaths or inadequate breathing			

3. List six goals achieved by endotracheal intubation during ACLS.

_____

_____

_____

4. List four approaches to providing artificial ventilation.

_____

_____

_____

5. If available, hook up an AED to a mannequin. Simulate pulseless ventricular tachycardia. Working in groups of two or three, operate the AED by following all prompts. Have your partners ensure that CPR is always performed correctly.

6. Working with two or three students, use the following algorithms to run scenarios on a mannequin or human patient simulator. Make sure to run scenarios where you achieve return of spontaneous circulation and ones in which your patient remains pulseless despite resuscitation attempts. Have a student sign below once you have completed the task. This should be done as a group.

a.

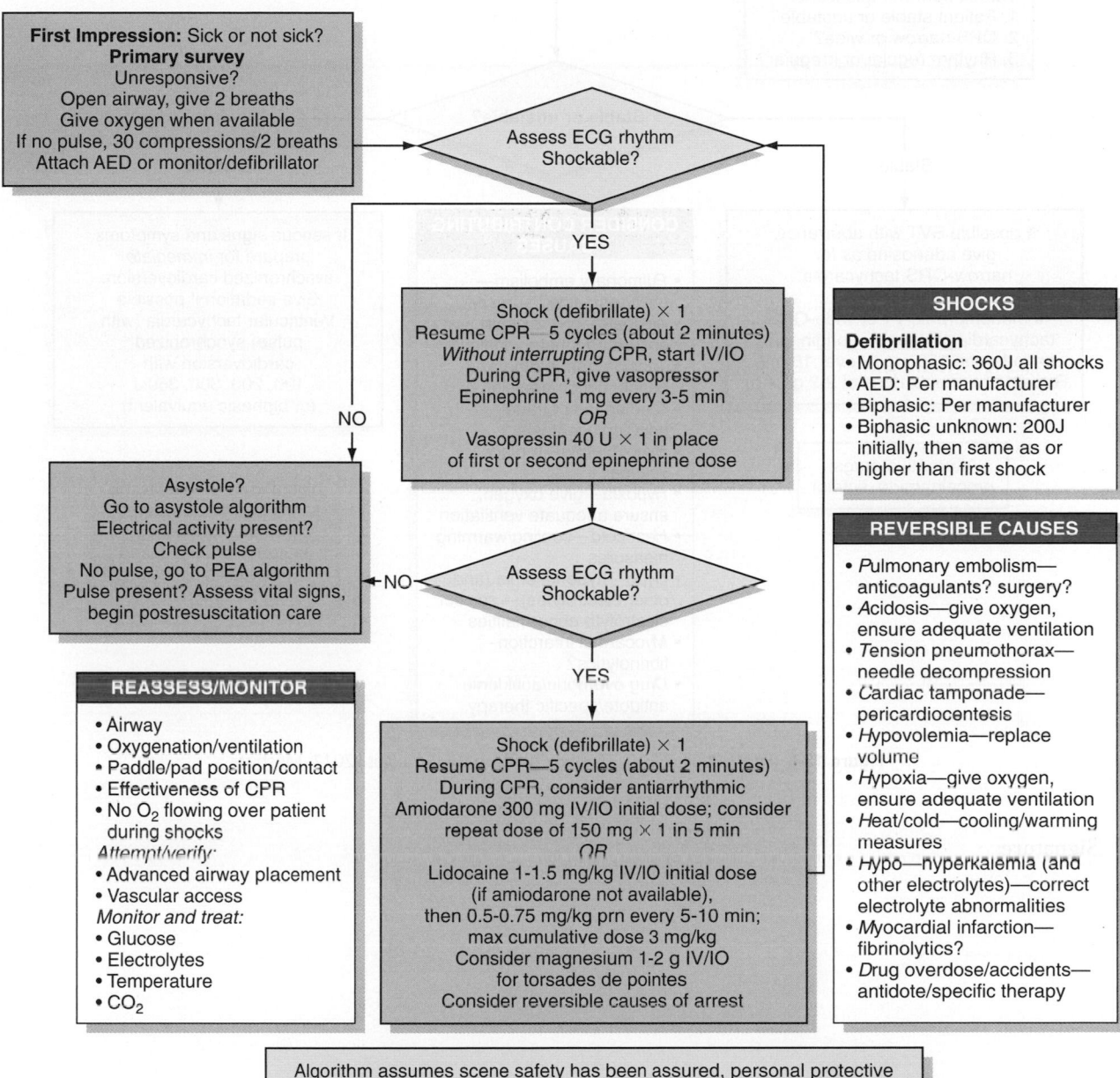

Figure 12-5 (From Aehlert B: ACLS study guide, ed 4, St. Louis, 2012, Mosby.)

Signature:_____

b.

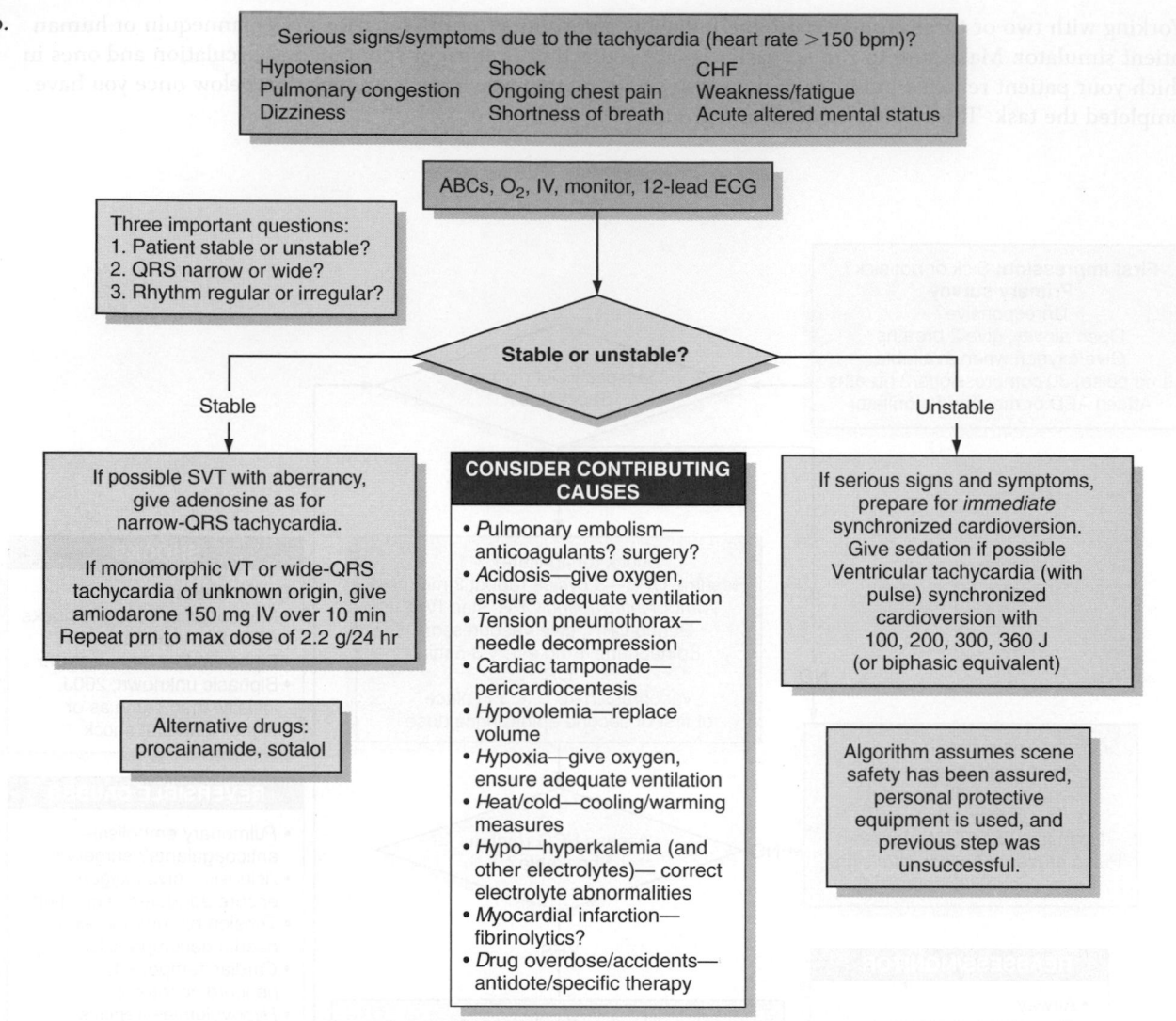

Figure 12-6 (From Aehlert B: ACLS study guide, ed 4, St. Louis, 2012, Mosby.)

Signature:_____

c.

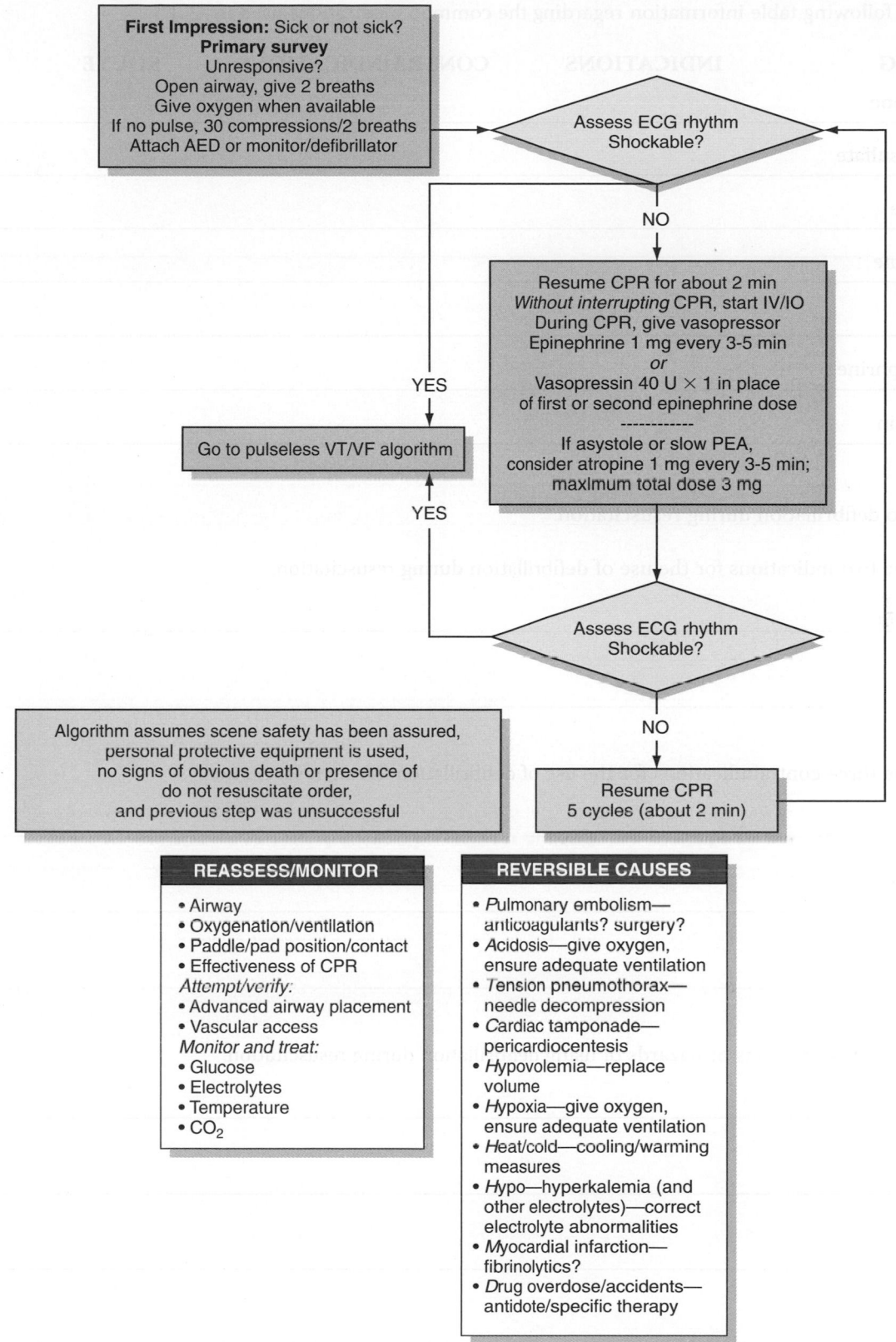

First Impression: Sick or not sick?
Primary survey
Unresponsive?
Open airway, give 2 breaths
Give oxygen when available
If no pulse, 30 compressions/2 breaths
Attach AED or monitor/defibrillator

Assess ECG rhythm
Shockable?

NO

Resume CPR for about 2 min
Without interrupting CPR, start IV/IO
During CPR, give vasopressor
Epinephrine 1 mg every 3-5 min
or
Vasopressin 40 U × 1 in place
of first or second epinephrine dose

If asystole or slow PEA,
consider atropine 1 mg every 3-5 min;
maximum total dose 3 mg

YES

Go to pulseless VT/VF algorithm

YES

Assess ECG rhythm
Shockable?

NO

Algorithm assumes scene safety has been assured,
personal protective equipment is used,
no signs of obvious death or presence of
do not resuscitate order,
and previous step was unsuccessful

Resume CPR
5 cycles (about 2 min)

REASSESS/MONITOR

• Airway
• Oxygenation/ventilation
• Paddle/pad position/contact
• Effectiveness of CPR
Attempt/verify:
• Advanced airway placement
• Vascular access
Monitor and treat:
• Glucose
• Electrolytes
• Temperature
• CO_2

REVERSIBLE CAUSES

• *P*ulmonary embolism—
anticoagulants? surgery?
• *A*cidosis—give oxygen,
ensure adequate ventilation
• *T*ension pneumothorax—
needle decompression
• *C*ardiac tamponade—
pericardiocentesis
• *H*ypovolemia—replace
volume
• *H*ypoxia—give oxygen,
ensure adequate ventilation
• *H*eat/cold—cooling/warming
measures
• *H*ypo—hyperkalemia (and
other electrolytes)—correct
electrolyte abnormalities
• *M*yocardial infarction—
fibrinolytics?
• *D*rug overdose/accidents—
antidote/specific therapy

Figure 12-7 (From Aehlert B: ACLS study guide, ed 4, St. Louis, 2012, Mosby.)

Signature:_____

7. Fill in the following table information regarding the common medications used in ACLS:

DRUG	INDICATIONS	CONTRAINDICATIONS	ROUTE	DOSE
Amiodarone				
Atropine sulfate				
Dopamine				
Epinephrine				
Lidocaine				
Norepinephrine				
Vasopressin				

8. Relating to defibrillation during resuscitation:

a. List the two indications for the use of defibrillation during resuscitation.

   1. _____

   2. _____

b. List the three contraindications for the use of defibrillation during resuscitation.

   1. _____

   2. _____

   3. _____

c. List the 10 precautions or hazards of using defibrillation during resuscitation.

   1. _____

   2. _____

   3. _____

   4. _____

   5. _____

   6. _____

7. _____

8. _____

9. _____

10. _____

Self-Assessment Questions

1. Correctly order the steps for administering basic life support by a single rescuer:

   1. Open the airway, and check breathing.
   2. Check for lack of movement or response, and check for pulse.
   3. Start chest compressions.
   4. Activate the emergency response system.

   A. 3, 1, 4, 2
   B. 2, 1, 3, 4
   C. 2, 4, 3, 1
   D. 1, 2, 3, 4

2. Which major artery is used to evaluate pulselessness in infants?
   A. Carotid artery
   B. Femoral artery
   C. Popliteal artery
   D. Brachial artery

3. Compared to normal cardiac output, the cardiac output produced by external chest compressions is approximately:
   A. One fourth
   B. One third
   C. One half
   D. The same

4. Successful resuscitation from sudden cardiac arrest caused by ventricular fibrillation depends on:
   A. Placement of an endotracheal tube
   B. Pharmacologic management
   C. Immediate CPR and delivery of a shock
   D. The etiology of the ventricular fibrillation

5. The most common complication(s) that occur with CPR include:

   1. Gastric inflation
   2. Vomiting
   3. Trauma during chest compressions
   4. Worsening of existing neck or spine injuries

   A. 3 only
   B. 1, 2, and 4 only
   C. 2, 3, and 4 only
   D. 1, 2, 3, and 4

6. CPR is contraindicated when:
   A. Rigor mortis is apparent
   B. Following cold water drowning
   C. The patient is pregnant
   D. The patient attempted suicide

7. Airway management during advanced cardiac life support includes:

   1. Pharyngeal airways
   2. Nasopharyngeal airways
   3. Masks
   4. Endotracheal tubes

   A. 4 only
   B. 1 and 4 only
   C. 1, 2, and 3 only
   D. 1, 2, 3, and 4

8. Bag-mask volumes obtained with a 1-second inspiratory squeeze typically result in tidal volumes of:
   A. 250 mL
   B. 500 mL
   C. 750 mL
   D. 1000 mL

9. Rescuers should hyperventilate victims of cardiac arrest.
   A. True
   B. False

10. Pulseless electrical activity is a shockable rhythm.
    A. True
    B. False

You walk into a patient's room and see the tracing in Figure 12-8 on the electrocardiography (ECG) monitor:

1. What is the first thing you would do?

_____

_____

2. Following a quick patient assessment, you note your patient is complaining of dizziness and fatigue and is hypotensive with a weak carotid pulse. What is your interpretation of the rhythm?

_____

_____

3. What are some contributing causes of this rhythm?

_____

_____

4. What should you do to immediately treat your patient?

_____

_____

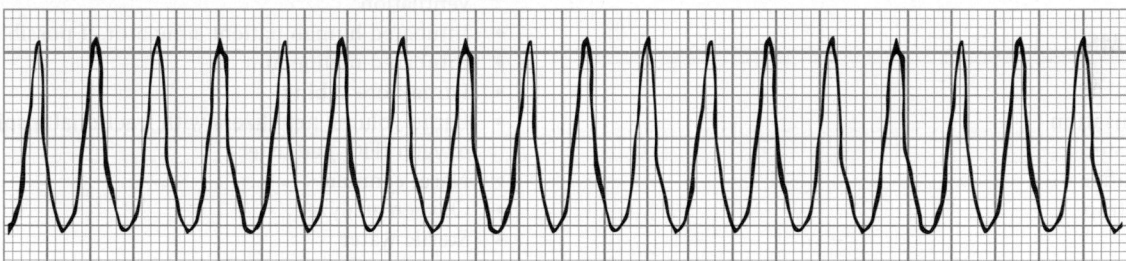

Figure 12-8 (From Kacmarek RM, Stoller JK, Heuer AJ: *Egan's fundamentals of respiratory care*, ed 10, St. Louis, MO, 2013, Mosby.)

Humidity and Bland Aerosol Therapy

■ OBJECTIVES

Upon the completion of the chapter activities and content review topics, the student will be able to:

1. Identify the goals of humidification and their clinical application.
2. Identify hazards and complications to bland aerosol therapy.
3. Use a bubble humidifier.
4. Use a large-volume nebulizer.
5. Perform sputum induction.
6. Use humidification during mechanical ventilation.
7. Compare and contrast the indications for heat and humidification versus heat moisture exchange use in the mechanically ventilated patient.

■ KEY TERMS

- Aerosol
- Condensation
- Inspissated
- Humidifier
- Water trap

■ CONTENT REVIEW TOPICS

- American Society for Testing and Materials (ASTM)
- Isothermic saturation boundary (ISB)
- Body temperature pressure saturated (BTPS)

■ PROCEDURAL ASSESSMENTS

13-1 Using a Bubble Humidifier
13-2 Using a Large-Volume Nebulizer
13-3 Sputum Induction
13-4 Humidification during Mechanical Ventilation

■ EQUIPMENT

- Aerosol face mask
- Bubble humidifiers
- Disposable gloves
- Heat moisture exchangers
- Heated humidification device used for mechanical ventilation
- Intubated human patient simulator, if possible
- Intubated mannequin
- Large-bore tubing
- Large-volume nebulizers with fractional inspired oxygen (FiO_2) adjusters
- Nasal cannula
- Oxygen analyzer
- Sterile water

The primary function of the upper respiratory tract is to heat and humidify the air we breathe. Clinical signs and symptoms of inadequate airway humidification may be noticed during routine patient assessment or reported by a patient as dryness of the nose or cough (Box 13-1). With numerous devices available, the respiratory therapist (RT) must be knowledgeable about how these devices work to be able to administer therapy to patients in the most appropriate and effective ways.

> → **Reality Check** Patients may get a nosebleed (epistaxis) with the use of a nasal cannula.

Determination of the most appropriate way to condition a patient's inspired medical gas requires patient assessment and evaluation of the goal of the therapy. An algorithm to assist in selecting the appropriate humidification delivery device is provided in Figure 13-1. This chapter will cover pertinent information relating to the equipment and clinical applications of humidification and bland aerosol therapy. Use of small-volume nebulizers for medication delivery will be covered in Chapter 19.

›› SKILL CHECK LISTS

13-1 Using a Bubble Humidifier

With the nose being the main participant in the process of filtering, heating, and humidifying inspired air, the additional flow of supplemental oxygen may impede its effectiveness. Humidification of oxygen is indicated for flow rates over 4 L/min. However, if the patient is complaining or displaying signs or symptoms of inadequate humidification, any amount of flow should be humidified. Bubble humidifiers should be used with oxygen flow rates under 10 L/min. The following is the step-by-step process for using a bubble humidifier.

> ✱ **Tip** Bubble humidifiers integrate pop-off relief valves. These valves prevent against build up when flow is obstructed. Typically, the spring-loaded valve releases and provides both audible and visible alarms for pressures greater than 2.

Procedural Preparation

1. Review the patient's chart.
2. Verify the physician's order or the facility's protocol for standard of care.
3. Obtain, clean, and inspect appropriate equipment prior to entering the patient's room.
4. Follow personal protective equipment (PPE) requirements, and observe standard precautions for any transmission-based isolation procedure.
5. Identify the patient using two patient identifiers.
6. Introduce yourself to the patient and to the family.

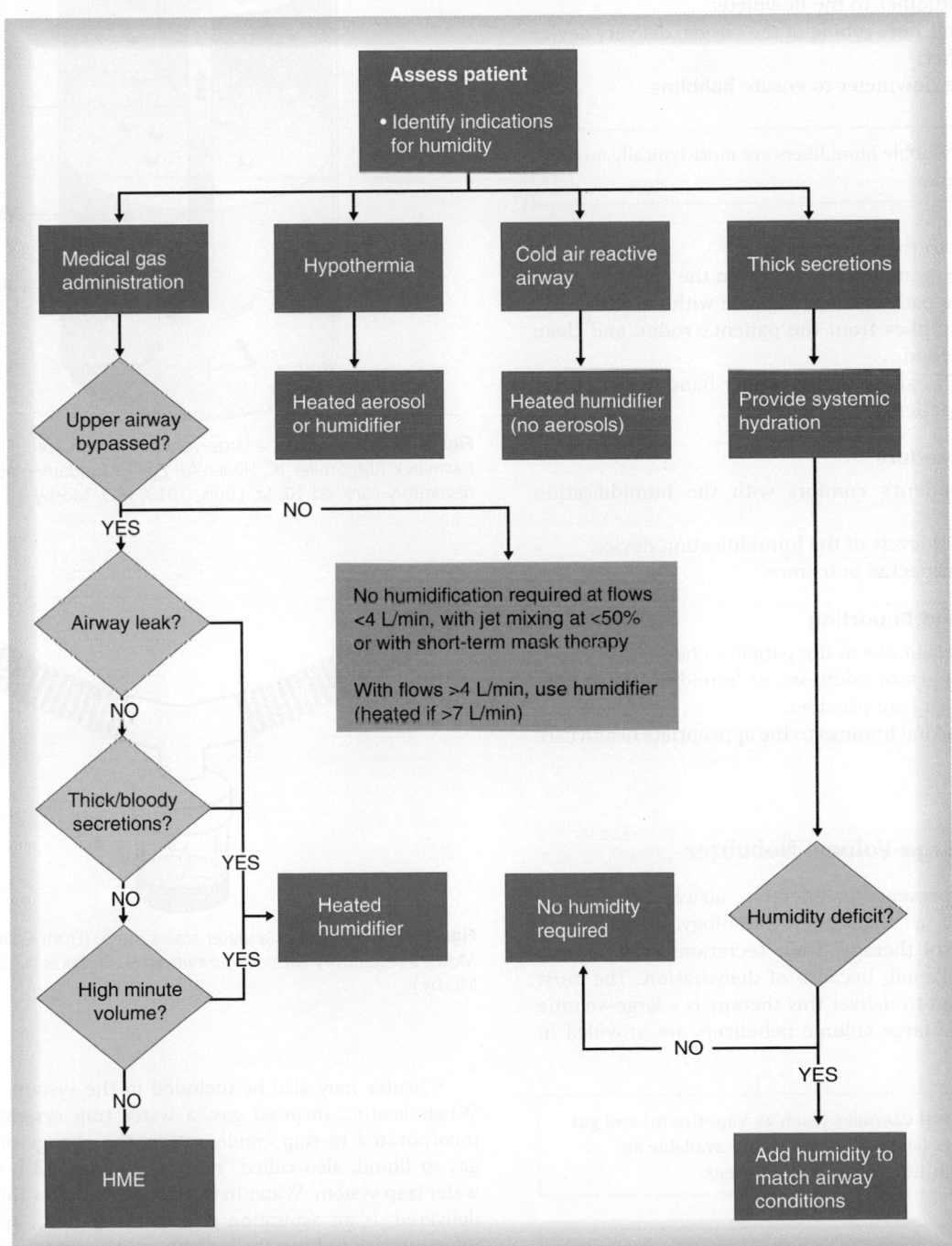

Figure 13-1 Selection algorithm for humidity and bland aerosol therapy. (From Kacmarek RM, Stoller JK, Heuer AJ: *Egan's fundamentals of respiratory care*, ed 10, St. Louis, 2013, MO, Mosby.)

7. Explain the procedure to the patient and to the family, and acknowledge the patient's understanding.
8. Perform proper hand hygiene, and put on gloves, mask, and protective eyewear, as appropriate for the procedure.

Implementation

1. Place the patient in a comfortable position.
2. Assess vital signs.
3. Assess the need for humidification:
   a. Determine if heated humidification is needed.
4. Fill the reservoir with sterile water:
   a. Snap off the connection port for prefilled bubble humidifiers.
5. Attach the humidifier to the flowmeter.
6. Attach the small-bore tubing of the oxygen delivery device to the humidifier:
   a. Turn on the flowmeter to ensure bubbling.

> **Reality Check** Bubble humidifiers are most typically used with nasal cannulas.

7. Adjust oxygen to the desired flow.
8. Position the oxygen delivery device on the patient.
9. Ensure that the patient is comfortable with the device.
10. Remove the supplies from the patient's room, and clean the area, as needed.
11. Remove the PPE, and perform proper hand hygiene prior to leaving the patient's room.

Evaluation of Procedure

1. Evaluate the patient's comfort with the humidification device.
2. Monitor the fluid levels of the humidification device.
3. Identify any unexpected outcomes.

Documentation and Reporting

1. Record humification use in the patient's chart.
2. Report any changes or additions of humidification to the appropriate health care provider.
3. Report any abnormal findings to the appropriate health care provider.

13-2 Using a Large-Volume Nebulizer

Frequently, in the presence of infection, airway adjunct use, or exacerbation of a respiratory pathology, patients will require bland aerosol therapy. Their secretions may become inspissated, or thickened, because of dehydration. The most common device used to deliver this therapy is a large-volume nebulizer. Images of large volume nebulizers are provided in Figure 13-2.

> * **Tip** High-flow nasal cannulas (such as Vapotherm) and gas injected nebulizers (such as MistyOx) are available as high-flow and high-humidity output devices.

> **Reality Check** Disposable large-volume nebulizers typically have F$_I$O$_2$ adjustment devices on the top.

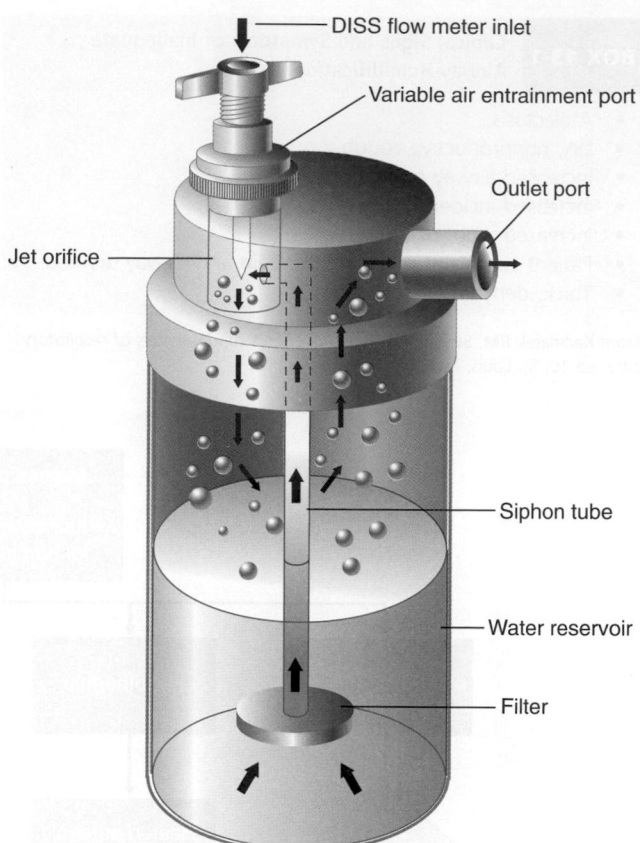

Figure 13-2 Diagram of a large-volume jet nebulizer. (From Kacmarek RM, Stoller JK, Heuer AJ: *Egan's fundamentals of respiratory care*, ed 10, St. Louis, 2013, MO, Mosby.)

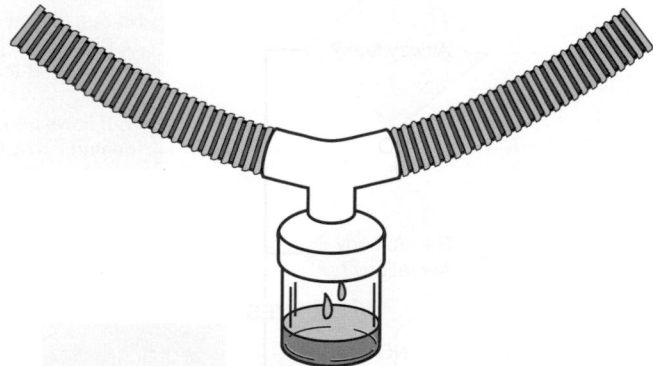

Figure 13-3 Example of a water trap system. (From Cairo JM: *Mosby's respiratory care equipment*, ed 9, St. Louis, MO, 2014, Mosby.)

A heater may also be included in the system, if required. When heating inspired gas, a water trap system should be incorporated to trap condensation, the change of state from gas to liquid, also called "rain-out." Figure 13-3 illustrates a water trap system. Water in the circuit may alter the FiO$_2$ being delivered, is an aspiration risk to the patient, and poses an infection risk to both the patient and the caregiver.

The following is the step-by-step process for using a large-volume nebulizer.

Procedural Preparation

1. Review the patient's chart.
2. Verify the physician's order or the facility's protocol for standard of care.
3. Obtain, clean, and inspect appropriate equipment prior to entering the patient's room.
4. Follow PPE requirements, and observe standard precautions for any transmission-based isolation procedure.
5. Identify the patient using two patient identifiers.
6. Introduce yourself to the patient and to the family.
7. Explain the procedure to the patient and to the family, and acknowledge the patient's understanding.
8. Perform proper hand hygiene, and put on gloves, mask, and protective eyewear, as appropriate for the procedure.

Implementation

1. Place the patient in a comfortable position.
2. Assess vital signs.
3. Assess the need for humidification:
a. Determine if heated humidification is needed.
4. Fills the reservoir with sterile water:
   a. Snap off the connection port for prefilled bubble humidifiers.
5. Attach the humidifier to the flowmeter.
6. Attach the large-bore tubing of the oxygen delivery device to the humidifier:
   a. Turn on the flowmeter to ensure bubbling.
7. Adjust oxygen to the desired flow and F_IO_2.
8. Position the oxygen delivery device on the patient.
9. Ensure that the patient is comfortable with the device.
10. Remove the supplies from the patient's room, and clean the area, as needed.
11. Remove PPE, and performs proper hand hygiene prior to leaving the patient's room.

Evaluation of Procedure

1. Evaluate the patient's comfort with the humidification device.
2. Monitor the fluid levels of the humidification device.
3. Analyze the F_IO_2 delivery per your facility's protocol.
4. Evaluate the need for a water trap.
5. Identify any unexpected outcomes.

Documentation and Reporting

1. Record the humidification use in the patient's chart.
2. Report any changes or additions to humidification therapy to the appropriate health care provider.
3. Report any abnormal findings to the appropriate health care provider.

13-3 Sputum Induction

When dealing with pulmonary infection, determination of the pathogen causing the illness is crucial to ensure that the proper antibiotic therapy is administered. Sputum induction is a diagnostic procedure utilized to obtain a sample of sputum for microbial testing of diseases such as tuberculosis or pneumocystis pneumonia. The following is the step-by-step process for sputum induction.

→ **Reality Check** Assessment of vital signs *always* includes breath sounds.

✱ **Tip** Sputum induction may cause bronchospasm. A short-acting β-agonist such as albuterol or levalbuterol should be available. Sputum induction with hypertonic saline should be used cautiously, if at all, on patients with a history of reactive airway disease.

✱ **Tip** Sputum induction should last about 15 to 30 minutes.

Procedural Preparation

1. Review the patient's chart.
2. Verify the physician's order or the facility's protocol for standard of care.
3. Obtain, clean, and inspect appropriate equipment prior to entering the patient's room.
4. Follow PPE requirements, and observe standard precautions for any transmission-based isolation procedure.
5. Identify the patient using two patient identifiers.
6. Introduce yourself to the patient and to the family.
7. Explain the procedure to the patient and to the family, and acknowledge the patient's understanding.
8. Perform proper hand hygiene, and put on gloves, mask, and protective eyewear, as appropriate for the procedure.

Implementation

1. Place the patient in a comfortable position.
2. Assess vital signs.
3. Provide the patient with the opportunity to rinse the mouth with water before taking the sample.
4. Ensure that the patient has an effective cough:
   a. Instruct the patient on how to cough correctly, if necessary.
   b. Instruct the patient to cough into a sterile specimen container.
5. Fill the appropriate delivery device with hypertonic saline:
   a. Use either a small-volume nebulizer or an ultrasonic nebulizer.

✱ **Tip** An ultrasonic nebulizer is electrically powered and uses a piezoelectric crystal to generate an aerosol.

   b. Instruct the patient to breathe through the mouth, if an aerosol face mask is used.
6. Position the delivery device on the patient.
7. Assess the patient for bronchospasm or any adverse reaction to therapy:
   a. Stop the therapy if any adverse reaction occurs.
   b. Deliver the bronchodilator per protocol, or obtain a physician's order.
   c. Inform the proper health care provider.
8. Instruct the patient to periodically stop to cough.
9. Attach the correct patient identification label and laboratory requisition to the side of the specimen container.

10. Place the specimen container in a plastic biohazard bag.
11. Offer the patient tissue to wipe the mouth, and provide mouth care, if needed.
12. Remove the supplies from the patient's room, and clean the area, as needed.
13. Remove PPE, and perform proper hand hygiene prior to leaving the patient's room.
14. Send the specimen immediately to the laboratory, according to your facility's protocols.

Evaluation of Procedure

1. Assess the patient frequently during therapy for bronchospasm.
2. Develop an appropriate respiratory care plan based on sputum data.
3. Identify any unexpected outcomes.

Documentation and Reporting

1. Record the time the sample was obtained in the patient's chart.
2. Report any abnormal findings to the appropriate health care provider.

13-4 Humidification during Mechanical Ventilation

During mechanical ventilation, the RT must provide all of the patient's heat and humidification requirements. Heat moisture exchangers (HMEs) and heated humidification are two of the most common options. HMEs are passive humidification devices that capture the patient's own expired air and gives it back to them in their next breath. Contraindications for their use are listed in Box 13-2. Most heated humidification devices used with mechanical ventilation utilize a hot plate element at the base of the humidifier to heat the inspired gas. Examples of both HMEs and a heated humidifier are provided in Figure 13-4. The following is the step-by-step process for humidification during mechanical ventilation.

→ **Reality Check** Active heat moisture exchangers, which add humidity by chemical and electrical means, do exist but are not frequently used in the United States.

✱ **Tip** HME is sometimes referred to as an "artificial nose."

Procedural Preparation

1. Review the patient's chart.
2. Verify the physician's order or the facility's protocol for standard of care.
3. Obtain, clean, and inspect appropriate equipment prior to entering the patient's room.
4. Follow PPE requirements, and observe standard precautions for any transmission-based isolation procedure.
5. Identify the patient using two patient identifiers.
6. Introduce yourself to the patient and to the family.
7. Explain the procedure to the patient and to the family, and acknowledge the patient's understanding.

BOX 13-2	Contraindications for Heat Moisture Exchanger Use

- Patients with thick, copious, or bloody secretions
- Patients with an expired tidal volume less that 70% of the delivered tidal volume
- Patients whose body temperature is <32°C
- Patients with spontaneous minute volumes >10 liters per minute (L/min)

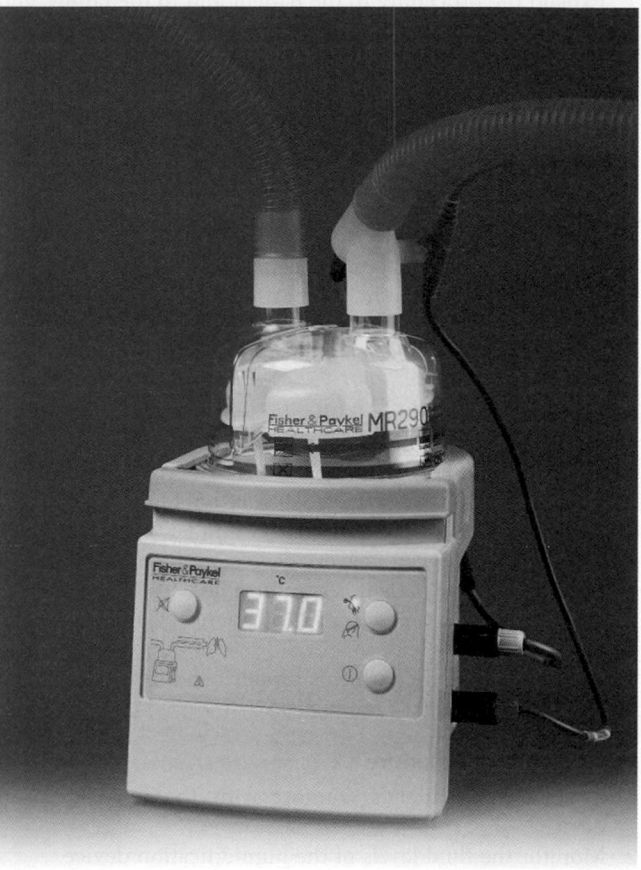

Figure 13-4 Fisher and Paykel MR 850 heated humidifier. (Courtesy of Fisher & Paykel Healthcare, Irvine, CA.)

8. Perform proper hand hygiene, and put on gloves, mask, and protective eyewear, as appropriate for the procedure.

Implementation

1. Assess vital signs.
2. Determine the appropriate humidification device.
   Heat Moisture Exchanger (HME)
   a. Rule out any contraindications for use.
   b. Attach a 15-mm ID opening to endotracheal or tracheostomy tube.
   c. Attach a 22-mm ID opening to the ventilator circuit.
   d. Ensure that all connections are secure.
   Heated Humidification (HH)
   a. Set up the equipment, per manufacturer's specifications.
   b. Maintain the water level.

c. Secure both temperature probes in place.

d. Set to deliver inspired gas at 33°C ± 2°C measured at airway opening.

e. Insert the water trap at the lowest point in the circuit (both inspiratory and expiratory limbs).

f. Ensure that the connections are secure.

g. Set the high (no higher than 37°C) and low (no lower than 30°C) temperature alarms.

Heated Wire Circuits

a. Place the temperature probe outside the incubator or away from the radiant warmer.

3. Perform patient–ventilator system assessment, as needed.

4. Remove the supplies from the patient's room, and clean the area, as needed.

5. Remove PPE, and perform proper hand hygiene prior to leaving the patient's room.

Evaluation of Procedure

1. Evaluate the choice of humidification device.

2. Ensure proper conditioning of the inspired gas.

3. Identify any unexpected outcomes.

Documentation and Reporting

1. Record the humidification device used in the patient's chart.

2. Record the quality, consistency, and characteristics of secretions in the patient's chart.

3. Report any abnormal findings to the appropriate health care provider.

Bibliography

Cairo JM, Pilbeam S: *Mosby's respiratory care equipment*, ed 8, St. Louis, MO, 2011, Mosby.

Cairo JM: *Pilbeam's mechanical ventilation*, ed 5, St. Louis, MO, 2012, Mosby.

Kacmarek RM, Stoller JK, Heuer AJ: *Egan's fundamentals of respiratory care*, ed 10, St Louis, MO, 2013, Mosby.

1. What is the primary goal of humidification?

_____

2. List the five indications for bland aerosol administration.

a. _____

b. _____

c. _____

d. _____

e. _____

3. List the two contraindications to bland aerosol administration.

a. _____

b. _____

4. List the nine hazards and complications associated with bland aerosol administration.

a. _____

b. _____

c. _____

d. _____

e. _____

f. _____

g. _____

h. _____

i. _____

j. _____

5. List the seven clinical signs and symptoms of inadequate airway humidification.

a. _____

b. _____

c. _____

d. _____

e. _____

f. _____

g. _____

6. What four factors may affect the quality of a humidifier's performance?

a. _____

b. _____

c. _____

d. _____

7. Name the piece of equipment in Figure 13-5.

_____

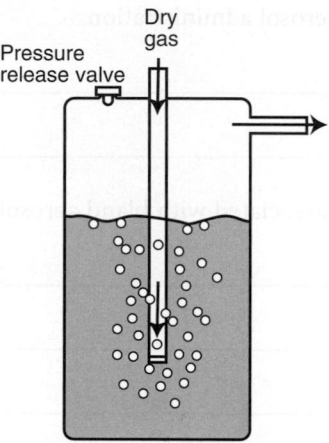

Figure 13-5 (From Cairo JM: *Mosby's respiratory care equipment*, ed 9, St. Louis, MO, 2014, Mosby.)

a. Explain how it works.

b. List three factors that will affect the amount of humidity this device will produce. Will each factor increase or decrease humidity output of the device?

1. _____

2. _____

3. _____

c. If this device is operated unheated, approximately what absolute humidity level can it produce?

_____

d. At what flow range is this device most effective?

_____

e. Give a clinical situation in which use of this device is indicated.

_____

8. Locate a bubble humidifier in the laboratory, and set it up. Identify all of its components, and explain its operation to your lab partner. Have the partner sign off that this has been done properly.

Signature: _____

9. Name the device in Figure 13-6.

_____

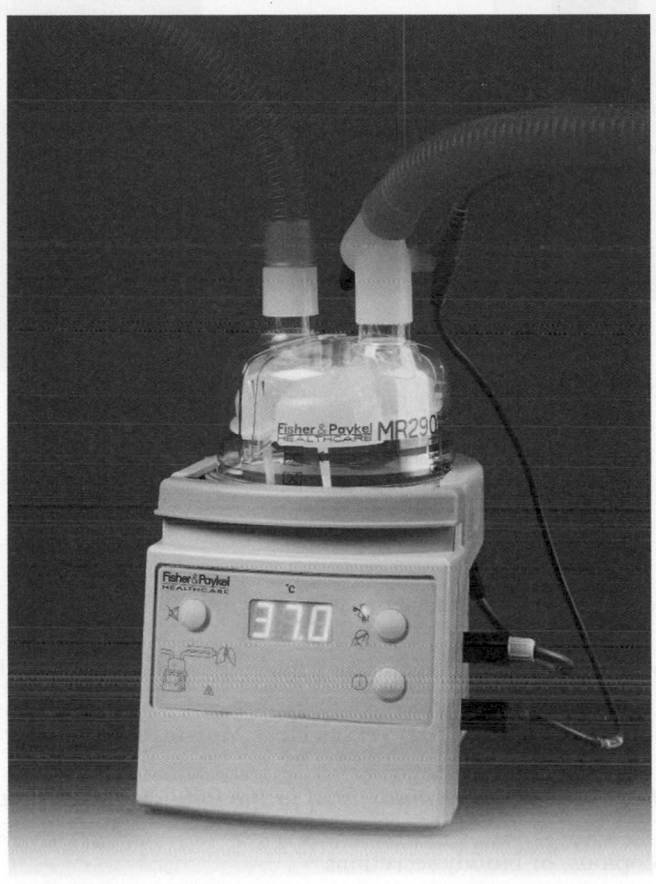

Figure 13-6 (From Fisher & Paykel Healthcare, Irvine, CA).)

a. Explain how it works.

_____

b. List a clinical situation where this device would be used.

_____

10. Using a mannequin or artificial lung, set up the device from question 9.

a. Have your instructor sign off that you assembled it correctly.

Instructor signature:_____

11. Identify the device in Figure 13-7.

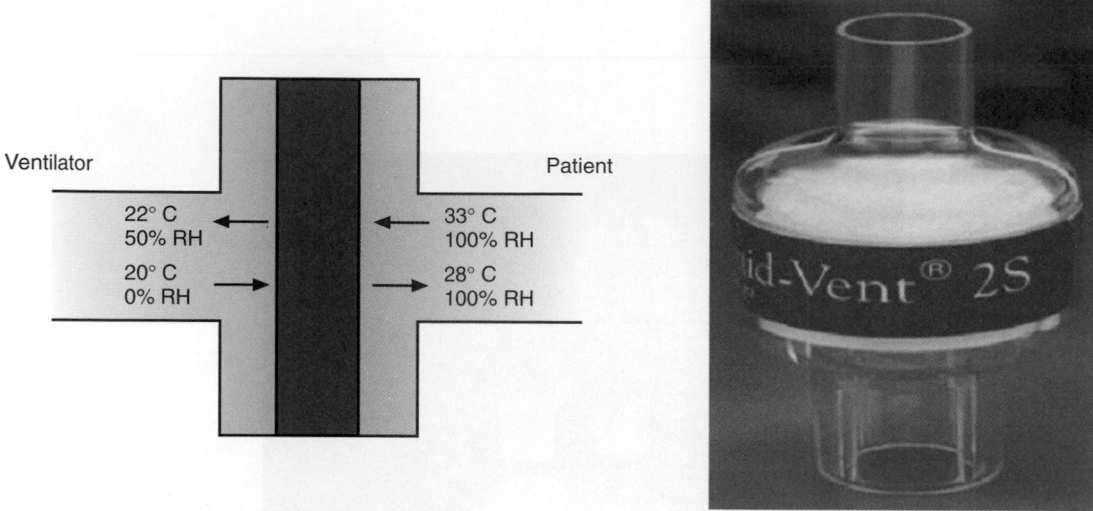

Figure 13-7 (From Cairo JM: *Mosby's respiratory care equipment*, ed 9, St. Louis, MO, 2014, Mosby and Teleflex Medical, Research Triangle Park, NC.)

a. Explain how it works.

b. List a clinical situation where this device may be used.

c. Compare and contrast heated humidification and heat moisture exchanger use. Fill in the table below:

Heated Humidification (HH) versus Heat Moisture Exchanger (HME)

(Circle which is contraindicated in the following situations.)

For patients with thick, copious, or bloody secretions	HH or HME
For patients with an expired tidal volume less that 70% of the delivered tidal volume	HH or HME
For patients whose body temperature is <32°C	HH or HME
For patients with spontaneous minute volumes >10 L/min	HH or HME
(For HH or HME, circle one or both that can cause the following hazard or complication.)	
Hypoventilation caused by increased dead space	HH or HME
Increased work of breathing	HH or HME
Potential electrical shock	HH or HME
Elevated airway pressures from condensate	HH or HME

12. Obtain a mannequin or artificial lung, and set it up with an HME in-line. Have your instructor sign off that you assembled it correctly.

Instructor signature:_____

13. With a partner, set up a large-volume nebulizer with an air entrainment device with F_1O_2 set to 0.4. Using an oxygen analyzer, measure the F_1O_2 the device is delivering.

Record it here: _____

14. Using the setup from question #14, add water to the large-bore tubing. Repeat the FiO_2 analysis.

Record it here: _____

15. Why did the F_1O_2 change in the set up in question 15?

_____

Self-Assessment Questions

1. A HME is contraindicated in:

   1. Patients with thick, copious secretions
   2. Patients whose body temperature is less than 32°C
   3. Patients with expired tidal volumes of less than 70% of delivered tidal volume
   4. Patients with low spontaneous minute volumes (<10 L/min)

   A. 1 only
   B. 1 and 3 only
   C. 1, 2, and 3 only
   D. 1, 2, 3, and 4

2. Heat and moisture exchange is a primary function of the:
   A. Lungs
   B. Upper respiratory tract
   C. Alveoli
   D. Mouth

3. Indications for heated humidification therapy include:

   1. Managing hypothermia
   2. Bypassed upper airway during mechanical ventilation
   3. Acute epiglottitis

   A. 2 only
   B. 3 only
   C. 1 and 2 only
   D. 1, 2, and 3

4. The most effective way to increase the output of a humidification device is to:
   A. Increase the flow of gas
   B. Increase the temperature
   C. Decrease the surface area
   D. Decrease the thermal mass

5. A recently extubated patient is experiencing mild shortness of breath with stridor. Which of the following would you recommend as the best way to treat this problem?
   A. Use heated humidification
   B. Use cool, bland aerosol
   C. Use salmeterol
   D. Use DuoNeb (albuterol and ipratropium)

6. What monitoring parameters should you utilize when using humidification during mechanical ventilation?

   1. Consistency of secretions
   2. High-temperature alarms if using HH
   3. Low-temperature alarms if using HH
   4. Water levels and function of the feed system

   A. 1 only
   B. 2 and 3 only
   C. 2, 3, and 4 only
   D. 1, 2, 3, and 4

7. Which of the following are types of passover humidifiers

   1. Heat moisture exchanger
   2. Wick type
   3. Membrane type
   4. Bubble type

   A. 1 and 2 only
   B. 2 and 3 only
   C. 1, 2, and 4 only
   D. 2, 3, and 4 only

8. What type of nebulizers use a piezoelectric crystal to generate aerosol?

   1. Small-volume nebulizer
   2. Large-volume nebulizer
   3. Ultrasonic nebulizer

   A. 1 only
   B. 3 only
   C. 1 and 3 only
   D. 1, 2, and 3

9. When heated, the amount of water that a large-volume nebulizer may produce is:
   A. 15–20 mg H_2O/L
   B. 26–35 mg H_2O/L
   C. 33–55 mg H_2O/L
   D. 50–60 mg H_2O/L

10. Recommended levels for gas delivered to the trachea include:
    A. Temperature range of 20°C–22°C and a relative humidity of 100%
    B. Temperature range of 20°C–22°C and a relative humidity of 50%
    C. Temperature range of 32°C–35°C and a relative humidity of 100%
    D. Temperature range of 32°C–35°C and a relative humidity of 50%

▶▶ CASE STUDY 13-1

You are a respiratory therapist assigned to the general floors of a small rural hospital. A nurse calls you to assess a patient with chronic obstructive pulmonary disease (COPD) who is complaining of nasal dryness and irritation. When you arrive, you find the patient receiving oxygen via nasal cannula at 4 L/min and resting comfortably, and vital signs are within normal limits.

1. How should you treat the patient's complaint?

_____

_____

2. What is the most appropriate device to accomplish this?

_____

_____

Storage and Delivery of Medical Gases

■ OBJECTIVES

Upon the completion of the chapter activities and content review topics, the student should be able to:

1. Identify common therapeutic medical gases.
2. Describe how to store, transport, and safely use compressed gas cylinders.
3. Describe how oxygen is produced.
4. Use the oxygen cylinder safely.
5. Calculate the duration of flow of a compressed oxygen cylinder.
6. Describe common safety indexing safety systems.
7. Use liquid oxygen safely.
8. Calculate the duration of flow of a liquid oxygen cylinder.

■ KEY TERMS

- American Standard Safety System (ASSS)
- Characteristics of medical gases

- Diameter-index safety systems (DISS)
- Fractional distillation
- Pin-indexing safety system (PISS)
- Therapeutic gases

■ CONTENT REVIEW TOPICS

- Compressed Gas Association (CGA)
- National Fire Protection Agency (NFPA)

■ PROCEDURAL ASSESSMENTS

14-1 Using an Oxygen Cylinder
14-2 Using a Liquid Oxygen System

The therapeutic use of medical gases is a fundamental part of respiratory care. Many gases are commercially produced, but only a few are used in the respiratory care of patients. The most common ones are listed in Box 14-1. Therapeutic gases are used daily by the respiratory therapist (RT) to relieve symptoms and improve the oxygenations of patients. Oxygen is the most commonly used medical gas by RTs, and its uses are described in detail in Chapter 15.

Care must be taken when dealing with medical gases. Understanding how cylinders work, how to safely store and appropriately use them will be discussed in this chapter. Oxygen concentrators will be discussed in Chapter 29.

≫ SKILL CHECK LISTS

14-1 Using an Oxygen Cylinder

The National Fire Protection Agency (NFPA) and the Compressed Gas Association (CGA) have guidelines for safe cylinder storage, transport, and use. RTs are frequently responsible for various aspects of the use of compressed gas cylinders and must be attentive to these guidelines. Safety aspects include how and where to store containers and how to safely transport them using carts with securing mechanisms. These tasks most frequently fall under the RT's duties.

→ **Reality Check** Large hospitals often have a facilities department that is responsible for bulk systems.

Ensuring the correct gas is given to the patient is a safety priority. Gas cylinders are identified from their label and

color. If the label and color do not match, the cylinder should not be used. The color codes for medical gas cylinders in the United States are given in Table 14-1. Reducing valves are needed to decrease the pressure of the cylinder to 50 pounds per square inch (psi), the standard working pressure for respiratory equipment. The American Standard Safety System (ASSS) provides standards for threaded high-pressure connections between large compressed gas cylinders and their attachments. Smaller cylinders (up to and including E size tanks) utilize a division of the ASSS, called the pin-indexing safety system (PISS), which helps avoid unintended misconnections between pieces of equipment. Figure 14-1 illustrates the different cylinder sizes available. Typically found at the station outlets of central piping and at the inlets of blenders, flowmeters, ventilators, and pneumatically powered equipment, the diameter-index safety system (DISS) helps prevent the interchange of medical connectors that are less than 200 pounds per square inch gauge (psig). To determine the duration of gas flow (also referred to as *duration of supply*) for a compressed oxygen cylinder a calculation must be done. The cylinder factors for common cylinder sizes are provided in Table 14-2. This formula is given in Box 14-2. The following is the step-by-step process for using an oxygen cylinder.

→ **Reality Check** When taking care of patients, a safety factor should be used when calculating duration of flow. Subtract 500 psi before calculating duration of flow to ensure that the tank is changed before it runs out completely.

TABLE 14-1 Color Code for Medical Gas Cylinders for the United States

Oxygen	Green
Air	Yellow
Nitrogen	Black
Helium	Brown
Nitric oxide	Teal and black
Carbon dioxide	Gray
Helium–oxygen	Brown and green
Carbon dioxide–oxygen	Gray and green

TABLE 14-2 Cylinder factors for Calculation of Cylinder Duration of Flow

Content	Size (Minutes)			
	D	E	G	H and K
O_2, O_2–N_2, air	0.16	0.28	2.41	3.14
O_2–CO_2	0.20	0.35	2.94	3.84
He–O_2	0.14	0.23	1.93	2.50

CO_2, Carbon dioxide; *He*, helium; *O_2*, oxygen; *N_2*, nitrogen.

BOX 14-1 Common Therapeutic Medical Gases

Air
Oxygen (O_2)
Helium–oxygen (He/O_2)
Carbon dioxide–oxygen (CO_2)
Nitric oxide (NO)

BOX 14-2 Duration of Oxygen Cylinder Gas Flow Formula

$$\text{Duration of gas (minutes)} = \frac{pressure(psig) \times cylinder\ factor}{Flow(L/min)}$$

Procedural Preparation

1. Obtain the appropriate medical gas cylinder based on need.
2. Verify the content based on the label and color.
3. Obtain the correct regulator for the cylinder.

Implementation

1. Release the safety strap or chain.
2. Move the cylinder onto the cart safely, and secure it.
3. Move the cart to the desired location for delivery of gas.
4. Secure the cylinder in the new location, if removing it from the cart.
5. Remove the protective cap or wrap.
6. Ensure the safety of bystanders by turning the valve away from the persons present.
7. Give a verbal warning of cylinder being cracked.
8. Visualize the valve or regulator inlet to confirm that it is contaminant-free.
9. Crack the cylinder.
10. Connect the regulator to the cylinder firmly, and open the cylinder.
11. Fix any leaks.
12. Following use, close the cylinder valve, bleed, and disconnect the regulator.

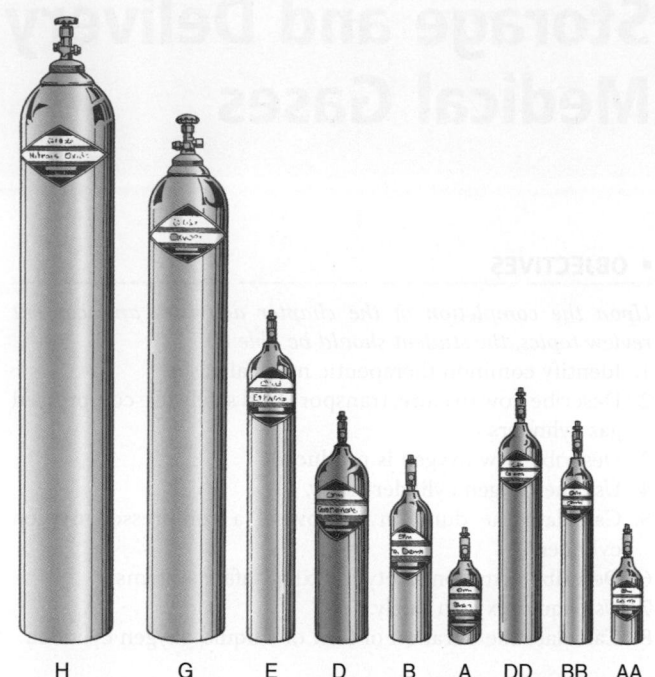

Figure 14-1 Cylinder sizes are identified by letter designations. (From Kacmarek RM, Stoller JK, Heuer AJ: Egan's fundamentals of respiratory care, ed 10, St. Louis, 2013, Mosby.)

13. Place the safety cap back on the cylinder, and return it to the appropriate storage location.

Evaluation of Procedure

1. Correctly calculate the duration of flow.
2. Identify any unexpected outcomes.

Documentation and Reporting

1. Record the beginning pressures and the time cylinder use began in the patient's chart.

14-2 Using a Liquid Oxygen System

Oxygen is colorless, odorless, transparent, and tasteless, with most of it produced by a process called fractional distillation. This process filters atmospheric air, liquefies it by compression, and cools it by rapid expansion. Then the mixture is heated slowly in a distillation tower, where the nitrogen is boiled off first, followed by the trace gases. The liquid left is pure oxygen. It must be stored in insulated cryogenic storage containers. Fractional distillation produces oxygen that is about 99.5% pure, which is above the United States Food and Drug Administration (FDA) requirement of 99% purity for medical-grade oxygen.

> **✳ Tip** It may be helpful to patients if you make a chart with certain weights and durations of flow so that they do not have to do the calculation.

Liquid-filled storage containers (Figure 14-2) must be weighed to determine the volume contained. The calculation for duration of flow of gas in the cylinder is given in Box 14-3.

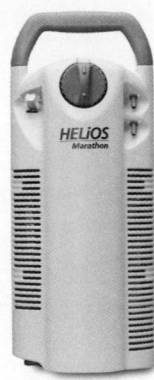

Figure 14-2 Portable liquid oxygen containers. (Courtesy of AirSep, A Chart Industries Company, Buffalo, NY.)

BOX 14-3	Duration of a Liquid Oxygen Storage Container Formula

$$\text{Amount of gas (liters)} = \frac{Liquid\ 02\ weight(lb) \times 860}{2.5\ lb/L}$$

$$\text{Duration of gas (minutes)} = \frac{amount\ of\ gas\ (liters)}{Flow(L/min)}$$

The following is the step-by-step process for using a liquid oxygen system.

Procedural Preparation

1. Weigh the portable system to determine if any refilling is needed.
2. Confirm that all safety rules are followed.

Implementation

1. Connect the portable system to the stationary system.
2. Open the gas vent valve.
3. Observe the venting through the gas vent port; close the gas vent valve.
4. Disconnect the portable system from the stationary system.
5. Confirm that the portable system is full.

Evaluation of Procedure

1. Calculate the duration of flow.
2. Identify any unexpected outcomes.

Documentation and Reporting

1. Record the amount of flow and the oxygen delivery device used in the patient's chart, if applicable.

Bibliography

Cairo JM: *Mosby's respiratory care equipment*, ed 9, St. Louis, MO, 2014, Mosby.

Kacmarek RM, Stoller JK, Heuer AJ: *Egan's fundamentals of respiratory care*, ed 10, St. Louis, MO, 2013, Mosby.

Lab Activities

1. What gas would be in your cylinder if the color was:

   a. Green:_____

   b. Yellow: _____

   c. Brown:_____

   d. Black:_____

   e. Gray and green:_____

   f. Gray:_____

   g. Teal and black:_____

   h. Brown and green:_____

2. What are laboratory gases used for?

   _____

3. What are therapeutic gases used for?

   _____

4. What are anesthetic gases used for?

   _____

5. Circle the best choice for the description of the gas use in the table below:

Gas	Description of Gas Use		
Nitrogen	Laboratory	Therapeutic	Anesthetic
Heliox	Laboratory	Therapeutic	Anesthetic
Nitrous oxide	Laboratory	Therapeutic	Anesthetic
Oxygen	Laboratory	Therapeutic	Anesthetic
Carbon dioxide	Laboratory	Therapeutic	Anesthetic
Helium	Laboratory	Therapeutic	Anesthetic
Air	Laboratory	Therapeutic	Anesthetic

6. Obtain an H-cylinder.

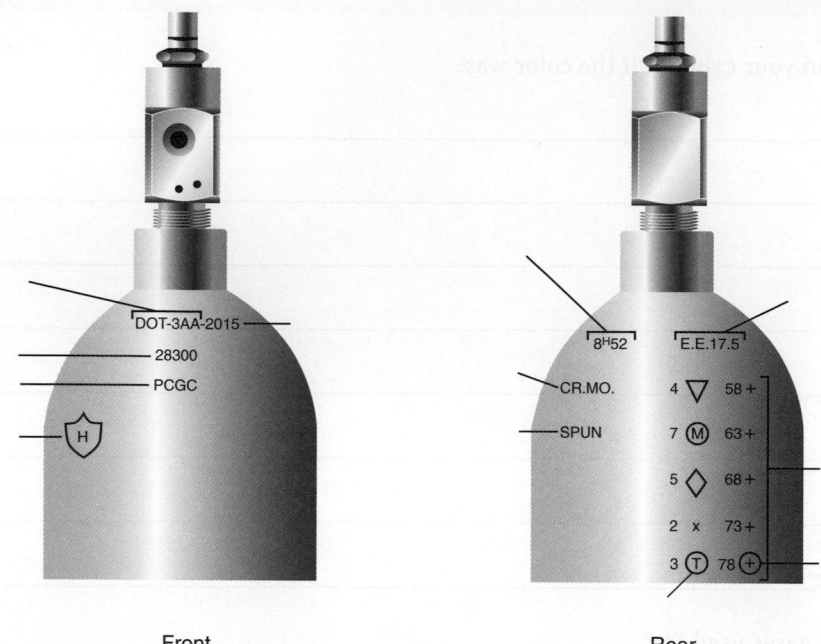

Front   Rear

Figure 14-3 (From Kacmarek RM, Stoller JK, Heuer AJ: *Egan's fundamentals of respiratory care*, ed 10, St. Louis, MO, 2013, Mosby.)

  a. Identify the typical markings on the cylinders using the image Figure 14-3.

  b. Obtain an oxygen regulator used for an H-tank. Describe all its safety components to a lab partner. Attach it and then take it off the H-tank following the skill check list in the beginning of the chapter. Have your partner sign once you have correctly performed the tasks.

    Signature: _____

7. Repeat the steps in question 6 for an E-tank. Have your partner sign once you have correctly performed the tasks.

  Signature: _____

8. Look at an H-cylinder and an E-cylinder.

  a. What is each made of?

    H cylinder_____

    E cylinder_____

  b. How do you determine this?

  _____

9. Fill in the section of the chart below regarding duration of flow.

Cylinder Size	Pressure (in psi)	Liter Flow (in liters/minute)	Duration of Flow (in minutes)
H	2200	15	
E	2200	15	
H	2200	2	
E	2200	2	
H	1000	15	
E	1000	15	
H	1000	2	
E	1000	2	

10. Describe the following cylinder high-pressure relief valves:

a. Frangible metal disk: _____

b. Fusible plug:_____

c. Spring-loaded valve:_____

11. What safety system is featured in Figure 14-4?

_____

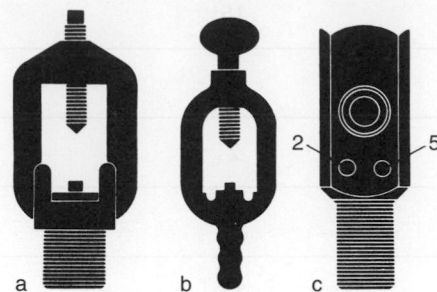

Figure 14-4 (Courtesy of Datex-Ohmeda, A GE Company, Madison, WI.)

12. What prevents the wrong gas from being connected to the equipment?

_____

_____

13. Label the Figure 14-5 with the appropriate gases.

14. Circle the one in Figure 14-5 that illustrates the pin position for oxygen.

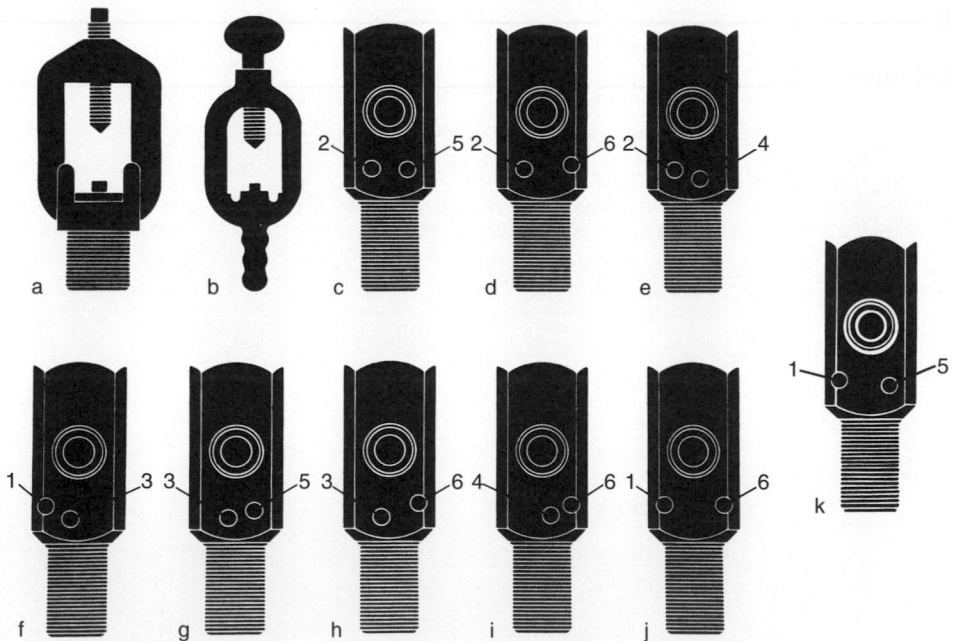

Figure 14-5 (Courtesy of Datex-Ohmeda, Madison, A GE Company, WI.)

15. Locate a quick connect system used for attaching a Thorpe tube flowmeter. Obtain a Thorpe tube for both oxygen and air.

a. Are they the same?

_____

b. How are they similar?

_____

c. How are they different?

_____

d. What safety feature do they incorporate?

_____

16. Attach oxygen tubing to either an air-compensated or oxygen-compensated Thorpe tube flowmeter that measures liter flows up to 15 L/min. Using a Wright respirometer (Figure 14-6) and a stop watch (or wrist watch), measure the volume of gas delivered in 1 minute with the flowmeter set at:

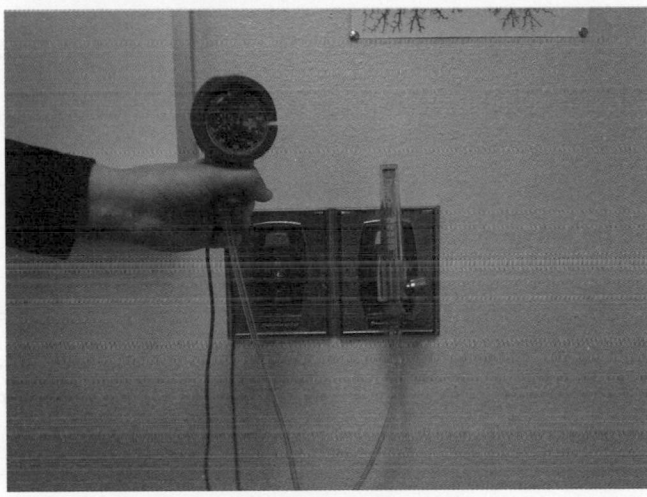

Figure 14-6

a. 5 L/min, and record your volume:_____

b. 10 L/min, and record your volume:_____

c. 15 L/min, and record your volume:_____

d. Now put the flowmeter to flush, and record your volume:_____

e. On the basis of the above data, is it safe to place your patient on an oxygen delivery device and set the flowmeter to flush?

_____

17. What is the device pictured in Figure 14-7?

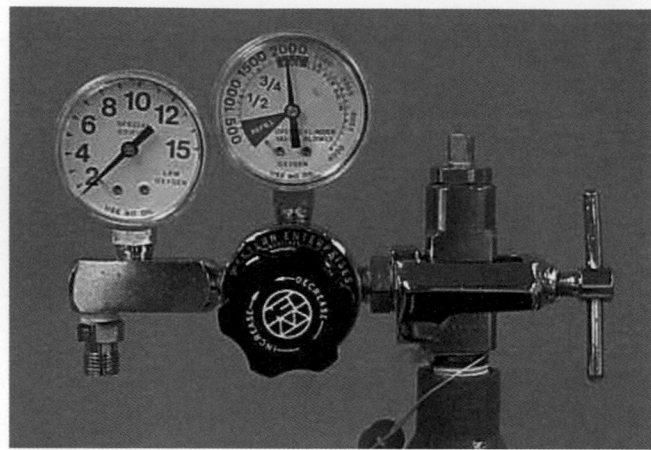

Figure 14-7 (From Kacmarek RM, Stoller JK, Heuer AJ: *Egan's fundamentals of respiratory care*, ed 10, St. Louis, MO, 2013, Mosby.)

a. What are the two components used for?

b. Give a clinical situation where it would be appropriate to use this device.

c. List a safety feature located on the device.

18. If available in you lab, locate H-tanks filled with contents other than oxygen; carbon dioxide and nitrogen are examples. Attempt to attach an oxygen regulator to them. Do they fit? Why, or why not?

Self-Assessment Questions

1. The most commonly used gas in respiratory care is:
   A. Oxygen
   B. Heliox
   C. Nitric oxide
   D. Nitrous oxide

2. What is the fire risk classification for oxygen?
   A. Flammable
   B. Nonflammable
   C. Supports combustion
   D. Acidic

3. Which of the following gases is the lightest?
   A. Nitrogen
   B. Air
   C. Oxygen
   D. Helium

4. During inspection of the shoulder of a compressed gas cylinder, you note an asterisk (*) next to the test date. This indicates:
   A. Department of Transportation (DOT) approval for 10-year testing
   B. DOT approval for 5-year testing
   C. It contains an anesthetic gas
   D. It contains a flammable gas

5. To estimate the duration of flow of a compressed gas cylinder, you must have:

   1. The weight of the cylinder
   2. The gas flow
   3. The cylinder size
   4. The pressure in the cylinder

   A. 1, 2, and 3 only
   B. 4 only
   C. 2, 3, and 4 only
   D. 1 only

6. What is the pin index hole position for oxygen?
   A. 2–5
   B. 2–4
   C. 1–5
   D. 3–5

7. What is the standard working pressure for respiratory equipment in the United States?
   A. 50 pounds psig
   B. 100 psig
   C. 150 psig
   D. It depends on the device you are using

8. The combination of a flowmeter with a reducing valve is called:
   A. A compensated Thorpe tube
   B. An uncompensated Thorpe tube
   C. A regulator
   D. Multistage reducing valve

9. A factor limiting the use of a pressure compensated Thorpe tube with oxygen is:
   A. Flow requirements
   B. Working pressure requirements
   C. Gas being used
   D. Gravity

10. Your cylinder is a DOT type 3A cylinder. What is it made of?
    A. Fiberglass
    B. Carbon steel
    C. Steel alloy
    D. Aluminum

> **CASE STUDY 14-1**

You are transporting a patient for computed tomography (CT) scanning from the intensive care unit (ICU). You anticipate the trip will take a total time of 20 minutes. Allowing for delays, you estimate it will be 30 minutes. You have an E-cylinder of oxygen at 2000 psi, and you must use a self-inflating manual resuscitator at a flow of 10 L/min.

1. Will one E-cylinder be enough for the trip?

_____

_____

A homecare patient is living in rural Minnesota where electric power outages for several hours to several days are common during the winter months. You determine that for his needs, an H-cylinder backup system is needed.

1. If your patient loses power for 3 days, how many H-cylinders will be needed at an oxygen flow of 3 L/min using a full pressure of 2200 psi?

_____

_____

2. You discuss the use of liquid oxygen for portable oxygen delivery for him when he travels to his doctor's appointments in the city. You have a portable liquid oxygen container that weighs 3 lbs. He runs his oxygen at 4 L/min. How long will this container last?

_____

_____

A patient in a skilled nursing facility is using an H-cylinder as the source of oxygen delivery through a nasal cannula during sleep at a flow of 2 L/min. She uses the cylinder an average of 10 hours per day.

1. How many days will the H-cylinder at 2200 psi last?

_____

_____

Medical Gas Therapy

▪ OBJECTIVES

Upon the completion of the chapter activities and content review topics, the student should be able to:

1. Describe the difference between hypoxemia and hypoxia.
2. Describe the basic goals of oxygen therapy.
3. Identify basic oxygen delivery devices.
4. Identify levels of hypoxemia.
5. Identify clinical signs of hypoxia.
6. Describe how to select an oxygen delivery system.
7. Administer oxygen therapy with a nasal cannula or mask.
8. Describe how to modify therapy to meet patient needs.
9. Administer oxygen therapy to a patient with an artificial airway.
10. Identify indications complications, and hazards of oxygen therapy.
11. Perform high-flow oxygen therapy.
12. Perform blender setup.

▪ KEY TERMS

- High-flow oxygen delivery systems
- Hypoxemia
- Hypoxia
- Low-flow oxygen delivery systems

▪ CONTENT REVIEW TOPICS

- Heliox therapy
- Humidity and bland aerosol therapy

- Hyperbaric oxygen (HBO) therapy
- Nitric oxide
- Oxygen-conserving devices
- Oxygen enclosures

▪ PROCEDURAL ASSESSMENTS

15-1 Administering Oxygen Therapy with a Nasal Cannula or Mask

15-2 Administering Oxygen Therapy to a Patient with an Artificial Airway

15-3 Administering high-Flow Oxygen Therapy

▪ EQUIPMENT

- Oxygen gas source
- Nasal cannula
- Simple face mask
- Nonrebreathing mask
- Aerosol face mask
- Face tent
- T-piece
- Tracheostomy collar
- Disposable gloves
- High-flow oxygen delivery system
- Mannequin with tracheostomy tube airway setup

As a respiratory care student, clinical decision making with regard to medical gas therapy plays a major role in your practice in becoming a high-quality clinician. This starts with extensive knowledge about medical gas therapy and its use in your goals and clinical objectives related to your patient's needs. Instructors and preceptors should facilitate your thought process when you are determining who needs oxygen, as well as when and how are you going to deliver it. This course of action requires you to compile data on numerous aspects, including the patient's chief complaint, history of present illness, and past medical history. This is why learning to perform an accurate patient assessment and then building a case for a particular therapy based on your interpretation of subjective and objective data are so imperative.

When delivering oxygen to a patient, it is important that you understand oxygen is a drug and its administration requires standing orders, protocols, or consultation with a physician. Just like other drugs, it may be misused in patient care. Respiratory therapists (RTs) must be knowledgeable about all aspects of the delivery devices and the complications that may result

in the oxygen therapy modality. This chapter will cover basic concepts in delivering oxygen therapy to patients.

> → **Reality Check** If you do not understand the operating characteristics of your medical gas therapy devices, you will not be able to choose the most appropriate device for your patient.

⟫ SKILL CHECK LISTS

15-1 Administering Oxygen Therapy with a Nasal Cannula or Mask

Correcting hypoxemia and decreasing the symptoms associated with it, as well as minimizing cardiopulmonary workload, should be the main concerns when deciding how to treat your patient. The two terms *hypoxemia* and *hypoxia* are used commonly when referring to conditions and symptoms affecting pulmonary patients. Hypoxemia is the abnormal deficiency of oxygen in the arterial blood, and hypoxia is the abnormal condition in which the oxygen available to the body cells is inadequate to meet the metabolic needs. These terms are frequently used interchangeably, but they do not mean the same thing, and they should be used appropriately when describing patient presentation.

Treating your patient begins with a thorough assessment to assess the need for oxygen therapy. Three basic ways to determine oxygen need include (1) lab measurements (Table 15-1), (2) the patient's clinical problem, and (3) its presentation during the bedside assessment (Table 15-2). Determination of the oxygen delivery device depends not only on the patient's oxygen needs but also on his or her level of cooperation with the use of the device. Common oxygen delivery devices are illustrated in Figure 15-1.

> → **Reality Check** If a patient feels claustrophobic because of an oxygen mask, you will have to find a device that works. A little oxygen via a nasal cannula is better than no oxygen because the patient keeps taking the mask off.

Real-life practice and experience will improve clinical judgment. Use your time as a student to learn from your instructors and preceptors' experiences, as well as from case study presentations by your classmates to build a solid foundation. The

TABLE 15-1 Hypoxemia/Hypoxia Classifications of PaO$_2$ and SpO$_2$

Classification	PaO$_2$	SpO$_2$
Normal	80–100 mm Hg	Greater than 95%
Mild hypoxemia	60–80 mm Hg	90%–94%
Moderate hypoxemia	40–60 mm Hg	75%–89%
Severe hypoxemia	Less than 40 mm Hg	Less than 75%

PaO$_2$, Partial pressure of oxygen; *SpO$_2$*, saturation of peripheral oxygen.

TABLE 15-2 Clinical Signs of Hypoxia

Finding	Mild to Moderate	Severe
Respiratory	Tachypnea Dyspnea Paleness	Tachypnea Dyspnea Cyanosis
Cardiovascular	Tachycardia Mild hypertension Peripheral vasoconstriction	Tachycardia, eventual bradycardia Arrhythmia Hypertension and eventual hypotension
Neurologic	Restlessness Disorientation Headaches Lethargy	Somnolence Confusion Distressed appearance Blurred vision Tunnel vision Loss of coordination Impaired judgment Slow reaction time Manic-depressive activity Coma

following is the step-by-step process for administering oxygen therapy with a nasal cannula or mask.

Procedural Preparation

1. Review the patient's chart, and note patient's most recent ABG results.
2. Verify the physician's order or the facility's protocol for standard of care.
3. Obtain, clean, and inspect the appropriate equipment prior to entering the patient's room.
4. Follow personal protective equipment (PPE) requirements, and observe standard precautions for any transmission-based isolation precaution.
5. Identify the patient using two patient identifiers.
6. Introduce yourself to the patient and to the family.
7. Explain the procedure to the patient and to the family, and acknowledge the patient's understanding.
8. Perform proper hand hygiene, and put on gloves, mask, and protective eyewear, as appropriate for the procedure.

Implementation

1. Place the patient in a comfortable position.
2. Assess vital signs.
3. Observe for signs and symptoms associated with hypoxemia.
4. Monitor pulse oximetry.
5. Choose the appropriate oxygen delivery device based on assessment and patient need.
6. Attach the nasal cannula or mask to the oxygen tube, and attach the oxygen tube to the oxygen source.
7. Turn on the flow.
8. Apply the oxygen delivery device properly, and adjust for the patient's comfort.
9. Allow sufficient slack on the oxygen tube.
10. Adjust the oxygen flow rate, as needed.
11. Remove the supplies from the patient's room, and clean the area, as needed.
12. Remove the PPE, and perform proper hand hygiene prior to leaving the patient's room.

Evaluation of Procedure

1. Establish a baseline, or compare with previous measurements.
2. Assess the patient's response to the procedure.
3. Develop an appropriate respiratory care plan based on assessment data.
4. Ensure proper functioning of the oxygen delivery device.
5. Consider humidification.
6. Identify any unexpected outcomes.

Documentation and Reporting

1. Record and report in the patient's chart the respiratory assessment findings, the method of oxygen delivery, and the patient's response before and during oxygen therapy.
2. Report any abnormal findings to the appropriate health care provider.

15-2 Administering Oxygen Therapy to a Patient with an Artificial Airway

Many patients have temporary or permanent artificial airways, and at times, they will require medical gas therapy. Besides

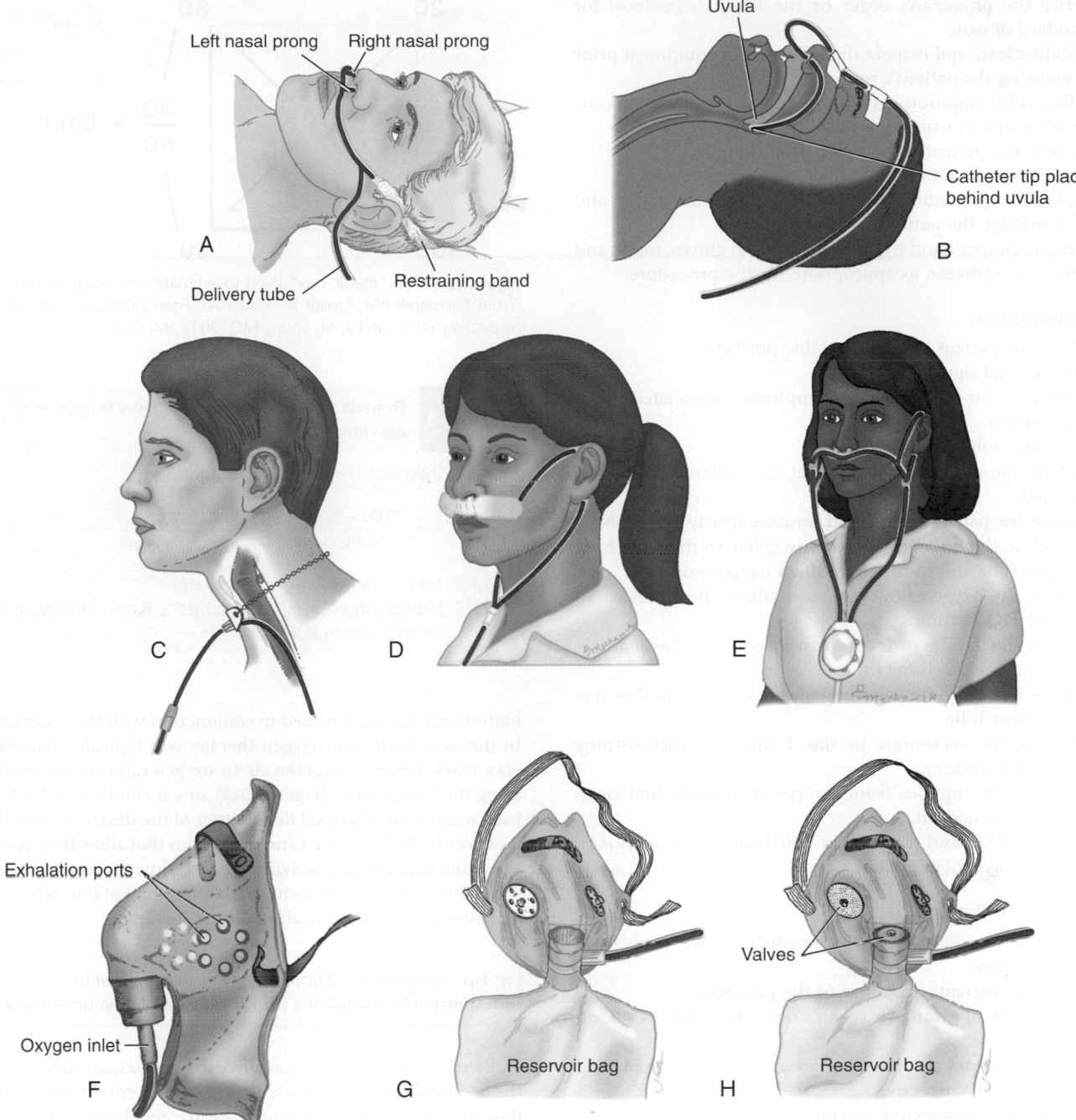

Figure 15-1 A, Nasal cannula. **B,** Nasal catheter. **C,** Transtracheal oxygen catheter. **D,** Reservoir cannula. **E,** Pendant reservoir cannula. **F,** Simple oxygen mask. **G,** Partial rebreathing mask. **H,** Nonrebreathing mask. (From Kacmarek RM, Stoller JK, Heuer AJ: *Egan's fundamentals of respiratory care*, ed 10, St. Louis, MO, 2013, Mosby.)

determining how to deliver the oxygen therapy, you must also consider the aspect of heating and humidifying the gas. All patients with endotracheal tubes or tracheostomy tubes receiving mechanical ventilation require some form of heat and humidification of the medical gas. Patients with permanent tracheostomy tubes, however, require heat and humidification on a case-by-case basis. It is the RT's responsibility to recognize the signs and symptoms of inadequate humidification and deliver the appropriate therapy, as needed.

Humidity and bland aerosol therapy are frequently needed, and this topic is covered in Chapter 13. The following is the step-by-step process for administering oxygen therapy to a patient with an artificial airway.

Procedural Preparation

1. Review the patient's chart, and note patient's most recent ABG results.

2. Verify the physician's order or the facility's protocol for standard of care.
3. Obtain, clean, and inspect the appropriate equipment prior to entering the patient's room.
4. Follow PPE requirements, and observe standard precautions for any transmission-based isolation precaution.
5. Identify the patient using two patient identifiers.
6. Introduce yourself to the patient and to the family.
7. Explain the procedure to the patient and to the family, and acknowledge the patient's understanding.
8. Perform proper hand hygiene, and put on gloves, mask, and protective eyewear, as appropriate for the procedure.

Implementation

1. Place the patient in a comfortable position.
2. Assess vital signs.
3. Observe for signs and symptoms associated with hypoxemia.
4. Monitor pulse oximetry.
5. Set up the suction equipment at the patient's bedside, if needed.
6. Assess for patent airway, and remove airway secretions.
7. Attach a T-tube or tracheostomy collar to the large-bore oxygen tube and to the humidified oxygen source.
8. Adjust the oxygen flow rate, and adjust the nebulizer to proper FiO_2 setting.
9. Attach the T-tube or tracheostomy collar to the endotracheal or tracheostomy tube.
10. Check if the T-tube is pulling on the endotracheal or tracheostomy tube.
11. Suction the secretions in the T-tube or tracheostomy collar, if necessary.
12. Remove the supplies from the patient's room, and clean the area, as needed.
13. Remove PPE, and perform proper hand hygiene prior to leaving the patient's room.

Evaluation of Procedure

1. Establish a baseline, or compare with previous measurements.
2. Assess the patient's response to the procedure.
3. Develop an appropriate respiratory care plan based on assessment data.
4. Observe the oxygen tube for accumulation of fluid, and drain the tube correctly.
5. Identify any unexpected outcomes.

Documentation and Reporting

1. Record and report in the patient's chart the respiratory assessment findings, the method of oxygen delivery, and the patient's response before and during oxygen therapy.
2. Report any abnormal findings to the appropriate health care provider.

15-3 Administering high-Flow Oxygen Therapy

High-flow oxygen delivery systems have the ability to deliver a precise and stable oxygen concentration to patients with flows that meet or exceed peak inspiratory flow needs. Heating and humidification must be taken into consideration when exposing the nasopharynx to high-flow rates. As a result,

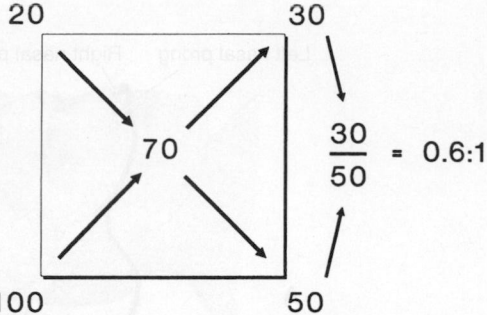

Figure 15-2 The "magic box" used to estimate air-to-oxygen ratio. (From Kacmarek RM, Stoller JK, Heuer AJ: *Egan's fundamentals of respiratory care*, ed 10, St. Louis, MO, 2013, Mosby.)

BOX 15-1	Formula to Calculate the Total Flow Output to an Air-Entrainment Device

Step 1: Calculate the air-to-oxygen ratio:

$$\frac{100 - \% \, Oxygen}{\% \, Oxygen - 21} = \frac{liters \; of \; air}{liters \; of \; oxygen}$$

Step 2: Add the air-to-oxygen ratio parts.
Step 3: Multiply the sum of the ratio parts times the flow set on the oxygen flowmeter.

humidification is often used in conjunction with these devices. In the past, high-flow oxygen therapy was typically delivered via a mask. Estimation of the air-to-oxygen ratio is obtained by using the "magic box" (Figure 15-2), or a formula (Box 15-1) is used to calculate the total flow output of the device. Currently, however, high-flow nasal cannula systems that allow the patient to eat and drink while receiving the high-flow therapy are available. These systems are comfortable for the patient, who has an easier time communicating during therapy.

> **Tip** A patient's total inspiratory flow demand can be estimated by multiplying their minute ventilation times three.

Blenders are devices typically used for oxygen delivery to the neonatal patient. As both air and oxygen enter the blender, they are passed through dual-pressure regulators, flow to a precision proportioning valve, and the gases are precisely mixed to the desired FiO_2 by varying the size of the air and oxygen inlets.

The following is the step-by-step process for high-flow oxygen delivery.

Procedural Preparation

1. Review the patient's chart.
2. Verify the physician's order or the facility's protocol for standard of care.
3. Obtain, clean, and inspect the appropriate equipment prior to entering the patient's room.
4. Follow PPE requirements, and observe standard precautions for any transmission-based isolation precaution.
5. Identify the patient using two patient identifiers.
6. Introduce yourself to the patient and to the family.

7. Explain the procedure to the patient and to the family, and acknowledge the patient's understanding.
8. Perform proper hand hygiene, and put on gloves, mask, and protective eyewear, as appropriate for the procedure.

Implementation

1. Place the patient in a comfortable position.
2. Assess vital signs.
3. Determine the appropriate FiO_2 and flow requirements needed to obtain the desired SaO_2 or SpO_2.
4. Attach the device to 50-psi gas source(s).

Air Entrainment System Using a Mask or Tracheostomy Collar

1. Attach the device to the flow meter.
2. Heat, if necessary.
3. Set to the predetermined FiO_2 and flow rate.
4. Ensure proper functioning of the device and aerosol production, if humidified.
5. Apply the device on the patient using a mask or tracheostomy collar.
6. Adjust FiO_2 and flow to maintain appropriate SpO_2.
7. Add a water trap to the system, if necessary.

Vapotherm System

1. Attach the disposable patient circuit.
2. Start up the device.
3. Adjust the flow.
4. Adjust the FiO_2.
5. Adjust the temperature.
6. Connect the device to the patient.

Fisher and Paykel Optiflow System

1. Attach the patient circuit to the high-flow device.
2. Warm the appropriate heating device.
3. Connect the high-pressure oxygen and air hoses to the wall outlet.
4. Attach the cannula to the patient:
   a. Set the flow at 20 to 60 L/min in the adult patient, working to meet the patient's inspiratory demand.
   b. Set the flow at 10 L/min or above for the pediatric patient, depending on the requirements of the patient.

5. Set the FiO_2 to obtain the appropriate oxygen saturation.
6. Reassess vital signs.
7. Remove the supplies from the patient's room, and clean the area, as needed.
8. Remove the PPE, and perform proper hand hygiene prior to leaving the patient's room.

Evaluation of Procedure

1. Ensure that the patient is comfortable with the high-flow device.
2. Ensure that the patient's FiO_2 and flow requirements are being met.
3. Develop an appropriate respiratory care plan based on assessment data.
4. Correlate SpO_2, if ABG values are available.
5. Identify any unexpected outcomes.

Documentation and Reporting

1. Record your findings in the patient's chart.
2. Report any abnormal findings to the appropriate health care provider.

Bibliography

Cairo JM: *Mosby's respiratory care equipment*, ed 9, St. Louis, MO, 2014, Mosby.

Des Jardins T: *Cardiopulmonary anatomy and physiology: essentials of respiratory care*, ed 6, Stamford, CT, 2012, Cengage Learning.

Kacmarek RM, Stoller JK, Heuer AJ: *Egan's fundamentals of respiratory care*, ed 10, St. Louis, MO, 2013, Mosby.

Khemani RG, Thomas NJ, Venkatachalam V, et al; Pediatric Acute Lung Injury and Sepsis Network Investigators (PALISI): Comparison of SpOs to PaOs based markers of lung disease severity for children with acute lung injury, *Crit Care Med* 40(4):1309–1316, 2012.

1. List the four indications for oxygen therapy.

   1. _____

   2. _____

   3. _____

   4. _____

2. List some possible complications of oxygen therapy.

   _____

   _____

   _____

   _____

   _____

   _____

   _____

3. Fill in the blanks for the timing of clinical assessment in the following scenarios:

   a. Within _____ hours of initiation with F_IO_2 less than 0.40

   b. Within _____ hours of with F_IO_2 greater than 0.40

   c. Within _____ hours in acute myocardial infarction

   d. Within _____ hours for any patient with a principal diagnosis of COPD

   e. Within _____ hours for the neonate

4. Identify the oxygen device illustrated in Figure 15-3. _____

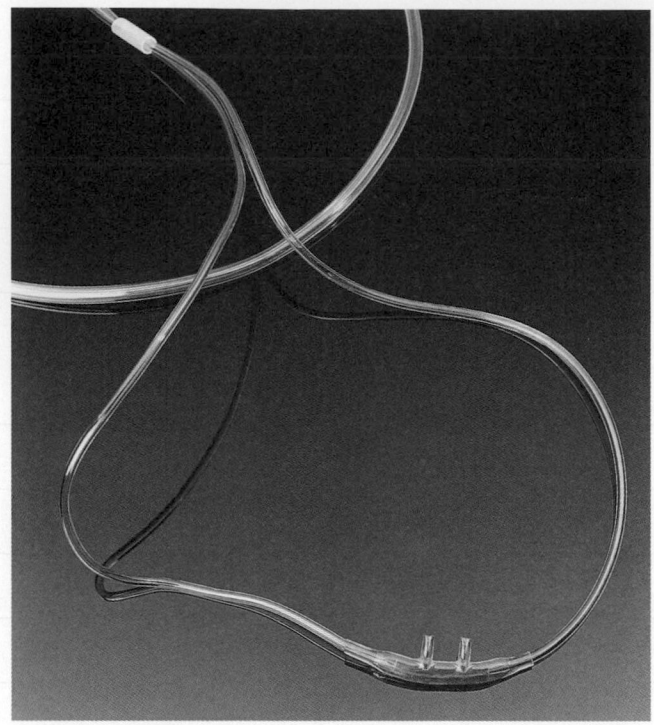

Figure 15-3 (From Cairo JM: *Mosby's respiratory care equipment*, ed 9, St. Louis, MO, 2014, Mosby.)

5. What is the F_IO_2 range for this device? _____

6. What is the operating liter flow range for this device? _____

7. What reservoir capacity does this device make use of? _____

8. What estimated F_IO_2 would be delivered at: _____

   a. 1 L/min _____

   b. 2 L/min _____

   c. 3 L/min _____

   d. 4 L/min _____

   e. 5 L/min _____

   f. 6 L/min _____

9. The device is running on a patient at 2 L/min.

    a. What estimated F_1O_2 is the patient receiving?

         _____

    b. If the patient began to breathe exclusively through his or her nose, what would happen to the delivered F_1O_2? Why?

         _____

    c. If the patient began to breathe exclusively through his or her mouth, what would happen to the delivered F_1O_2? Why?

         _____

10. Identify the oxygen device illustrated in Figure 15-4. _____

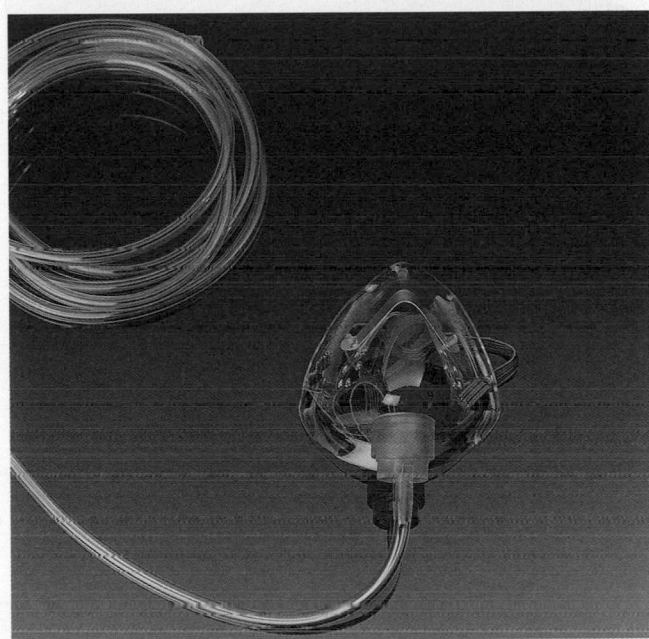

Figure 15-4 (From Cairo JM: *Mosby's respiratory care equipment*, ed 9, St. Louis, MO, 2014, Mosby.)

11. What is the F_1O_2 range for this device? _____

12. What is the operating liter flow range for this device? _____

13. What reservoir capacity does this device make use of? _____

14. The device is running on a patient at 8 L/min. _____

    a. If the patient began to breathe low tidal volumes, what would happen to the delivered F_1O_2? Why?

         _____

    b. If the patient began to breathe at a very fast rate, what would happen to the delivered F_1O_2? Why?

         _____

15. Identify the oxygen device illustrated in Figure 15-5._____

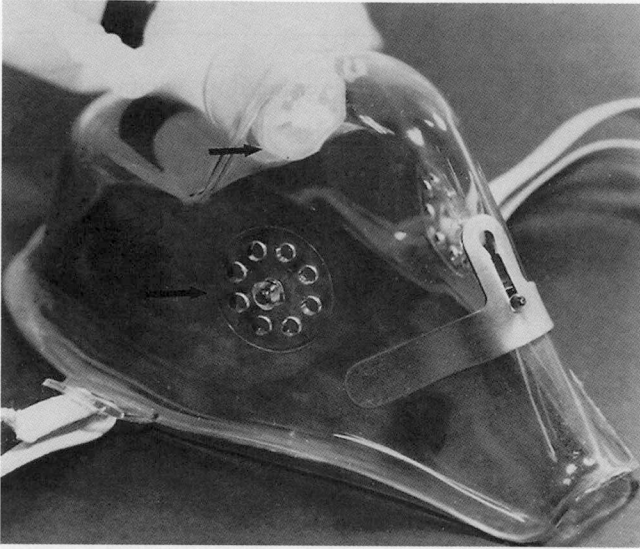

Figure 15-5 (From Gilmore TJ, Shoup CA: Laboratory exercises in respiratory care, ed 3, St. Louis, 1988, Mosby.)

16. What is the F_IO_2 range for this device? _____

17. What is the operating liter flow range for this device? _____

18. What reservoir capacity does this device make use of? _____

19. The device is running on a patient at 10 L/min. _____

    a. If the liter flow is lowered to 6 L/min, what would happen to the delivered F_IO_2? Why?

      _____

    b. If the liter flow is lowered to 6 L/min and the patient began to breathe at a very fast rate, what would happen to the delivered F_IO_2? Why?

      _____

    c. What would you do if the reservoir bag was collapsing during patient inspiration by more than one third?

      _____

20. Identify the oxygen device illustrated in Figure 15-6. _____

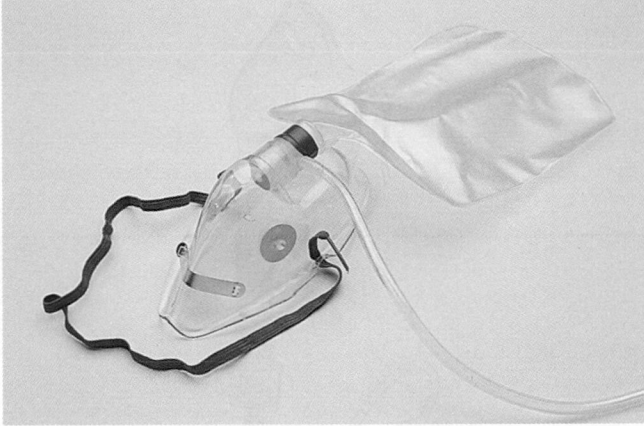

Figure 15-6 (From Sorrentino S, Gorek B: *Mosby's textbook for long-term care nursing assistants*, ed 6, St. Louis, MO, 2011, Mosby.)

21. What is the FiO$_2$ range for this device? _____

22. What is the operating liter flow range for this device? _____

23. What reservoir capacity does this device make use of? _____

24. The device is running on a patient at 10 L/min and the bag completely deflates at the peak of inspiration with each patient breath. _____

    a. How will this affect the patient clinically? _____

    b. How would you correct the problem? _____

25. Fill in the table below listing the variables that affect the FiO$_2$ delivery of a low-flow system:

Increases FiO$_2$	Decreases FiO$_2$

26. Identify the device in Figure 15-7. _____

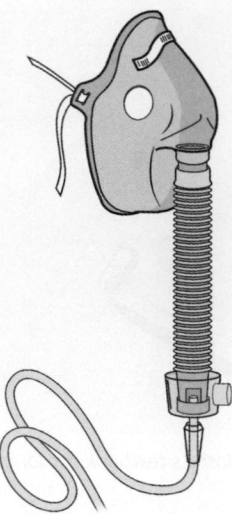

Figure 15-7 (From deWit SC: *Fundamental nursing concepts and skills*, ed 3, St. Louis, 2009, Saunders.)

27. What is the definition of a high-flow device? _____

28. What FiO_2 ranges are available for this device? _____

29. What is part B in Figure 15-7? When and why is it used? _____

30. What are the common liter flows for this device? _____

31. The device is running at 24% and 4 L/min. _____

    a. If the patient began to breathe in a shallow manner, what would happen to the FiO_2?

        _____

    b. If the patient began to breathe fast, what would happen to the FiO_2?

        _____

32.

FIO₂ Magic Box	Air-to-Oxygen Ratio	Total Flow of the Device at 4 L/min
FiO₂ 0.24		
FiO₂ 0.28		
FiO₂ 0.31		
FiO₂ 0.35		
FiO₂ 0.60		

33. Identify all the devices illustrated in Figure 15-8 on lines below.

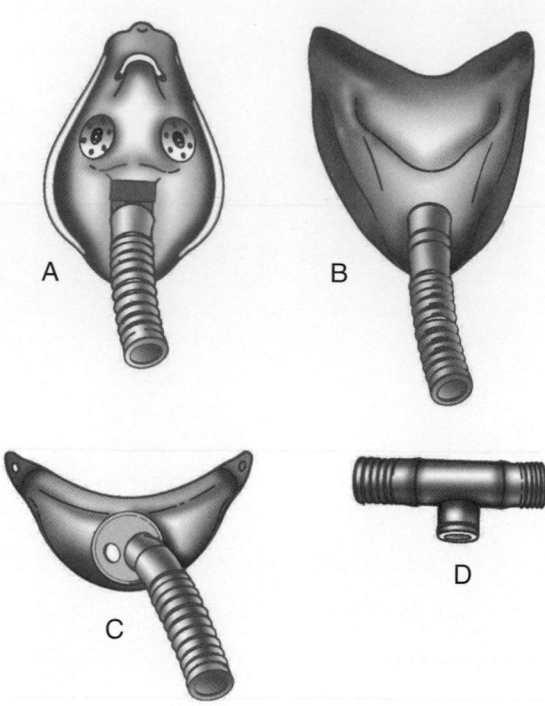

Figure 15-8 (From Kacmarek RM, Stoller JK, Heuer AJ: *Egan's fundamentals of respiratory care*, ed 10, St. Louis, MO, 2013, Mosby.)

A. _____

B. _____

C. _____

D. _____

34. Working with a lab partner, set up the above delivery devices using an air entrainment system and humidification. Using an oxygen analyzer, set each device at a specific FiO_2, and check its accuracy. Have your lab partner sign once you have completed the exercise.

Aerosol mask setup complete. Signature:_____

Face tent setup complete. Signature:_____

Tracheostomy setup complete. Signature:_____

T-tube setup complete. Signature:_____

35. Using one of the setups from question 34, add water to the corrugated tubing to simulate excess condensation and analyzer oxygen concentration from the device. What happened? Why?

_____

_____

_____

36. Give a clinical situation when each would be used.

a. Aerosol mask _____

b. Face tent _____

c. Tracheostomy _____

d. T-tube _____

37. Fill in the following table. Assume that the patient is breathing room air (FIO_2 0.21)

PaO₂	Level of Hypoxemia	Device/Liter Flow
80–100 mm Hg		
60–79 mm Hg		
40–59 mm Hg		
<40 mm Hg		

38. Determine the level of hypoxemia (if present) and what oxygen device at what liter flow or FIO_2 is needed to treat each of the following patients. Make sure you can explain your choice.

a. A patient complaining of chest pain with a normal ventilatory pattern and a PaO_2 of 67 mm Hg.

_____

b. A patient in respiratory distress with an unstable respiratory rate and a PaO_2 of 52 mm Hg.

_____

c. A patient with his upper airway bypassed by a tracheostomy tube and a PaO_2 of 56 mm Hg.

_____

d. A postoperative patient in respiratory distress, with a respiratory rate of 45 breaths per minute and a PaO_2 of 80 mm Hg, who is currently on a nasal cannula at 6 L/min.

_____

39. Set up all oxygen delivery devices available to you in your lab, and get your lab partner's signature.

Signature:_____

Signature:_____

Signature:_____

Signature:_____

40. Identify the device in Figure 15-9. _____

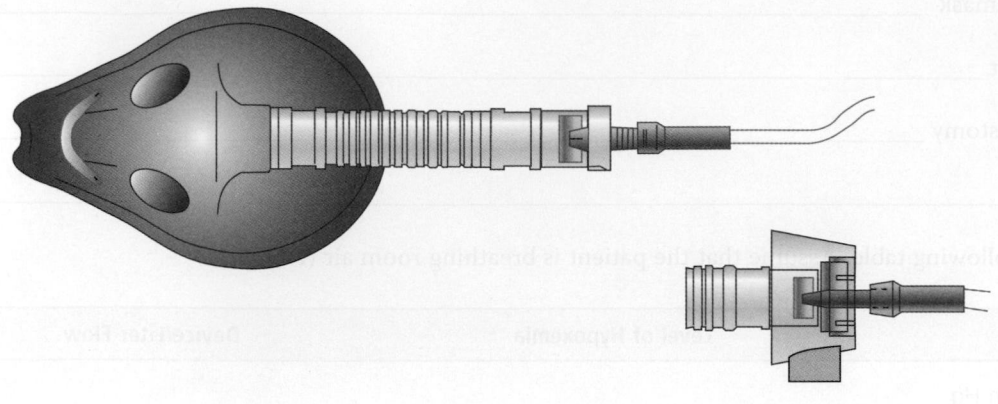

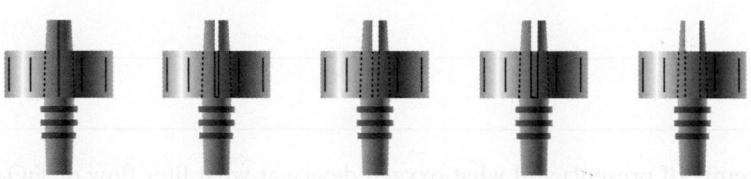

Figure 15-9 (From Kacmarek RM, Stoller JK, Heuer AJ: *Egan's fundamentals of respiratory care*, ed 10, St. Louis, MO, 2013, Mosby.)

41. Explain how the device in Figure 15-9 works.

_____

_____

42. Find this piece of equipment in the lab, and set it up with your lab partner. Have him or her sign off when this is completed.

Lab partner's signature:_____

43. Disconnect either the oxygen or the air to the blender. What happens?

_____

44. Give two clinical circumstances in which you would use the equipment in Figure 15-9.

a. _____

b. _____

Self-Assessment Questions

1. Goals of oxygen therapy include all of the following except:
   A. Correcting documented or suspected acute hypoxemia
   B. Improving a patient's carbon dioxide removal
   C. Decreasing symptoms associated with chronic hypoxemia
   D. Decreasing myocardial workload

2. Precautions and hazards of supplemental oxygen delivery include:

   1. Oxygen toxicity
   2. Depression of ventilation
   3. Absorption atelectasis
   4. Fire hazard

   A. 1 and 3 only
   B. 1, 2, and 3 only
   C. 2, 3, and 4 only
   D. 1, 2, 3, and 4

3. Unless a specialized device is used, flows delivered to newborns and infants should not exceed:
   A. 0.25 L/min
   B. 0.5 L/min
   C. 1 L/min
   D. 2 L/min

4. Your patient requires full-time oxygen therapy for chronic hypoxemia and is on a nasal cannula running at 4 L/min. The patient is complaining of soreness over the ears. What action should you take?
   A. Explain that it is part of wearing a nasal cannula and that the patient has to get used to it
   B. Loosen the straps or place cotton balls at pressure points
   C. Switch to a simple mask at 4 L/min
   D. Discontinue the oxygen because it is causing discomfort to the patient

5. A patient wearing a nasal cannula is exclusively nose breathing. What will happen to the FiO_2 being delivered by the device?
   A. It will go up.
   B. It will go down.
   C. It will remain the same.
   D. It depends on the patient's medical diagnosis.

6. To qualify as a high-flow device, a system should provide at least:
   A. 30 L/min
   B. 40 L/min
   C. 50 L/min
   D. 60 L/min

7. A patient is receiving 10 L/min oxygen through a partial rebreathing mask. The reservoir bag collapses completely before the end of each inspiration. What should you do to correct this?
   A. Increase the flow
   B. Decrease the flow
   C. Place the patient on humidified therapy via a nasal cannula at 10 L/min
   D. Place the patient on a simple mask at 15 L/min

8. What is the minimum liter flow range for an oxyhood?
   A. ≥ 7 L/min
   B. ≥ 10 L/min
   C. ≥ 12 L/min
   D. ≥ 15 L/min

9. Which of the following statements about an Isolette is false?
   A. It provides a temperature controlled environment.
   B. It is inexpensive and allows for patient mobility.
   C. It is best used in infants who need supplemental oxygen.
   D. It is not used in the adult population.

10. Which of the following variables will increase the delivered FiO_2 of a low-flow system?
    A. High inspiratory flow
    B. High tidal volume
    C. Short inspiratory time
    D. Slow rate of breathing

CASE STUDY 15-1

You have a patient that requires oxygen therapy. You choose a simple face mask at 5 L/min. The patient keeps removing the mask.

1. What should you do? Why?

_____

_____

CASE STUDY 15-3

A woman who was just pulled out of a house fire is admitted. She has soot around her nares, tachypnea, tachycardia, and clear lung sounds in all fields, with a pulse oxygen reading of 99% on room air.

1. What (if any) oxygen delivery device would you choose for this patient? Why, or why not?

_____

_____

CASE STUDY 15-2

You have a confused postoperative male patient breathing room air and exhibiting tachypnea, tachycardia, and mild peripheral cyanosis. His pulse oxygen reading is 96%.

1. What (if any) oxygen therapy would you recommend to his surgeon? Why, or why not?

_____

_____

CAST STUDY 15-4

You are treating a patient with COPD, who is hospitalized following a wrist injury. She is on 2 L/min oxygen therapy via a nasal cannula at home at all times. With regard to her respiratory status, she is complaint-free.

1. What, if any, oxygen delivery device should she be placed on? Why, or why not?

_____

_____

Lung Expansion Therapy

▪ OBJECTIVES

Upon the completion of the chapter activities and content review topics, the student should be able to:

1. Identify clinical signs of atelectasis.
2. Describe chest radiographic indications of atelectasis.
3. Identify the indications, contraindications, and hazards associated with incentive spirometry.
4. Perform patient teaching on the correct techniques for incentive spirometry.
5. Identify the indications, contraindications, and hazards associated with intermittent positive pressure breathing.
6. Perform patient teaching on the correct techniques for intermittent positive pressure breathing.
7. Identify the indications and steps for administering EzPAP.
8. Identify the indications and steps for the use of the MetaNeb System.

▪ KEY TERMS

- Atelectasis
- Flow-oriented device
- Incentive spirometry (IS)
- Intermittent positive pressure breathing (IPPB)
- Sustained maximal inspiration (SMI)
- Volume-oriented device

▪ CONTENT REVIEW TOPICS

- Intermittent use of continuous positive airway pressure (CPAP)
- Use of the MetaNeb system in-line with patients receiving invasive mechanical ventilation

▪ PROCEDURAL ASSESSMENTS

- 16-1 Performing Incentive Spirometry
- 16-2 Performing Intermittent Positive Pressure Breathing
- 16-3 Administering EzPAP
- 16-4 Using the MetaNeb system

▪ EQUIPMENT

- 50-psi air source
- 50-psi oxygen source
- Disposable IPPB circuit
- Disposable mouthpieces
- Disposable nose clips
- EzPAP device
- Incentive spirometry device
- IPPB machine (Bird 7, 8, or both; Bennett PR-1, PR-2, or both)
- MetaNeb
- MetaNeb Circuit
- Mouthpiece or mask
- MetaNeb Nebulizer Attachment
- Respirometer
- Stopwatch
- Test lung

Treating and preventing atelectasis, the collapse of distal lung parenchyma, should always be a main concern of a respiratory therapist (RT), especially when dealing with postoperative and bedridden patients. Correct therapy must be implemented early before atelectasis leads to deterioration of the patient's pulmonary status. A patient's medical history should provide the RT with the first indication that atelectasis may be present. Clinical signs of atelectasis, when recognized, often indicate considerable pulmonary involvement. Boxes 16-1 and 16-2 list these signs and chest radiography findings, which help confirm the presence of atelectasis. If the atelectasis becomes significant, hypoxemia may manifest clinically with tachycardia. Respiratory therapists must be vigilant in their assessments of patients to ensure that even the subtlest signs are not overlooked.

In the hospital setting, patients capable of ambulation will be assisted out of bed and encouraged to walk. This exercise has a dramatic influence and facilitates improvement in their pulmonary status. In cases with suspected or confirmed atelectasis, additional lung expansion modalities may also be supplemented to a patient's treatment regimen.

This chapter will discuss the concept of lung expansion and includes incentive spirometry (IS) and intermittent positive pressure breathing (IPPB) therapies. Understanding clinical signs and identifying patients at risk for developing atelectasis are also discussed.

≫ SKILL CHECK LISTS

16-1 Performing Incentive Spirometry

IS is used to treat and prevent atelectasis. Devices, illustrated in Figure 16-1, may be flow-oriented devices, which measure and visually indicate the inspiratory flow and equate it with volume, or volume-oriented devices, which measure and indicate visually the volume the patient is achieving during a

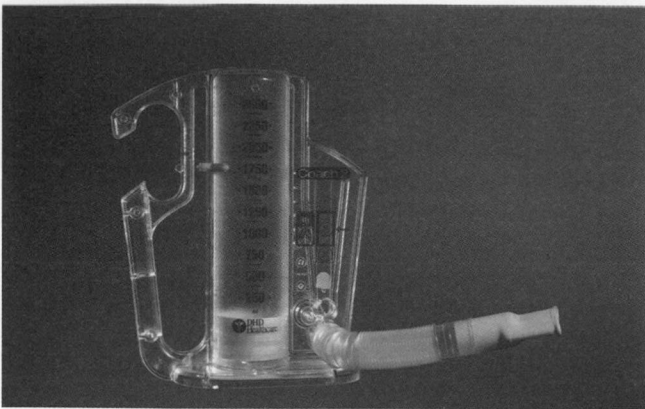

Figure 16-1 Volumetric incentive spirometer. (Smiths Medical, Dublin OH.)

BOX 16-1 **Clinical Signs of Atelectasis**

- Fine, late-inspiratory crackles
- Bronchial-type breath sounds
- Diminished lung sounds
- Tachycardia
- Abnormalities in respiratory and heart rates

BOX 16-2 **Chest Radiography Findings Indicating Atelectasis**

- Increased opacity in atelectatic region
- Evidence of volume loss
- Direct signs:
  - Displacement of the interlobar fissures
  - Crowding of the pulmonary vessels
  - Air bronchograms
- Indirect signs:
  - Elevation of diaphragm
  - Shift of trachea, heart, or mediastinum toward atelectasis
  - Pulmonary opacification
  - Narrowing of space between ribs
  - Compensatory hyperexpansion of surrounding lung

---

sustained maximal inspiration (SMI). To attain a SMI, the patient must breathe in slowly and deeply to total lung capacity (TLC) and then hold the breath for about 5 to 10 seconds. A comparison of alveolar and pleural pressure changes during a normal, spontaneous breath and during an SMI are illustrated in Figure 16-2.

Success and beneficial outcomes with IS are dependent on competent instruction regarding the use of the device.

> **Reality Check** IS does not help a patient if it just sits on the hospital bed-side table and is not used or is improperly used by the patient.

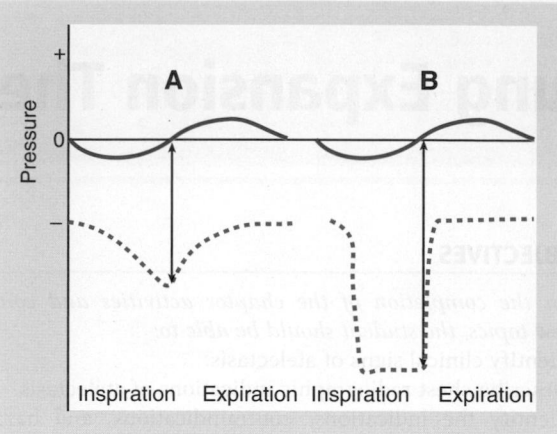

Figure 16-2 Alveolar (*solid lines*) and pleural (*dotted lines*) pressure during spontaneous breathing (*A*) and sustained maximal inspiration (SMI) (*B*). Note the difference in posterolateral gradients (*double arrows*). (From Kacmarek RM, Stoller JK, Heuer AJ: *Egan's fundamentals of respiratory care*, ed 10, St. Louis, MO, 2013, Mosby.)

BOX 16-3 **Incentive Spirometry: Patient Monitoring**

- Observe patient performance, and use the following:
  - Frequency of sessions
  - Number of breaths per session
  - Volume and flow goals achieved
  - Breath-hold maintained
  - Effort and motivation
  - Device within reach of patient and patient encouraged to perform independently
  - New and increasing inspiratory volumes established each day
  - Vital signs and breath sounds
- Periodically observe patient compliance; give additional instruction, as needed

(Modified from Kacmarek RM, Stoller JK, Heuer AJ: *Egan's fundamentals of respiratory care*, ed 10, St. Louis, MO, 2013, Mosby.)

Box 16-3 lists the assessment tools and monitoring parameters that help evaluate a patient's performance with the IS device.

The following is the step-by-step process for the use of incentive spirometry.

Procedural Preparation

1. Review the patient's chart.
2. Verify the physician's order or the facility's protocol for standard of care.
3. Obtain, clean, and inspect the appropriate equipment prior to entering the patient's room.
4. Follow personal protective equipment (PPE) requirements, and observe standard precautions for any transmission-based isolation procedure.
5. Identify the patient using two patient identifiers.
6. Introduce yourself to the patient and to the family.
7. Explain the procedure to the patient and to the family, and acknowledge the patient's understanding.
8. Perform proper hand hygiene, and put on gloves, mask, and protective eyewear, as appropriate for the procedure.

Implementation

1. Place the patient in the semi-Fowler position, and instruct the patient to breathe normally.
2. Assess vital signs.
3. Demonstrate how to place the mouthpiece and hold the device.
4. Instruct the patient to inhale slowly and deeply to a maximal inspiration while maintaining a constant flow through the device.
5. Instruct the patient to hold the breath for 5 to 10 seconds.
6. Instruct the patient to exhale passively through pursed lips (see PA 27-2).
7. Encourage the patient to cough.
8. Advise the patient to perform the maneuver 5 to 10 times every hour while awake.
9. Remove the supplies from the patient's room, and clean the area, as needed.
10. Remove PPE, and perform proper hand hygiene prior to leaving the patient's room.

Evaluation of Procedure

1. Establish a baseline, or compare with previous measurements.
2. Assess the patient's performance of maneuver, and coach the patient to improve proficiency with the device.
3. Identify any unexpected outcomes.
4. Correlate patient progress with chest radiographs and blood gas values, if available.

Documentation and Reporting

1. Record in the patient's chart the predicted goal volume and actual volume attained.
2. Report any abnormal findings to the appropriate health care provider.

16-2 Performing Intermittent Positive Pressure Breathing

IPPB is a treatment modality in which inspiratory positive pressure is applied to the airway of a spontaneously breathing patient on a short-term basis, usually lasting about 15 minutes per treatment to treat atelectasis. Figure 16-3 illustrates pressure changes during spontaneous breathing compared with IPPB.

In the past, IPPB was a widely accepted and commonly implemented therapy used for lung expansion by RTs. However, with little evidence of benefit for many patients and increasing cost-consciousness in respiratory departments, the use of IPPB has diminished. The American Association for Respiratory Care (AARC) has established comprehensive guidelines for the use of IPPB therapy.

> ✳ **Tip** IPPB is likely to be an infrequently performed procedure. Continuing education and refreshers on its use may be necessary before utilizing it on a patient. Always ask for help if you have not performed IPPB in the clinical setting.

Patients selected for IPPB therapy must be carefully chosen and the indications for therapy and goals clearly understood.

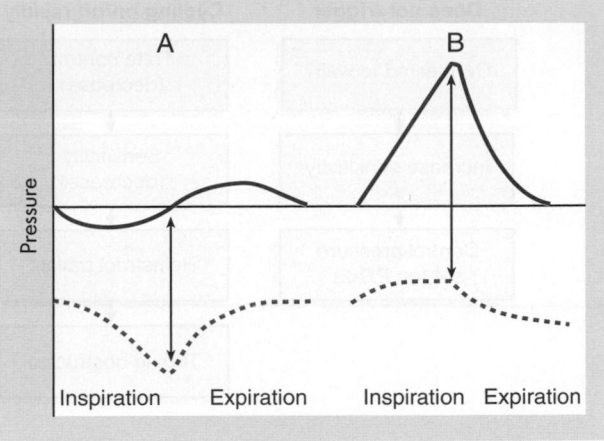

Figure 16-3 Alveolar (*solid lines*) and pleural (*dotted lines*) pressure changes during spontaneous breathing (*A*) and intermittent positive pressure breathing (IPPB) (*B*). Note the difference in posterolateral gradients (*double arrows*). (From Kacmarek RM, Stoller JK, Heuer AJ: *Egan's fundamentals of respiratory care*, ed 10, St. Louis, MO, 2013, Mosby.)

Troubleshooting the machine is important to ensure the best patient outcomes. The chart in Figure 16-4 illustrates some common problems and how to correct them. When determining the effectiveness of the therapy, the RT should evaluate for improved breath sounds, increased tidal volume by 25%, and an increase in the vital capacity to 15 mL/kg. The following is the step-by-step process for the use of IPPB as a lung expansion therapy.

> ✳ **Tip** IPPB may be utilized as a learning tool and an introduction for the concepts involved in invasive mechanical ventilation.

Procedural Preparation

1. Review the patient's chart.
2. Verify the physician's order or the facility's protocol for standard of care.
3. Obtain, clean, and inspect the appropriate equipment prior to entering the patient's room.
4. Follow PPE requirements, and observe standard precautions for any transmission-based isolation procedure.
5. Identify the patient using two patient identifiers.
6. Introduce yourself to the patient and to the family.
7. Explain the procedure to the patient and to the family, and acknowledge the patient's understanding.
8. Perform proper hand hygiene, and put on gloves, mask, and protective eyewear, as appropriate for the procedure.

Implementation

1. Place the patient in the semi-Fowler position, and instruct the patient to breathe normally.
2. Assess vital signs.
3. Obtain baseline values for inspiratory capacity, expiratory tidal volume, and peak expiratory flow rate.
4. Check machine sensitivity:
    a. Increase sensitivity control until the machine self-cycles.
    b. Return to the sensitivity level if it does not self-cycle.

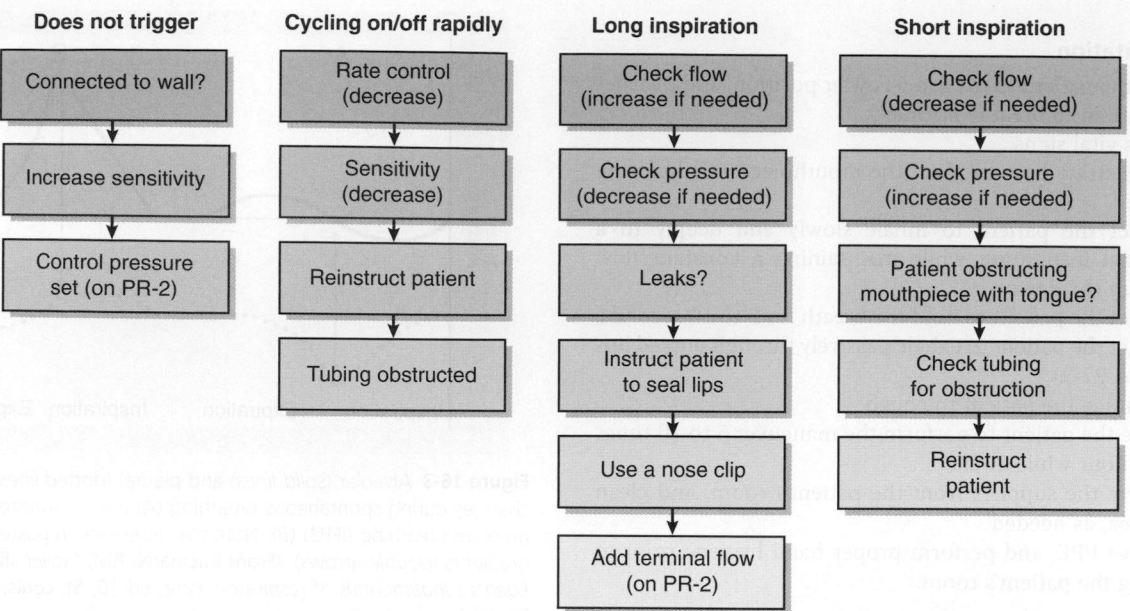

Does not trigger	Cycling on/off rapidly	Long inspiration	Short inspiration
Connected to wall?	Rate control (decrease)	Check flow (increase if needed)	Check flow (decrease if needed)
Increase sensitivity	Sensitivity (decrease)	Check pressure (decrease if needed)	Check pressure (increase if needed)
Control pressure set (on PR-2)	Reinstruct patient	Leaks?	Patient obstructing mouthpiece with tongue?
	Tubing obstructed	Instruct patient to seal lips	Check tubing for obstruction
		Use a nose clip	Reinstruct patient
		Add terminal flow (on PR-2)	

Figure 16-4 IPPB critical thinking flow chart.

5. Check the machine and circuit for leaks:
   a. Occlude the outlet, and observe the pressure cycling.
6. Instruct the patient on how to breathe correctly:
   a. Explain to the patient how to initiate a breath and how expiration occurs; expiration occurs passively and should be two to three times as long as inspiration.
7. Adjust the machine as required by the patient's ventilatory patterns:
   a. Use flow, pressure, or sensitivity.
8. Monitor inspiratory capacity, respiratory rate, heart rate, and blood pressure midway through the procedure.
9. Encourage the patient to cough.
10. Reassess vital signs.
11. Remove the supplies from the patient's room, and clean the area, as needed.
12. Remove PPE, and perform proper hand hygiene prior to leaving the patient's room.

Evaluation of Procedure

1. Establish a baseline, or compare with previous measurements.
2. Monitor the effectiveness of therapy.
3. Develop an appropriate respiratory care plan based on assessment data.
4. Return the patient to the previous oxygen modality.
5. Identify any unexpected outcomes.

Documentation and Reporting

1. Record your findings in the patient's chart.
2. Report any abnormal findings to the appropriate health care provider.

16-3 Administering EzPAP

Another device used for lung expansion therapy to aid in the treatment and prevention of atelectasis is EzPAP Positive

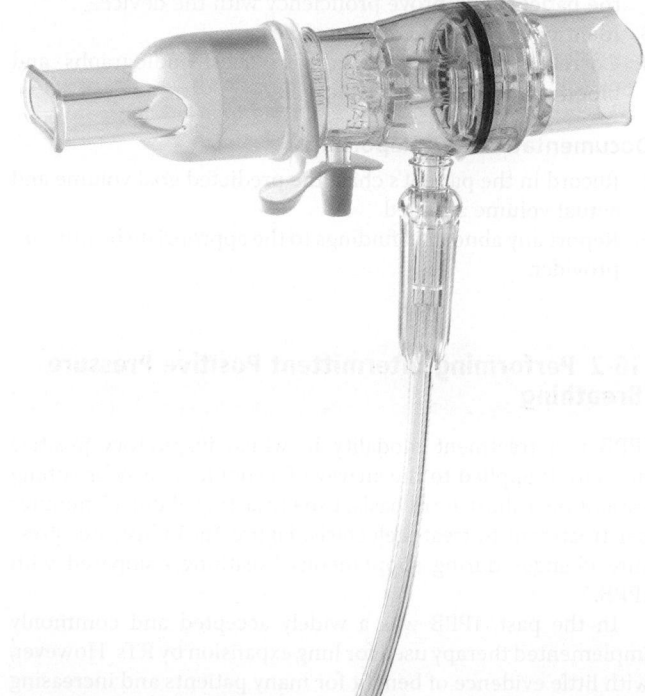

Figure 16-5 EzPAP® Positive Airway Pressure System. (Courtesy of Smiths Medical, Norwell, MA.)

Airway Pressure System (Smiths Medical, Norwell, MA) (Figure 16-5). It is often used when a patient has difficulties with incentive spirometry. It may be administered using a mouthpiece or a mask, and it allows for the addition of an in-line nebulizer during use. Positive airway pressure is produced via a flowmeter, using oxygen or air, throughout the patient's breathing cycle. The following is the step-by-step process for the use of EzPAP.

Procedural Preparation

1. Review the patient's chart.
2. Verify the physician's order or the facility's protocol for standard of care.
3. Obtain, clean, and inspect the appropriate equipment prior to entering the patient's room.
4. Follow PPE requirements, and observe standard precautions for any transmission-based isolation procedure.
5. Identify the patient using two patient identifiers.
6. Introduce yourself to the patient and to the family.
7. Explain the procedure to the patient and to the family, and acknowledge the patient's understanding.
8. Perform proper hand hygiene, and put on gloves, mask, and protective eyewear, as appropriate for the procedure.

Implementation

1. Place the patient in the semi-Fowler position.
2. Assess vital signs.
3. Assemble the unit:
   a. Connect the tube to the flowmeter.
   b. Connect the other end to the EzPAP device's gas inlet port.
   c. Connect one end of the second tube to the pressure port.
   d. Connect the other end to a pressure monitoring device such as a pressure monometer or high and low pressure indicator (if no pressure monitoring device is available, seal the pressure port).
4. Attach the mouthpiece or the face mask to the rounded end of the device.
5. Instruct the patient to relax while performing diaphragmatic breathing (see PA 27-3).
6. Set the initial flow rate to 5 L/min on the air or oxygen flowmeter.
7. Attach the appliance to the patient.
8. Monitor the airway pressure while slowly increasing the flowmeter until the desired expiratory airway pressure is reached (10–20 cmH$_2$O).
9. Instruct the patient to inhale and exhale slowly, as this will assist in maintaining adequate airway pressure during the breathing cycle.
10. Reassess vital signs.
11. Remove the supplies from the patient's room, and clean the area, as needed.
12. Remove PPE, and perform proper hand hygiene prior to leaving the patient's room.

Evaluation of Procedure

1. Establish a baseline, or compare with previous measurements.
2. Assess the patient's performance of the maneuver, and coach the patient to improve proficiency with the device.
3. Identify any unexpected outcomes.
4. Correlate patient progress with chest radiographs and blood gas values, if available.

Documentation and Reporting

1. Record pressure, flow rates, and patient's tolerance to the procedure in the patient's chart.
2. Report any abnormal findings to the appropriate health care provider.

16-4 Using the MetaNeb® System

The MetaNeb® system is used to aid in the treatment and prevention of atelectasis as well as enhance secretion removal (Figure 16-6). It has three available modes including; aerosol mode which is used to deliver aerosolized medication, continuous high frequency oscillation (CHFO) mode which is a pneumatic form of chest physiotherapy, and continuous positive expiratory pressure (CPEP) mode which provides a constant airway pressure which aids in splinting open and expanding airways. Box 16-4 lists the possible adverse reactions a patient can experience when receiving therapy with the MetaNeb system. Aerosolized medication can be delivered in all three modes. Box 16-5 lists patients who may benefit from the MetaNeb system. The following is the step-by-step process for use of the MetaNeb system.

BOX 16-4	Possible Adverse Reactions

- Hyperventilation
- Gastric distention
- Decreased cardiac output
- Increased intracranial pressure
- Increased air trapping
- Hyperoxygenation
- Pneumothorax
- Pulmonary air leak
- Pulmonary hemorrhage

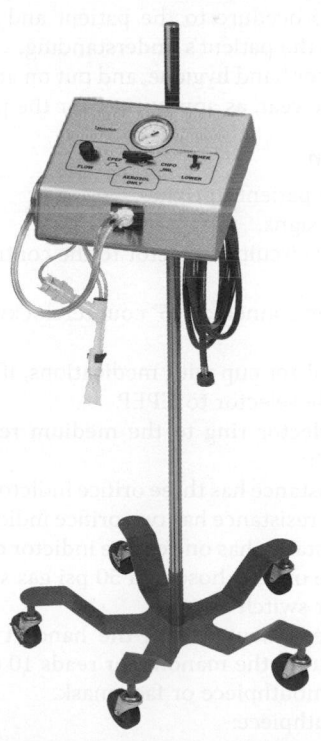

Figure 16-6 The MetabNeb® System (The MetaNeb System User Manual (162902 Rev 2) © 2010 Hill-Rom Services, Inc. REPRINTED WITH PERMISSION—ALL RIGHTS RESERVED)

BOX 16-5 Disease States Which May Benefit from MetaNeb

- Bronchiolitis
- Cystic fibrosis
- Asthma
- Chronic bronchitis
- Bronchiectasis
- Neuromuscular disorders
- Emphysema
- Patients in need of postoperative airway management

✱ **Tip** Aerosol mode is used for medication administration only, CPEP mode aids in the mobilization of secretions while splinting the airways open, and CHFO mode can be used to enhance mucus clearance and resolve atelectasis.

→ **Reality Check** Absolute contraindications for the use of MetaNeb include untreated tension pneumothorax or an untrained or unskilled operator.

Procedural Preparation

1. Review the patient's chart.
2. Verify the physician's order or the facility's protocol for standard of care.
3. Obtain, clean, and inspect the appropriate equipment prior to entering the patient's room.
4. Follow PPE requirements, and observe standard precautions for any transmission-based isolation procedure.
5. Identify the patient using two patient identifiers.
6. Introduce self to the patient and the family.
7. Explain the procedure to the patient and the family, and acknowledge the patient's understanding.
8. Perform proper hand hygiene, and put on gloves, mask, and protective eyewear, as appropriate for the procedure.

Implementation

1. Position the patient upright.
2. Assess vital signs.
3. Connect the circuit connector to the controller connector port.
   a. Rotate the connector 45° counterclockwise to lock it in position.
4. Fill the nebulizer cup with medications, if applicable.
5. Set the mode selector to CPEP.
6. Turn the selector ring to the medium resistance setting (Figure 16-7).
   a. High resistance has three orifice indictor dots.
   b. Medium resistance has two orifice indictor dots.
   c. Low resistance has one orifice indictor dot.
7. Connect the oxygen hose to a 50 psi gas source.
8. Turn master switch on.
9. Occlude the patient end of the handset and adjust the CPEP flow until the manometer reads 10 cmH₂O.
10. Attach the mouthpiece or face mask.
    For the mouthpiece:
    a. Attach the mouthpiece to the handset (Figure 16-8)
    b. Connect the nebulizer cup to the nebulizer port on the bottom of the handset.

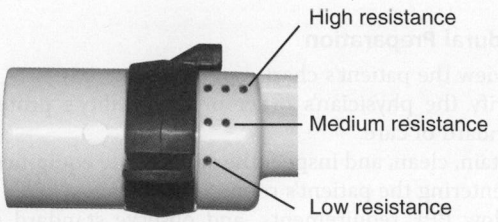

Figure 16-7 Turn the selector ring to the medium resistance setting: align the selector ring tab with the two orifice indicator dots (medium opening and medium resistance). (The MetaNeb System User Manual (162902 Rev 2) © 2010 Hill-Rom Services, Inc. REPRINTED WITH PERMISSION—ALL RIGHTS RESERVED)

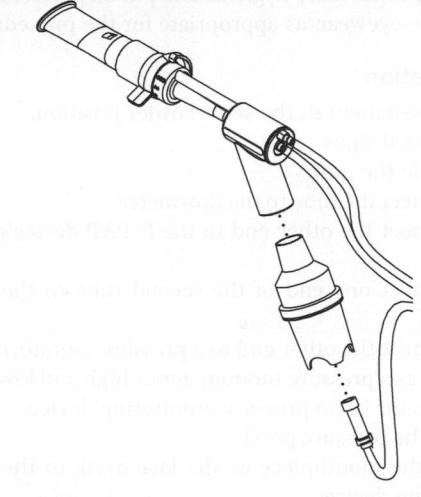

Figure 16-8 Attach the mouthpiece to the handset: insert at a 45° angle and gently push in and twist to the proper orientation. Then, connect the nebulizer port in the bottom of the handset. (The MetaNeb System User Manual (162902 Rev 2) © 2010 Hill-Rom Services, Inc. REPRINTED WITH PERMISSION—ALL RIGHTS RESERVED)

   c. Without twisting the green hose of the tubing, connect it to the bottom of the nebulizer.
   d. If using the mouthpiece, instruct patient to inhale and exhale through the mouthpiece.
   e. Ensure the patient creates a tight seal around the mouthpiece.
For the mask:
   a. Remove the 22 mm × 22 mm adapter from the package (Figure 16-9).
   b. Inset the adapter at a 45° angle, lightly put it in and twist.
   c. Without twisting the green hose of the tubing, connect it to the bottom of the nebulizer.
11. Encourage slow exhalation.
12. Adjust the ring selector as applicable for the patient.
   a. Three dots is the highest resistance.
   b. One dot is the lowest resistance.
13. Continue CPEP for about 2 ½ minutes.
14. Inform the patient that they are about to feel a pulsating flow of gas.
15. Move the Higher/Lower switch to the Higher position and change the mode to CHFO.
   a. The Lower setting switch reduces the percussion rate and the pressure.
   b. This may be used as an introductory mode.
   c. The Higher switch position can be used to enhance the therapy.

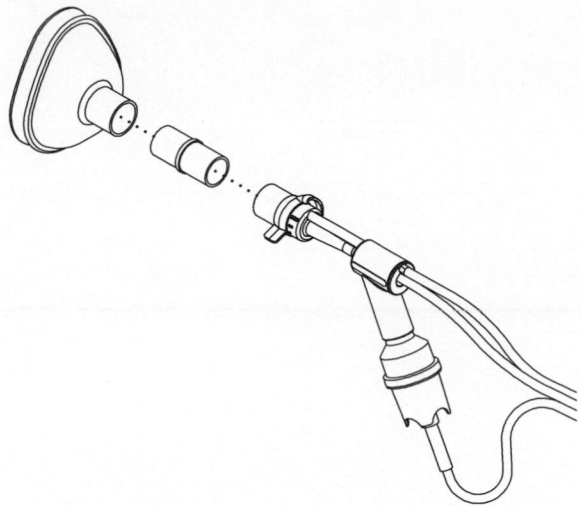

Figure 16-9 For mask configuration, insert the adapter at a 45° angle and gently push it in and twist. (The MetaNeb System User Manual (162902 Rev 2) © 2010 Hill-Rom Services, Inc. REPRINTED WITH PERMISSION—ALL RIGHTS RESERVED)

16. Encourage slow exhalation.
17. Continue CHFO for about 2 ½ minutes.
18. Alternate between CPEP and CHFO until therapy is complete.
    a. Therapy lasts about 10 minutes.
19. Turn Metaneb machine off.
    a. Disconnect nebulizer from Metaneb.
    b. Empty nebulizer cup of residual medication.
    c. Put nebulizer in bag so that it is available for the next treatment.
    d. Detach oxygen tubing from wall outlet.
20. Remove the supplies from the patient's room, and clean the area, as needed.
21. Remove PPE, and perform proper hand hygiene prior to leaving the patient's room.

Evaluation of Procedure

1. Establish a baseline, or compare with previous measurements.
2. Identify any unexpected outcomes.
3. Correlate the patient's progress with chest radiographs and blood gas values, if available.

Documentation and Reporting

1. Record the settings, medications, and the patient's tolerance to the procedure in the patient's chart.
2. Report any abnormal findings to the appropriate health care provider.

Bibliography

American Association for Respiratory Care: The pros and cons of IPPB: AARC provides an assessment on its effectiveness, *AARC Times* 10:48, 1986.

American Thoracic Society statement on the use of intermittent positive pressure breathing, *Respiratory Care* 24(8):398–699, 1979.

Cairo JM: *Mosby's respiratory care equipment*, ed 9, St. Louis, MO, 2014, Mosby.

Celli BR, Rodriguez KS, Snider GL: A controlled trial of intermittent positive pressure breathing, incentive spirometry, and deep breathing exercises in preventing pulmonary complication after abdominal surgery, *Am Rev Respir Dis* 130(1):12–5, 1984.

Kacmarek RM, Stoller JK, Heuer AJ: *Egan's fundamentals of respiratory care*, ed 10, St. Louis, MO, 2013, Mosby.

MetaNeb® System User Manual. (162902), © 2010 by Hill-Rom Services, Inc. MetaNeb® is a registered trademark of Comedica, Inc.

Restrepo RD, Wettstein R, Wittnelbel L, et al: Incentive spirometry, *Respir Care* 56(10):1600–1604, 2011.

1. List three indications for incentive spirometry (IS) and how it could help treat or prevent atelectasis.

   a. _____

   b. _____

   c. _____

2. List five contraindications for IS and explain why it would be contraindicated.

   _____

   _____

   _____

   _____

   _____

3. List five hazards or complications of IS and how to prevent them.

   _____

   _____

   _____

   _____

   _____

4. Teach IS to two classmates. Get their signatures once you have correctly set up their goal volumes and have given the instructions.

   Signature #1: _____

   Signature #2: _____

5. List five indications for intermittent positive pressure breathing (IPPB) and how it could help treat or prevent atelectasis.

   _____

   _____

   _____

   _____

6. List five contraindications for IPPB and explain why it would be contraindicated.

_____

_____

_____

_____

_____

7. List five hazards or complications of IPPB and how to prevent them.

_____

_____

_____

_____

_____

8. List nine possible adverse reactions a patient receiving MetaNeb thearapy could experience.

_____

_____

_____

_____

_____

_____

_____

_____

_____

Exercises 9 to 17 should be completed using a Bennett PR-1 ventilator, PR-2 ventilator, or both.

9. Label Figure 16-10:

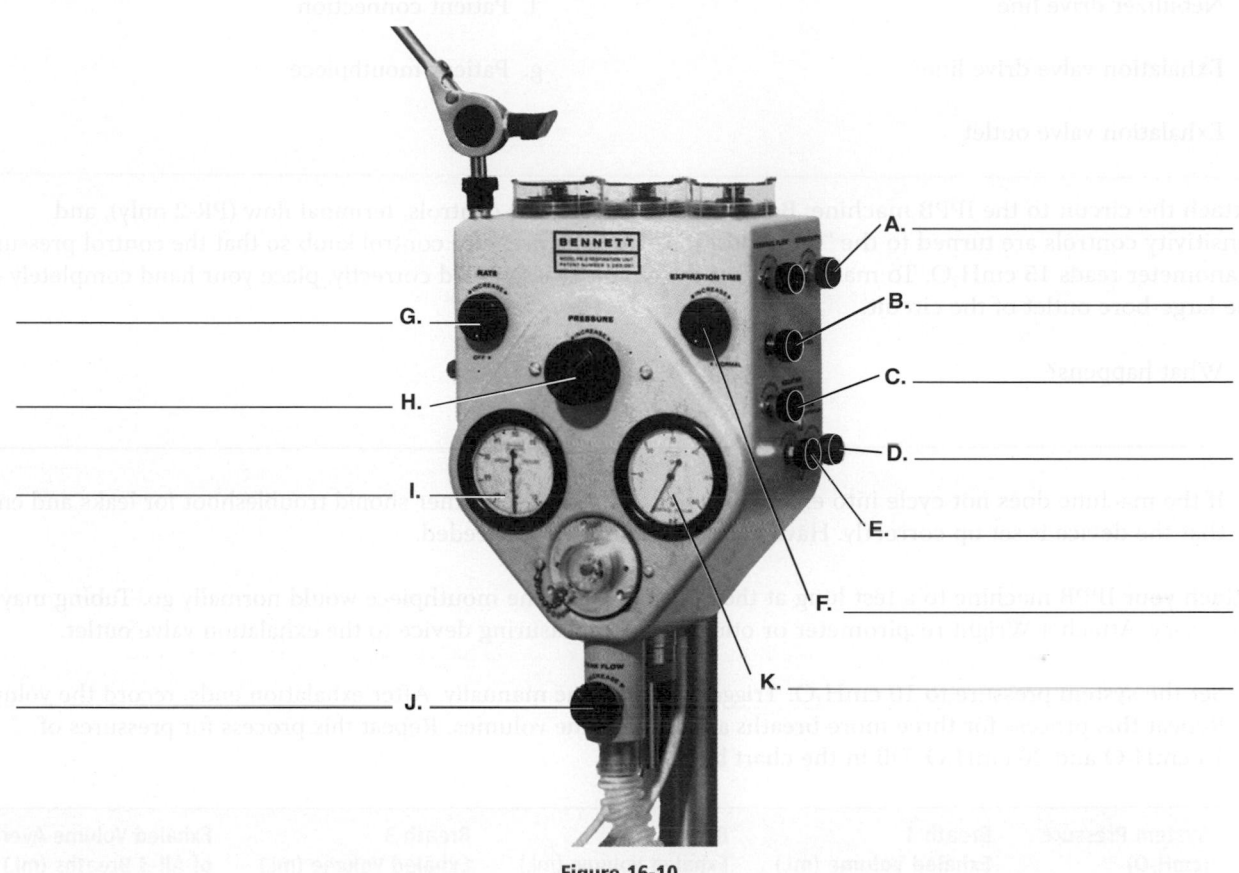

A. _____

B. _____

C. _____

D. _____

E. _____

F. _____

G. _____

H. _____

I. _____

J. _____

K. _____

Figure 16-10

10. With a lab partner, identify the following features on the Bennett PR-1 ventilator, PR-2 ventilator, or both:

a. Gas inlet

b. Gas outlet to patient

c. Bennett valve and housing

d. Adjustable pressure regulator

e. Control pressure gauge

f. System pressure gauge

g. Sensitivity control

h. Oxygen/air diluter control

i. Nebulizer controls

j. Valve driveline connection

k. Nebulizer driveline connection

l. Terminal flow control (PR-2 only)

m. Peak flow control (PR-2) only

11. Obtain an IPPB circuit from your lab instructor. Identify the following features:

   a. Main bore outlet connection

   b. Nebulizer drive line

   c. Exhalation valve drive line

   d. Exhalation valve outlet

   e. Nebulizer cup

   f. Patient connection

   g. Patient mouthpiece

12. Attach the circuit to the IPPB machine. Be sure that the nebulizer controls, terminal flow (PR-2 only), and sensitivity controls are turned to the "OFF" position. Turn the pressure control knob so that the control pressure manometer reads 15 cmH$_2$O. To make sure that the circuit is assembled correctly, place your hand completely over the large-bore outlet of the circuit.

   a. What happens?

   _____

   b. If the machine does not cycle into expiration, you and your lab partner should troubleshoot for leaks and ensure that the device is set up correctly. Have your instructor help, if needed.

13. Attach your IPPB machine to a test lung at the position where the mouthpiece would normally go. Tubing may be necessary. Attach a Wright respirometer or other volume-measuring device to the exhalation valve outlet.

   a. Set the system pressure to 10 cmH$_2$O. Trigger the machine manually. After exhalation ends, record the volume. Repeat this process for three more breaths and average the volumes. Repeat this process for pressures of 15 cmH$_2$O and 20 cmH$_2$O. Fill in the chart below:

System Pressure (cmH$_2$O)	Breath 1 Exhaled Volume (mL)	Breath 2 Exhaled Volume (mL)	Breath 3 Exhaled Volume (mL)	Exhaled Volume Average of All 3 Breaths (mL)
10				
15				
20				

   b. What happens to the exhaled volume if the pressure is increased?

   _____

14. On the IPPB machine, set the system pressure to 15 cmH$_2$O. Rotate the inspiratory nebulizer control knob at least two full turns counter-clockwise to open. Measure the exhaled volumes in the chart below:

Pressure of 15 cmH$_2$O

Volume with nebulizer off _____ mL   Volume with nebulizer on _____ mL

   a. Did the tidal volume increase, decrease, or stay the same? _____

   b. Why?

   _____

15. Connect a circuit to IPPB machine and a test lung. Set the sensitivity to the "OFF" position by turning the knob clockwise, until it stops. Rapidly squeezing your test lung will manually trigger the device.

   a. Manually trigger the machine, and note the deflection of the manometer needle just prior to the beginning of inspiration.

   b. Rotate the knob one full turn, and repeat step *a*.

   c. Continue to rotate the knob one full turn, and manually trigger after each breath until you notice the machine goes into inspiration automatically without having to touch the test lung.

   d. How many turns of the knob does it take until the device self-triggers? _____

   e. What is the sensitivity control used for?

   _____

16. On the IPPB machine, set the pressure to 15 cmH$_2$O. Make sure that the nebulizer, terminal flow (set on PR-2 only), and sensitivity controls are all turned to the "OFF" position.

   a. Trigger the machine several times manually using the Bennett valve. Measure the inspiratory time:

      _____seconds

   b. Keep the pressure at 15 cmH$_2$O but turn on the terminal flow two to three full turns. Cycle the machine several times by manually using the Bennett valve. Measure the inspiratory time: _____seconds

   c. Is there a difference? Why, or why not?

   _____

   _____

   d. What can the terminal flow control help with?

   _____

   _____

17. What is the peak flow control used for?

   _____

   _____

Questions 18 to 24 should be completed using a Bird Mark 7, Bird Mark 8, or both.

18. With a lab partner, thoroughly inspect the machine(s), and identify the following features:

a. Gas outlet to patient

b. Pressure manometer

c. Sensitivity

d. Pressure control

e. Flow control

f. Air mix control

g. Expiratory timer

h. Nebulizer/exhalation drive line connector

19. Label the Bird Mark 7 ventilator in Figure 16-11.

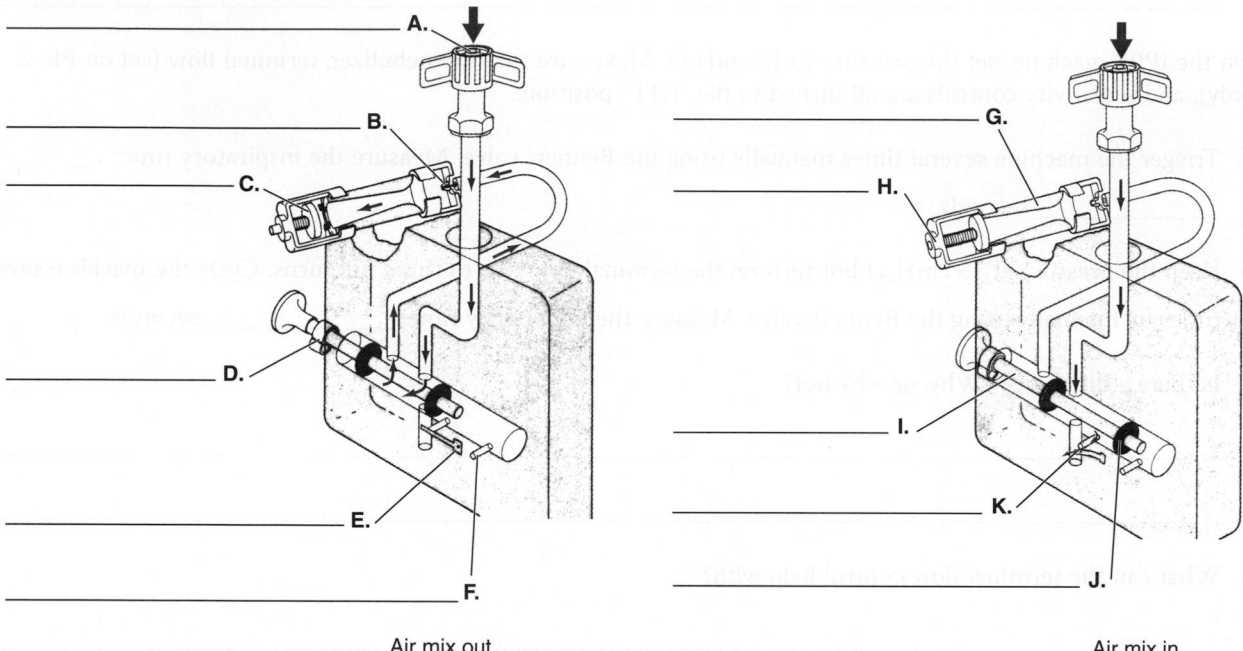

Air mix out   Air mix in

Figure 16-11 Bird Mark 7. (Modified from Cairo JM: *Mosby's respiratory care equipment*, ed 9, St. Louis, MO, 2014, Mosby.)

20. Label the Bird Mark 8 ventilator in Figure 16-12.

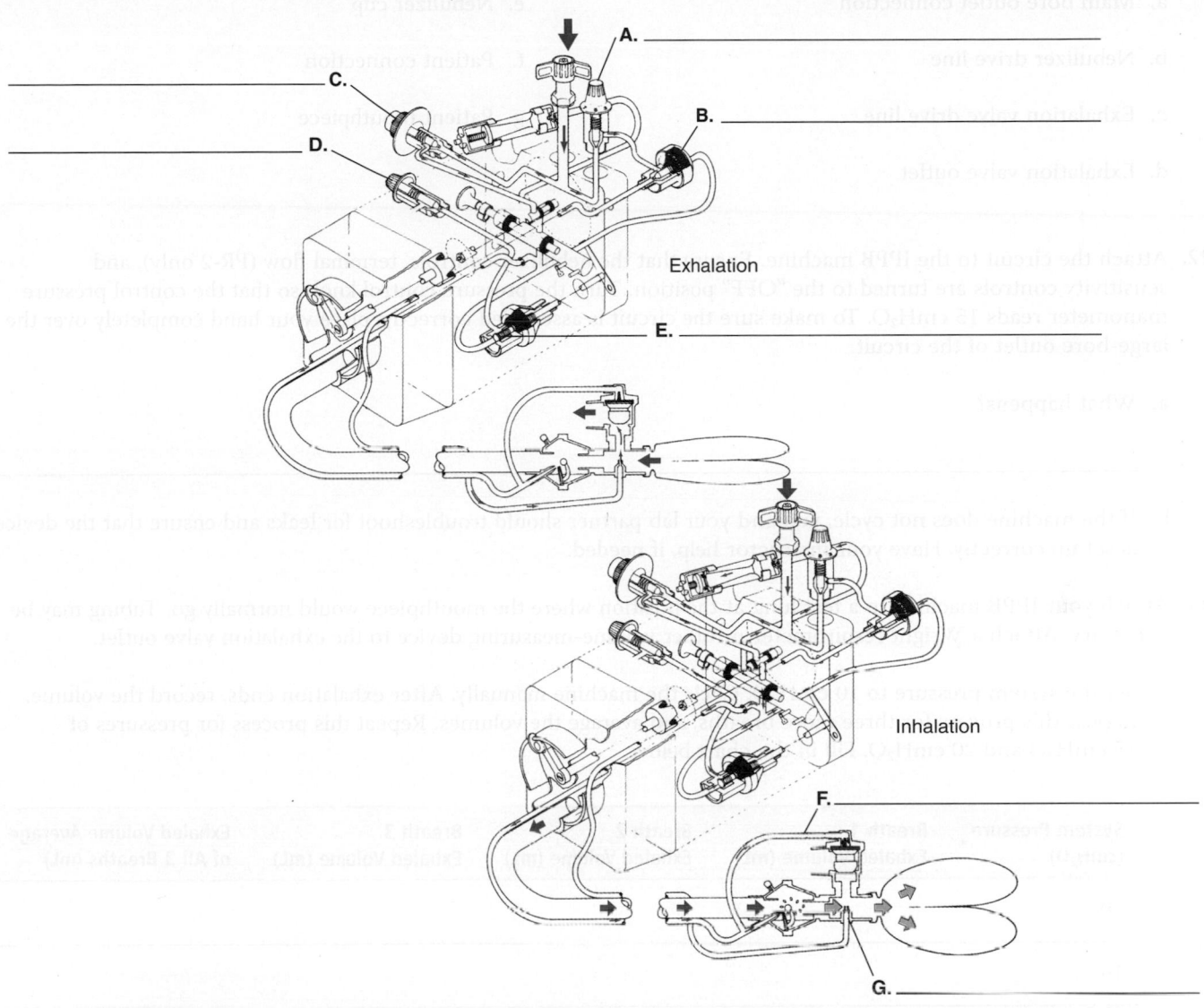

Figure 16-12 Bird Mark 8. (Modified from Cairo JM: *Mosby's respiratory care equipment*, ed 9, St. Louis, MO, 2014, Mosby.)

21. Obtain an IPPB circuit from your lab instructor. Identify the following features:

    a. Main bore outlet connection

    b. Nebulizer drive line

    c. Exhalation valve drive line

    d. Exhalation valve outlet

    e. Nebulizer cup

    f. Patient connection

    g. Patient mouthpiece

22. Attach the circuit to the IPPB machine. Ensure that the nebulizer controls, terminal flow (PR-2 only), and sensitivity controls are turned to the "OFF" position. Turn the pressure control knob so that the control pressure manometer reads 15 cmH$_2$O. To make sure the circuit is assembled correctly, place your hand completely over the large-bore outlet of the circuit.

    a. What happens?

    _____

    b. If the machine does not cycle, you and your lab partner should troubleshoot for leaks and ensure that the device is set up correctly. Have your instructor help, if needed.

23. Attach your IPPB machine to a test lung at the position where the mouthpiece would normally go. Tubing may be necessary. Attach a Wright respirometer or other volume-measuring device to the exhalation valve outlet.

    a. Set the system pressure to 10 cmH$_2$O. Cycle the machine manually. After exhalation ends, record the volume. Repeat this process for three more breaths, and average the volumes. Repeat this process for pressures of 15 cmH$_2$O and 20 cmH$_2$O. Fill in the chart below.

System Pressure (cmH$_2$O)	Breath 1 Exhaled Volume (mL)	Breath 2 Exhaled Volume (mL)	Breath 3 Exhaled Volume (mL)	Exhaled Volume Average of All 3 Breaths (mL)
10				
15				
20				

    b. What happens to the exhaled volume if the pressure is increased?

    _____

24. What does the air mix control do?

_____

_____

25. Attach your IPPB machine to a test lung at the position where the mouthpiece would normally go. Tubing may be necessary. Attach a Wright respirometer or other volume-measuring device to the exhalation valve outlet.

a. Set the system pressure to 15 cmH$_2$O and the flow to 15 L/min. Trigger the machine manually. After each exhalation ends, record the exhaled volume and the time for inspiration in the chart below making the appropriate flow changes.

System Pressure (cmH$_2$O)	Flow Rate (L/min)	Exhaled Volume (mL)	I-Time (seconds)
15	15		
15	30		
15	45		

b. What is the relationship between I-time and flow?

_____

c. Make the following changes and fill in the chart below:

System Pressure (cmH$_2$O)	Flow Rate (L/min)	Exhaled Volume (mL)	I-Time (seconds)
10	40		
15	40		
20	40		

d. What is the relationship of pressure to I-time when the flow stays the same?

_____

Self-Assessment Questions

1. Two primary types of atelectasis associated with postoperative or bedridden patients include:

   1. Gas absorption atelectasis
   2. Compression atelectasis
   3. Postoperative atelectasis
   4. Sedation atelectasis

   A. 1 and 3
   B. 2 and 3
   C. 1 and 2
   D. 1 and 4

2. Factors associated with causing atelectasis include all of the following except:
   A. Taking deep breaths
   B. Obesity
   C. Heavy sedation
   D. Upper abdominal surgery

3. All modes of lung expansion therapy aid lung expansion by:
   A. Increasing the transpulmonary pressure gradient
   B. Decreasing the transthoracic pressure gradient
   C. Increasing the pressure in the pleural space
   D. Decreasing the pressure in the alveoli

4. Hazards and complications of incentive spirometry include:

   1. Hyperventilation
   2. Fatigue
   3. Barotrauma
   4. Exacerbation bronchospasm

   A. 1 and 2 only
   B. 2, 3, and 4 only
   C. 1, 2, and 3 only
   D. 1, 2, 3, and 4

5. Beneficial results from IS therapy requires:
   A. State of the art equipment
   B. Effective patient teaching
   C. Setting low goals for patients
   D. Fast and shallow inspirations by the patient

6. Hazards and complications of IPPB include:

   1. Air trapping
   2. Increased airway resistance
   3. Gastric distension
   4. Increased cough and secretion clearance

   A. 1 and 2 only
   B. 2 and 3 only
   C. 1, 2, and 3 only
   D. 1, 3, and 4 only

7. If a leak is present in a pressure-cycled IPPB device:
   A. The device will not cycle into the expiratory phase
   B. The device will continuously cycle
   C. The patient will be more comfortable
   D. A working pressure above 45 to 55 psig will be required to operate the device

8. The parameters of monitoring IPPB machine performance include:

   1. Sensitivity
   2. Flow settings
   3. I:E ratio
   4. Peak pressure

   A. 1 only
   B. 1 and 3 only
   C. 1, 2, and 4 only
   D. 1, 2, 3, and 4

9. Which therapy can be administered to a postoperative patient with atelectasis who is unable to cooperate?
   A. Flutter
   B. ExPAP
   C. CPT
   D. Autogenic drainage

10. Adding a nebulizer to an IPPB circuit may increase the flow to the patient and alter the tidal volume the machine is delivering.
    A. True
    B. False

> ## CASE STUDY 16-1

While evaluating your patient receiving IPPB treatment with a Bennett PR-2 ventilator, you detect a longer-than-necessary inspiratory phase.

1. What are some factors you should assess?

_____

_____

2. How would you correct these factors?

_____

_____

›› CASE STUDY 16-2

You are administering IPPB treatment to a patient with atelectasis. The patient has a history of chronic obstructive pulmonary disease (COPD) diagnosed 15 years ago and currently is on 2 liters per minute (L/min) oxygen. The patient was admitted 2 days ago for shortness of breath. The most recent vital signs and lab values are as follows:

RR: 28 breaths/min
HR: 110 beats/min
BP: 152/88 mm Hg
Lung sounds: Diminished in the bases
Arterial blood gas: During last routine pulmonologist visit while patient on 2 L/min oxygen via nasal cannula, pH was 7.32; $PaCO_2$: 59 mm Hg; HCO_3^-: 39 mEq/L; PaO_2: 67 mm Hg; BE: +7

1. The IPPB machine is set up and powered with oxygen as a gas source. After about 1 minute of therapy, the patient becomes lethargic, and his respiratory rate drops to 8. What should you do?

_____

_____

2. How can you correct this problem during future IPPB treatments?

_____

_____

›› CASE STUDY 16-3

Mrs. Damico is a 47-year-old female patient you are evaluating. She is in the general ward and is recovering from a hysterectomy she had yesterday. Her vital signs are within normal limits, and she has no significant pulmonary history.

1. Is lung expansion therapy indicated for this patient? Why, or why not?

_____

_____

Three days later, she is up and walking and has been performing her incentive spirometry diligently as prescribed following her surgery. She is currently feeling well and is walking much more than in the previous days. She has no complaints, and her vital signs are all within normal limits.

2. What assessment criteria would you look at to determine if IS is still indicated for her at this time?

_____

_____

Airway Clearance Therapy

▪ OBJECTIVES

Upon the completion of the chapter activities and content review topics, the student should be able to:

1. Describe normal airway clearance mechanisms and factors that may impair their function.
2. Describe the cough reflex.
3. Identify pulmonary pathologies associated with abnormal section clearance.
4. Perform and properly instruct the patient regarding the following airway clearance activities:
   a. Chest physical therapy
   b. Directed cough
   c. Forced expiratory technique
   d. Mechanical insufflation–exsufflation
   e. Positive airway pressure adjuncts
   f. High-frequency chest wall compression

▪ KEY TERMS

- Chest physical therapy (CPT)
- Forced expiratory technique (FET)
- Inspissation of secretions
- Oscillation
- Postural drainage, percussion, and vibration (PDPV)
- Splinting

▪ CONTENT REVIEW TOPICS

- Active cycle of breathing technique (ACBT)
- Autogenic drainage (AD)

- Ciliary dyskinetic syndromes
- Diaphragmatic breathing
- Pursed lip breathing

▪ PROCEDURAL ASSESSMENTS

17-1 Administering Chest Physical Therapy
17-2 Teaching Directed Cough
17-3 Teaching Forced Expiratory Technique
17-4 Using a Mechanical Insufflation–Exsufflation Device
17-5 Administering Positive Airway Pressure Therapy
17-6 Using High-frequency Chest Wall Oscillation
17-7 Using an Intrapulmonary Percussive Ventilation Device

▪ EQUIPMENT

- Hospital bed or surface adequate for CPT
- Mechanical insufflation–exsufflation
- Mannequin
- Positive airway pressure adjuncts
- Interfaces for positive airway pressure adjuncts
- High-frequency chest wall oscillation device
- Intrapulmonary percussive ventilation device
- Disposable gloves

A patient's pulmonary status may deteriorate quickly if airway secretions are not removed. Thickening of secretions from inadequate humidification, also termed inspissation of secretions, may result from the use of oxygen therapy during illness (Box 17-1). For normal mucus clearance to occur, a patient must have a patent airway, a functional mucociliary escalator, and, perhaps most important, an effective cough. The four phases of the cough reflex are illustrated in Figure 17-1.

These phases together contribute to mucus progression along the airways, and a problem in one or more of these phases may result in a patient's inability to remove the secretions (Box 17-2).

Airway clearance therapies are a vital component of patient care when an acute pathologic condition is preventing secretion removal or as an element of a patient's treatment regimen for a chronic condition. Tailoring therapy to suit the patient's needs and pulmonary goals should be the objective of airway clearance therapy.

This chapter contains information relating to airway clearance therapies and their application in respiratory care. Breathing techniques, autogenic drainage, and the 6-minute walk test will be covered in the chapter on "Cardiopulmonary Rehabilitation."

❯❯ SKILL CHECK LISTS

17-1 Administering Chest Physical Therapy

Chest physical therapy (CPT) integrates an airway clearance routine to aid in the removal of secretion and improve lung efficiency. CPT entails five distinct elements:
1. Postural drainage
2. Percussion
3. Vibration
4. Deep breathing
5. Coughing

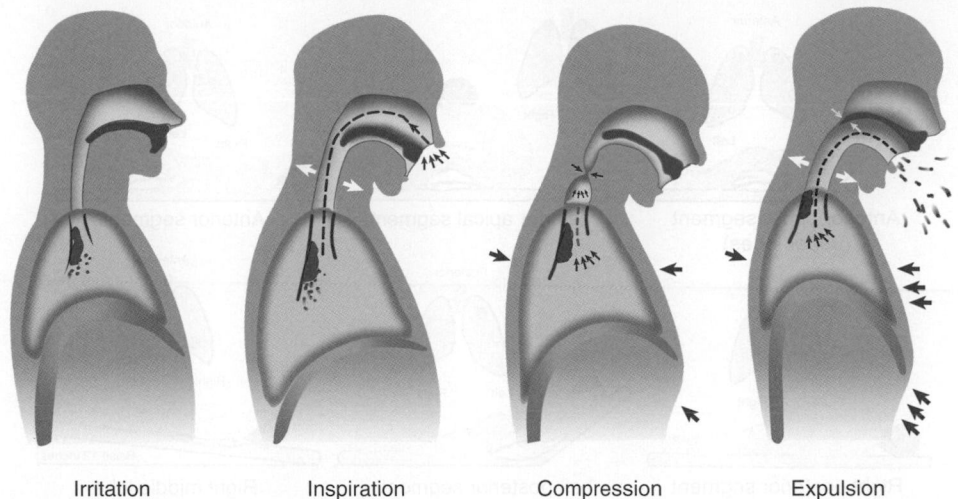

| Irritation | Inspiration | Compression | Expulsion |

Figure 17-1 The cough reflex. (From Kacmarek RM, Stoller JK, Heuer AJ: *Egan's fundamentals of respiratory care*, ed 10, St. Louis, MO, 2013, Mosby.)

<table>
<tr><td>BOX 17-1</td><td>Causes of Impaired Mucociliary Clearance in Intubated Patients</td></tr>
</table>

- Endotracheal or tracheostomy tube
- Tracheobronchial suction
- Inadequate humidification
- High fractional inspired oxygen FiO_2
- Drugs
- General anesthetics
- Opiates
- Narcotics
- Underlying pulmonary disease

<table>
<tr><td>BOX 17-2</td><td>Indications for Airway Clearance Therapy</td></tr>
</table>

Acute Conditions
- Copious secretions
- Acute respiratory failure
- Acute lobar atelectasis
- V/Q abnormalities caused by unilateral lung disease

Chronic Conditions
- Cystic fibrosis (CF)
- Bronchiectasis
- Ciliary dyskinetic syndromes
- Chronic bronchitis

Disorders Associated with Retention of Secretions
- Acute disease
- Immobile patients
- Postoperative patients—related to the effects of general anesthetics, opiates, and narcotics
- Inadequate humidification
- Acute exacerbations of chronic obstructive pulmonary disease (COPD), CF, or bronchiectasis
- Chronic disease: CF or neuromuscular disorders

It is important to convey to the patient how these distinct "parts" function as a "whole" and its influence on airway clearance therapy. For example, percussion without coughing is not beneficial.

> ✳ **Tip** Guidelines for positioning the patient during airway clearance have changed, and some suggest that the Trendelenburg position may have adverse effects in the patient with cystic fibrosis (CF).

During a session of CPT, the patient may be placed in any of 10 to 12 different positions (Figure 17-2). Secretions are mobilized through postural drainage, percussion, and vibration (PDPV). Clearance is augmented with deep breathing and coughing. Complete therapy includes all the five elements listed above. However, breathing techniques will be covered in detail in Chapter 27.

> → **Reality Check** Many patients feel significantly better following CPT and would not be able to function and perform activities of daily living without it.

Knowledge of a patient's medical history, anatomy of the lungs, and all the indications, contraindications, and hazards of CPT is central when determining the need for and performing CPT. Figure 17-2 illustrates the postural drainage positions incorporated in percussion and vibrations.

The following is the step-by-step process for administering chest physical therapy, including postural drainage, chest percussion and vibration, which are also referred to as postural drainage, percussion, and vibration (PDPV).

> → **Reality Check** CPT is performed by the physical therapy (PT) department at some facilities, so you will have to coordinate with them to ensure the best patient care.

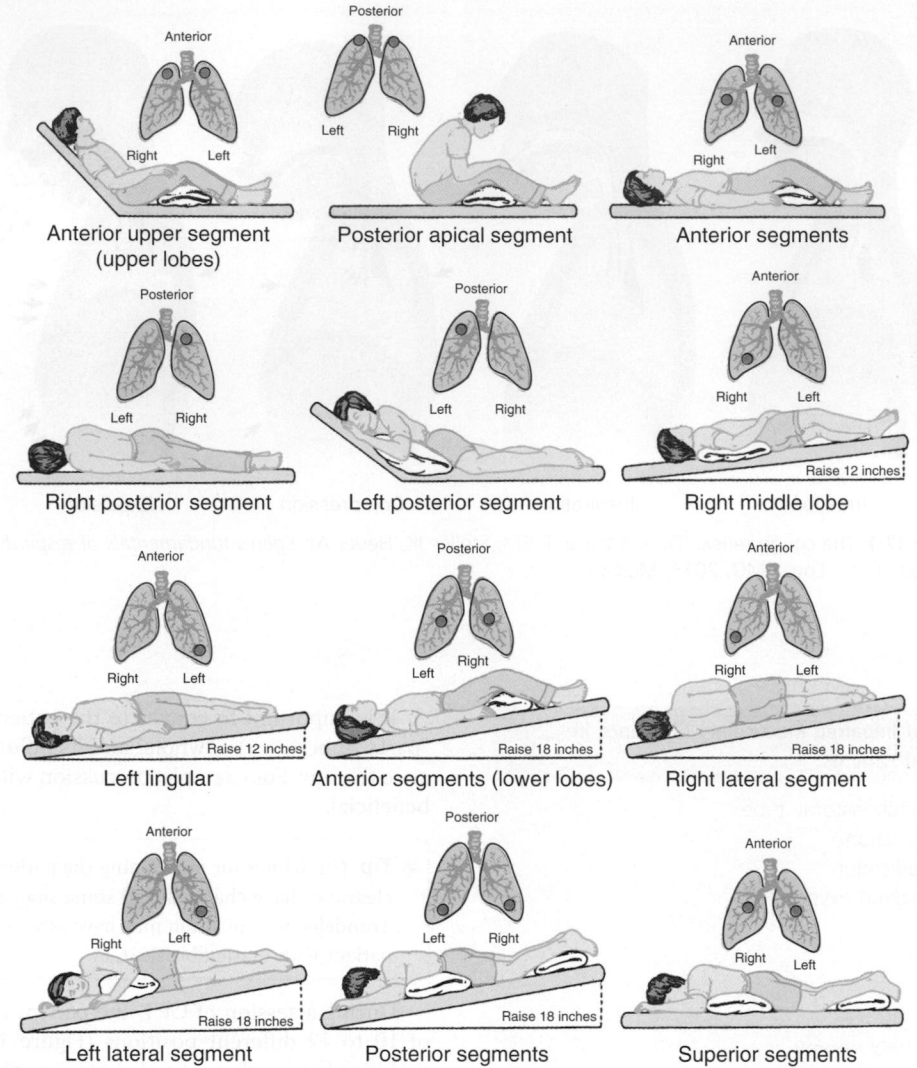

Figure 17-2 Patient positions for postural drainage. (From Kacmarek RM, Stoller JK, Heuer AJ: *Egan's fundamentals of respiratory care*, ed 10, St. Louis, MO, 2013, Mosby.)

Procedural Preparation

1. Review the patient's chart, and identify the appropriate lobe(s) and segment(s) for drainage.
2. Verify the physician's order or the facility's protocol for standard of care.
3. Obtain, clean, and inspect the appropriate equipment prior to entering the patient's room.
4. Follow personal protective equipment (PPE) requirements, and observe standard precautions for any transmission-based isolation procedure.
5. Identify the patient using two patient identifiers.
6. Introduce yourself to the patient and to the family.
7. Explain the procedure to the patient and to the family, and acknowledge the patient's understanding.
8. Perform proper hand hygiene, and put on gloves, mask, and protective eyewear, as appropriate for the procedure.

Implementation

1. Assess vital signs.
2. Place the patient in the proper position for drainage.

3. Confirm patient comfort in the drainage position.
4. Percuss the patient over the proper segment for 3 to 5 minutes.
5. Instruct the patient to exhale through pursed lips during vibrations (see PA 27-2).
6. Instruct the patient to cough.
7. Reassess vital signs, and continuously observe the patient for any adverse effects or complications during the procedure.
8. Restore the patient to the pretreatment position of comfort.
9. Ensure the patient's stability and comfort.
10. Remove the supplies from the patient's room, and clean the area, as needed.
11. Remove PPE, and perform proper hand hygiene.

Evaluation of Procedure

1. Establish a baseline, or compare with previous measurements.
2. Develop an appropriate respiratory care plan based on assessment data.

3. Note any need for oxygen therapy during the procedure.
4. Identify any unexpected outcomes.

Documentation and Reporting

1. Record your findings in the patient's chart, including position used, time in position, patient tolerance, and subjective and objective indicators of treatment effectiveness.
2. Report any abnormal findings to the appropriate health care provider.

17-2 Teaching Directed Cough

It may seem strange to have to "teach" a patient how to cough, but coaching a patient to deliberately cough may aid in effective removal of his or her secretions and prevent further pulmonary compromise. Indications for directed cough therapy are listed in Box 17-3. The following is the step-by-step process for instruction on directed cough.

Procedural Preparation

1. Review the patient's chart.
2. Verify the physician's order or the facility's protocol for standard of care.
3. Obtain, clean, and inspect the appropriate equipment prior to entering the patient's room.
4. Follow PPE requirements, and observe standard precautions for any transmission-based isolation procedure.
5. Identify the patient using two patient identifiers.
6. Introduce yourself to the patient and to the family.
7. Explain the procedure to the patient and to the family, and acknowledge the patient's understanding.
8. Perform proper hand hygiene, and put on gloves, mask, and protective eyewear, as appropriate for the procedure.

Implementation

1. Assess vital signs.
2. Instruct the patient to assume the sitting position with one shoulder rotated inward and the head and spine slightly flexed; elevate the head of the bed, if necessary.
3. Instruct the patient to use diaphragmatic breathing techniques (see PA 27-3).
4. Confirm that the patient can take a deep breath.
5. Instruct the patient to bear down against the glottis, followed by a slight breath-hold, and then to cough.
6. Supply tissue for sputum removal.

BOX 17-3   **Indications for Directed Cough**

- Need for aid in the removal of retained secretions for central airways
- Presence of atelectasis
- Prophylaxis against postoperative pulmonary complications
- Routine part of bronchial hygiene in patients with CF, bronchiectasis, chronic bronchitis, necrotizing pulmonary infection, spinal cord injury
- Integral part of postural drainage, positive airway pressure (PAP), and incentive spirometry therapies
- To obtain sputum samples for diagnostic analysis

---

7. Remove the supplies from the patient's room, and clean the area, as needed.
8. Remove the PPE, and perform proper hand hygiene prior to leaving the patient's room.

Evaluation of Procedure

1. Establish a baseline, or compare with previous measurements.
2. Develop an appropriate respiratory care plan based on assessment data.
3. Evaluate the color, consistency, volume, and odor of sputum.
4. Note any use of oxygen therapy.
5. Identify any unexpected outcomes.

Documentation and Reporting

1. Record your findings in the patient's chart.
2. Report any abnormal findings to the appropriate health care provider.

17-3 Teaching Forced Expiratory Technique

Patients with COPD and neuromuscular disorders and postoperative patients may require additional coughing techniques to aid in the mobilization of retained secretions. In the postoperative patient, it is important to minimize the anxiety he or she may experience associated with pain.

> ✳ **Tip** Coordinate with the nurse so that you can perform bronchial hygiene therapies following administration of pain medications to the patient.

The mere thought of sneezing, laughing, coughing, even taking a deep breath brings with it anxiety about how much it may hurt. Shallow tidal volumes caused by pain and fear of taking a deep breath further complicate a patient's pulmonary recovery and may lead to retained secretions and atelectasis.

> → **Reality Check** Splinting, support over the area of incision during the expiratory phase of a cough, may seem unimportant but makes a remarkable difference in patient comfort.

The following is the step-by-step process for instruction on the forced expiratory technique (FET), also called the *"Huff" cough.*

Procedural Preparation

1. Review the patient's chart.
2. Verify the physician's order or the facility's protocol for standard of care.
3. Obtain, clean, and inspect the appropriate equipment prior to entering the patient's room.
4. Follow PPE requirements, and observe standard precautions for any transmission-based isolation procedure.
5. Identify the patient using two patient identifiers.
6. Introduce yourself to the patient and to the family.
7. Explain the procedure to the patient and to the family, and acknowledge the patient's understanding.

8. Perform proper hand hygiene, and put on gloves, mask, and protective eyewear, as appropriate for the procedure.

Implementation

1. Place the patient in a comfortable position.
2. Assess vital signs.
3. Instruct the patient to assume the sitting position with one shoulder rotated inward and the head and spine slightly flexed:
   a. If the patient is unable to do this, elevate the head of the bed.
   b. Explain splinting to the postsurgical patient.
4. Confirm that the patient can take a moderate to deep breath.
5. Instruct the patient to take a moderate to deep breath followed by a short breath-hold.
6. Instruct the patient to perform three uninterrupted forced exhalations while saying "huff":
   a. Huff cough #1, with lung deflation
   b. Huff cough #2, with further lung deflation
   c. Huff cough #3, with still further lung deflation
7. Instruct the patient to take one deep breath in, followed by a single abrupt Huff cough, for final expectoration.
8. Repeat, as necessary, after a brief rest, if clearance is not complete.
9. Instruct the patient to use diaphragmatic breathing techniques following FET.
10. Remove the supplies from the patient's room, and clean the area, as needed.
11. Remove PPE, and perform proper hand hygiene prior to leaving the patient's room.

Evaluation of Procedure

1. Establish a baseline, or compare with previous measurements.
2. Develop an appropriate respiratory care plan based on assessment data.
3. Evaluate the color, consistency, volume, and odor of sputum.
4. Note any use of oxygen therapy.
5. Identify any unexpected outcomes.

Documentation and Reporting

1. Record your findings in the patient's chart.
2. Report any abnormal findings to the appropriate health care provider.

17-4 Using a Mechanical Insufflation–Exsufflation Device

For simulating a normal cough, a device called a *mechanical insufflation–exsufflation* (MIE) is used to produce an artificial cough by delivering positive pressures with an abrupt reversal to negative pressures. The generated cough may achieve peak expiratory flows in the mean range of 7.5 liters per second. This electronically powered device helps patients with neuromuscular disorders such as amyotrophic lateral sclerosis, spinal muscular atrophy, muscular dystrophy, myasthenia gravis, and spinal cord injuries clear retained secretion. The Respironics Coughassist MIE is illustrated in Figure 17-3.

The following is the step-by-step process for the use of an MIE.

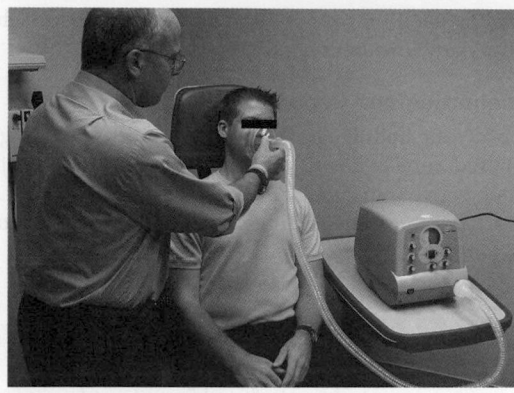

Figure 17-3 Respironics Coughassist. (From Mason R, Broaddus V, Martin T, et al: *Murray and Nadel's textbook of respiratory care*, ed 10, Philadelphia, PA, 2010, Saunders.)

Procedural Preparation

1. Review the patient's chart.
2. Verify the physician's order or the facility's protocol for standard of care.
3. Obtain, clean, and inspect the appropriate equipment prior to entering the patient's room.
4. Follow PPE requirements, and observe standard precautions for any transmission-based isolation procedure.
5. Identify the patient using two patient identifiers.
6. Introduce yourself to the patient and to the family.
7. Explain the procedure to the patient and to the family, and acknowledge the patient's understanding.
8. Perform proper hand hygiene, and put on gloves, mask, and protective eyewear, as appropriate for the procedure.

Implementation

1. Place the patient in a comfortable position.
2. Assess vital signs.
3. Assemble the equipment.
4. Set correct pressures:
   a. Positive pressure from 30 to 50 cmH$_2$O
   b. Negative pressures from −30 to −50 cmH$_2$O
5. Set correct interval times:
   a. Positive pressures for 1 to 3 seconds
   b. Negative pressures for 2 to 3 seconds
6. Inform the patient about the intended session time and the subsequent period of normal spontaneous or assisted breathing.
7. Repeat the session until secretions are cleared.
8. Reassess vital signs.
9. Remove the supplies from the patient's room, and clean the area, as needed.
10. Remove PPE, and perform proper hand hygiene prior to leaving the patient's room.

Evaluation of Procedure

1. Establish a baseline, or compare with previous measurements.
2. Develop an appropriate respiratory care plan based on assessment data.
3. Note any use of oxygen therapy.

4. Monitor the patient for any adverse reactions to the procedure.
5. Identify any unexpected outcomes.

Documentation and Reporting

1. Record your findings in the patient's chart.
2. Report any abnormal findings to the appropriate health care provider.

17-5 Administering Positive Airway Pressure Therapy

Positive airway pressure (PAP) adjuncts are devices with a mouthpiece (or mask) and an expiratory valve that creates a resistance of 10 to 20 cmH$_2$O on exhalation. This generates a positive pressure in the patient's airway, which, in turn, prevents airway collapse and aids in the mobilization of secretions during the expiratory phase.

> ✳ **Tip** Flutter valves provide both high-frequency oscillations and positive expiratory pressure throughout exhalation.

Images of the numerous devices available are provided in Figure 17-4. Depending on the patient and his or her tolerance to the therapy, after about 10 to 20 breaths, the device should be removed from the mouth. The patient should then be coached to perform two to three forced expirations, followed by a forced expiratory technique (see PA 17-3). This procedure should be repeated until the patient feels improvement in secretion mobilization but should not exceed 20 minutes. The following is the step-by-step process the instruction and use of a PAP therapy device.

Procedural Preparation

1. Review the patient's chart, and determine the need for PAP therapy.
2. Verify the physician's order or the facility's protocol for standard of care.

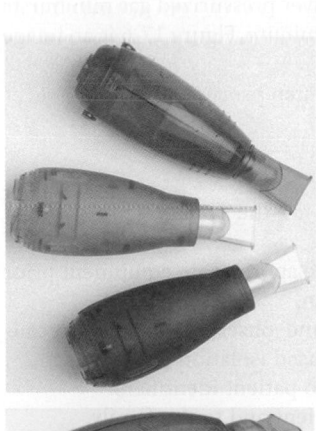
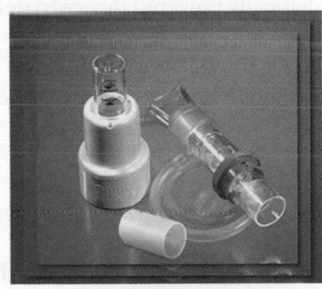
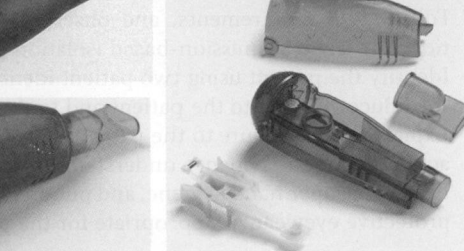

Figure 17-4 Positive airway pressure (PAP) devices. (From Frownfelter D, Dean E: *Cardiovascular and pulmonary physical therapy, evidence and practice*, ed 4, St. Louis, MO, 2007, Mosby.)

3. Obtain, clean, and inspect the appropriate equipment prior to entering the patient's room.
4. Follow PPE requirements, and observe standard precautions for any transmission-based isolation procedure.
5. Identify the patient using two patient identifiers.
6. Introduce yourself to the patient and to the family.
7. Explain the procedure to the patient and to the family, and acknowledge the patient's understanding.
8. Confirm the patient's knowledge of FET (see PA 17-3).
9. Perform proper hand hygiene and put on gloves, mask, and protective eyewear, as appropriate for procedure.

Implementation

1. Place the patient in a comfortable position.
2. Assess vital signs.
3. Bring the equipment to the bedside, and provide initial therapy after adjusting pressure settings to meet the patient's need and determining treatment pressure (between 10 and 20 cmH$_2$O).
4. Apply the mask or mouthpiece:
   a. If using a mask, apply it tightly over the patient's mouth and nose; confirm that the patient is comfortable.
   b. If using a mouthpiece, instruct the patient to place the lips firmly around it and breathe through the mouth.
5. Instruct the patient to do the following:
   a. Take in a larger than normal breath, but do not fill the lungs.
   b. Exhale actively, not forcefully, to obtain the treatment pressure.
   c. Perform 10 to 20 breaths.
6. Remove the mask or mouthpiece.
7. Instruct the patient to perform two to three FETs.
8. Repeat the above cycle four to eight times, but do not exceed 20 minutes.
9. Reassess vital signs.
10. Assess the patient's ability for self-administration.
11. Remove the supplies from the patient's room, and clean the area, as needed.
12. Remove PPE, and perform proper hand hygiene prior to leaving the patient's room.

Evaluation of Procedure

1. Establish a baseline, or compare with previous measurements.
2. Develop an appropriate respiratory care plan based on assessment data.
3. Evaluate for PAP therapy to be used in conjunction with bronchodilator aerosol therapy.
4. Identify any unexpected outcomes.

Documentation and Reporting

1. Record your findings in the patient's chart.
2. Report any abnormal findings to the appropriate health care provider.

17-6 Using a High-Frequency Chest Wall Oscillation

High-frequency chest wall oscillation (HFCWO) devices such as The Vest are mechanical devices that rapidly inflate and deflate. These small gas volumes being alternately introduced

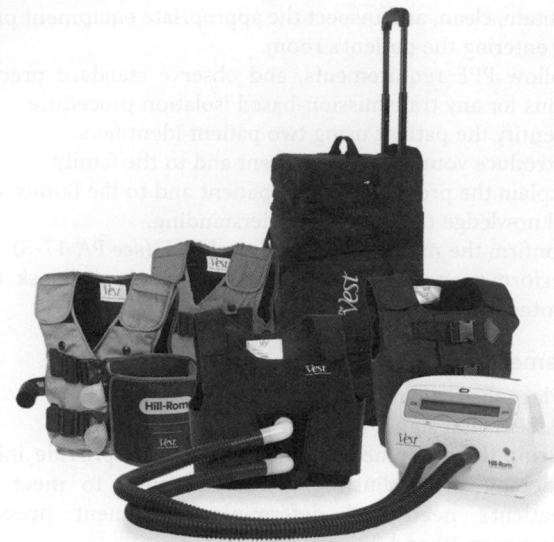

Figure 17-5 The Vest Airway Clearance System for high-frequency chest wall oscillation. (Courtesy of Hill-Rom Services, Inc., Reprinted with permission. All rights reserved.)

and withdrawn from the vest create an oscillatory motion on the patient's thorax. This oscillation results in mobilization of secretions. An HFCWO device consists of a nonstretchable, inflatable vest, which is attached to an air-pulse generator. An example of this device is provided in Figure 17-5. Therapy session times and the device's oscillatory frequencies depend on physician orders, patient response, and comfort. Breathing and coughing techniques must be incorporated to move secretions along the airways and expel them once they have been loosened during HFCWO therapy.

HFCWO therapy allows the patient some freedom and autonomy because he or she does not need someone to perform manual CPT. The following is the step-by-step process for HFCWO therapy.

Procedural Preparation

1. Review the patient's chart.
2. Verify the physician's order or the facility's protocol for standard of care.
3. Obtain, clean, and inspect the appropriate equipment prior to entering the patient's room.
4. Follow PPE requirements, and observe standard precautions for any transmission-based isolation procedure.
5. Identify the patient using two patient identifiers.
6. Introduce yourself to the patient and to the family.
7. Explain the procedure to the patient and to the family, and acknowledge the patient's understanding.
8. Perform proper hand hygiene, and put on gloves, mask, and protective eyewear, as appropriate for the procedure.

Implementation

1. Place the patient in a comfortable position.
2. Assess vital signs.
3. Assemble the equipment, plug it in, and place it near the patient.
4. Place the patient's vest or disposable single-patient-use, nonstretchable vest on the patient.

5. Secure the straps:
   a. Have the patient take a deep breath in.
   b. Tighten the straps before exhalation occurs.
   c. Repeat this until all the straps have been secured.
6. Set the controls appropriately:
   a. Frequency: Typically ranges from 10 to 14
   b. Pressure: Typically ranges from 4 to 6
   c. Time: Typically ranges from 10 to 30 minutes
7. Inform the patient that therapy will begin.
8. Pause the therapy to instruct the patient to clear the secretions.
9. Reassess vital signs when the therapy has been completed.
10. Remove the supplies from the patient's room, and clean the area, as needed.
11. Remove PPE, and perform proper hand hygiene prior to leaving the patient's room.

Evaluation of Procedure

1. Establish a baseline, or compare with previous measurements and settings.
2. Develop an appropriate respiratory care plan based on assessment data.
3. Note any use of oxygen or medications during therapy.
4. Identify any unexpected outcomes.

Documentation and Reporting

1. Record your findings in the patient's chart.
2. Report any abnormal findings to the appropriate health care provider.

17-7 Using an Intrapulmonary Percussive Ventilation Device

Oscillation refers to the rapid vibratory movements of small volumes of air back and forth in the respiratory tract. This type of oscillation is applied in an airway clearance technique called *intrapulmonary percussive ventilation (IPV)*. IPV uses a pneumatically powered device to deliver pressurized gas minibursts at rates of 100 to 225 cycles per minute. Figure 17-6 is an image of a type of IPV device.

The following is the step-by-step process for IPV.

Procedural Preparation

1. Review the patient's chart.
2. Verify the physician's order or the facility's protocol for standard of care.
3. Obtain, clean, and inspect the appropriate equipment prior to entering the patient's room.
4. Follow PPE requirements, and observe standard precautions for any transmission-based isolation procedure.
5. Identify the patient using two patient identifiers.
6. Introduce yourself to the patient and to the family.
7. Explain the procedure to the patient and to the family, and acknowledge the patient's understanding.
8. Perform proper hand hygiene, and put on gloves, mask, and protective eyewear, as appropriate for the procedure.

Implementation

1. Place the patient in a comfortable position.
2. Assess vital signs.

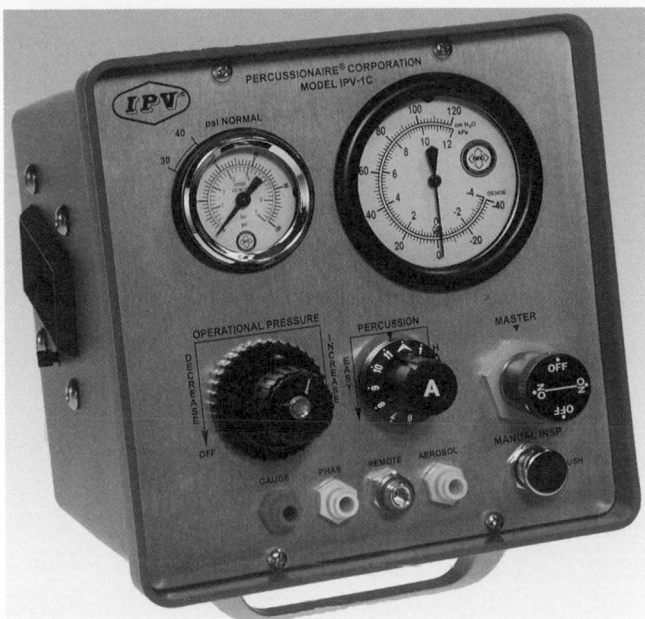

Figure 17-6 Intrapulmonary percussive ventilator (IPV). (Courtesy of Percussionaire, Sandpoint, ID.)

3. Select the appropriate interface.
4. Fill the reservoir with the ordered solution or medication.
5. Turn the device on, and adjust amplification and frequency to generate sufficient percussion and aerosol.

6. Attach the device to the patient, and ensure patient comfort.
7. Instruct the patient to cough.
8. Stop the therapy after 20 minutes or after the drug has been completely nebulized.
9. Reassess vital signs, for efficacy of therapy, and for tolerance.
10. Remove the supplies from the patient's room, and clean the area, as needed.
11. Remove the PPE, and perform proper hand hygiene prior to leaving the patient's room.

Evaluation of Procedure

1. Establish a baseline, or compare with previous measurements.
2. Develop an appropriate respiratory care plan based on assessment data.
3. Identify any unexpected outcomes.

Documentation and Reporting

1. Record your findings in the patient's chart.
2. Report any abnormal findings to the appropriate health care provider.

Bibliography

Kacmarek RM, Stoller JK, Heuer AJ: *Egan's fundamentals of respiratory care*, ed 10, St. Louis, MO, 2013, Mosby.

1. List the four distinct phases to a normal cough and explain each.

   a. _____

   b. _____

   c. _____

   d. _____

2. Fill in the chart below:

   Causes of Impaired Mucociliary Clearance in Intubated Patients

   1. _____

   2. _____

   3. _____

   4. _____

   5. _____

   6. _____

   7. _____

   8. _____

   9. _____

3. Review the different types of airway clearance therapy devices listed below, and fill in the chart.

Device	Indications for Use and Patient Population Used for	Source of Information
Acapella		
Flutter valve		
Mechanical insufflation–exsufflation (MIE)		

4. Explain the operation of the following devices, or explain the procedure while demonstrating their correct use to three different student peers. Have them sign once you have correctly explained each.

a. Flutter valve:

Signature:_____

Signature:_____

Signature:_____

b. Acapella (or PEP device):

Signature:_____

Signature:_____

Signature:_____

c. 10–12 postural drainage positions:

Signature:_____

Signature:_____

Signature:_____

d. HFCWO (The Vest):

Signature:_____

Signature:_____

Signature:_____

Self-Assessment Questions

1. Place the cough reflex phases in the proper order.
   A. Inspiration, irritation, compression, expulsion
   B. Irritation, expulsion, compression, inspiration
   C. Irritation, inspiration, compression, expulsion
   D. Inspiration, compression, irritation, expulsion

2. The components of normal airway clearance include:

   1. Patent airway
   2. Functional mucociliary escalator
   3. Undamaged neuromuscular system
   4. Effective cough

   A. 1 and 4 only
   B. 1, 2, and 3 only
   C. 2, 3, and 4 only
   D. 1, 2, and 4 only

3. The term used to describe the retention of secretions that results in complete airway obstruction is:
   A. $\dot{V}/\dot{Q}$ mismatch
   B. Mucus plugging
   C. Ciliary dyskinetic syndrome
   D. Inspissations

4. Airway clearance therapy is indicated for:

   1. Asthma
   2. Bronchiectasis
   3. Cystic fibrosis
   4. Ciliary dyskinetic syndromes

   A. 1 and 4 only
   B. 2 and 4 only
   C. 2, 3, and 4 only
   D. 1, 2, 3, and 4

5. The primary goal of airway clearance is:
   A. To help mobilize and remove retained secretions
   B. To improve exercise tolerance in patients with asthma
   C. To improve the effects of aerosol drug therapy
   D. To decrease the time a patient spends intubated on mechanical ventilation

6. Chest physical therapy typically includes:

   1. Postural drainage
   2. Mechanical insufflation–exsufflation
   3. Percussion
   4. Vibration

   A. 1, 2, and 3 only
   B. 1, 2, and 4 only
   C. 1, 3, and 4 only
   D. 1, 2, 3, 4

7. The two absolute contraindications for postural drainage as indicated by therapy guidelines are:
   A. Active hemoptysis and empyema
   B. A confused and anxious patient
   C. Unstable head injury and hemodynamic instability with active bleeding
   D. Recently placed pacemaker and bronchopleural fistula

8. A patient receiving postural drainage, percussion, and vibration (PDPV) is on 2 L/min oxygen via a nasal cannula. His normal SpO_2 readings are 89%. During therapy, his SpO_2 drops to 86%. What would you suggest to the physician to help remedy the situation?
   A. Discontinue the therapy.
   B. Increase his oxygen flow during therapy to maintain his normal saturations.
   C. Change the oxygen delivery device to an air entrainment mask at an FiO_2 of 0.28.
   D. Discuss with the patient the addition of steroids to his daily medications.

9. Complications of postural drainage include vomiting and aspiration.
   A. True
   B. False

10. The MIE device delivers positive pressure breaths followed by an abrupt reversal to negative pressures.
    A. True
    B. False

▶▶ CASE STUDY 17-1

Mr. Cee is a 67-year-old patient recovering from upper abdominal surgery. He had a complete pulmonary function test performed prior to surgery, and all values were within normal limits. Currently, his cough is adequate, and sputum production is moderate.

1. Determine an appropriate course of action to maintain proper bronchial hygiene for your patient. More than one choice of treatment is possible, so be sure to explain your rationale, goals, and the equipment you will use for treatment.

_____

_____

▶▶ CASE STUDY 17-3

Miss Teener is an 18-year-old patient with a history of cystic fibrosis and has had mucus production of about 20 mL per day for the past 2 years. She uses The Vest at home. Currently, she is being hospitalized for an upper respiratory infection, with her daily mucus production increased to about 50 mL per day.

1. Determine an appropriate course of action to maintain proper bronchial hygiene for your patient. More than one choice of treatment is possible, so be sure to explain your rationale, goals, and the equipment you will use for treatment.

_____

_____

▶▶ CASE STUDY 17-2

Lucy T is a 59-year-old female recovering from open heart surgery and is on postoperative day 6. She has a 50-pack-year smoking history, is alert and oriented, but is reluctant to cough. Auscultation of her lungs reveals minimal expiratory wheezing in the apices, with bilateral, coarse, expiratory crackles throughout.

1. Determine an appropriate course of action to maintain proper bronchial hygiene for your patient. More than one choice of treatment is possible, so be sure to explain your rationale, goals, and the equipment you will use for treatment.

_____

_____

▶▶ CASE STUDY 17-4

Mr. Petes is a 52-year-old male with myasthenia gravis, who is at your pulmonary rehabilitation center recovering from pneumonia. His cough is weak and nonproductive despite coarse inspiratory and expiratory crackles on auscultation of his lungs.

1. Determine an appropriate course of action to maintain proper bronchial hygiene for your patient. More than one choice of treatment is possible, so be sure to explain your rationale, goals, and the equipment you will use for treatment.

_____

_____

Airway Pharmacology

Douglas S. Gardenhire

▪ OBJECTIVES

Upon the completion of the chapter activities and content review topics, the student should be able to:

1. Administer drugs.
2. Describe the three phases that constitute the course of drug action from dose to effect.
3. Describe the classes of drugs that are delivered via the aerosol route.
4. Compare the available aerosol formulations, brand names, and dosages for each specific drug class.
5. Select the appropriate drug class for a given patient or clinical situation.

▪ KEY TERMS

- Drug administration phase
- Pharmacokinetic phase
- Pharmacodynamic phase
- Six rights of medication administration

▪ CONTENT REVIEW TOPICS

- Computerized Physician Order Entry (CPOE)
- Global Initiative for Chronic Obstructive Lung Disease (GOLD)
- Institute for Safe Medication Practice (ISMP)
- National Asthma Education and Prevention Program (NAEPP)
- Pulmonary medications

▪ PROCEDURAL ASSESSMENT

18-1 Medication Administration

▪ EQUIPMENT

- Mock medication ampoules
- Small-volume nebulizer

The primary objective of airway pharmacology is the delivery of inhaled aerosols to the respiratory tract for the diagnosis and treatment of pulmonary diseases. Because the administration of medications is such an important part of the daily activities of a respiratory therapist (RT), a deep understanding of them is essential. How medications work is an important part of the assessment process and in choosing the right medication to treat the pulmonary needs of your patients.

Three phases constitute the course of drug action from dose to effect: (1) the drug administration phase, (2) the pharmacokinetic phase, and (3) the pharmacodynamic phase. These three phases of drug action may be applied to treatment of the respiratory tract with bronchoactive inhaled agents and are defined in Box 18-1. Devices that are most commonly used to administer orally inhaled aerosols are the metered-dose inhaler (MDI), the small-volume nebulizer (SVN), and the dry-powder inhaler (DPI). They will be discussed in more detail in Chapter 19.

> → **Reality Check** Some facilities utilize computerized physician order entry (CPOE), which eliminates the need for written orders. Still, errors such as juxtaposition errors (choosing the wrong medication or dosage that is next on the list) could be made.

Treatment of the respiratory tract with inhaled aerosols offers many advantages such as: (1) Doses are usually smaller than doses for systemic administration, (2) the onset of drug action is rapid, (3) delivery is targeted to the organ requiring treatment, and (4) systemic side effects are often fewer and less severe.

The delivery of inhaled aerosols in treating respiratory disease also has some disadvantages, and these include (1) a number of variables affecting the delivered dose and (2) lack of adequate knowledge about device performance and use among patients and caregivers. Although other drug classes are used in respiratory care, this chapter will focus on medication administration and a review of bronchoactive inhaled aerosols.

≫ SKILL CHECK LISTS

18-1 Medication Administration

With RTs being responsible for the administration of numerous pulmonary medications, it may be a complex and demanding part of their daily responsibilities. Patients may be receiving several different inhaled medications during their hospital stay. Consequently, it is important to always practice safe medication administration. In the United States, The Joint Commission (TJC) accredits health care organizations, and improving patient safety must be a constant goal of the organizations. Medication safety aspects of the national patient safety goals are listed in Box 18-2.

Safe medication administration begins with the six rights of medication administration:

1. Right medication
2. Right dose

> ### BOX 18-1   Phases of Drug Action
>
> - Drug administration phase: describes the method by which a drug dose is made available to the body
> - Pharmacokinetic phase: describes the time course and disposition of a drug in the body based on its absorption, distribution, metabolism, and elimination
> - Pharmacodynamic phase: describes the mechanisms of drug action by which a drug molecule causes its effects in the body

> ### BOX 18-2   Joint Commission 2011 National Patient Safety Goals: Implications for Medication Administration
>
> - Use at least two patient identifiers when providing care, treatment, and services.
> - Improve the effectiveness of communication among caregivers.
> - Improve safety in using medications.
> - Accurately and completely reconcile medications across the continuum of care.

3. Right patient
4. Right route
5. Right time
6. Right documentation

Regardless of how you receive an order (verbal, written, protocol), you should always compare it with the medication administration record (MAR; eMAR for electronic versions) to ensure that the right medication is being administered. Many respiratory medications come in ampoules with measured doses. This does not negate the responsibility of the therapist to confirm that the right dose is being given. Concentration differences and the addition of a combination medication may result in a dose error if the RT is not careful. Two patient identifiers are mandatory before giving medication to a patient. The majority of respiratory medications are given via aerosolization. However, the order always has a designated route. The RT should assess the patient and make sure that the ordered route is the best for the patient's current condition. The Institute for Safe Medication Practice (ISMP) compiled a list of error-prone abbreviations. Table 18-1 lists some abbreviations that are commonly misinterpreted. The right time for respiratory medications to be delivered may help the patient control his or her symptoms, as with delivery of inhaled corticosteroids, or used to relieve current complaints such as shortness of breath caused by bronchospasm.

> ✳ **Tip** Albuterol may be given via several different routes. The RT should ensure that the route ordered is appropriate for the patient's current condition.

Documentation is a vital component of patient safety and is important for evaluating the efficacy of the drug therapy. The following is the step-by-step process for medication administration.

> → **Reality Check** Unlabeled medications should never be carried in the RT's pocket.

> → **Reality Check** Truly, memorization is the only way for you to learn all the generic and trade names of inhaled pulmonary medications.

Procedural Preparation

1. Review the patient's chart.
2. Verify the physician's order or the facility's protocol for standard of care.
3. Compare the order with the MAR or the eMAR.
4. Avoid any distractions during medication preparation.
5. Read the label on the medication container, and compare the instructions with the MAR three times:
   a. Before removing the container from the supply drawer
   b. When placing it in the nebulizer, reservoir device, or MDI adapter for the endotracheal tube (ETT)
   c. Just before administering the medication to the patient
6. Use aseptic technique when preparing the medication.
7. Ensure compatibility if mixing medications for simultaneous delivery.
8. Do not use the medication if the label is illegible or the container is unmarked.
9. Follow personal protective equipment (PPE) requirements, and observe standard precautions for any transmission-based isolation procedure.
10. Identify the patient using two patient identifiers.
11. Introduce yourself to the patient and to the family.
12. Explain the procedure to the patient and to the family, and acknowledge the patient's understanding.
13. Perform proper hand hygiene, and put on gloves, mask, and protective eyewear, as appropriate for the procedure.

Implementation

1. Place the patient in a comfortable position.
2. Assess vital signs.
3. Follow the six rights of medication administration.
4. Remain with the patient until all of the medication has been administered.
5. Reassess vital signs.
6. Remove the supplies from the patient's room, and clean the area, as needed.
7. Remove PPE, and perform proper hand hygiene prior to leaving the patient's room.

Evaluation of Procedure

1. Monitor the patient's response to the medication.
2. Identify any unexpected outcomes.

Documentation and Reporting

1. Record all the required information in the patient's chart.
2. Document patient refusal of medication and reason.
3. Report any adverse medication reactions to the appropriate health care provider.

TABLE 18-1 Institute for Safe Medication Practice List of Error-Prone Abbreviations*

Abbreviation	Intended Meaning	Misinterpretation	Correction
μg	Microgram	Mistaken as "mg"	Use "mcg"
AD, AS, AU	Right ear, left ear, each ear	Mistaken as OD, OS, OU (right eye, left eye, each eye)	Use "right ear," "left ear," or "each ear"
OD, OS, OU	Right eye, left eye, each eye	Mistaken as AD, AS, AU (right ear, left ear, each ear)	Use "right eye," "left eye," or "each eye"
BT	Bedtime	Mistaken as "BID" (twice daily)	Use "bedtime"
cc	Cubic centimeters	Mistaken as "u" (units)	Use "mL"
D/C	Discharge or discontinue	Premature discontinuation of medication if D/C (intended to mean "discharge") has been misinterpreted as "discontinued" when followed by a list of discharge medications	Use "discharge" and "discontinue"
IJ	Injection	Mistaken as "IV" or "intrajugular"	Use "injection"
IN	Intranasal	Mistaken as "IM" or "IV"	Use "intranasal" or "NAS"
HS	Half-strength	Mistaken as bedtime	Use "half-strength"
hs	At bedtime, hour of sleep	Mistaken as half-strength	Use "bedtime"
IU**	International unit	Mistaken as IV (intravenous) or 10 (ten)	Use "units"
o.d. or OD	Once daily	Mistaken as "right eye" (OD—oculus dexter), leading to oral liquid medications administered in the eye	Use "daily"
OJ	Orange juice	Mistaken as OD or OS (right or left eye); drugs meant to be diluted in orange juice may be given in the eye	Use "orange juice"
Per os	By mouth, orally	The "os" can be mistaken as "left eye" (OS—oculus sinister)	Use "PO," "by mouth," or "orally"
q.d. or QD**	Every day	Mistaken as q.i.d., especially if the period after the "q" or the tail of the "q" is misunderstood as an "i"	Use "daily"
qhs	Nightly at bedtime	Mistaken as "qhr" or every hour	Use "nightly"
qn	Nightly or at bedtime	Mistaken as "qhr" or every hour	Use "nightly" or "at bedtime"
q.o.d. or QOD**	Every other day	Mistaken as q.d. (daily) or q.i.d. (4 times daily) if the "o" is poorly written	Use "every other day"
q1d	Daily	Mistaken as q.i.d. (4 times daily)	Use "daily"
q6PM, etc.	Every evening at 6 PM	Mistaken as every 6 hours	Use "6 PM nightly" or "6 PM daily"
SC, SQ, sub q	Subcutaneous	SC mistaken as SL (sublingual); SQ mistaken as "5 every"; the "q" in "sub q" has been mistaken for "every" (e.g., a heparin dose ordered "sub q 2 hours before surgery" misunderstood as every 2 hours before surgery)	Use "subcut" or "subcutaneously"
ss	Sliding scale (insulin) or ½ (apothecary)	Mistaken as "55"	Spell out "sliding scale"; use "one-half" or "½"
SSRI	Sliding scale regular insulin	Mistaken as selective-serotonin reuptake inhibitor	Spell out "sliding scale (insulin)"
SSI	Sliding scale insulin	Mistaken as Strong Solution of Iodine (Lugol's)	Spell out "sliding scale (insulin)"
i/d	One daily	Mistaken as "tid"	Use "1 daily"
TIW or tiw	3 times a week	Mistaken as "3 times a day" or "twice a week"	Use "3 times weekly"
U or u**	Unit	Mistaken as the number 0 or 4, causing a 10-fold overdose or greater (e.g., 4U seen as 40 or 4u seen as 44); mistaken as "cc" so dose given in volume instead of units (e.g., 4u seen as 4cc)	Use "unit"

*These abbreviations, symbols, and dose designations have been reported to ISMP though the USP-ISMP Medication Error Reporting Program for being frequently misinterpreted and involved in harmful medication errors. They should never be used when communicating medical information. The Joint Commission has established a National Patient Safety Goal that specifies that certain abbreviations must appear on an accredited organization's do-not-use list; those items are indicated with a double asterisk (**). These abbreviations are included on The Joint Commission's "minimum list" of dangerous abbreviations, acronyms, and symbols that must be included on an organization's "Do Not Use" list, effective January 1, 2004. Report medication errors or near misses to the ISMP Medicaton Errors Reporting (MERP) at 1-800-FAILSAF(E) or online at www.ismp.org.
Used with permission, Institute for Safe Medication Practice (ISMP): http://www.ismp.org.

Pharmacology Review

As an RT, it will be your responsibility to remember all of the pulmonary medicines you learned about in school as well as to keep current with the pulmonary medications that become available for your patients as a result of new research. As a student RT, this can be a daunting task. To begin, start with the most common medications you will come across, and once you have a solid understanding of them, go on to a new medication. Keep this up, and soon knowledge of all the pulmonary medications will become second nature. The following is a review of common classes of pulmonary medications (see also Table 18-2).

> ✱ **Tip** It is difficult to memorize medications when you are not in the clinical environment. Once you begin administering medications several times a day, it will become much easier.

Adrenergic Bronchodilators

Adrenergic bronchodilators, such as β_2-agonists, represent the largest group of drugs among the aerosolized agents used for oral inhalation. The general indication for use of an adrenergic bronchodilator is the presence of reversible air flow obstruction. The most common therapeutic use of these agents is to improve flow rates in asthma (including exercise-induced asthma), acute and chronic bronchitis, emphysema, bronchiectasis, cystic fibrosis, and other obstructive airway states.

Anticholinergic Bronchodilators

The second method of producing airway relaxation is through blockade of cholinergic-induced bronchoconstriction. An important difference between β_2-agonists and anticholinergic bronchodilators is the active stimulatory action of the former versus the passive blockade of the latter. A cholinergic blocking agent is only effective if bronchoconstriction exists because of

TABLE 18-2 Common Agents Used in Respiratory Therapy

Drug Group	Therapeutic Purpose	Agents
Adrenergic agents	*β-Adrenergic:* Relaxation of bronchial smooth muscle and bronchodilation, to reduce *Raw* and to improve ventilatory flow rates in airway obstruction resulting from COPD, asthma, CF, acute bronchitis	Albuterol Arformoterol Formoterol Levalbuterol Pirbuterol Salmeterol
	α-Adrenergic: Topical vasoconstriction and decongestion Used to treat upper airway swelling	Racemic epinephrine
Anticholinergic agents	Relaxation of cholinergically induced bronchoconstriction to improve ventilatory flow rates in COPD and asthma	Ipratropium bromide Tiotropium bromide
Mucoactive agents	Modification of properties of respiratory tract mucus; current agents reduce viscosity and promote clearance of secretions	Acetylcysteine Dornase alfa
Corticosteroids	Reduction and control of airway inflammatory response usually associated with asthma (lower respiratory tract) or with seasonal or chronic rhinitis (upper respiratory tract)	Beclomethasone dipropionate Budesonide Ciclesonide Flunisolide Fluticasone propionate Mometasone furoate Triamcinolone acetonide
Antiasthmatic agents	Prevention of onset and development of the asthmatic response, through inhibition of chemical mediators of inflammation	Cromolyn sodium Montelukast Omalizumab Zafirlukast Zileuton
Antiinfective agents	Inhibition or eradication of specific infective agents, such as *Pneumocystis carinii (jiroveci)* (pentamidine), RSV (ribavirin), *Pseudomonas aeruginosa* in CF or influenza A and B	Aztreonam Pentamidine Ribavirin Tobramycin Zanamivir
Exogenous surfactants	Approved clinical use is by direct intratracheal instillation, for the purpose of restoring more normal lung compliance in respiratory distress syndrome of newborns	Beractant Calfactant Lucinactant Poractant alfa
Prostacyclin analogues	Clinically indicated to treat pulmonary hypertension for the purpose of decreasing shortness of breath and increasing walking distance	Iloprost Treprostinil

CF, Cystic fibrosis; *COPD,* chronic obstructive pulmonary disease; *Raw,* airway resistance; *RSV,* respiratory syncytial virus.
From Gardenhire, D: *Rau's respiratory care pharmacology,* ed 8, St. Louis, MO, 2012, Mosby.

cholinergic activity. Generally, anticholinergic agents have been found to be as effective as β_2-agonists in air flow improvement in patients with COPD but less so in those with asthma. A combination anticholinergic and β-agonist, such as ipratropium bromide and albuterol (Combivent; Combivent Respimat; Duoneb), is indicated for use in patients with COPD who are on regular treatment and require additional bronchodilation for relief of air flow obstruction.

Mucolytics

The two mucus-controlling agents currently approved in the United States for oral inhalation with an effect on mucus are *N*-acetyl-l-cysteine (NAC) and Dornase alfa. Both agents are mucolytic, although their modes of action differ.

Inhaled Corticosteroids

Corticosteroids are endogenous hormones produced in the adrenal cortex which regulate basic metabolic functions in the body and exert an antiinflammatory effect. Inhaled corticosteroid (ICS) agents are used to treat inflammation in the pulmonary system. Primarily, ICSs are used as maintenance therapy for persistent asthma and severe COPD.

> ✱ **Tip** Patients should always rinse the mouth following administration of ICSs.

Nonsteroidal Antiasthma Agents

Nonsteroidal antiasthma agents constitute a growing class of drugs in the treatment of asthma. These include cromolyn sodium, antileukotrienes, also termed *leukotriene modifiers* (zafirlukast, zileuton, and montelukast), and monoclonal antibodies or anti-immunoglobulin E (IgE) agents (omalizumab). Antileukotrienes are administered orally, and monoclonal antibody agents are given parenterally but are included as bronchoactive drugs. The general indication for the clinical use of these medications is prophylactic management (control) of persistent asthma.

Aerosolized Antiinfective Agents

Multiple aerosolized antiinfective agents are available in the market today. Some may be used less often than others in respiratory therapy. Medications, such as Tobramycin and Aztreonam, are commonly given to manage chronic *Pseudomonas aeruginosa* infection in patients with cystic fibrosis.

Bibliography

Gardenhire DS: *Rau's respiratory care pharmacology*, ed 8, St. Louis, MO, 2012, Elsevier.

Institute for Safe Medication Practice (ISMP): http://www.ismp.org. Accessed 7/8/12.

Kacmarek RM, Stoller JK, Heuer AJ: *Egan's fundamentals of respiratory care*, ed 10, St. Louis, MO, 2013, Mosby.

The Joint Commission: Accreditation program: national patient safety goals: http://www.jointcommission.org/assets/1/6/2011_NPSGs_HAP.pdf. Accessed 7/8/12.

1. What are the six rights of medication administration?

_____

_____

2. Obtain an ampoule of medication for administration using a small-volume nebulizer. Demonstrate how you would obtain it from a medication area for a lab partner by using the six rights. Once correctly performed, obtain your partner's signature.

Signature: _____

3. Fill in the "Effect" column of the following chart pertaining to airway receptors:

Airway Receptors and Their Effects in the Cardiopulmonary System*

Location	Receptor	Effect
Heart	β_1-adrenergic	
	M_2-cholinergic	
Bronchiolar smooth muscle	β_2-adrenergic	
	M_3-cholinergic	
Pulmonary blood vessels	β_1-adrenergic	
	β_2-adrenergic	
	M_3-cholinergic	
Bronchial blood vessels	β_1-adrenergic	
	β_2-adrenergic	
Submucosal glands	β_1-adrenergic	
	β_2-adrenergic	
	M_3-cholinergic	

4. Fill in the following chart pertaining to adrenergic bronchodilators:

Adrenergic Bronchodilator Agents Currently Available in the United States

Drug	Brand Name	Receptor Preference	Adult Dosage	Time Course (Onset, Peak, Duration)
ULTRA SHORT-ACTING ADRENERGIC BRONCHODILATOR AGENTS				
Racemic epinephrine				Onset:
				Peak:
				Duration:
SHORT-ACTING ADRENERGIC BRONCHODILATOR AGENTS				
Albuterol				Onset:
				Peak:
				Duration:
Pirbuterol				Onset:
				Peak:
				Duration:
Levalbuterol				Onset:
				Peak:
				Duration:
LONG-ACTING ADRENERGIC BRONCHODILATOR AGENTS				
Salmeterol				Onset:
				Peak:
				Duration:
Formoterol				Onset:
				Peak:
				Duration:
Arformoterol				Onset:
				Peak:
				Duration:

Drug	Brand Name	Receptor Preference	Adult Dosage	Time Course (Onset, Peak, Duration)
Indacaterol				Onset:
				Peak:
				Duration:

5. What are the indications for short-acting adrenergic bronchodilators?

_____

6. What are the indications for long-acting adrenergic bronchodilators?

_____

7. Fill in the following chart pertaining to inhaled anticholinergic bronchodilators:

Inhaled Anticholinergic Bronchodilator Agents

Drug	Brand Name	Adult Dosage
Ipratropium bromide		
Ipratropium bromide and albuterol		
Tiotropium bromide		

8. What are the indications for anticholinergic bronchodilators?

_____

9. What are the indications for combined anticholinergic and β_2-agonist bronchodilators?

_____

10. Fill in the following chart pertaining to mucoactive agents:

Mucoactive Agents Available for Aerosol Administration

Drug	Brand Name	Adult Dosage	Use
Acetylcysteine 10%			
Acetylcysteine 20%			
Dornase alfa			

11. What are the indications for Dornase alfa?

_____

12. Fill in the following chart pertaining to corticosteroids and combination products available by aerosol:

Corticosteroids and Combination Products Available by Aerosol

Drug	Brand Name	Formulation and Dosage
Beclomethasone dipropionate HFA		
Ciclesonide		
Flunisolide hemihydrate HFA		
Fluticasone propionate		
Budesonide		
Mometasone furoate		
Fluticasone propionate/salmeterol		
Budesonide/formoterol fumarate HFA		
Mometasone furoate/formoterol fumarate HFA		

13. What is the indication for use of inhaled corticosteroids?

14. Fill in the following chart pertaining to currently available inhaled antiinfective agents:

Currently Available Inhaled Antiinfective Agents

Drug	Brand Name	Formulation and Dosage	Clinical Use
Pentamidine			
Ribavirin			
Tobramycin			
Aztreonam			
Zanamivir			

15. Use 3 × 5 index cards to make drug flash cards for the drugs indicated using the following format:

Front of card: Generic name

Back of card: Trade name, drug class, indications, contraindications, dose, route, mode of action, and receptor preference (if applicable)

- Racemic epinephrine

- Albuterol

- Pirbuterol

- Levalbuterol

- Salmeterol

- Formoterol

- Arformoterol

- Indacaterol

- Ipratropium bromide

- Tiotropium bromide

- Aclidinium bromide

- Ipratropium bromide and albuterol

- *N*-Acetylcysteine (NAC)

- Dornase alfa

- Beclomethasone diproprionate HFA

- Flunisolide hemihydrates HFA

- Fluticasone propionate

- Budesonide

- Mometasone furoate

- Ciclesonide

- Fluticasone propionate/salmeterol

- Budesonide/formoterol fumarate HFA

- Mometasone furoate/formoterol fumarate HFA

- Pentamidine isethionate

- Ribavirin

- Tobramycin

- Aztreonam

- Zanamivir

Self-Assessment Questions

1. Aerosolized aztreonam is most commonly given for:
   A. Asthma
   B. CF
   C. COPD
   D. CHF

2. Three phases that constitute the course of drug action from dose to effect are:
   A. Drug administration, pharmacokinetic, and pharmacodynamic phases
   B. Drug administration, distribution, and elimination phases
   C. Drug absorption, pharmacokinetic, and pharmacodynamic phases
   D. Drug absorption, elimination, and pharmacodynamic phases

3. The devices most commonly used to administer orally inhaled aerosols are:

   1. MDI
   2. SVN
   3. DPI
   4. Endotracheal tubes (ETT)

   A. 1 and 3 only
   B. 2, 3, and 4 only
   C. 1, 2, and 3 only
   D. 1, 2, 3, and 4

4. In the United States, what agency accredits health care organizations and strives to improve patient safety?
   A. NBRC
   B. AARC
   C. TJC
   D. RRT-NPS

5. Short-acting β_2-agonists are indicated for:
   A. Reduction of airway edema
   B. Relief of acute reversible air flow limitation
   C. Maintenance only for bronchodilation
   D. Thinning of secretions

6. In what percent solution should racemic epinephrine be delivered?
   A. 0.9%
   B. 2.25%
   C. 3%
   D. 7%

7. Treatment of the respiratory tract with inhaled aerosols offers many advantages such as:

   1. Doses are usually smaller than doses for systemic administration.
   2. Onset of drug action is slow.
   3. Delivery is targeted to the organ requiring treatment.
   4. Systemic side effects are often fewer and less severe.

   A. 1 and 4 only
   B. 1, 2, and 3 only
   C. 1, 3, and 4 only
   D. 1, 2, 3, and 4 only

8. Your patient is an 18-year-old female complaining of shortness of breath, and severe wheezing on auscultation is noted in her assessment. What medication would you administer?
   A. Xopenex
   B. Atrovent
   C. Foradil
   D. Serevent

9. An indication for anticholinergic bronchodilator therapy is:
   A. Maintenance treatment in COPD
   B. Treatment of infection in patients with CF
   C. First-line therapy in acute asthma exacerbations
   D. All of the above

10. The combination of albuterol and atrovent is called:
    A. Duoneb
    B. Combivent
    C. A and B are correct
    D. None of the above is correct

▶▶ CASE STUDY 18-1

You have administered an aerosol treatment of albuterol using a MDI to a 67-year-old patient with newly diagnosed COPD who was admitted for an acute exacerbation and shortness of breath. When you return for the second treatment that day, he informs you that he began to feel very shaky and nervous, beginning about 30 minutes after the previous treatment. He had also noticed a tremor when he held his water cup and took a drink. His heart rate during the earlier treatment was 84 beats/min. Your clinical assessment shows that he is alert and oriented to person, place, and time, has good color, is not diaphoretic, and is in no respiratory distress. His respiratory rate (RR) is 16 breaths/min and regular. Auscultation reveals mild wheezing in the apices anteriorly with little change from earlier breath sounds. You observe a mild tremor when he holds his hand out. On questioning, he states that he is now feeling better.

1. What are some effects of adrenergic bronchodilators?

   _____

   _____

2. What are some choices you can make with regard to medication delivery and patient education?

   _____

   _____

3. How would you assess the efficacy of this patient's bronchodilator therapy?

   _____

   _____

Medication Delivery Devices

Douglas S. Gardenhire

■ OBJECTIVES

Upon the completion of the chapter activities and content review topics, the student should be able to:
1. Define aerosol therapy.
2. Select an appropriate aerosol medication nebulizer on the basis of particle size distributions.
3. Differentiate among the types of aerosol devices.
4. Describe the clinical applications of aerosol devices.
5. Perform therapy using a small-volume nebulizer.
6. Perform therapy using a pressurized metered-dose inhaler.
7. Perform therapy using a dry-powder inhaler.
8. Perform therapy using the Combivent Respimat inhaler.

■ KEY TERMS

- Aerosol therapy
- Combivent Respimat
- Dry-powder inhaler (DPI)
- Pressurized metered-dose inhaler (pMDI)
- Small-volume nebulizer (SVN)

■ CONTENT REVIEW TOPICS

- Pulmonary airway pharmacology

■ PROCEDURAL ASSESSMENTS

19-1   Using a Small-Volume Nebulizer
19-2   Using a Pressurized Metered-Dose Inhaler
19-3   Using a Dry-Powder Inhaler
19-4   Using a Combivent Respimat

■ EQUIPMENT

- 50 psi gas source
- Combivent Respimat inhaler
- Demonstrator DPIs
- Demonstrator pMDIs
- Mock medication ampoules or saline ampoules
- Small-volume nebulizers

Aerosol generation and delivery to the lungs is a complex topic. Development of both the technology and the scientific basis of inhaled aerosol administration is an ongoing process. Respiratory therapists (RTs) are the primary health care providers responsible for this modality. The term aerosol therapy may be defined as the delivery of aerosol particles to the respiratory tract. At present, the three main uses of aerosol therapy in respiratory care are as follows:
1. Humidification of dry inspired gases, using bland aerosols
2. Improved mobilization and clearance of respiratory secretions, including sputum induction, using bland aerosols of water, and hypertonic or hypotonic saline
3. Delivery of aerosolized drugs to the respiratory tract
   Lung deposition is dependent on a variety of factors such as the aerosol generator, the patient, the drug, and the disease. Depending on the type of the small-volume nebulizer (SVN) used, most of the drug loss with an SVN occurs in the device, whereas the main drug loss with the pressurized metered dose inhaler (pMDI) and dry-powder inhaler (DPI) occurs in the oropharyngeal airways. Adding a reservoir device to a pMDI or using a nonelectrostatic valved holding chamber shifts the loss from the throat to the reservoir and increases aerosol deposition in the lungs. Figure 19-1 indicates the percentages of drug deposition for different aerosol generators and shows that oropharyngeal loss, device loss, and exhalation or ambient loss differ among aerosol device types, as do lung doses.
   It should be noted that the overall efficiency in lung deposition of 10% to 15% of the total drug dose is not significantly

better than with most pMDI or DPI devices used clinically in the past. Nebulizers, as well as pMDIs and DPIs, are evolving to greater efficiency. One of the major factors influencing aerosol deposition in the lungs is particle size. The effect of particle size on deposition in the respiratory tract is illustrated in Figure 19-2. This chapter will focus on the physical principles of aerosol delivery to the airways and on aerosol-generating devices for the inhalation of drugs.

≫ SKILL CHECK LISTS

19-1 Using a Small-Volume Nebulizer Therapy

The term *nebulizer* encompasses a variety of devices that operate on different physical principles to generate an aerosol from a drug solution. The SVN is a type of aerosol generator converting liquid drug solutions or suspensions into aerosol. Because SVNs are often used in infants or in patients in acute respiratory distress, slow breathing and an inspiratory pause may not be feasible or obtainable. One of the main advantages of SVNs is that dose delivery occurs over 60 to 90 breaths rather than in one or two inhalations, as with pMDIs. Thus, a single ineffective breath will not undermine the efficacy of the treatment. Box 19-1 summarizes the advantages and disadvantages of SVNs. SVNs may be classified into three categories: (1) jet (pneumatic) nebulizers, (2) mesh nebulizers, and (3) ultrasonic nebulizers. Box 19-2 lists the nebulizers that have specific applications. The following is the step-by-step process for the use of an SVN.

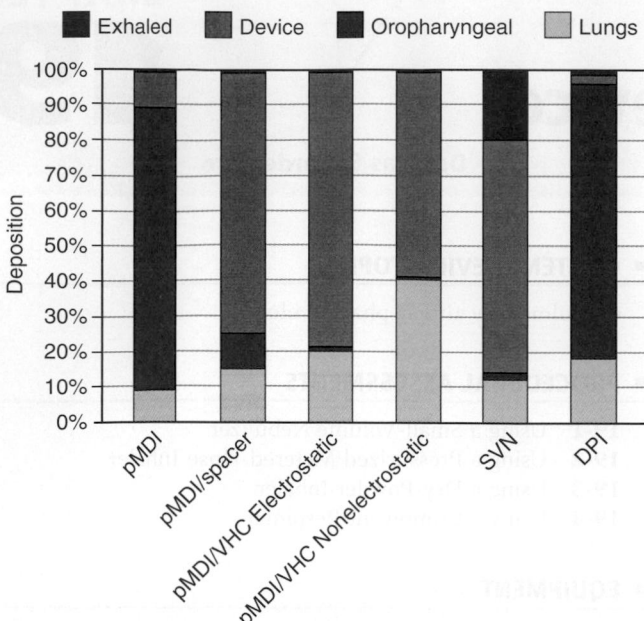

Figure 19-1 Drug deposition with common aerosol inhaler devices. (Modified from Ari A, Hess DR, Myers TR, Rau JL: *A guide to aerosol delivery devices for respiratory therapists*, ed 2, Dallas TX, 2009, American Association for Respiratory Care.)

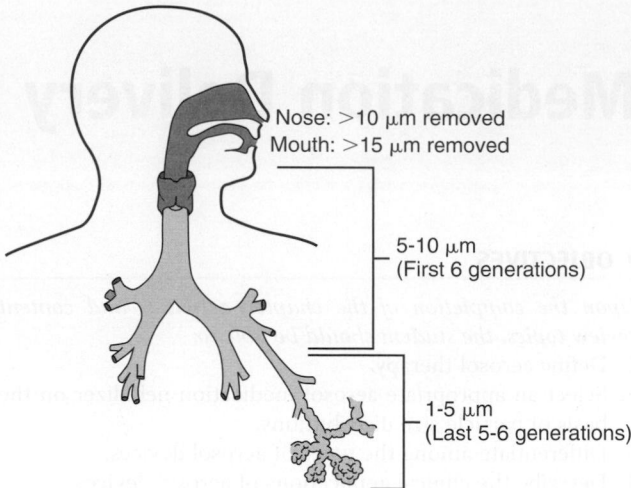

Figure 19-2 Effect of aerosol particle size on area of preferential deposition within the airway. (From Gardenhire DS: *Rau's respiratory care pharmacology*, ed 8, St. Louis, MO, 2012, Mosby.)

BOX 19-1	Advantages and Disadvantages of Small-Volume Nebulizers

Advantages
- Many drug solutions can be aerosolized with SVNs.
- Drug mixtures (i.e., more than one drug) can be aerosolized, with suitable testing of drug activity.
- Minimal cooperation or coordination is required for inhalation.
- They are useful in the very young or the very old, debilitated patients, or those in acute distress.
- They are effective with low inspiratory flows or volumes.
- Normal breathing pattern can be used, and inspiratory pause (breathhold) is not required for efficacy.
- Drug concentrations and dose can be modified, if desired.

Disadvantages
- The equipment required for use is expensive and cumbersome.
- Treatment times are somewhat lengthy and may range from 5 to 25 minutes, depending upon the type of SVN used for aerosol drug delivery.
- Performance characteristics vary among different types, brands, and models.
- Contamination is possible with inadequate cleaning.
- Assembly and cleaning are required.
- A wet, cold spray occurs with mask delivery.
- A power source, battery, electricity, or compressed gas, is needed.
- Aerosol drug administration with a face mask may inadvertently deposit the medication in the eyes and result in eye irritation.

BOX 19-2	Specific Nebulizer Applications

Nebulizer for Ribavirin Administration
The small-particle aerosol generator (SPAG) device is a large reservoir nebulizer, capable of holding 300 mL of solution for long periods of nebulization. It operates on a jet-shearing principle.

Nebulizer for Pentamidine Administration
A SVN fitted with inspiratory and expiratory one-way valves and with expiratory filter is used for the administration of aerosolized pentamidine. The one-way valves used with the SVN prevent second-hand exposure of pentamidine by eliminating the contamination of the ambient environment with exhaled aerosol.

Nebulizer for Aztreonam Administration
The Altera Nebulizer System has been customized to deliver aztreonam (Cayston). It is an active vibrating mesh nebulizer. The nebulizer produces aerosols with a very high density of drug, a precisely defined droplet size, and a high proportion of respirable aerosol.

 Reality Check Breath-enhanced nebulizers allow more aerosol release during inspiration with decreased output during exhalation or breath-hold through two one-way valves used to prevent the loss of aerosol to environment.

✳ Tip Here are some recommendations that apply to all nebulizers:
- Read and follow the instructions on the nebulizer before using it.
- Make sure that the nebulizer is properly assembled according to the manufacturer's instructions.
- Make sure that the nebulizer is cleaned and dried between treatments.
- Make sure that the nebulizer is operated in its proper orientation.

Procedural Preparation

1. Review the patient's chart.
2. Verify the physician's order or the facility's protocol for standard of care.
3. Obtain, clean, and inspect the appropriate equipment prior to entering the patient's room.
4. Follow personal protective equipment (PPE) requirements, and observe standard precautions for any transmission-based isolation procedure.
5. Identify the patient using two patient identifiers.
6. Introduce yourself to the patient and to the family.
7. Explain the procedure to the patient and to the family, and acknowledge the patient's understanding.
8. Perform proper hand hygiene, and put on gloves, mask, and protective eyewear, as appropriate for the procedure.

Implementation

1. Place the patient in the upright position.
2. Assess vital signs.
3. Select mask or mouthpiece delivery.
4. Place the medication in the nebulizer.
5. Attach the equipment to the appropriate gas for pneumatic power and proper liter flow (6–10 L/min, depending on the device).
6. Check for proper function.
7. Coach the patient to breath slowly through their mouth.
8. Reassess pulse rate, respiratory rate, and lung sounds half way through the treatment.
9. Continue the treatment until the nebulizer sputters.
10. Disconnect the nebulizer from the gas source.
11. Rinse the nebulizer with sterile water and leave it to air-dry or discard it, between treatments.
12. Instruct the patient to rinse their mouth following the treatment.
13. Reassess pulse rate, respiratory rate, and lung sounds after the treatment.
14. Remove the supplies from the patient's room, and clean the area, as needed.
15. Remove PPE, and perform proper hand hygiene prior to leaving the patient's room.

Evaluation of Procedure

1. Establish a baseline, or compare with previous measurements.
2. Reassess the patient for any adverse response.
3. Discontinue the treatment if any adverse reaction occurs.
4. Develop an appropriate respiratory care plan based on assessment data.
5. Identify any unexpected outcomes.

Documentation and Reporting

1. Record your findings in the patient's chart.
2. Report any abnormal findings to the appropriate health care provider.

19-2   Using a Pressurized Metered-Dose Inhaler

pMDIs, or MDIs are the most common aerosol generators prescribed for patients with asthma or chronic obstructive pulmonary disease (COPD). These devices are small, pressurized canisters for oral inhalation of aerosol drugs and contain multiple doses of accurately metered medication. The drug in a pMDI is either a suspension of micronized powder in a liquefied propellant or a solution of the active ingredient in a co-solvent (usually ethanol) mixed with the propellant hydrofluoroalkanes (HFAs). Advantages and disadvantages of drug delivery by pMDI are listed in Box 19-3.

The conventional pMDI has a press-and-breathe design. When the canister is depressed into the actuator, the drug–propellant mixture in the metering valve is released under pressure. The liquid propellant rapidly expands and vaporizes, or "flashes," as it ejects from the pressurized valve into ambient pressure. This expansion and vaporization shatters the liquid stream into an aerosol. The initial vaporization of propellant causes cooling of the liquid–gas aerosol suspension, which can be felt if discharged onto skin (with the older versions of pMDIs, chlorofluorocarbons [CFCs] were used); however, HFA versions have a much "warmer" spray temperature. On release, the metering valve refills with the mixture of drug and propellant from the bulk of the canister and is ready for the next discharge. The accuracy and consistency of dose from pMDIs may be more sensitive to handling practices than previously thought. Research on the drug content of sprays of albuterol via pMDIs has shown that various factors affect dose consistency. These factors are listed in Box 19-4.

Extension, or reservoir, devices were introduced primarily to simplify the complex coordination of aiming, actuation, and breathing with a pMDI. Figure 19-3 is an illustration of a generic reservoir device. Using accessory devices with pMDIs improves the effectiveness of aerosol drug administration because pMDI accessory devices can modify the aerosol discharged from a pMDI in the following three ways:

BOX 19-3   Advantages and Disadvantages of Pressurized Metered-Dose Inhalers

Advantages
- Pressurized metered-dose inhalers (pMDIs) are portable, light, and compact.
- Drug delivery is efficient.
- Treatment time is short.
- They are easy to use.
- More than 100 doses per device are possible.
- Fine particle sizes are available in hydrofluoroalkanes (HFA) formulations.
- They are difficult to contaminate.
- No drug preparation is needed.
- It is possible to reproduce emitted doses.

Disadvantages
- Complex hand–breathing coordination, proper inhalation pattern, and breath-hold are required.
- Drug concentrations and doses are fixed.
- Canister depletion is difficult to determine accurately.
- Reactions to the propellants may occur in a small percentage of patients.
- High oropharyngeal impaction and loss occur if an extension device is not used.
- Foreign body aspiration of coins and debris from the mouthpiece may occur.
- It is difficult to determine the dose remaining in the canister without a dose counter.

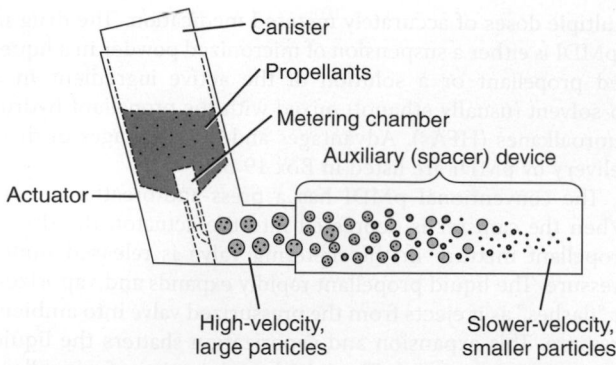

Figure 19-3 A pMDI with a spacer. See the effect of a reservoir device on aerosol particle size and velocity from the pMDI. (From Gardenhire DS: *Rau's respiratory care pharmacology*, ed 8, St. Louis, MO, 2012, Mosby.)

BOX 19-4	Factors That Affect Dose Consistency in Pressurized Metered-Dose Inhalers

Loss of Dose
Loss of dose refers to the loss of drug content in the valve even though propellant may seem to discharge a normal dose.

Shaking the Canister
Many of the drugs in pMDI formulation are suspensions that may separate from the propellants on standing (*creaming*).

Timing of Actuation Intervals
A pause of 1 to 5 minutes between each puff of a bronchodilator from a pMDI has been advocated to improve distribution of the inhaled drug in the lungs.

Loss of Prime
Loss of prime refers to the loss of propellant from the metering valve of the pMDI; when this occurs, little or no drug will be discharged on actuation.

Storage Temperature
Data indicate that dose delivery from CFC–propelled pMDIs of albuterol decreases at lower temperatures; in contrast, HFA–propelled albuterol remains constant in total dose over the range of −20°C to 20°C

Nozzle Size and Cleanliness
Aerosol drug delivery with a pMDI is dependent on nozzle size, cleanliness, and lack of moisture.

Breathing Technique
Techniques for using a pMDI without a spacer include the *open-mouth* technique and the *closed-mouth* technique and the use of a reservoir device.

Patient Characteristics
The characteristics of the patient using the pMDI cause variability of aerosol deposition.

---

1. Such devices allow space and time for more vaporization of the propellants and evaporation of initially large particles to smaller sizes.
2. Reservoirs allow the high initial velocity of particles released from a pMDI to slow before reaching the oropharynx. Particles discharged from the actuator nozzle have velocities exceeding 30 m/sec. By holding the actuator 4 cm in front

---

BOX 19-5	Advantages and Disadvantages of Pressurized Metered-Dose Inhaler Accessory Devices

Advantages
- Reduced oropharyngeal drug loss
- Separation of pMDI actuation and inhalation
- Ability to use MDI during acute air flow obstruction with dyspnea
- Available with mask for children
- No drug preparation required
- Increased inhaled dose by twofold or fourfold compared with pMDI alone

Disadvantages
- Large and cumbersome (some brands)
- Additional expense compared with pMDI alone
- Some assembly required
- Possible source of bacterial contamination with inadequate cleaning
- Patient errors in use of pMDI accessory devices such as firing multiple puffs into the chamber before inhaling or a delay between actuation and inhalation

MDI, Metered dose inhaler; *pMDI*, pressurized metered dose inhaler.
(From Gardenhire, DS: *Rau's respiratory care pharmacology*, ed 8, St. Louis, MO, 2012, Mosby.)

---

of the mouth or by using an extension device, this velocity is allowed to slow.

3. As holding chambers for the aerosol cloud released, reservoir devices separate the actuation of the canister from the inhalation and simplify the coordination required for effective use.

The combined effect of the first two advantages reduces oropharyngeal deposition. This will reduce the amount of drug swallowed, and thereby absorbed from the gastrointestinal (GI) tract, and also reduce any local oropharyngeal side effects such as those seen with inhaled corticosteroids. Box 19-5 summarizes the advantages and disadvantages of accessory devices.

The following is the step-by-step process for the procedural assessment for using a pMDI.

→ **Reality Check** CFCs and HFAs are the two types of propellants used with pMDIs. The U.S. Food and Drug Administration (FDA) banned the use of CFC-pMDIs because one CFC molecule can destroy 100,000 molecules of stratospheric ozone.

Procedural Preparation

1. Review the patient's chart.
2. Verify the physician's order or the facility's protocol for standard of care.
3. Obtain, clean, and inspect the appropriate equipment prior to entering the patient's room.
4. Follow PPE requirements, and observe standard precautions for any transmission-based isolation procedure.
5. Identify the patient using two patient identifiers.
6. Introduce yourself to the patient and to the family.

7. Explain the procedure to the patient and to the family, and acknowledge the patient's understanding.
8. Perform proper hand hygiene, and put on gloves, mask, and protective eyewear, as appropriate for the procedure.

Implementation

1. Place the patient in the upright position, and instruct the patient to breathe normally.
2. Assess vital signs.
3. Shake the pMDI vigorously.
4. Before the first use of a new pMDI, and when the pMDI has not been used for several days, have the patient prime the pMDI by pointing it into the air (away from people) and actuate.
5. Assemble the apparatus, and uncap the mouthpiece, ensuring that no loose objects are present in the device
6. For the open-mouth technique:
   a. Instruct the patient to open their mouth wide, keep their tongue down, hold the pMDI with the canister oriented downward, and aim the outlet at their mouth approximately two fingerbreadths away from mouth.
   b. Instruct the patient to breathe out normally.
   c. Instruct the patient to slowly begin to breathe in and then actuate the pMDI.
   d. Instruct the patient to continue inspiration to total lung capacity.
7. For the closed-mouth technique:
   a. Instruct the patient to place their mouthpiece between the lips, with the tongue out of the path of the outlet.
   b. Instruct the patient to breathe out normally.
   c. Instruct the patient to slowly begin to breathe in and actuate the pMDI.
   d. Instruct the patient to continue inspiration to total lung capacity.
8. For using a reservoir device (preferred method):
   a. Instruct the patient to breathe out normally.
   b. Instruct the patient to place the mouthpiece of the reservoir device between their lips, with the tongue out of the path of the outlet.
   c. Instruct the patient to actuate the pMDI.
   d. Instruct the patient to slowly breathe in.
9. Instruct the patient to hold their breath up to, but no longer than, 10 seconds and then to relax and breathe normally.
10. Instruct the patient to wait 1 minute between puffs.
11. Disassemble the apparatus, and recap the mouthpiece.
12. Reassess vital signs.
13. Remove the supplies from the patient's room, and clean the area, as needed.
14. Remove PPE, and perform proper hand hygiene prior to leaving the patient's room.

Evaluation of Procedure

1. Have the patient demonstrate the proper use of the pMDI.
2. Evaluate the patient for any side effects of the therapy.
3. Identify any unexpected outcomes.

Documentation and Reporting

1. Record your findings in the patient's chart.
2. Report any abnormal findings to the appropriate health care provider.

BOX 19-6 Advantages and Disadvantages of DPI Devices

Advantages
- Small and portable
- Short preparation and administration times
- Breath actuation; no need for hand–breathing coordination
- No inspiratory hold or head tilt needed
- No CFC propellants (environmentally friendly)
- No cold Freon effect to cause bronchoconstriction or inhibit full inspiration
- Simple determination of remaining drug doses
- Built-in dose counter

Disadvantages
- Only a limited range of drugs available to date
- Patients not as aware of the dose inhaled as with an MDI and may distrust delivery
- Moderate to high inspiratory flow rates needed for powder dispersion
- Relatively high oropharyngeal impaction and deposition may occur
- A device such as the Aerolizer, which is a single-dose device, must be loaded before each use
- Vulnerable to ambient humidity or exhaled humidity into mouthpiece
- Different DPIs with different drugs
- Easy for patient to confuse directions for use with other devices

CFC, Chlorofluorocarbon; *MDI*, metered dose inhaler.
(From Gardenhire, DS: Rau's Respiratory Care Pharmacology, ed 8, St. Louis, 2012, Mosby-Elsevier)

19-3 Using a Dry-Powder Inhaler

A DPI is similar to a pMDI except that the drug is in powder form. The main advantage is that the DPI is breath actuated; that is, hand–breathing coordination is not needed. The main disadvantage is that it requires a high inspiratory flow rate from the patient to dispense the drug. The flow rate needed is usually between 30 and 90 L/min. A list of advantages and disadvantages is provided in Box 19-6.

→ **Reality Check** Children and patients with respiratory disease may not be able to generate the flow needed to use a DPI.

DPIs may be divided into three categories based on the design of their dose containers:
1. Unit-dose DPIs
2. Multiple unit-dose DPIs
3. Multiple-dose DPIs

All types of DPIs have the same components incorporated into the inhaler, including a drug holder, an air inlet, an agglomeration compartment, and a mouthpiece. Figure 19-4 provides diagrammatic representations of the types of DPIs. Factors that affect DPI performance and drug delivery are listed in Box 19-7.

The following is the step-by-step process for using a DPI.

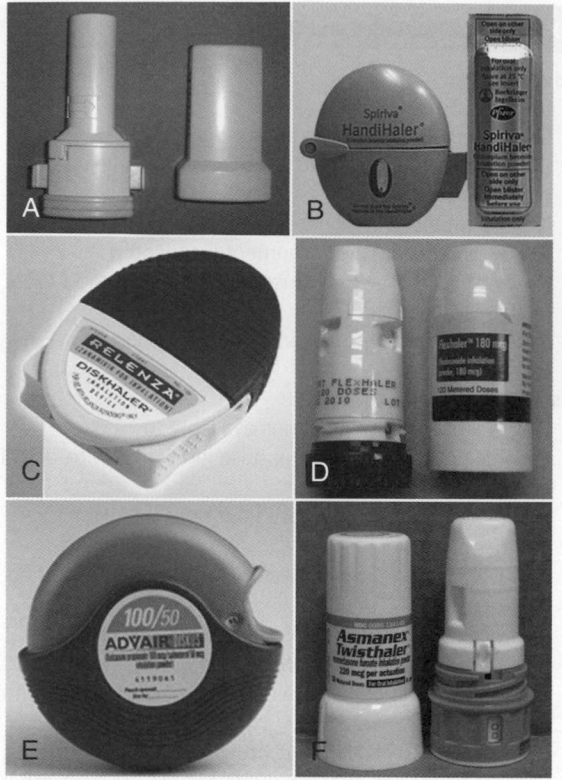

Figure 19-4 Diagrammatic representation of types of dry-powder inhalers (DPIs). **A,** Unit-dose DPI: Aerolizer (Merck & Co Inc., Whitehouse Station, NJ). **B,** Handihaler (Boeheringer Ingelheim Pharmaceuticals Inc., Ridgefield, CT). C, Multiple unit-dose DPI: Diskhaler (GlaxoSmithKline, used with permission). **D,** Flexhaler (AstraZeneca LP, Wilmington, DE). **E,** Multiple-dose DPI: Diskus inhaler (GlaxoSmithKline, used with permission). **F,** Twisthaler (Merck & Co. Inc., Whitehouse Station, NJ). (**A and F,** The Foradil Aerolizer and the Asmanex Twisthaler are registered trademarks of the Schering Corporation, a subsidiary of Merck &Co., Inc. All rights reserved.)

BOX 19-7   Factors Affecting DPI Performance and Drug Delivery

Intrinsic Resistance
Intrinsic resistance of the DPI determines how much inspiratory flow is needed to be created in the device to release the correct amount of drug.

Inspiratory Flow Rate
Dispersal of drug powder depends on the energy of the inspiratory flow.

Humidity
Humidity and moisture may cause powder clumping and reduce deaggregation, as well as a fine particle mass in the dose.

Procedural Preparation

1. Review the patient's chart.
2. Verify the physician's order or the facility's protocol for standard of care.
3. Obtain, clean, and inspect the appropriate equipment prior to entering the patient's room.

4. Follow PPE requirements, and observe standard precautions for any transmission-based isolation procedure.
5. Identify the patient using two patient identifiers.
6. Introduce yourself to the patient and to the family.
7. Explain the procedure to the patient and to the family, and acknowledge the patient's understanding.
8. Perform proper hand hygiene, and put on gloves, mask, and protective eyewear, as appropriate for the procedure.

Implementation

1. Place the patient in the upright position, and instruct the patient to breathe normally.
2. Assess vital signs.
3. Assemble the apparatus.
4. Load a dose while keeping the device upright.
5. Instruct the patient to exhale slowly and completely.
6. Instruct the patient to seal their lips around the mouthpiece and inhale deeply and forcefully.
7. Instruct the patient to repeat the process until the dose is complete.
8. Instruct the patient to rinse their mouth once the treatment is complete.
9. Reassess vital signs.
10. Remove the supplies from the patient's room, and clean the area, as needed.
11. Remove PPE, and perform proper hand hygiene prior to leaving the patient's room.

Evaluation of Procedure

1. Have the patient demonstrate the proper use of the DPI during the next scheduled treatment.
2. Evaluate the patient for any side effects of the therapy.
3. Identify any unexpected outcomes.

Documentation and Reporting

1. Record your findings in the patient's chart.
2. Report any abnormal findings to the appropriate health care provider.

19-4 Using a Combivent Respimat

The Respimat is a soft mist inhaler developed and licensed by Boehringer Ingelheim International (Figure 19-5). The device is similar to a pMDI in that it provides a soft metered dose of drug for each actuation. Currently, in the United States, it is only available as Combivent. Combivent Respimat is a sterile, aqueous solution of ipratropium bromide and albuterol sulfate filled into a 4.5-mL plastic container crimped into an aluminum cylinder. The device does not have a propellant. It provides the patient with 120 doses of the drug.

Combivent Respimat inhalation spray is for the treatment of patients with COPD. The following is the step-by-step process for using of Combivent Respimat.

Procedural Preparation

1. Review the patient's chart.
2. Verify the physician's order or the facility's protocol for standard of care.
3. Obtain, clean, and inspect the appropriate equipment prior to entering the patient's room.

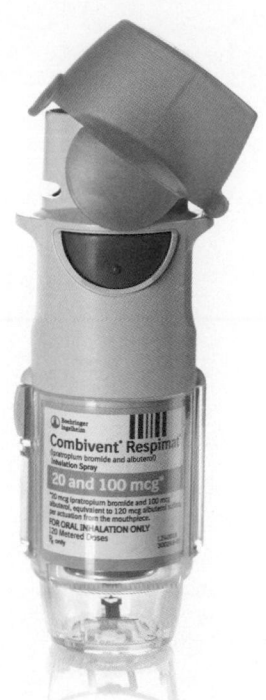

Figure 19-5 Combivent Respimat. Copyright © Boehringer Ingelheim Pharmaceuticals, Inc. or one of its affiliated companies. 2013. All Rights Reserved.

4. Follow PPE requirements, and observe standard precautions for any transmission-based isolation procedure.
5. Identify the patient using two patient identifiers.
6. Introduce yourself to the patient and to the family.
7. Explain the procedure to the patient and to the family, and acknowledge the patient's understanding.
8. Perform proper hand hygiene, and put on gloves, mask, and protective eyewear, as appropriate for the procedure.

Implementation

1. Place the patient in a comfortable position, and instruct the patient to breathe normally.
2. Assess vital signs.
3. For the first-time use of Combivent Respimat:
   a. With the orange cap closed, press the safety catch while pulling off the clear base.
      Be cautious not to touch the piercing element located inside the bottom of the clear base.
   b. Write a *discard by* date on the label of the inhaler.
      The *discard by* date should be 3 months from the date the cartridge is inserted into the inhaler.
   c. Remove the cartridge from the box.
   d. Push the *narrow* end of the cartridge into the inhaler.
      The base of the cartridge will not sit flush with the inhaler, and about one eighth of an inch will remain visible when the cartridge is correctly inserted.

   e. Do not remove the cartridge once it has been inserted into the inhaler.
   f. Put the clear base back in its place.
   g. Do not remove the clear base again.
      The inhaler should not be taken apart after inserting the cartridge. Put the clear base back in its place.
4. For priming:
   a. Hold the inhaler upright, with the orange cap closed.
   b. Turn the clear base in the direction of the white arrows on the label until it clicks (one half turn).
   c. Flip the orange cap until it snaps fully open.
   d. Point the inhaler toward the floor.
   e. Press the dose release button.
   f. Close the orange cap.
   g. Repeat steps *a* through *f* until a spray is visible.
   h. Once the spray is visible, repeat steps *a* through *f* three more times to make sure that the inhaler is prepared for use.
5. For daily use:
   a. Hold the inhaler upright, with the orange cap closed.
   b. Turn the clear base in the direction of the white arrows on the label until it clicks (one half turn).
   c. Flip the orange cap until it snaps fully open.
   d. Instruct the patient to breathe out slowly and fully and then close their lips around the end of the mouthpiece without covering the air vents.
   e. Instruct the patient to point the inhaler to the back of their throat.
   f. Instruct the patient to take in a slow, deep breath through the mouth, press the dose release button, and continue to breathe in slowly.
   g. Instruct the patient to hold their breath for 5-10 seconds.
   h. Close the orange cap.
6. Remove the supplies from the patient's room, and clean the area, as needed.
7. Remove PPE, and perform proper hand hygiene prior to leaving the patient's room.

Evaluation of Procedure

1. Establish a baseline, or compare with previous measurements.
2. Develop an appropriate respiratory care plan based on assessment data.
3. Identify any unexpected outcomes.

Documentation and Reporting

1. Record your findings in the patient's chart.
2. Report any abnormal findings to the appropriate health care provider.

Bibliography

Gardenhire DS: *Rau's respiratory care pharmacology*, ed 8, St. Louis, MO, 2012, Mosby.
Kacmarek RM, Stoller JK, Heuer AJ: *Egan's fundamentals of respiratory care*, ed 10, St. Louis, MO, 2013, Mosby.

1. Understanding aerosol drug therapy and choosing the proper device requires comprehension of terminology. Define the following terms. Explain them to a lab partner.

a. Aerodynamic diameter of a particle

_____

b. Aerosol

_____

c. Aerosol therapy

_____

d. Cascade impactor

_____

e. Chlorofluorocarbons (CFCs)

_____

f. Dead volume

_____

g. Deposition

_____

h. Heterodisperse

_____

i. Hydrofluoroalkane (HFA)

_____

j. In vitro

_____

k. In vivo

_____

l. Monodisperse

_____

m. Nebulizer

_____

n. Penetration

_____

o. Polydisperse

_____

p. Reservoir device

_____

q. Spacer

_____

r. Stability

_____

s. Valved holding chamber

_____

2. Fill in the table below pertaining to the advantages and disadvantages of aerosol delivery of drugs:

Advantages	Disadvantages

3. Fill in the table below pertaining to the advantages and disadvantages of SVNs:

Advantages	Disadvantages

4. Locate an SVN in the lab. Explain its operation, and identify its parts to a classmate. Get his or her signature.

Signature:_____

5. What are the eight questions you should ask when selecting an aerosol delivery device?

a. _____

b. _____

c. _____

d. _____

e. _____

f. _____

g. _____

h. _____

6. List the seven factors to consider when selecting the proper aerosol device.

a. _____

b. _____

c. _____

d. _____

e. _____

f. _____

g. _____

7. Fill in the table below pertaining to the advantages and disadvantages of pMDIs:

Advantages	Disadvantages

8. Locate a pMDI in the lab. Explain its operation, and identify its parts to a classmate. Get his or her signature.

Signature:_____

9. Fill in the table below pertaining to the advantages and disadvantages of DPIs.

Advantages	Disadvantages

10. Locate a DPI in the lab. Explain its operation, and identify its parts to a classmate. Get his or her signature.

Signature:_____

11. List the eight factors associated with reduced aerosol drug deposition in the lungs.

a. _____

b. _____

c. _____

d. _____

e. _____

f. _____

g. _____

h. _____

12. Aerosol particles produced for inhalation into the lungs by inhalant devices such as the MDI, SVN, or DPI include a range of sizes (polydisperse or heterodisperse) rather than a single size (monodisperse). Define the terms below related to aerosol particle size distributions:

a. Count mode _____

b. Count median diameter (CMD) _____

c. Mass median diameter (MMD) or mass median aerodynamic diameter (MMAD)_____

d. Geometric standard deviation (GSD)_____

13. Locate a Combivent Respimat inhaler in the lab. Explain its operation, and identify its parts to a classmate. Get his or her signature.

Signature:_____

Self-Assessment Questions

1. Which of the following is a disadvantage of aerosol delivery of drugs?
   A. Aerosol doses are smaller than those for systemic treatment.
   B. Onset of drug action is rapid.
   C. Drug delivery is targeted to the respiratory system for local pulmonary effect.
   D. Many physicians, nurses, and therapists lack knowledge about device use and administration protocols.

2. What is the recommended MMAD for delivery of medication to the lower airways?
   A. 5 to 50 μm
   B. 2 to 5 μm
   C. 1 to 3 μm
   D. <0.1 μm

3. What is the primary hazard of aerosol drug therapy?
   A. Adverse reaction to the medication being administered
   B. Onset of the medication's action too rapid
   C. Pulmonary infection
   D. Second hand exposure to the medication being aerosolized

4. The most commonly prescribed method of aerosol delivery in the United States is:
   A. pMDI
   B. DPI
   C. SVN
   D. Altera nebulizer

5. The current propellant used in a pMDI is:
   A. CFCs
   B. HFAs
   C. Dry powder
   D. Soy lecithin

6. Your patient has an order for albuterol, and the physician asks for your suggestion regarding the delivery device. Currently, your patient has a respiratory rate of 26 breaths per minute and an inspiratory flow of 50 L/min. What device(s) would you suggest?

   1. DPI
   2. pMDI
   3. SVN

   A. 1, 2 and 3
   B. 2 only
   C. 1 and 2 only
   D. 2 and 3 only

7. DPIs may be:
   A. Unit-dose DPIs
   B. Multiple unit-dose DPIs
   C. Multiple dose drug reservoir DPIs
   D. All of the above

8. Spacers and valved holding chambers are pMDI accessory devices designed to:
   A. Reduce oropharyngeal deposition
   B. Increase oropharyngeal deposition
   C. Increase the initial forward velocity of the droplets
   D. Increase particle size

9. The particle size above and below which 50% of the mass of the particles is found is called:
   A. Count mode
   B. Count median diameter
   C. Mass median aerodynamic diameter
   D. Geometric standard deviation

10. The advantages of using a DPI include:

    1. Breath actuation
    2. Small and portable
    3. Short preparation and administration times
    4. HFA propellants are safe for environment

    A. 1 and 2 only
    B. 1, 2, and 3 only
    C. 1, 2, and 3 only
    D. 1, 2, 3, and 4

>> **CASE STUDY 19-1**

You are taking over from the off-going RT and getting report on a 69-year-old male patient who is currently hospitalized following an exacerbation of his COPD. The off-going RT reports that the patient has been refusing his Combivent MDI because "it doesn't work as good as my one at home." So the off-going RT suggests that you not even try. As you introduce yourself, the patient explains that he cannot "feel the cold" from the inhaler so he might as well not take it.

1. What would be your explanation to your patient?

_____

_____

2. You notice that your patient is having a difficult time coordinating actuation and inhalation. What would you suggest to him?

_____

_____

Mechanical Ventilators

Edward Hoskins

▪ OBJECTIVES

Upon the completion of the chapter activities and content review topics, the student should be able to:

1. Prepare a mechanical ventilator for use.
2. Place the ventilator in the various modes of ventilation.
3. Identify various modes using wave forms.

▪ KEY TERMS

- Baseline pressure
- Continuous positive airway pressure (CPAP)
- End expiratory flow
- Peak airway pressure
- Peak inspiratory flow
- Plateau pressure ($P_{plateau}$)
- Positive end expiratory pressure (PEEP)

▪ CONTENT REVIEW TOPICS

- Airway trapping
- Auto-PEEP
- Barotrauma
- Inspiration-to-expiration (I:E) ratio
- Mean airway pressure
- Static pressure
- Time constants

- Transairway pressure
- Volutrauma

▪ PROCEDURAL ASSESSMENTS

20-1   Preparing a Mechanical Ventilator for Use
20-2   Wave Form Analysis

▪ EQUIPMENT

- Compressed gases (oxygen, air)
- Gloves
- Hand hygiene products
- One or more critical care mechanical ventilators
- Test lungs with varying compliance and airway resistance
- Ventilator tubing circuit

echanical ventilators have been in use for many decades. The recent advances in technology have provided the respiratory therapist (RT) with highly sophisticated computerized life support devices with capabilities we could only have dreamed of 40 years ago.

Management of a patient on ventilatory support is one of the most difficult tasks a respiratory therapist will have to execute. An understanding of the information provided by wave forms will help the RT recognize problems with the patient–ventilator system and make quick changes. It is essential for the RT to be knowledgeable in anatomy, physiology, pathophysiology, clinical assessment, pharmacology, science, and technology. Also, it is important to remember the patient's life and safety are our most important responsibility, and the ventilator is a tool to help achieve that goal. This chapter will focus on the science and technology aspects involved in the proper setup of a mechanical ventilator, as well as modes of ventilation with wave form analysis.

→ **Reality Check** As a RT, you must be current on all aspects of professional practice relating to your clinical responsibilities. No one else in the clinical environment will have the depth of knowledge to provide the patient the best chances of survival once placed on mechanical ventilation. The health care system demands that our practice be evidence based. The best sources to maintain currency and provide evidence-based practices are peer-reviewed journals.

❯❯ SKILL CHECK LISTS

20-1 Preparing a Mechanical Ventilator for Use

It is critically important to ensure that each mechanical ventilator is cleaned, that a new circuit is applied, and that the ventilator has passed an internal diagnostic test before its use and it is available and ready to go when needed. When a patient is in need of ventilatory support, delays in the initiation of ventilatory support increase the patient's risk of complications. It is imperative that the RT understands and knows how to complete this process correctly. The following is the step-by-step process for preparing a mechanical ventilator for use.

Procedural Preparation

1. Clean the exterior surface of the ventilator according to the manufacturer's specifications.
2. Attach the appropriate inspiratory and expiratory filters.
3. Attach a clean ventilator tubing circuit to the ventilator.
4. Connect the ventilator to compressed oxygen and air outlets.
5. Plug the ventilator into the appropriate electrical outlet.

Implementation

1. Follow the ventilator manufacturer's instructions to initiate the diagnostic process of the ventilator.
2. Follow the ventilator instructions to complete the diagnostic process.
3. Cover the ventilator until use.

Evaluation of Procedure

1. Establish that all pressure tests have been completed successfully.
2. Establish that all flow tests have been completed successfully.
3. Establish that all volume tests have been completed successfully.
4. Establish that all tubing compliance tests have been completed successfully.
5. Establish that all oxygen sensor tests have been completed successfully
6. Establish that all leak tests have been completed successfully.

Documentation and Reporting

1. Record the successful tests in the appropriate log and on the ventilator.
2. Report any failure to the appropriate health care provider.

20-2 Wave Form Analysis

Several different modes of ventilation exist, and it is important for the RT to select the appropriate mode of ventilation based on the patient's condition and the physician's orders. The most common wave forms seen together on the screen of critical care ventilators are *pressure*, *volume*, and *flow*. RTs must also be able to recognize the output wave form associated with each mode and how the wave forms are affected with change in compliance and resistance. We will be using scalar graphics with three different wave forms: (1) volume-time, (2) flow-time, and (3) pressure-time to represent each breath of the patient. The beginning of inspiration, the end of inspiration, the beginning of exhalation, and the end of exhalation can be seen on each of the waveforms.

Spontaneous Modes
Continuous Positive Airway Pressure

Continuous positive airway pressure (CPAP) is a spontaneous mode of ventilation.

> → **Reality Check** In CPAP it is very important to set the apnea alarm appropriately. In addition, the low tidal volume and low respiratory rate alarms should be set closely to the patient's actual tidal volume and rate so that deviations or patient failure on CPAP are detected sooner rather than later when apnea ventilation sets in.

In this mode, the RT sets a pressure level that is maintained by the ventilator throughout breathing, and the patient's tidal volume and respiratory rate are totally dependent on his or her effort. Therefore, the baseline on the pressure-time scalar graphic will be above atmospheric pressure. The baseline pressure is raised to cause an increase in the patient's functional residual capacity (FRC). It should look similar to the graphics in Figure 20-1, which shows an illustrations of eight breaths. At the beginning of each breath on the graphic, a slight drop in pressure is seen. This is the patient's inspiratory effort. The pressures during this mode ideally will fluctuate plus or minus 2 or 3 cm H_2O in relation to the set baseline pressure.

Pressure Support Ventilation

Pressure support ventilation (PSV) is often used in conjunction with CPAP and provides assistance to a spontaneous breath. A pressure support (PS) level is set by the RT, and once the patient's inspiratory effort surpasses the trigger threshold, the PS is delivered. Parameters that the RT may adjust in PSV are the PS level, the trigger sensitivity threshold, the inspiratory rise time, and, occasionally, the terminal flow value. As in CPAP, the patient in PSV can initiate a breath as often as desired, and the PS breath will augment the patient's inspiratory effort. This is illustrated in Figure 20-2. The breath is controlled by the patient, and inspiration ends or cycles off as a result of terminal inspiratory flow. The terminal inspiratory flow is set to an amount based on a percentage of the patient's peak inspiratory flow. Some ventilators have a fixed value of 25% of the patient's peak inspiratory flow. In addition, some ventilators will allow the operator to adjust the percent of terminal inspiratory flow to higher or lower values, depending on the patient's needs. The changes in the parameters of a PSV are illustrated in Figure 20-3. A PS breath results in a descending flow pattern.

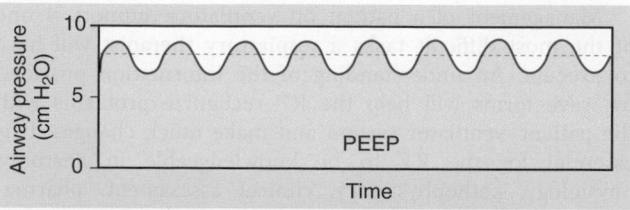

Figure 20-1 With continuous positive airway pressure (CPAP) a caregiver-defined level of pressure within the ventilatory circuit is maintained. Changes in the airway pressure with inspiration and expiration are constantly compensated for by pressure generated by the ventilator. *PEEP,* positive end-expiratory pressure. (From Spiro SG, Silvestri GA, Agustí A: *Clinical respiratory medicine,* ed 4, Philadelphia, PA, 2012, Saunders.)

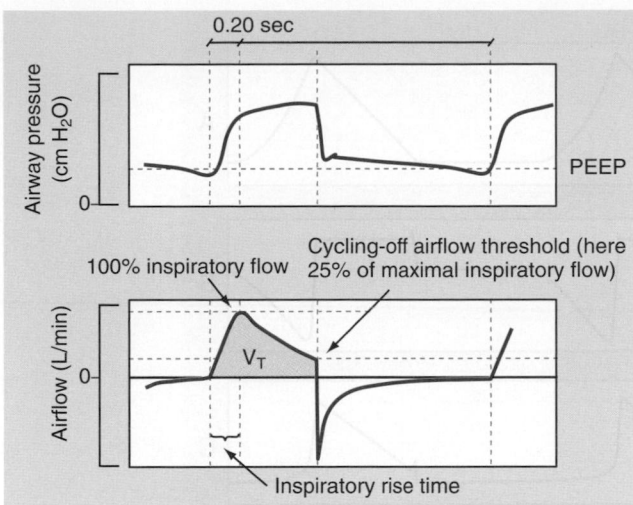

Figure 20-2 Pressure support ventilation (PSV). The delivered tidal volume (V_T) is calculated by integrating the area under the flow curve (*shaded area*). The inspiratory rise time defines how fast the maximal airflow (100%) is achieved. Thereafter, the inspiratory airflow continuously decreases because once the pressure target is reached, maintaining this level requires progressively less air to flow into the lungs. As soon as the cycling-off air flow threshold (i.e., a preset percentage of maximal air flow) is reached, the ventilator ceases to deliver inspiratory flow, and the expiratory valve is opened to allow passive exhalation (From Spiro SG, Silvestri GA, Agustí A: *Clinical respiratory medicine*, ed 4, Philadelphia, PA, 2012, Saunders.)

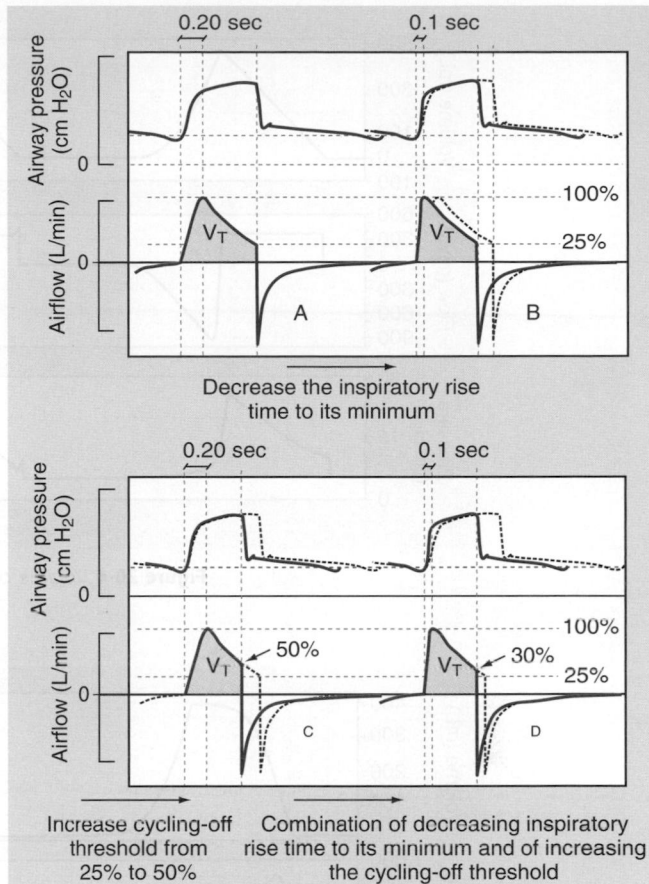

Figure 20-3 Changes in the parameters of PSV result in characteristic changes of the pressure and volume curves. Panels "A" to "D" demonstrate isolated changes of parameters, assuming that all other ventilatory parameters and the mechanical characteristics of the respiratory system remain unchanged. **A,** PSV breath with an inspiratory rise time of 0.20 second. **B,** After reducing the inspiratory rise time to its minimum, the peak inspiratory flow and consequently also the cycling-off air flow threshold are both reached earlier. Decreasing the inspiratory rise time results in a shorter inspiratory time, while the tidal volume (V_T) remains unchanged. Note that although the inspiratory rise time is decreased to 0 seconds, the peak inspiratory flow is reached with a small delay. **C,** Increasing the cycling-off air flow threshold from 30% to 50% similarly shortens the inspiratory time; however, V_T decreased in this case. **D,** A combination of a maximal decrease in the inspiratory time and a moderate increase in the cycling-off air flow threshold shortens the inspiratory time, whereas the loss of V_T is only minimal. Such an approach may be used to achieve a prolongation of the expiratory time in patients at risk for dynamic hyperinflation because of the expiratory flow limitation (e.g., patients with chronic obstructive pulmonary disease [COPD]). (From Spiro SG, Silvestri GA, Agustí A: *Clinical respiratory medicine*, ed 4, Philadelphia, PA, 2012, Saunders.)

Controlled Modes
Volume Control

Volume control ventilation is a mandatory mode, in which the tidal volume and flow rate remain constant breath to breath, and the airway pressure applied varies, depending on the patient's airway resistance and lung thorax compliance. This mode is represented in the scalar graphic in Figure 20-4. For the graphic "A," the tidal volume peaks at 0.5 liters (L) and does not vary. For the graphic "B," the peak flow is 400 liters per second (L/s) and does not vary. This inspiratory flow time wave form is most often described as square. The inspiratory time (I-time) is 1.3 seconds and does not vary. Graphic "C" reflects a peak airway pressure of 25 cmH$_2$O. This wave form is described as exponential, accelerating, or a shark-fin pattern. Remember that volume and flow will not vary, causing an increase in peak airway pressure, if the patient's airway resistance increases, lung compliance decreases, or both. Conversely, the peak airway pressure will decrease if the patient's airway resistance decreases or lung compliance increases. During volume control, the base line pressure may be increased, which will, in turn, increase the patient's FRC. This effect may be seen on graphic "C." At the end of each breath, the baseline pressure is held to 5 cmH$_2$O. This indicates the amount of PEEP set.

In assist control–volume control–ventilation (AC/VC), a minimum respiratory rate is set on the ventilator, but the patient can initiate and receive more than that set rate. This is done by patient effort reaching the trigger sensitivity. Each subsequent breath will be the set mandatory breath, as in the example on the scalar graphic in Figure 20-4, and each and every tidal volume will be 0.5 L.

Pressure Control Ventilation

Pressure control ventilation is a mandatory mode, in which the amount of pressure applied during each breath is controlled and does not vary with patient characteristics (see Figure 20-5). As a result, the patient's tidal volume and peak inspiratory flow rate vary, depending on airway resistance, lung compliance, or both. During this mode, if the patient airway resistance increases or lung compliance decreases, the tidal volume the

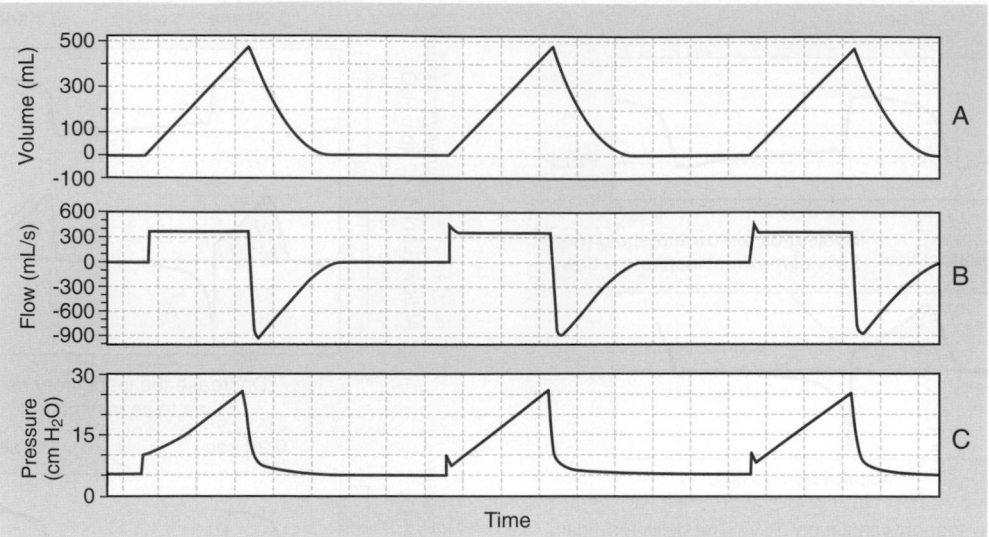

Figure 20-4 Volume control ventilation with PEEP.

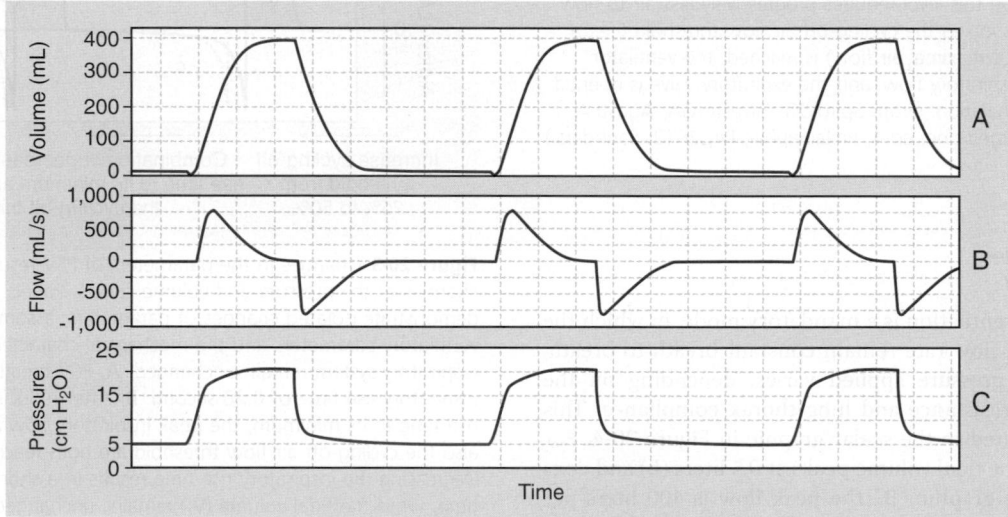

Figure 20-5 Pressure Control with PEEP.

patient receives decreases. The peak inspiratory pressure (PIP) is considered to be constant during inspiration and is described as a square wave form. This is shown on the pressure-time scalar graphic "C" in Figure 20-5. The flow pattern is described as descending and is illustrated on the scalar graphic "B" in Figure 20-5. As in the other modes, PEEP may be added. The amount of PEEP illustrated in Figure 20-5 is 5 cm H_2O. During this mode, the operator sets the PIP, respiratory rate, I-time, fractional inspired oxygen FiO_2, and PEEP, and the patient receives these settings with each breath. If the patient's effort reaches the trigger sensitivity, the patient can initiate additional breaths above the set respiratory rate.

Generally, the operator cannot control the patient's peak inspiratory flow rate, but most intensive care unit (ICU) ventilators being used these days allow control of the speed at which the flow rises to its peak. This is called the *rise time*, *rise time %*, or *slope*. A modification to this parameter is used to alter the inspiratory flow rate at the beginning of

the breath. The effect on the patient is dependent on airway dynamics. Usually, as the flow is decreased at the beginning of the breath, it results in a change in tidal volume delivered to the patient.

Synchronized Intermittent Mandatory Ventilation

Synchronized intermittent mandatory ventilation (SIMV) is a mode of ventilation that allows the RT to set either a volume-targeted or pressure-targeted breath (mandatory breaths) in addition to the unassisted spontaneous breaths a patient is able to take. The patient receives a minimum set tidal volume (or pressure), respiratory rate, and I-time on the mandatory breaths, set inspiratory flow rate on mandatory breaths, FiO_2, and PEEP. During a mandatory breath, each breath is a volume-controlled or pressure-controlled breath, where the tidal volume (or pressure) is the same breath to breath. If the patient chooses to breathe above the set mandatory rate, each additional breath will be spontaneous. As in the other modes, a baseline pressure may be used to increase the patient's FRC. In SIMV-volume control, the mandatory breaths have square flow patterns with exponential pressure patterns, while the spontaneous breaths are taken between the mandatory breaths with CPAP. An example of SIMV-volume control is provided in Figure 20-6. Pressure support may be added to the additional spontaneous breaths.

Dual-Control Mode

Dual-control mode is a mandatory mode, in which the ventilator uses a pressure-controlled breath delivery with a targeted tidal volume. Various manufacturers' nomenclature for dual-control ventilation are continuous mandatory ventilation (CMV) with autoflow, pressure-regulated volume control (PRVC), and AC/VC+. The RT sets a tidal volume, which becomes the targeted amount. Once the ventilator is attached to the patient, a few volume-targeted breaths are delivered at a low pressure level. Then a measure of the pressure applied to achieve the tidal volume is calculated by the ventilator, and the inspiratory pressure is adjusted to obtain the set tidal volume in the subsequent breaths. The ventilator delivers the volume breath as a pressure-controlled breath. If the PIP that is required to deliver the breath changes a specified amount, the ventilator recalculates and applies the new PIP based on the changes in the system compliance. These calculations are done breath to breath to achieve the targeted tidal volume. During this mode, if the patient's airway resistance increases or lung compliance decreases severely, the tidal volume the patient receives may decrease momentarily while the ventilator adjusts the PIP to achieve the targeted tidal volume over the next few breaths. If the opposite occurs, the tidal volume delivered may

increase momentarily. See Figure 20-7 for an illustration of a dual-control mode of ventilation. The peak airway pressure is considered to be constant during inspiration; it is described as a square wave form and looks like the pressure-time graphic in "A" in Figure 20-7. The flow pattern is described as

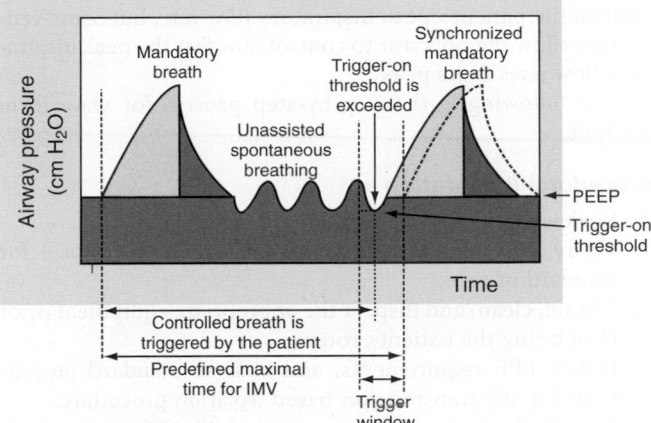

Figure 20-6 SIMV with unassisted spontaneous breathing between two volume-targeted breaths. Within a short period before starting the next mandatory breath, a trigger window allows synchronization of the controlled breath to the patient's breathing effort. When the patient's breathing effort does not exceed the trigger-on threshold, the ventilator delivers a mandatory breath (either volume-targeted or pressure-targeted, as defined by the RT) after the maximal interval for intermittent mandatory ventilation (IMV) had elapsed. This interval is defined by the preset rate for IMV. (From Spiro SG, Silvestri GA, Agustí A: *Clinical respiratory medicine*, ed 4, Philadelphia, PA, 2012, Saunders.)

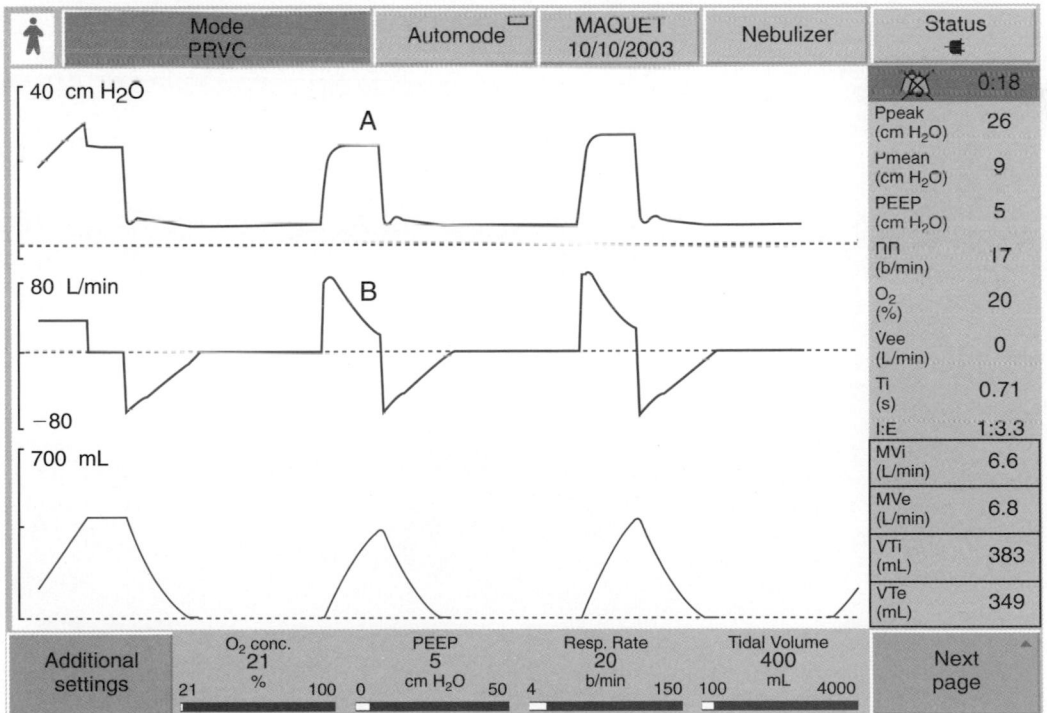

Figure 20-7 A screen capture of pressure-regulated volume control (PRVC) in an adult patient on the Maquet Servo[i] ventilator. The first breath (left) is a volume-targeted test breath with an inspiratory hold to measure $P_{plateau}$. The second breath (middle) is a pressure-targeted breath with a pressure equal to the measured Pplateau. Set tidal volume is 400 mL. Measured exhaled tidal volume is about 350 mL. Note how the pressure is increased by a few centimeters of H2O on the third breath (far right) for the ventilator to achieve the set tidal volume. (Cairo JM: *Pilbeam's Mechanical Ventilation*, ed 5, St. Louis, 2012, Mosby.)

descending and is represented in the graphic in "B" in Figure 20-7. As in the other control modes, PEEP may be added. The RT will set the tidal volume, respiratory rate, I-time, F$_1$O$_2$, and PEEP. If the patient's effort reaches the trigger sensitivity, the patient can initiate additional breaths above the set respiratory rate. As with pressure control, the operator usually cannot control the patient's peak inspiratory flow rate, but some ventilators allow the operator to control how fast the peak inspiratory flow rises to its peak.

The following is the step-by-step process for wave form analysis.

Procedural Preparation

1. Review the patient's chart.
2. Verify the physician's order or the facility's protocol for standard of care.
3. Obtain, clean, and inspect the appropriate equipment prior to entering the patient's room.
4. Follow PPE requirements, and observe standard precautions for any transmission-based isolation procedure.
5. Identify the patient using two patient identifiers.
6. Introduce yourself to the patient and to the family.
7. Explain the procedure to the patient and to the family, and acknowledge the patient's understanding.
8. Perform proper hand hygiene, and put on gloves, mask, and protective eyewear as appropriate for the procedure.

Implementation

1. Identify the desired wave form for analysis:
   a. Pressure-time
   b. Flow-time
   c. Volume-time

2. Analyze the wave form for the following:
   a. Changes in resistance
   b. Leaks
   c. Air trapping
   d. Inadequate inspiratory flow
3. Calculate static compliance, if applicable for the mode.
4. Adjust the ventilator per protocols, as needed.
5. Remove the PER, and perform proper hand hygiene prior to leaving the patient's room.

Evaluation of Procedure

1. Establish a baseline, or compare with previous wave form analyses.
2. Develop an appropriate respiratory care plan based on assessment data.
3. Identify any unexpected outcomes.

Documentation and Reporting

1. Record the changes and findings in the patient's chart or on the ventilator flow sheet.

Bibliography

Cairo JM: *Mosby's respiratory care equipment*, ed 9, St. Louis, MO, 2014, Mosby.

Spiro SG, Silvestri GA, Agustí A: *Clinical respiratory medicine*, ed 4, Philadelphia, PA, 2012, Saunders.

1. With a lab partner, select a mechanical ventilator, and perform the following steps. Write your signature after each step once you have completed it.

> **✴ Tip** The internal diagnostic test will vary with each ventilator manufacturer. The purpose of the process is to test and calibrate the ventilator. This usually includes calibrations for compressed gas pressures, airway pressures, volume, flow, and oxygen concentration, as well as internal calculations for ventilator resistance, compliance, and compression and a leak test.

a. Remove all items that were used on the last patient.

Signature _____

b. Clean and sanitize the exterior surface of the ventilator, including hoses and wires, with institutionally approved solutions and according to the manufacturer's specifications.

Signature _____

c. Inspect the ventilator to ensure that both oxygen and air-compressed hoses are attached to the ventilator with the correct connections.

Signature _____

d. Inspect to make sure that the compressed gas dryers are attached correctly to the air and oxygen and inlet hoses.

Signature _____

e. Attach clean inlet and outlet filters appropriate for the selected ventilator.

Signature _____

f. Attach the new exterior patient tubing circuit without contaminating the system.

Signature _____

g. Attach the ventilator to a compressed source for oxygen and air and to an electrical outlet.

Signature _____

h. Turn on the ventilator, and initiate the procedure as specified by the ventilator manufacturer. Then follow the instructions given to you on screen by the ventilator. Make sure to verify that each step has been completed successfully.

Signature _____

i. Once the procedure is completed, attach the appropriate tag, and write the date of test completion and your signature. In some facilities, a log is kept on the date and times each ventilator undergoes this process.

Signature _____

*The following exercises will use the terminology from the Covidien PB 840. However, you may use **any ventilator** to complete the exercise. It is suggested that you select a different ventilator for each mode, if possible.*

With a lab partner, select a mechanical ventilator, and perform the following steps. Write your signature after each step once you have completed it.

2. CPAP Mode: If not using the Covidien PB 840, list the name of the equivalent mode:

_____

a. Connect the selected ventilator to the compressed gases and the electric power source.

Signature _____

b. Turn on the ventilator.

Signature _____

c. Once the ventilator has gone through its initial internal checks, select the mode that represents CPAP.

Signature _____

d. Set the parameters: CPAP of 0 cmH$_2$O, and FIO$_2$ of 0.21. Set the apnea alarm at 20 seconds in AC/VC with a tidal volume of 0.4 L frequency of 14 breaths/min and flow to attain an I-time of 1 second (only if possible on your selected ventilator)

Signature _____

e. Attach a test lung with airway resistance and compliance similar to what would be expected in normal lungs.

Signature _____

f. Wait for some time, and observe the screen on the ventilator; confirm that the baseline is 0 on the pressure-time graphic.

Signature _____

g. Confirm that the measured value for respiratory rate is 0 and that the ventilator will not provide a breath to the test lung.

Signature _____

h. When the set time for apnea has expired, the ventilator alarm will go off and provide a predetermined tidal volume and respiratory rate.

Signature _____

i. Reset the alarm.

Signature _____

j. Increase the CPAP setting to 5 cmH$_2$O. At this point, you should see the test lung volume increase and hold and the pressure at 5 cm H$_2$O.

k. Manually compress and release the test lung to create a respiratory rate of 12 breaths/min. View the ventilator screens to confirm that the graphic correctly reflects the expected wave forms.

Signature _____

l. Increase the CPAP to 10 cm H_2O, and observe the increase in the residual volume of the test lung. Confirm that the baseline on the pressure-time graphic increases to 10 cm H_2O.

Signature _____

> → **Reality Check** *The effects that you have observed with the test lung will similarly occur in patients when CPAP is applied.*

3. AC/PC Mode: If not using the Covidien PB 840, list the name of the equivalent mode:

_____

a. Connect the selected ventilator to the compressed gases and the electric power source.

Signature _____

b. Turn on the ventilator. Once the ventilator has gone through its initial internal checks, select the mode AC/PC.

Signature _____

c. Set the parameters: PIP of 15 cm H_2O, frequency 12 breaths/min, I-time 1 second, PEEP 0 cmH_2O, FiO_2 0.21.

Signature _____

d. Attach a test lung with airway resistance and compliance similar to what would be expected in normal lungs.

Signature _____

e. Wait and watch the screen on the ventilator, and confirm that the baseline is 0 cmH_2O on the pressure-time graphic.

Signature _____

f. Change the PEEP to 5 cmH_2O, and make no other adjustments. What happens to the PIP?

Signature _____

g. View the ventilator screens to confirm that the graphics correctly reflect a square pressure-time wave form.

Signature _____

h. Does the particular ventilator you are using adjust the inspiratory pressure to a "pressure above PEEP"?

Signature _____

i. Increase the PIP to 20 cmH_2O with no adjustment to PEEP. What happens to the delivered tidal volume?

Signature _____

j. How are the machine breaths cycled?

Signature _____

k. Simulate breaths by manually compressing and releasing the test lung to create a respiratory rate of 5 breaths/min above the set frequency.

Signature _____

4. AC/VC Mode: If not using the Covidien PB 840, list the name of the equivalent mode:

_____

a. Connect the selected ventilator to the compressed gases and the electric power source.

Signature _____

b. Turn on the ventilator. Once the ventilator has gone through its initial internal checks, select the mode AC/VC.

Signature _____

c. Set the parameters: tidal volume 0.4 L; frequency 12 breaths/min; flow rate 30 L/min, square wave form; PEEP 0 cmH$_2$O; and F$_I$O$_2$ 0.21.

Signature _____

d. Connect the ventilator to a test lung with compliance similar to normal lung values.

Signature _____

e. View the ventilator's monitoring screen, and identify the flow-time wave form for flow rate. The top of the wave form should indicate 30 L/min as set.

Signature _____

f. Review the shape of the wave form. The beginning of inspiration is marked by an upward deflection from the "X" axis to a flat line that continues till you get to a downward deflection back to baseline on the "X" axis marking the end of inspiration. This represents inspiratory time. On the bottom end of that line, at what looks to be the same moment in time, is the beginning of exhalation. The flow-time wave form proceeds back to baseline of zero flow at the end of exhalation.

Signature _____

g. Identify the volume-time wave form. The peak of the volume wave form should occur at the end of inspiration on the flow-time graphic.

Signature _____

h. Identify the peak of the pressure wave form on the pressure-time graphic. The peak of pressure should occur at the end of inspiration.

Signature _____

i. Press (may need to hold down for 1 second on some ventilators) the inspiratory pause button, or perform an inspiratory hold maneuver. Watch the pressure-time wave form while performing this procedure. During the pause or hold time, you will see a drop in airway pressure. The pressure during this time is called plateau pressure ($P_{plateau}$). The value of pressure difference between the PIP and $P_{plateau}$ is thought be created by the gas flow rate and the resistance of the ventilator tubing and circuit and the patient's airway to gas flow. The pressure difference from baseline pressure (PEEP) and $P_{plateau}$ is dependent on the volume held in the system and the ventilator system and patient lung thorax compliance. This is called "Delta P (ΔP)". This is illustrated in Figure 20-8.

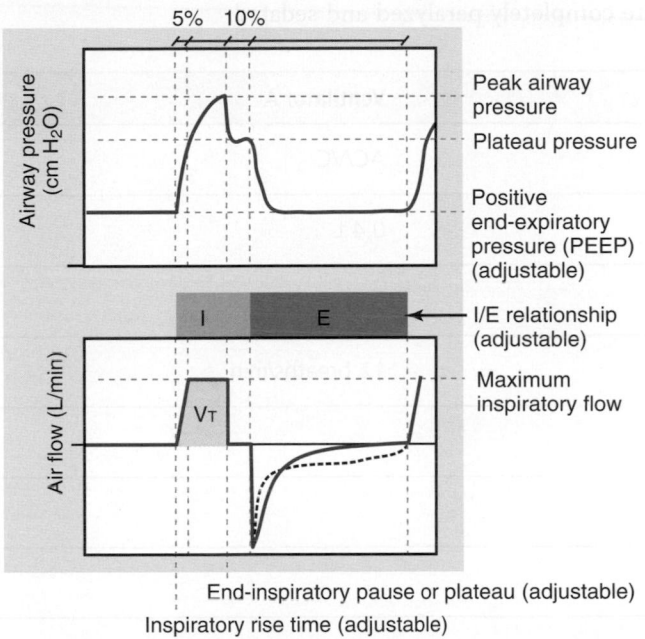

Figure 20-8 Volume-targeted (or volume-controlled) ventilation with a square-wave flow pattern. The delivered tidal volume (V_T) is calculated by integrating the area under the flow curve. During the end-inspiratory pause, the inspiratory and expiratory valves of the ventilator are closed for a predefined interval (expressed as a percentage of the entire breath period). Ideally, at the end of expiration, the full V_T applied during inhalation (minus what is lost during gas exchange) has left the lung, and the air flow is reduced to zero. (From Spiro SG, Silvestri GA, Agustí A: *Clinical respiratory medicine*, ed 4, Philadelphia, PA, 2012, Saunders.)

j. Increase the peak flow to 40 L/min. What happens to the PIP? What happens to the I-time?

Signature _____

k. Increase the frequency to 30 breaths/min. Review the pressure-time graphic. What happened to the interval between breaths?

Signature _____

l. Review the flow-time graphic, and identify the change in the interval between the end of exhalation and the beginning of the next breath.

Signature _____

m. Increase the frequency to 40 breaths/min. Review the intervals again.

Signature _____

n. Does the terminal expiratory flow return to the baseline value? This may result in what is called *air trapping*. The patient does not have enough time to exhale the tidal volume delivered. As a result, the amount of pressure remaining in the patient's lungs will be higher at the end of each subsequent exhaled breath. What is this called? Is there a way to quantify this value? *Hint: Use the expiratory pause button.*

Signature _____

5. If two ventilators are available, set both of them up to a test lung with identical characteristics for compliance and resistance, using the following parameters to simulate "patients." Fill in the following chart with the assumption the test lungs are patients who are completely paralyzed and sedated.

Parameter	Ventilator A	Ventilator B
Mode	AC/VC	SIMV-VC
Set tidal volume	0.4 L	0.4 L
Delivered tidal volume		
Set frequency	12 breaths/min	12 breaths/min
Delivered frequency		
Minute ventilation		
Measured PIP		
Flow rate	30 L/min	30 L/min
Flow pattern	Square	Square
PEEP	5 cmH$_2$O	5 cmH$_2$O
FiO$_2$	0.21	0.21
PS	N/A	8 cmH$_2$O

a. In the above "patients," does a difference exist is the volume-time graphic? Pressure-time graphic? Minute ventilation? Delivered tidal volume?

_____

_____

b. Now, simulate a patient triggering the ventilator to deliver breaths 10 above the set frequency. What changes are seen in the pressure-time and the volume-time graphics now between ventilator A and B? Has the minute ventilation changed? How are the PS breaths cycled?

_____

_____

Self-Assessment Questions

1. A patient is receiving treatment with a mechanical ventilator in the SIMV-VC mode with a set rate of 8 breaths/min. Which of the following wave forms would best describe the flow-time graphic for a mandatory breath?
   A. Exponential
   B. Ascending
   C. Square
   D. Shark fin

2. In the situation described in question #1, if pressure support was added to aid the patient with spontaneous breaths, how would those breaths be cycled?
   A. Pressure
   B. Volume
   C. Flow
   D. Time

3. In the situation described question #1, what kind of breaths are additional breaths delivered above the set 8 breaths/min considered to be?
   A. Supported
   B. Mandatory
   C. Volume control
   D. Dual control

4. When an inspiratory hold is initiated during volume control, the difference between PIP and $P_{plateau}$ is affected by:
   A. System lung compliance
   B. Tidal volume
   C. Height of patient
   D. System resistance

5. The inspiratory terminal flow does not reach the baseline during pressure control ventilation. What may be done to allow the terminal inspiratory flow to reach the baseline?
   A. Increase PIP
   B. Decrease PEEP
   C. Increase I-time
   D. Increase f

6. A patient receiving mechanical ventilation in the AC/PC mode experiences a decrease in lung compliance. Which of the following is expected to occur?
   A. PEEP decreases
   B. Tidal volume decreases
   C. I-time increases
   D. PIP increases

7. What causes inspiration to end during PS ventilation?
   A. Flow
   B. Pressure
   C. Time
   D. PIP

8. What determines the tidal volume the patient receives during CPAP?
   A. PIP set
   B. Tidal volume set
   C. Patient effort
   D. CPAP pressure set

9. A patient is on AC/VC and develops increased airway resistance as a result of reactive airway disease. Which of the following is expected to occur?
   A. PEEP decreases
   B. Tidal volume decreases
   C. I-time increases
   D. PIP increases

10. On the basis of the graphic in Figure 20-9, what mode of ventilation is the patient receiving?
    A. CPAP
    B. Pressure control
    C. Volume control
    D. SIMV

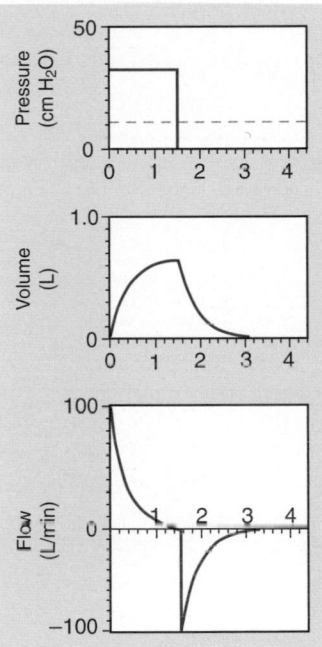

Figure 20-9 (From Kacmarek RM, Stoller JK, Heuer AJ: *Egan's fundamentals of respiratory care,* ed 10, St. Louis, MO, 2013, Mosby.)

CASE STUDY 20-1

You are the RT working in the intensive care unit on the overnight shift. The first patient you assess is intubated and receiving mechanical ventilation. The patient is a 23-year-old man who is on day 1 after surgery for repair of fractures to left and right femurs, has left and right chest contusions, and has no pneumothorax at this time. The patient is on AC/VC with PIP 20 cmH$_2$O, set frequency of 12 breaths/min, total frequency of 22 breaths/min, I-time of 0.8 seconds, PEEP of 5 cmH$_2$O, and FiO$_2$ of 0.6. The patient's last arterial blood gas was pH 7.44; PaCO$_2$ was 33 mm Hg; and PaO$_2$ was 50 mm Hg.

1. What changes would you recommend to the physician to improve the patient's oxygenation?

_____

_____

2. What kind of wave form should be seen on the pressure-time scalar graphic for inspirations for the additional 10 breaths above the set 12 breaths/min?

_____

_____

3. What kind of wave form should be seen on the flow-time scalar graphic for inspiration for all breaths?

_____

_____

Noninvasive Ventilatory Support

▪ OBJECTIVES

Upon the completion of the chapter activities and content review topics, the student should be able to:

1. Identify the goals and benefits of noninvasive ventilatory support.
2. List the indications, selection, and exclusion criteria for successful noninvasive ventilation (NIV).
3. List the predictive factors for successful NIV.
4. Identify types of interfaces used in conjunction with NIV and their complications during use.
5. Perform initiation of NIV.
6. Describe how NIV settings influence physiologic outcomes of the patient.
7. Perform a continuous positive airway pressure (CPAP) or bilevel positive airway pressure (BiPAP) patient-ventilator system assessment.

▪ KEY TERMS

- Bilevel positive airway pressure (BiPAP)
- Continuous positive airway pressure (CPAP)
- Delta P (ΔP)
- Driving pressure
- Interfaces
- Noninvasive ventilation (NIV)

▪ CONTENT REVIEW TOPICS

- Negative-pressure ventilation
- Polysomnography uses of NIV

▪ PROCEDURAL ASSESSMENTS

21-1 Initiating Noninvasive Ventilation: CPAP and BiPAP
21-2 Assessing a CPAP or BiPAP Patient-Ventilator System

▪ EQUIPMENT

- Circuits
- Compressed gas source
- CPAP or BiPAP ventilator
- Disposable gloves
- Interfaces
- Lung analog or simulator
- Oxygen source

Delivery of ventilatory support without using an invasive artificial airway is termed noninvasive ventilation (NIV). NIV may include the application of continuous positive airway pressure (CPAP) or bilevel positive airway pressure (BiPAP). NIV is used to maintain or improve oxygenation and ventilation and to provide respiratory muscle rest. A listing of the goals of NIV is provided in Box 21-1.

Typically, NIV is delivered via a nasal mask, a pillow, or a full face mask. Images of these devices, or interfaces, are provided in Figure 21-1. Selection of an interface device that fits properly and that the patient is comfortable with is important to help ensure patient compliance and use. Selection factors such as facial features, ease of use, patient preference, and, of course, availability, should all be taken into consideration when choosing an interface.

> → **Reality Check** It is important to know when to use NIV and equally as important to know when NOT to use it.

Complications such as pulmonary infection and tracheal injury, which are associated with invasive mechanical ventilation, make NIV highly advantageous as a ventilatory management therapy. However, some exclusions of its use include refractory asthma, hemodynamic instability, excessive secretions, severe agitation, inability to protect the airway, and

apnea. The patient's medical history, current respiratory complaints, and concurrent medical therapies must be evaluated when choosing NIV therapy to facilitate the best therapeutic outcomes for your patients. Disease processes for which treatment with NIV may be useful are listed in Box 21-2.

> ✳ **Tip** If you are currently working in an acute care facility, ask for the NIV protocols, if available, and review them.

NIV is used in many realms of respiratory care, ranging from the acute care, long-term care, and home care to polysomnography and sleep medicine. This chapter will focus on its use in the acute and long-term care settings. Its use in preventing airway obstruction during sleep will be discussed in Chapter 28.

≫ SKILL CHECK LISTS

21-1 Initiating Noninvasive Ventilation: CPAP and BiPAP

Over time, clinical judgment and experience will influence your choice of patients likely to benefit from NIV therapy. Until then, selection criteria and guidance from clinical preceptors, physicians, and instructors should be your foundation.

BOX 21-1   Goals of Noninvasive Ventilation

Acute Care Setting
Improve gas exchange
Avoid intubation
Decrease mortality
Decrease length of time on ventilator
Decrease length of hospitalization
Decrease incidence of ventilator-associated pneumonia
Relieve symptoms of respiratory distress
Improve patient-ventilator synchrony
Maximize patient comfort

Long-Term Care Setting
Relieve or improve symptoms
Enhance quality of life
Avoid hospitalization
Increase survival
Improve mobility

A comprehensive physical assessment is essential prior to application of NIV in the long-term setting. However, in the acute care setting and emergent situations, this may not be possible. Selection and exclusion criteria for NIV are provided in Box 21-3. The two forms of NIV discussed here are CPAP and BiPAP.

> **Reality Check** A patient with asthma typically requires very high inspiratory pressure, which leads to minimal success with NIV.

> **✳ Tip** Patient comfort and ability to tolerate the therapy are vital to compliance with therapy. Start the support setting lower than your goal settings, and gradually increase the pressures once the patient gets used to the feel of BiPAP. Holding the interface on the patient's face or having him or her hold it before securing it may also help.

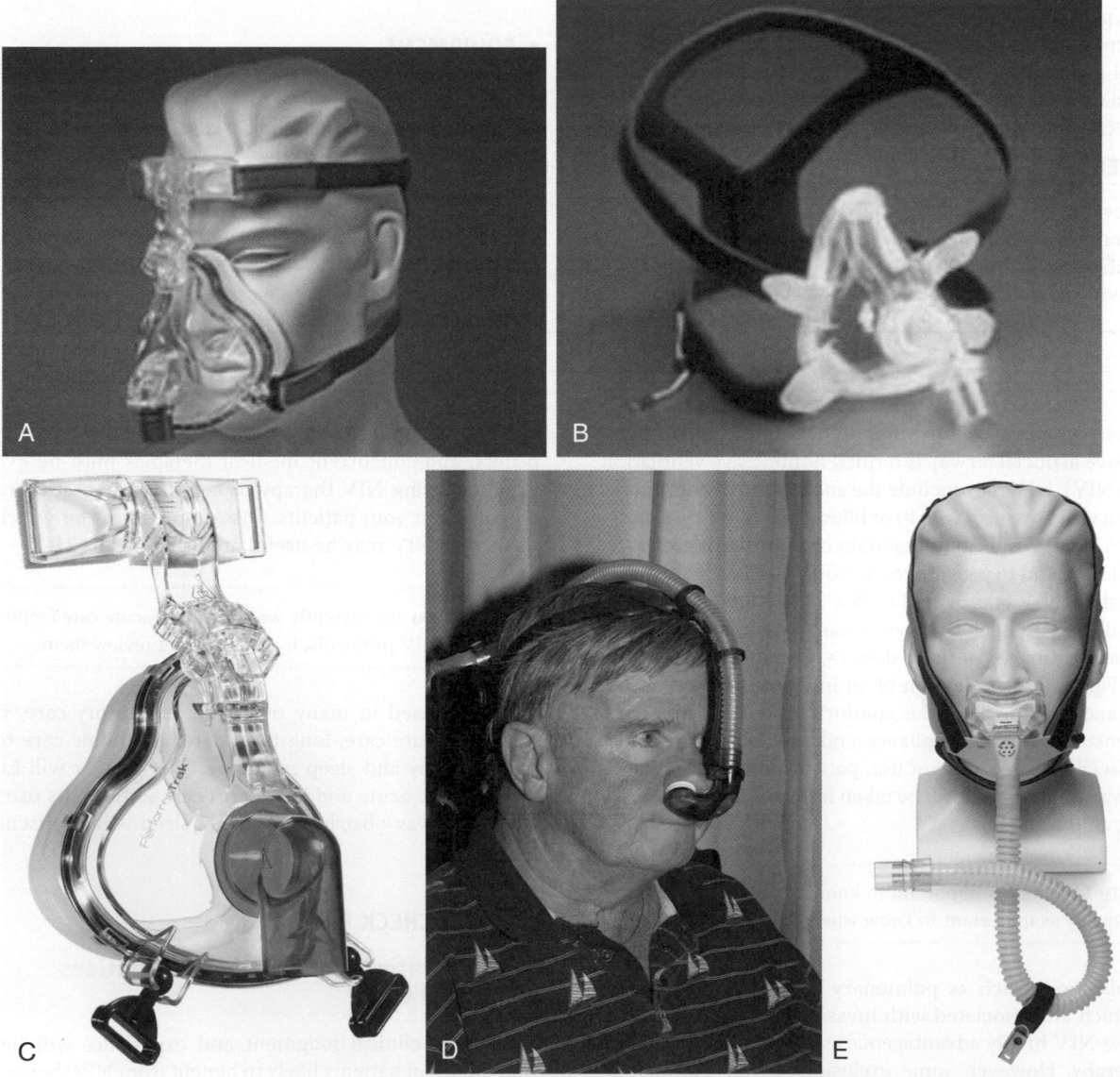

Figure 21-1 A and **B,** Nasal masks and head straps. **B, C,** Nasal mask with adjustable forehead support to minimize pressure on the bridge of nose. **D,** Nasal pillows. **E,** Hybrid mask.

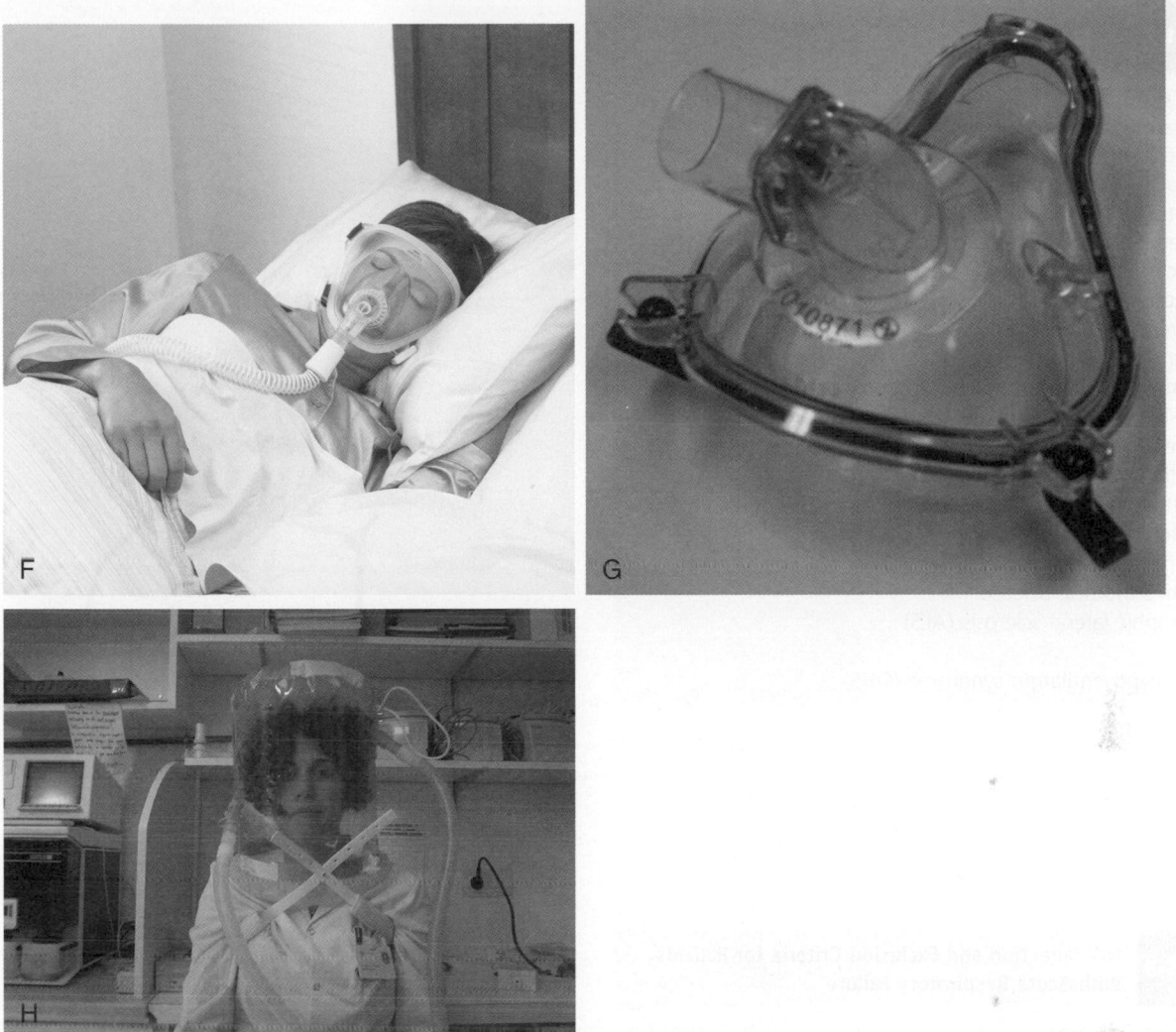

Figure 21-1 cont'd F, Total face mask. **G,** Full face mask used for NIV. **H,** Helmet providing continuous positive airway pressure (CPAP). (**A** and **F,** Courtesy of Philips Respironics, Murrysville, PA; **B,** From Albert R, Spiro S, Jett: *Clinical respirtory medicine,* ed 2, Philadelphia, PA, 2004, Mosby; **C,** From Kacmarek RM, Stoller JK, Heuer AJ: *Egan's fundamentals of respiratory care,* ed 10, St. Louis, MO, 2013, Mosby; **D,** From Panillo J, Dellinger R: *Critical care medicine: principles of diagnosis and management in the adult,* ed 3, Philadelphia, PA, 2007, Mosby; **F,** Courtesy of ResMed Corp, San Diego, CA; Philips; **G** and **H,** From Albert RK, Slutsky AS, Ranien VM, et al: *Clinical critical care medicine,* Philadelphia, PA, 2006, Mosby.)

CPAP is the noninvasive application of continuous pressure whereby the patient breathes spontaneously without mechanical assistance against threshold resistance, with pressures above atmospheric pressure maintained at the airway throughout breathing Examples of the devices used to deliver CPAP and BiPAP can be found in Figure 21-2. Initial CPAP pressure settings are generally around 8 to 12 cm H_2O, with various oxygen concentrations used to meet the patient's needs. BiPAP is a spontaneous breathing mode of support, which allows separate regulation of the inspiratory positive airway pressure (IPAP) and expiratory positive airway pressure (EPAP). The pressure difference between the IPAP and the EPAP, which is called the driving pressure or delta P (ΔP), determines the tidal volume being delivered. This concept is illustrated in Figure 21-3. IPAP is associated with ventilation, whereas the EPAP setting is used for oxygenation.

The following is the step-by-step process for initiation of noninvasive ventilation.

Procedural Preparation

1. Review the patient's chart.
2. Verify the physician's order or the facility's protocol for standard of care.
3. Obtain, clean, and inspect appropriate equipment prior to entering the patient's room.
4. Follow personal protective equipment (PPE) requirements, and observe standard precautions for any transmission-based isolation procedure.
5. Identify the patient using two patient identifiers.
6. Follow the facility's protocol for patient interaction, and introduce yourself to the patient and to the family.
7. Explain the procedure to the patient and to the family, and acknowledge the patient's understanding.
8. Perform proper hand hygiene, and put on gloves, mask, and protective eyewear, as appropriate for the procedure.

| BOX 21-2 | Acute and Chronic Disease Processes Indicating a Need for Noninvasive Ventilation |

Acute Conditions

Hypercapnic respiratory failure
Chronic obstructive pulmonary disease (COPD) exacerbation
Asthma
Facilitation of extubation in COPD
Hypoxemic respiratory failure
Acute cardiogenic pulmonary edema
Pneumonia
Acute respiratory distress syndrome (ARDS) or acute lung injury (ALI)
Respiratory failure in immunocompromised patients
End-of-life care and DNI (Do-Not-Intubate) orders
Postoperative respiratory failure
Prevention of reintubation in high-risk patients
Postextubation respiratory failure

Chronic Conditions

Nocturnal hypoventilation
Restrictive thoracic disease
Amyotrophic lateral sclerosis (ALS)
COPD
Obesity hypoventilation syndrome (OHS)

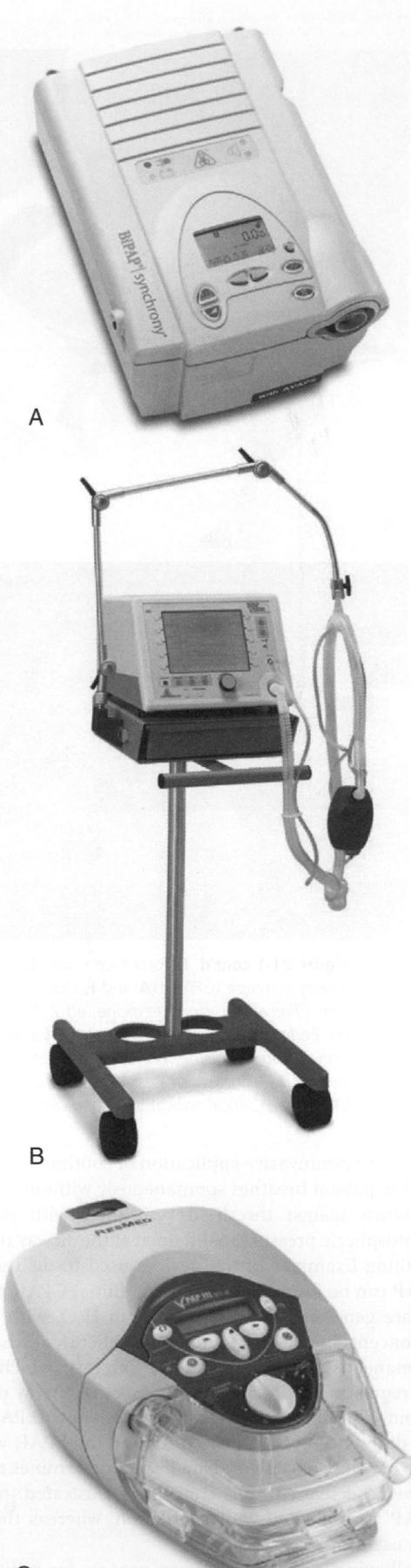

A

B

C

| BOX 21-3 | NIV Selection and Exclusion Criteria for Patients with Acute Respiratory Failure |

Selection Criteria

Use of accessory muscles
Paradoxical breathing
Respiratory rate ≥25 breaths/min
Moderate to severe dyspnea
$PaCO_2$ >45 mm Hg with pH <7.35
PaO_2 to FIO_2 ratio <200

Exclusion Criteria

Apnea
Inability to protect airway or high aspiration risk
Hemodynamic or cardiac instability
Lack of patient cooperation
Inability to use an interface
Excessive amounts of secretions

Figure 21-2 A to C, Examples of new generation noninvasive ventilators that include extensive monitoring and alarm capabilities. (**A** and **B,** Courtesy of Philips Respironics, Murryville, PA; **C,** Copyright ResMed, 2012, Used with permission.)

Implementation

1. Place the patient in a comfortable position.
2. Assess vital signs.
3. Determine the noninvasive interface for use with CPAP or BiPAP.
4. Ensure proper fit of the interface to prevent excessive leaks.
5. Assemble the circuit, plug it in, attach to the gas source(s), and test the device.

   For CPAP
   a. Select the CPAP mode or other vendor-specific setting.
   b. Select the appropriate CPAP level.
   c. Select the appropriate FiO_2 level.

   For BiPAP
   a. Select the BiPAP levels.
   b. Select any additional BiPAP options.
   c. Select the appropriate FiO_2 level

6. Connect the device to the patient, and readjust the interface, as needed, to prevent leaks.
7. Reassess vital signs, and monitor the patient.
8. Remove the supplies from the patient's room, and clean the area, as needed.
9. Remove PPE, and perform proper hand hygiene prior to leaving the patient's room.

Evaluation of Procedure

1. Establish a baseline, or compare with previous measurements.
2. Develop an appropriate respiratory care plan based on assessment data.

3. Obtain arterial blood gas values, and obtain the order for radiography, if indicated.
4. Identify any unexpected outcomes.

Documentation and Reporting

1. Record your findings in the patient's chart.
2. Report any abnormal findings to the appropriate health care provider.

21-2 Assessing a CPAP or BiPAP Patient-Ventilator System

To ensure patient safety and reduce the possibilities of unfavorable results, careful monitoring of the patient receiving NIV is essential. Assessment of the patient-ventilator system should begin with the patient. Familiarity with both the expected and unexpected outcomes that one may encounter during the assessment is important. Box 21-4 lists some of these outcomes. Assessing the interface is important to reduce the risk of skin damage and breakdown, which, in turn, influences patient comfort and compliance with therapy. Frequency of patient-ventilator assessment may be scheduled according to the protocol at your facility (q2hr, q4hr, etc.), but the schedule needs to be adjusted to meet the needs of your patient. A patient requiring NIV as a treatment for acute ventilatory failure will require repeated assessments and monitoring compared with the patient on CPAP for airway obstruction during sleep. Figure 21-4 is an example of a flow sheet used to document patient-ventilator assessment. The following is the

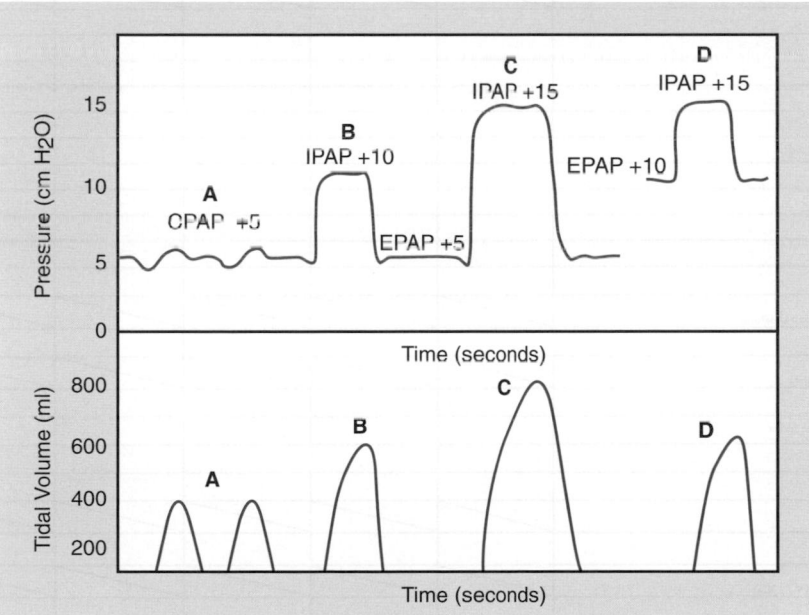

Figure 21-3 Changes in noninvasive ventilator settings (IPAP and EPAP) and corresponding effects on V_T. **A,** Spontaneous breathing on CPAP of 5 cm H_2O. **B,** Patient-triggered breath with the addition of 5 cm H_2O of pressure support (noninvasive ventilator settings are IPAP 10 cm H_2O and EPAP 5 cm H_2O). **C,** Pressure support was increased to 10 cm H_2O (NIV settings are IPAP 15 cm H_2O and EPAP 5 cm H_2O). Higher V_T occurs as pressure support is increased in A and B. **D,** IPAP 15 cm H_2O and EPAP 10 cm H_2O. Increasing EPAP setting results in lower V_T because pressure support was decreased to 5 cm H_2O. *EPAP,* Expiratory positive airway pressure; *IPAP,* inspiratory positive airway pressure; *NIV,* noninvasive ventilation; V_T, tidal volume. (From Kacmarek RM, Stoller JK, Heuer AJ: *Egan's fundamentals of respiratory care,* ed 10, St. Louis, MO, 2013, Mosby.)

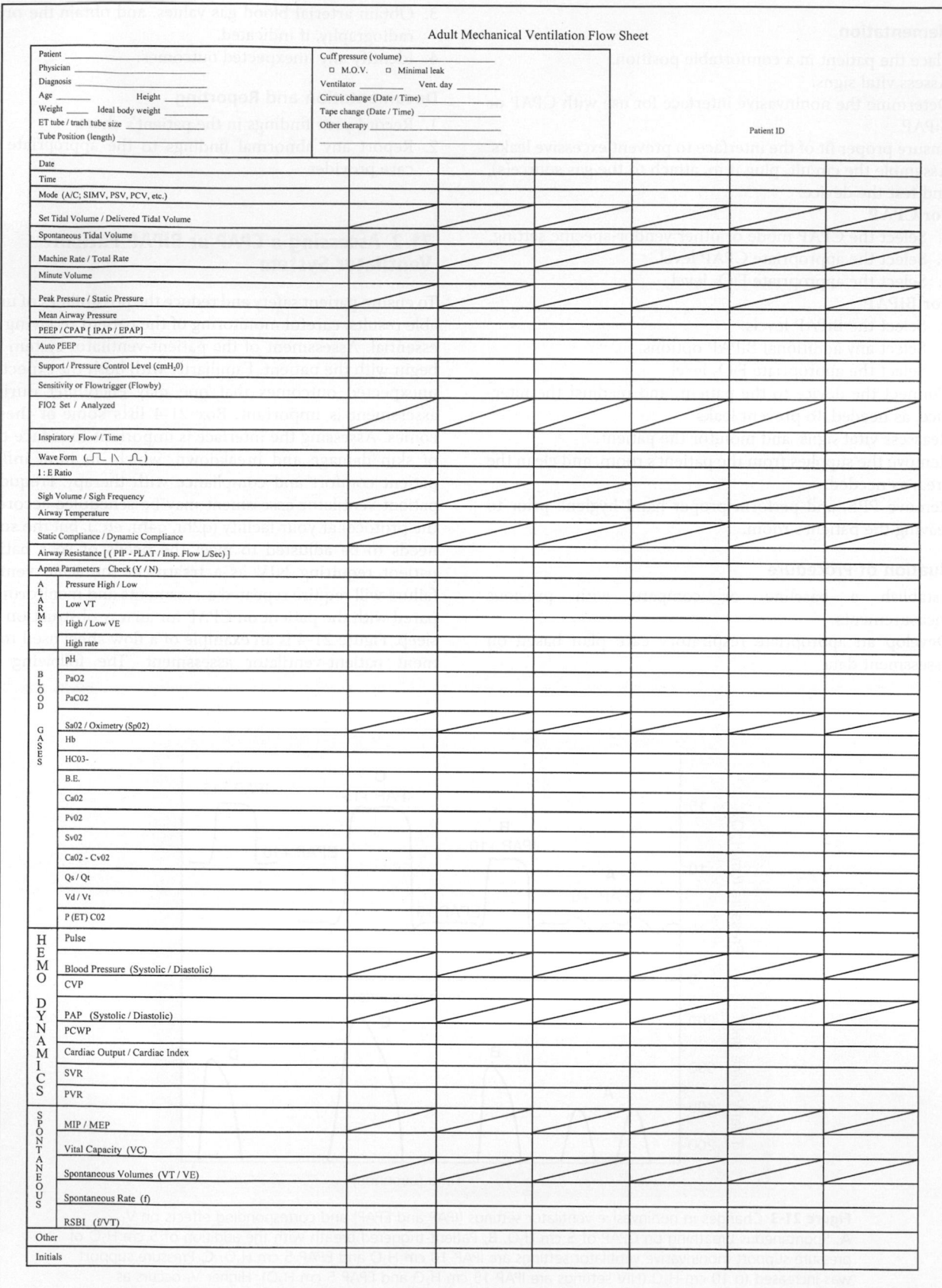

Adult Mechanical Ventilation Flow Sheet

Patient _____
Physician _____
Diagnosis _____
Age _____ Height _____
Weight _____ Ideal body weight _____
ET tube / trach tube size _____
Tube Position (length) _____

Cuff pressure (volume) _____
☐ M.O.V. ☐ Minimal leak
Ventilator _____ Vent. day _____
Circuit change (Date / Time) _____
Tape change (Date / Time) _____
Other therapy _____

Patient ID

Date							
Time							
Mode (A/C; SIMV, PSV, PCV, etc.)							
Set Tidal Volume / Delivered Tidal Volume							
Spontaneous Tidal Volume							
Machine Rate / Total Rate							
Minute Volume							
Peak Pressure / Static Pressure							
Mean Airway Pressure							
PEEP / CPAP [IPAP / EPAP]							
Auto PEEP							
Support / Pressure Control Level (cmH$_2$0)							
Sensitivity or Flowtrigger (Flowby)							
FIO2 Set / Analyzed							
Inspiratory Flow / Time							
Wave Form (⎍ \ ⎍)							
I : E Ratio							
Sigh Volume / Sigh Frequency							
Airway Temperature							
Static Compliance / Dynamic Compliance							
Airway Resistance [(PIP - PLAT / Insp. Flow L/Sec)]							
Apnea Parameters Check (Y / N)							

ALARMS								
	Pressure High / Low							
	Low VT							
	High / Low VE							
	High rate							

BLOOD GASES								
	pH							
	PaO2							
	PaC02							
	Sa02 / Oximetry (Sp02)							
	Hb							
	HC03-							
	B.E.							
	Ca02							
	Pv02							
	Sv02							
	Ca02 - Cv02							
	Qs / Qt							
	Vd / Vt							
	P (ET) C02							

HEMODYNAMICS								
	Pulse							
	Blood Pressure (Systolic / Diastolic)							
	CVP							
	PAP (Systolic / Diastolic)							
	PCWP							
	Cardiac Output / Cardiac Index							
	SVR							
	PVR							

SPONTANEOUS								
	MIP / MEP							
	Vital Capacity (VC)							
	Spontaneous Volumes (VT / VE)							
	Spontaneous Rate (f)							
	RSBI (f/VT)							

Other							
Initials							

A

Figure 21-4 Example of a ventilator flow chart.

Adult Mechanical Ventilation Flow Sheet

Respiratory Care Progress Notes

S: (pt Awareness, response, sedations / paralytics) Responds ☐ Non-responsive ☐ Sedated ☐ Paralytics ☐ See comment ☐ ☐

O: (WOB, Color, Chest Expansion, BBS, Sputum Production, latest x-ray, pertinent pt assessment concerns, lab values, fluids)

General Skin Color
☐ Pink
☐ Ashy
☐ Cyanotic
☐ Jaundice

Skin Characteristics
☐ Warm
☐ Dry
☐ Diaphoretic
☐ Cool
☐ Moist

Mucous Membranes
☐ Pink
☐ Ashy
☐ Cyanotic

Work of Breathing
☐ Normal
☐ Mild
☐ Moderate
☐ High
☐ Absent

Chest Excursion
☐ Bilateral
☐ Unilateral
☐ Diminished
☐ Paradoxical/Flail

Chest Configuration
☐ Normal
☐ Other _____

☐ Subcutaneous
   Emphysema

☐ Tactile Fremitus
☐ Tracheal Deviation
☐ Abdominal
   Distention

Nailbeds
☐ Pink
☐ Ashy
☐ Cyanotic

Capillary Refill
☐ Rapid
☐ Sluggish

Auscultation
1) Clear
2) Wheeze
3) Crackles
4) Rhonchi

Anterior

Posterior
A. Good Aeration
B. Diminished
C. Absent

A: (Pt history, Admit dx. & date, events leading to intubation/trach/ventilation, significant problems, etc.)

P: (Care plan, standing orders, treatments)

WEANING MECHANICS		
TIME		
VC		
I/E FORCES		
VT		
RR		
VE		
f/VT		

Pt. EVENTS/CHANGES	Time	(Reasons for changes, significant pt. events, CT Scan, chest tube placement, BP problems, codes, etc.)

Signature _____

Initials _____

B

Figure 21-4, cont'd

Noninvasive Ventilation CPAP or BiPAP Outcomes

Expected outcomes
Maintenance of adequate pH and $PaCO_2$
Maintenance of adequate PaO_2
Maintenance of adequate breathing patterns
Respiratory muscle rest
Unexpected Outcomes
Unacceptable pH, $PaCO_2$, and PaO_2
Hemodynamic instability
Pulmonary barotrauma
Respiratory muscle fatigue
Skin breakdown under mask

step-by-step process for the procedural assessment for assessing a CPAP or BiPAP patient-ventilator system.

Procedural Preparation

1. Review the patient's chart for the patient's current vital signs and ventilator settings.
2. Review the patient's most recent blood gases or SpO_2
3. Review the most recent chest radiograph.
4. Identify the patient's current sedation medications.
5. Verify the physician's order or the facility's protocol for standard of care.
6. Obtain, clean, and inspect the appropriate equipment prior to entering the patient's room.
7. Follow PPE requirements, and observe standard precautions for any transmission-based isolation procedure.
8. Identify the patient using two patient identifiers.
9. Introduce yourself to the patient and to the family.
10. Explain the procedure to the patient and to the family, and acknowledge the patient's understanding.
11. Perform proper hand hygiene, and put on gloves, mask, and protective eyewear, as appropriate for the procedure.

Implementation

1. Perform the patient assessment before conducting the ventilator assessment.
2. Examine the patient's appearance and comfort, as well as ventilator synchrony.
3. Confirm stabilization of the interface device.
4. Assess breath sounds; suction, if indicated.

5. Observe the chest-rise.
6. Evaluate the chest tubes.
7. Palpate the peripheral pulses.
8. Inspect the indwelling catheter(s).
9. Elevate the head of the bed to at least 30 degrees.
10. Perform oral care for the patient.
11. Assess the ventilator's function and settings:
    a. Security of circuit connections
    b. Heat and humidification device, airway temperature
    c. IPAP and EPAP levels, or CPAP level
    d. Rate
    e. Exhaled tidal volume and minute ventilation
    f. Inspiratory time
    g. Graphics
    h. FiO_2
    i. Monitor alarms
12. Ensure that the manual ventilation device and the suction equipment are available at the patient's bedside.
13. Remove the supplies from the patient's room, and clean the area, as needed.
14. Remove PPE, and perform proper hand hygiene prior to leaving the patient's room.

Evaluation of Procedure

1. Establish a baseline, or compare with previous measurements.
2. Develop an appropriate respiratory care plan based on assessment data.
3. Corrects any problems.
4. Consider discontinuation of noninvasive ventilation, if indicated.
5. Identify any unexpected outcomes.
6. Consider mechanical ventilation, if indicated.

Documentation and Reporting

1. Record your findings in the patient's chart.
2. Report any abnormal findings to the appropriate health care provider.

Bibliography

Cairo JM, *Mosby's respiratory care equipment*, ed 9, St. Louis, MO, 2014, Mosby.
Kacmarek RM, Stoller JK, Heuer AJ: *Egan's fundamentals of respiratory care*, ed 10, St. Louis, MO, 2013, Mosby.

1. List 15 disease processes for which NIV is indicated and the reasons.

_____

_____

_____

_____

_____

_____

_____

_____

_____

_____

_____

_____

_____

_____

_____

_____

_____

_____

2. Research in your textbooks some predictors of NIV success in the acute care setting. List them in the table below:

a. _____

b. _____

c. _____

d. _____

e. _____

f. _____

3. Obtain templates and mask interfaces commonly used in NIV. Get three lab partners, and fit each with an interface. Fit a nasal mask on each. Have each partner sign below, once the interface is fitted and applied properly.

Face Mask	Nasal Mask
Signature:	Signature:
Signature:	Signature:
Signature:	Signature:

4. What interfaces are commonly used in the application of NIV in the acute care setting?

_____

5. What is a potential risk for overtightening the head gear and straps on an interface?

_____

6. What are some characteristics of noninvasive ventilators?

_____

7. What must be present for an NIV to work properly?

_____

8. What physiologic effect occurs when EPAP is raised on a patient receiving NIV?

_____

9. Label Figure 21-5 of the control panel of the Respironics BiPAP Vision.

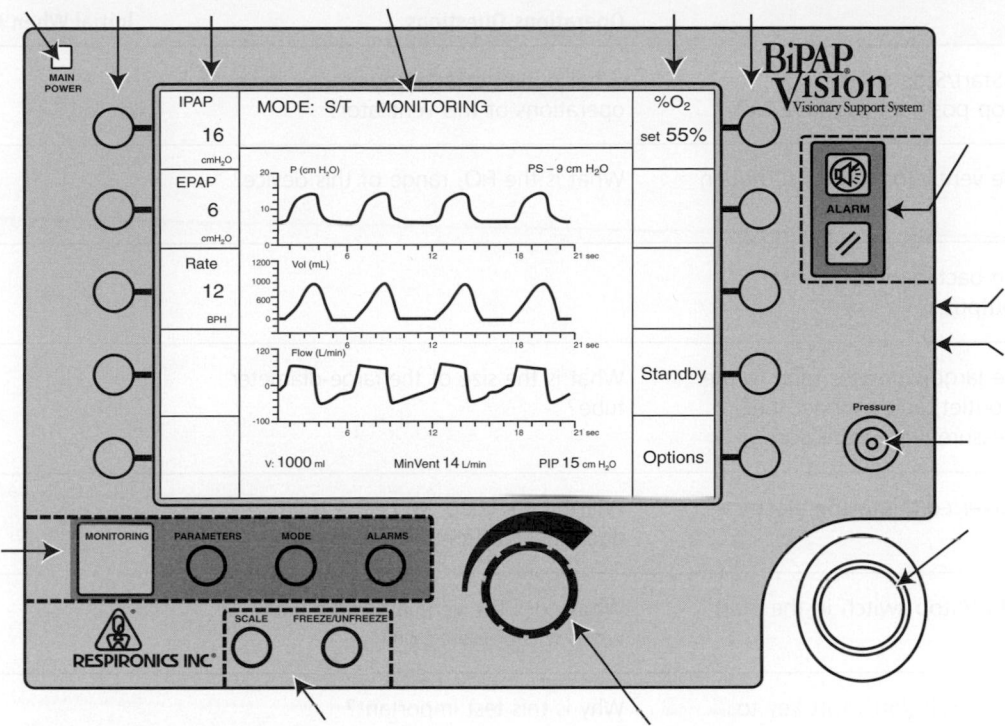

Figure 21-5 (Courtesy Philips Respironics, Murrysville, PA)

Obtain a Respironics BiPAP Vision, and use it for questions 10 through 16 (See Figure 21-2B).

If you do not have this particular NIV ventilator in your lab, adapt the exercise to suit your needs. The importance of the following activities is to understand the concepts involved in the application of NIV.

10. Fill in the following chart for the Respironics BiPAP ventilator set-up:

Task	Operations Questions	Initial When Completed
Locate the Start/Stop switch (place in Stop position) (Figure 21-6).	What outlet voltage powers the main operations of this ventilator?	
Connect the ventilator to 50 psi oxygen source.	What is the FiO_2 range of this device?	
Connect the bacteria filter to the ventilator output.		
Connect the large-diameter tube to the ventilator's outlet, and connect the proximal pressure line to the port.	What is the size of the large-diameter tube?	
Plug the power cord into the electrical outlet.	Will this ventilator work if it is disconnected from its power source?	
Place the Start/Stop switch in the Start position.	What does the ventilator do initially when it is powered on?	
Press the "Test Exh Port" soft key to begin the exhalation port test. Occlude the mask port on the circuit. Press the "Start Test" soft key.	Why is this test important? What would you do if the ventilator detected a leak?	

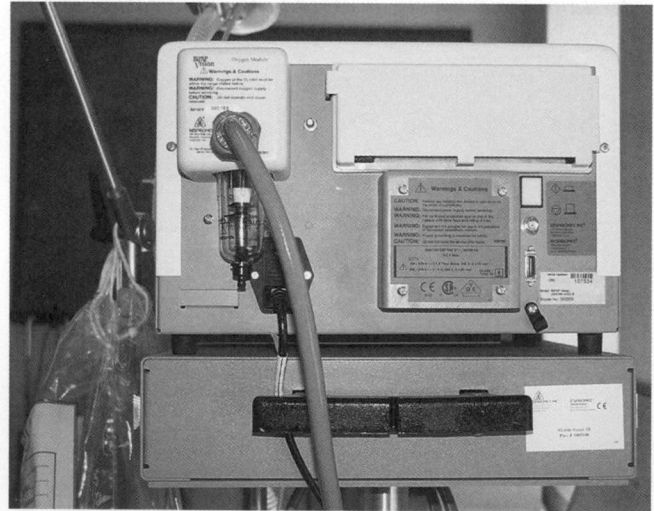

Figure 21-6 (Courtesy Philips Respironics, Murrysville, PA)

11. Fill in the following chart for the Respironics BiPAP ventilator control and display:

Hard Keys	Explanation of Key
Monitoring	
Parameters	
Mode	
Alarms	
Scale	
Freeze/Unfreeze	
Alarm silence	
Alarm reset	

12. Fill in the following chart for the Respironics BiPAP ventilator alarm control:

Alarm	Range and Purpose
High pressure	
Low pressure	
Low pressure delay	
Apnea	
Low minute volume	
Low rate/High rate	
Vent Inop	

13. Fill in the following chart pertaining to the setup of the Respironics BiPAP Vision using a lung analog or simulator (test lung). You will have to simulate breathing in your lung.

Task	Operation Questions	Initial When Completed
Assemble the ventilator's circuit.		
Select the CPAP mode using the correct soft key.	Where is the soft key located?	
Adjust the CPAP level to 8 cm H_2O.	How do you adjust the CPAP level?	
Select the "Activate New Mode" soft key.	Where is the soft key located?	
Simulate breathing with the test lung.	What does the display screen illustrate?	
Select the "%O_2" soft key.	How do you select the FiO_2 level?	
Press the "Alarms" hard key. A setup page should be displayed.	What alarms should you set?	

14. Obtain and set up the Respironics BiPAP Vision with a clean, new circuit. Perform the following activity using a partner, and fill in the chart provided. Make sure you use proper PPE during this activity. Always use FiO_2 settings of 0.21. When alarm goes off, it is important to remember that your facility may have protocols to use when setting alarms, or you may have very specific goals for your patient that require very tight alarm parameters. You will have to simulate breathing in your lung.

Task	Operation Questions	Initial When Completed
Assemble the ventilator's circuit.		
Select the correct size interface for your patient, and connect it to the circuit.	What size and type of interface did you use?	
Set the ventilator to a CPAP level of 8 cm H_2O and the FiO_2 to 0.21.	What are initial settings for a patient with acute cardiogenic pulmonary edema?	
Fit the interface to your patient.	Is there a leak? Is your patient comfortable?	
Observe and record the following: CPAP level: _____ Respiratory rate: _____ FiO_2: _____ Tidal volume: _____		
Set all the appropriate alarms.	What settings are appropriate for: High pressure: _____ Low pressure: _____ Low pressure delay: _____ Apnea: _____ Low minute volume: _____ Low rate/High rate: _____	
Adjust the CPAP level to 12 cm H_2O.	What happens to the tidal volume?	

15. Obtain and set up the Respironics BiPAP Vision using a lung analog or simulator (test lung). Fill in the chart below. You will have to simulate breathing in the lung.

Task	Operation Questions	Initial When Completed
Assemble the ventilator's circuit.		
Press the "Mode" key and then the S/T soft key.	Where is the Mode key located? What does S/T stand for?	
Set the following values. Be sure to push the "Activate New Mode" soft key to initiate the settings: Rate: 12 breaths/min IPAP: 12 cm H_2O EPAP: 6 cm H_2O Timed inspiration: 0.1 second FiO_2: 0.21 IPAP rise time: 0.1 second	Record the following values: Rate: _____ IPAP: _____ EPAP: _____ Timed inspiration: _____ FiO_2: _____ IPAP rise time: _____	
Note: Settings should be based on patient's underlying pathologies, physical assessment, goals of NIV, blood gases, other clinical tests, radiography, what the patient can tolerate, and protocols and standards of care.		
Connect the patient outlet port to the test lung, and observe the following displays and graphs: Pressure, volume, flow graphics: _____ Respiratory rate: _____ IPAP pressure: _____ EPAP pressure: _____	What is the ΔP? What ventilatory parameter does the ΔP influence?	
Change the IPAP to 14 and the EPAP to 8 cm H_2O. Leave all other settings the same.	What is the ΔP? Should the tidal volume increase, decrease, or stay the same? Why?	
Change the IPAP to 16, and leave all other settings the same.	What is the ΔP? Should the tidal volume increase, decrease, or stay the same? Why?	

Use any available noninvasive ventilator and test lung to complete the following questions. Use a different machine than you did for the previous exercises, if available. You can also use a critical care ventilator that has an NIV option.

16. Set up your machine properly using your textbooks or the machine's operation manual. Use an FiO_2 of 0.21 for all tasks. Attach the patient circuit to a test lung. Perform the following tasks and fill in the chart. Only change what is indicated in the task section. You will have to simulate breathing in your lung.

BiPAP

Task	What Happens?
Set: IPAP: 10 cm H_2O EPAP: 5 cm H_2O Rate: 10 breaths/min Timed inspiration: 0.2 seconds IPAP rise time: 0.2 seconds	Tidal volume: _____ ΔP: _____
IPAP to 15 cm H_2O EPAP: 5 cm H_2O	Tidal volume: _____ ΔP: _____
IPAP: 15 cm H_2O EPAP:10 cm H_2O	Tidal volume: _____ ΔP: _____
IPAP: 15 cm H_2O EPAP:5 cm H_2O Timed inspiration: 0.1 seconds IPAP rise time: 0.1 seconds	Tidal volume: _____ ΔP: _____
Increase the resistance on your test lung. If the equipment does not allow this, place a rubber band around the test lung to simulate an increase in the resistance	Tidal volume: _____ ΔP: _____
IPAP: 10 cm H_2O EPAP: 5 cm H_2O Rate: 10 breaths/min Timed inspiration: 0.2 seconds IPAP rise time: 0.2 seconds Loosen the circuit so that a large leak occurs.	What happens?

Switch to CPAP

Task	What Happens?
Switch to the CPAP mode, and return resistance to previous settings. Pressure: 5 cm H_2O	Tidal volume: _____
CPAP: 10 cm H_2O	Tidal volume: _____ What happened to the inspiratory time? _____

Self-Assessment Questions

1. Research strongly supports the use of NIV in the management of:
   A. Hypercapnic respiratory failure in a patient with COPD
   B. Status asthmaticus with a history of endotracheal intubations
   C. Hypercapnia in an apneic patient who had a drug overdose
   D. Pulmonary embolism

2. In acute cardiogenic pulmonary edema, initial pressures for CPAP are typically:
   A. 2–3 cm H_2O
   B. 4–5 cm H_2O
   C. 6–8 cm H_2O
   D. 8–12 cm H_2O

3. Successful application of NIV would present clinically in a patient with:
   1. Improvement of arterial blood gases
   2. Tidal volume increases
   3. Accessory muscle use increases
   4. Blood pressure stabilization

   A. 1 and 4 only
   B. 2 and 3 only
   C. 1, 2, and 4 only
   D. 1, 2, 3, and 4 only

4. Your patient has been receiving BiPAP for the past 2 hours for hypercapnic respiratory failure caused by COPD. The current settings are an IPAP of 14 cm H_2O and an EPAP of 8 cm H_2O. The patient's condition is not improving. What is your next step?
   A. Switch the patient to a CPAP of 10 cm H_2O
   B. Decrease the IPAP to 12 cm H_2O
   C. Increase the IPAP to 16 cm H_2O and the EPAP to 10 cm H_2O
   D. Intubate and mechanically ventilate the patient

5. Acute disease processes for which NIV may be indicated include:
   1. COPD exacerbation
   2. Pneumonia
   3. Hypercapnic respiratory failure
   4. Acute cardiogenic pulmonary edema

   A. 1 and 3 only
   B. 2 and 4 only
   C. 2, 3, and 4 only
   D. 1, 2, 3, and 4

6. Physical assessment of your patient reveals the following:
   - 28
   - pH: 7.32
   - $PaCO_2$: 56 mm Hg
   - Partial pressure of arterial oxygen (PaO_2): 67 mm Hg

   The patient, who is alert and oriented, has a past medical history of COPD and is complaining of shortness of breath. The physician asks for your suggestions to improve the patient's condition. What should you suggest?

   A. A nasal cannula at 2 L/min
   B. A nonrebreathing mask at 15 L/min
   C. NIV with a nasal mask interface
   D. Intubation and mechanical ventilation

7. When selecting an interface for NIV, factors that should be considered include:
   1. Patient comfort
   2. Volume of dead space and position of the exhalation port
   3. Fit of the interface
   4. Air leak associated with the interface

   A. 1 only
   B. 1 and 3 only
   C. 1, 3, and 4 only
   D. 1, 2, 3, and 4

8. A patient presents in the emergency department with acute pulmonary edema. The patient is alert, oriented, and is complaining of shortness of breath. First-line therapy should include:
   A. CPAP of 10 cm H_2O and FiO_2 of 1.0
   B. CPAP of 6 cm H_2O and FiO_2 of 0.4
   C. IPAP 16 cm H_2O, EPAP of 10 cm H_2O, and FiO_2 of 1.0
   D. Intubation and mechanical ventilation

9. Patients with acute exacerbation of COPD should be evaluated for NIV as an alternative to intubation and mechanical ventilation.
   A. True
   B. False

10. The terms CPAP and BiPAP are interchangeable.
    A. True
    B. False

›› CASE STUDY 21-1

Mr. T is a 68-year-old male patient with a long history of chronic COPD. He was rushed into the emergency department by his daughter. Vital signs and lab assessments are as follows:

HR: 118 beats/min
RR: 30 breaths/min
BP: 128/90 mm Hg
Lung sounds: Diminished throughout
The patient is alert and oriented.
Arterial blood gas interpretation suggests hypercapnic respiratory failure with moderate hypoxemia.

The physician asks for your suggestions regarding treatment for his respiratory complaint.

1. What would you suggest?

_____

_____

2. On the basis of your choice, what initial pressure settings would you choose?

_____

_____

3. If the patient is having initial difficulties tolerating the therapy, how could you resolve this issue?

_____

_____

4. How and when would you evaluate the efficacy of the treatment?

_____

_____

5. How would you describe a successful application of NIV relating to the patient's blood gases?

_____

_____

›› CASE STUDY 21-2

Miss Zash is a 23-year-old patient with a history of asthma. She is currently compliant with all her medications and up to date on her seasonal immunizations. She has been intubated and mechanically ventilated two times as a child for her asthma and has had no recent hospitalizations. Paramedics have brought her to the emergency department. She has received two albuterol treatments of 2.5 mg each via a small-volume nebulizer (SVN) with minimal improvement. She is currently on a nonrebreathing mask running at 15 L/min. Her vital signs are as follows:

HR: 128 beats/min
RR: 36 breaths/min
BP: 118/92 mm Hg
Lung sounds: Silent chest
The patient has an altered level of consciousness.
Chest radiography: Hyperinflation of lung fields with a flattened diaphragm
Arterial blood gas is pending.

The emergency medicine intern suggests a trial of NIV. The attending physician asks for your opinion about this suggested therapy.

1. Do you agree with the intern's suggestion? Why, or why not?

_____

_____

2. What would you suggest if you did not agree?

_____

_____

Invasive Ventilatory Support

▪ OBJECTIVES

Upon the completion of the chapter activities and content review topics, the student should be able to:

1. Describe the physiologic goals of mechanical ventilatory support.
2. Describe the clinical objectives of mechanical ventilatory support.
3. Distinguish between volume and pressure modes of mechanical ventilation.
4. Choose the appropriate initial ventilator settings and alarms.
5. Calculate dynamic and static compliances (C_D and C_S).

▪ KEY TERMS

- Dynamic compliance (C_D)
- Full ventilatory support
- Partial ventilatory support
- Plateau pressure ($P_{plateau}$)
- Pressure control ventilation
- Static compliance (C_S)
- Synchronized intermittent mandatory ventilation (SIMV)
- Volume control ventilation

▪ CONTENT REVIEW TOPICS

- Barotrauma
- Blood gas interpretation
- Type I respiratory failure
- Type II respiratory failure
- Ventilator bundles

▪ PROCEDURAL ASSESSMENTS

22-1   Initiating Invasive Mechanical Ventilation
22-2   Assessing a Patient-Ventilator System
22-3   Compliance Calculation

▪ EQUIPMENT

- 50-psi air source
- 50-psi oxygen source
- Adult circuits for ventilators
- Intubated human patient simulator, if available
- Mechanical ventilators
- Rubber bands
- Test lungs or lung simulator
- Ventilator bacterial filters

Mechanical ventilation is arguably the topic that causes the most apprehension for respiratory therapy students. With numerous different ventilators and inconsistent mode terminology adding to the complexity of this life-support technology, a strong foundation with regard to the pulmonary system and its cardiovascular overlap is imperative. A ventilator simply pushes air into the patient's lungs. A critical factor in successful mechanical ventilation depends on how skillfully the respiratory therapist (RT) can manipulate pressures, volumes, and flows in a way that will optimize a patient's oxygenation, ventilation, and acid–base balance. All of this must be accomplished while minimizing the possible adverse effects of mechanical ventilation.

> → **Reality Check** The most influential variable in the success of patients receiving mechanical ventilation is the knowledge of the therapists taking care of them!

While learning the art of mechanical ventilation, remember not to get caught up in all the "bells and whistles" that the technology of respiratory care offers you as a therapist. A ventilator is merely a very expensive piece of equipment at a patient's bedside if the RT operating it does not know how to effectively use it to benefit the patient. Initiation of mechanical

ventilation may be the result of countless patient scenarios, physiologic objectives, and clinical goals. Essentially, patients are intubated and mechanically ventilated because they cannot oxygenate, ventilate, protect their airway, or maintain their secretions. These circumstances are explained in Box 22-1. This chapter will discuss the aspects of initiation of mechanical ventilation as well as the care of the patient receiving mechanical ventilation.

≫ SKILL CHECK LISTS

22-1 Initiating Invasive Mechanical Ventilation

A majority of patients are placed in a volume control mode of ventilation following intubation and initiation of mechanical ventilation. In this mode, the RT selects a tidal volume for delivery based on the patient's ideal body weight (IBW), also referred to as *predicted body weight*. Two different formulas for both men and women are given in Table 22-1. The patient's current reason for mechanical ventilation along with any underlying pulmonary condition needs to be taken into consideration when choosing mode and settings for mechanical ventilation. Typical values for both volume and pressure control ventilation are provided in Table 22-2. The mode choice and the settings are different for the patient intubated

BOX 22-1   Goals and Objectives of Ventilatory Support

Physiologic Goals
- Support or manipulate gas exchange
- Alveolar ventilation ($PaCO_2$ and pH)
- Arterial oxygenation (PaO_2, SaO_2, SpO_2, CaO_2, and DO_2)
- Increase lung volumes
- End-inspiratory and end-expiratory lung inflation
- Functional residual capacity (FRC)
- Reduce or manipulate work of breathing (WOB)
- Minimize cardiovascular impairment
- Ensure patient-ventilator synchrony
- Avoid ventilator-induced lung injury

Clinical Objectives
- Reverse hypoxemia
- Reverse acute respiratory acidosis
- Relieve respiratory distress
- Prevent or reverse atelectasis
- Reverse ventilatory muscle dysfunction
- Allow sedation and neuromuscular blockade
- Decrease systemic or myocardial oxygen consumption
- Maintain or improve cardiac output
- Reduce intracranial pressure
- Stabilize the chest

CaO_2, Arterial oxygen; *DO_2*, oxygen delivery; *$PaCO_2$*, partial pressure of arterial carbon dioxide; *PaO_2*, partial pressure of arterial oxygen; *SaO_2*, saturation of arterial oxygen; *SpO_2*, saturation of peripheral oxygen.

TABLE 22-1   Ideal Body Weight Calculation in Kilograms (kg)

Men	[106 + 6(height in inches − 60)] ÷ 2.2
	or
	[(height in inches − 60) × 2.2] + 50
Women	[105 + 5(height in inches − 60)] ÷ 2.2
	or
	[(height in inches − 60) × 2.2] + 45

and mechanically ventilated for a surgical procedure with no pulmonary history, compared with the patient whose pulmonary status is deteriorating from pneumonia and exacerbation of chronic obstructive pulmonary disease (COPD).

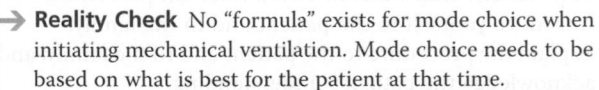

> **Reality Check** No "formula" exists for mode choice when initiating mechanical ventilation. Mode choice needs to be based on what is best for the patient at that time.

> **Reality Check** Lung protective therapy should be on your mind as soon as the decision is made to intubate and mechanically ventilate the patient.

The following is the step-by-step process for initiating mechanical ventilation.

Procedural Preparation
1. Review the patient's chart.
2. Verify the physician's order or the facility's protocol for standard of care.

TABLE 22-2 Typical Values for Initiation of Volume or Pressure Control Ventilation in the Adult Patient

Setting	Typical Value
Tidal volume	
For normal lungs	6–8 mL/kg IBW
For COPD	Begin at 6–8 mL/kg
For ALI/ARDS	4–8 mL/kg IBW to maintain $P_{plateau}$ <30 cmH_2O
Acute asthma	4–6 mL/kg IBW
Neuromuscular disease	6–10 mL/kg IBW
Peak inspiratory pressure	**Pressure level to achieve**
Frequency	**6–8 mL/kg IBW**
RESPIRATORY RATE	
For Normal Lungs	12–16 breaths/min
For COPD	10–12 breaths/min
For ALI/ARDS	20–35 breaths/min
Acute asthma	10–12 breaths/min
Neuromuscular disease	12–16 breaths/min
Inspiratory time	0.8–1.2 seconds
	Longer expiratory time for patients with obstructive disease
FLOW	
Inspiratory flow	60–100 L/min
Volume control flow pattern	Decreasing ramp
PEEP	
Most patients without ALI	5 cmH_2O
ALI	5–10 cmH_2O
ARDS	10–15 cmH_2O
COPD/Asthma	5 cmH_2O
TRIGGER SENSITIVITY	
Pressure	−0.5–2.0 cmH_2O
Flow	2–3 L/min
PRESSURE LIMIT	
Volume mode	40 cmH_2O
Pressure mode	30 cmH_2O
Peak pressure alarm	Once patient is connected and stabilized adjust to 10–15 cmH_2O above PIP
Initial FIO_2	1.0 and lower as quickly as possible based on patient's ABG values and condition
Humidification	H/H provide 35°C at the airway connection or appropriate HME

ALI, Acute lung injury; *ARDS*, acute respiratory distress syndrome; *COPD*, chronic obstructive pulmonary disease; *HH*, heat and humification; *IBW*, ideal body weight; *L/min*, liters per minute; *mL/kg*, milliliter per kilogram; *PEEP*, positive end-expiratory pressure; *PIP*, peak inspiratory pressure.

3. Obtain, clean, and inspect the appropriate equipment prior to entering the patient's room.
4. Follow personal protective equipment (PPE) requirements, and observe standard precautions for any transmission-based isolation procedure.
5. Identify the patient using two patient identifiers.
6. Introduce self to the patient and to the family.
7. Explain the procedure to the patient and to the family, and acknowledge the patient's understanding.

8. Perform proper hand hygiene, and put on gloves, mask, and protective eyewear, as appropriate for the procedure.

Implementation

1. Assess vital signs.
2. Establish and implement the appropriate settings for the following setup decisions:
   a. Type and method of artificial airway
   b. Partial versus full support
   c. Mode of ventilation
      i. Assist-control (volume vs. pressure)
      ii. Synchronized intermittent mandatory ventilation (SIMV; volume vs. pressure): with or without pressure support
3. Establish and implement the appropriate settings for the following ventilatory values:
   a. Trigger method (pressure vs. flow) and sensitivity
   b. Tidal volume or pressure level
   c. Frequency
   d. Inspiratory flow, inspiratory time, expiratory time, or I:E ratio
   e. Inspiratory flow wave form
   f. FIO_2
   g. PEEP or CPAP
4. Attach the patient to the ventilator.
5. Perform initial assessment of ventilatory support:
   a. Inspection, palpation, and auscultation
   b. Assess position of artificial airway and cuff pressure
   c. Assess pulse, blood pressure, oximetry, and electrocardiography (ECG)
   d. Inspect patient-ventilatory system breathing circuit, humidifier, and ventilator settings
6. Establish and implement the appropriate settings for the following alarms and backup values:
   a. Low-pressure, low PEEP alarms
   b. High-pressure limit and alarm
   c. Low and high tidal volume alarms
   d. Low and high minute ventilation alarms
   e. Low and high frequency alarms
   f. Apnea alarm and apnea ventilation values
   g. Low and high oxygen alarm
   h. Low and high airway temperature alarms
   i. I:E ratio limit and alarm
7. Allow enough slack on the circuit so that the artificial airway remains secure.
8. Confirm or place the manual ventilation device at the patient's bedside.
9. Remove the supplies from the patient's room, and clean the area, as needed.
10. Remove PPE, and perform proper hand hygiene prior to leaving the patient's room.

Evaluation of Procedure

1. Establish a baseline, or compare with previous measurements.
   a. Obtain arterial blood gas (ABG), and confirm that chest radiography has been ordered.
   b. Evaluate the radiograph when it becomes available.
2. Develop an appropriate respiratory care plan based on assessment data.
3. Identify any unexpected outcomes.

Documentation and Reporting

1. Record your findings in the patient's chart.
2. Report any abnormal findings to the appropriate health care provider.

22-2 Assessing a Patient-Ventilator System

With so many intricacies involved in the management of a patient receiving mechanical ventilation, the term "vent check" seems unimportant; however, it is a deceptively trivial expression of the contemplation and skill that actually go into a patient-ventilator system assessment. The evaluation procedure should begin with a careful patient assessment. All current laboratory values, chest radiographs, and the health care provider's progress notes should be reviewed prior to entering the patient's room.

Typically, patients are placed on an FIO_2 of 1.0 following intubation and initiation of mechanical ventilation. This should be one of the first parameters that need to be adjusted. Once the patient is stabilized a blood gas sample is drawn and interpreted, and the FIO_2 should be lowered slowly, if indicated. An FIO_2 adjustment formula is given in Box 22-2.

> → **Reality Check** Because many patients are on isolation precautions, manometers to measure cuff pressures will not always be readily available.

The following is the step-by-step process for assessing a patient-ventilator system.

Procedural Preparation

1. Review the patient's chart for patient's current vital signs and ventilator settings.
2. Review the patient's most recent blood gases or SpO_2.
3. Review the most recent chest radiograph.
4. Identify current sedation medications.
5. Verify the physician's order or the facility's protocol for standard of care.
6. Obtain, clean, and inspect the appropriate equipment prior to entering the patient's room.
7. Identify the patient using two patient identifiers.
8. Follow PPE requirements, and observe standard precautions for any transmission-based isolation procedure.
9. Introduce yourself to the patient and to the family.
10. Explain the procedure to the patient and to the family, and acknowledge the patient's understanding.

BOX 22-2 Adjusting FIO_2 of a Ventilated Patient

Adjusting oxygen percentage:

$$FIO_2 = \left(\frac{PaO_2 \text{ desired}}{PaO_2/PAO_2 \text{ ratio}} + PaCO_2 \times 1.25 \right) \times \frac{1}{P_B - P_{H2O}}$$

Simpler but less accurate:

$$\frac{PaO_2(\text{initial})}{FIO_2(\text{Initial})} = \frac{PaO_2(\text{Desired})}{FIO_2(\text{New})}$$

FIO_2, Fractional inspired oxygen; $PaCO_2$, partial pressure of arterial carbon dioxide; PaO_2, partial pressure of arterial oxygen.

11. Perform proper hand hygiene, and put on gloves, mask, and protective eyewear, as appropriate for the procedure.

Implementation

1. Approach the patient before you approach the ventilator.
2. Assess the patient for:
   a. Overall appearance, comfort, and ventilator synchrony
   b. Airway position, patency, and security
   c. Cuff pressure
   d. Breath sounds
   e. Suction, if indicated
   f. Chest-rise
   g. Peripheral pulses
   h. Indwelling catheter(s)
   i. Chest tubes
   j. Head of bed elevated to at least 30 degrees
   k. Oral care
3. Assess ventilator functions and settings:
   a. Security of circuit connections
   b. Heat and humidification device, airway temperature
   c. Mode
   d. Tidal volume or inspiratory pressure
   e. Exhaled tidal volume (V_T)
   f. Set frequency
   g. Spontaneous frequency
   h. Inspiratory time
   i. Flow rate
   j. Flow pattern
   k. Mean airway pressure
   l. PEEP level
   m. Set FIO_2
   n. Analyzed FIO_2 (most critical care ventilators do this automatically)
   o. Pressure support
   p. Trigger
   q. Alarms
   r. Calculation of C_S
4. Ensure that the manual ventilation device and the suction equipment are available at the patient's bedside.
5. Ensure that replacement tracheostomy tubes are available at the patient's bedside.
6. Remove the supplies from the patient's room, and clean the area, as needed.
7. Remove PPE, and perform proper hand hygiene prior to leaving the patient's room.

Evaluation of Procedure

1. Establish a baseline, or compare with previous measurements.
2. Develop an appropriate respiratory diagnosis based on assessment data.
3. Ensure that lung protective therapy is in place.
4. Consider mode change, discontinuation of mechanical ventilation, or weaning.
5. Identify any unexpected outcomes.

Documentation and Reporting

1. Record your findings in the patient's chart.
2. Report any abnormal findings to the appropriate health care provider.

BOX 22-3	Calculating Dynamic and Static Compliance

$$\text{Dynamic compliance } C_D = \frac{V_T}{PIP - PEEP}$$

$$\text{Static compliance } C_S = \frac{V_T}{P_{Plateau} - PEEP}$$

PIP, Peak inspiratory pressure; *PEEP*, positive end-expiratory pressure; V_T, tidal volume.

22-3   Compliance Calculations

Part of your patient-ventilator system assessment includes calculation of the patient's dynamic compliance (C_D) and obtaining a $P_{plateau}$ to calculate the static compliance (C_S) (Box 22-3). Evaluation and trending of these compliance values is a good way to monitor the progression of your patient's pulmonary status.

The following is the step-by-step process for compliance calculations.

> **Reality Check** The patient's family members are more interested in how the patient is doing than exactly what diagnostic test or procedure you are performing.

Procedural Preparation

1. Review the patient's chart.
2. Verify the physician's order or the facility's protocol for standard of care.
3. Obtain, clean, and inspect the appropriate equipment prior to entering the patient's room.
4. Follow PPE requirements, and observe standard precautions for any transmission-based isolation procedure.
5. Identify the patient using two patient identifiers.
6. Introduce yourself to the patient and to the family.
7. Explain the procedure to the patient and to the family, and acknowledge the patient's understanding.
8. Perform proper hand hygiene, and put on gloves, mask, and protective eyewear, as appropriate for the procedure.

Implementation

1. Perform a patient-ventilator system assessment (see PA 22-2).
2. Identify PIP.
3. Identify exhaled tidal volume.
4. Identify PEEP.
5. Identify auto-PEEP.
6. Identify total PEEP (PEEP + auto-PEEP).
7. Identify dynamic compliance (C_D):
   a. Subtract total PEEP from PIP.
   b. Divide exhaled tidal volume by the number obtained in step 7 a.
   c. Report C_D in mL/cmH_2O.
8. Identify static compliance (C_S):
   a. Observe several ventilator respiratory cycles.
   b. Perform an inspiratory hold maneuver to obtain plateau pressure.

c. Subtract total PEEP from plateau pressure.

d. Divide exhaled tidal volume by the number obtained in 8 c.

e. Report C_{stat} in mL/cm H_2O.

9. Remove supplies from the patient's room, and clean the area, as needed.

10. Remove the PPE, and perform proper hand hygiene prior to leaving the patient's room.

Evaluation of Procedure

1. Establish a baseline, or compare with previous measurements.

2. Develop an appropriate respiratory diagnosis based on assessment data.

3. Note any increasing FiO_2 requirements.

4. Observe trends in the C_{dyn} and C_{stat}, and use them to determine improvement or deterioration of the underlying disease process.

5. Identify any unexpected outcomes.

Documentation and Reporting

1. Record your findings in the patient's chart.

2. Report any abnormal findings to the appropriate health care provider.

Bibliography

Cairo JM: *Pilbeam's mechanical ventilation*, ed 5, St. Louis, MO, 2012, Mosby.

Kacmarek RM, Stoller JK, Heuer AJ: *Egan's fundamentals of respiratory care*, ed 10, St. Louis, MO, 2013, Mosby.

1. What is the definition of full ventilatory support?

   _____

2. What is the definition of partial ventilatory support?

   _____

3. What is the definition of volume-controlled ventilation?

   _____

4. What is the definition of pressure-controlled ventilation?

   _____

5. List the six complications of invasive mechanical ventilation.

   a. _____

   b. _____

   c. _____

   d. _____

   e. _____

   f. _____

6. List the seven factors that increase the mean airway pressure.

   a. _____

   b. _____

   c. _____

   d. _____

   e. _____

   f. _____

   g. _____

7. List the five beneficial effects of appropriate levels of PEEP.

   a. _____

   b. _____

   c. _____

d. _____

e. _____

8. List the five detrimental effects of inappropriate levels of PEEP.

a. _____

b. _____

c. _____

d. _____

e. _____

*The following exercises will use the terminology from the Covidien PB 840. You can use **any ventilator** to complete the exercise. The settings used are for the demonstration of concepts and may not be comparable with "real life" settings. Use an FIO_2 of 0.21 for all ventilator activities. Note that the oxygen sensor needs to be disabled on the PB 840. A similar step may need to be taken on the ventilator you are using if it is not PB 840.*

9. This is a wave form activity in volume control. Set the ventilator parameters as follows:
- Mode: AC/VC If not using the PB 840, list the equivalent mode name
- Tidal volume: 0.50 L
- Frequency: 12/min
- Inspiratory flow rate: 70 L/min
- PEEP: 0 cmH_2O
- Sensitivity: −1 cmH_2O

Record the following first with a square wave flow pattern followed by a decelerating flow pattern.

Recorded Values	Square Wave Form	Decelerating Wave Form
PIP (cmH_2O)		
Exhaled V_T (mL)		
I : E ratio		
Mean airway pressure (cmH_2O)		
Inspiratory time (seconds)		

10. What changes were seen between the different wave forms in each of the recorded values? When you switch from a square to a decelerating wave form:

_____

_____

11. This is a sensitivity activity. Now set the sensitivity setting to −2.0 cmH₂O. Gently lift or squeeze the test lung to initiate a ventilator breath to attain a total respiratory rate of 18 to 20 breaths/min.

a. What did the pressure-graph look like at the baseline at the beginning of inspiration with *machine breaths*? Draw it on Figure 22-1.

_____

_____

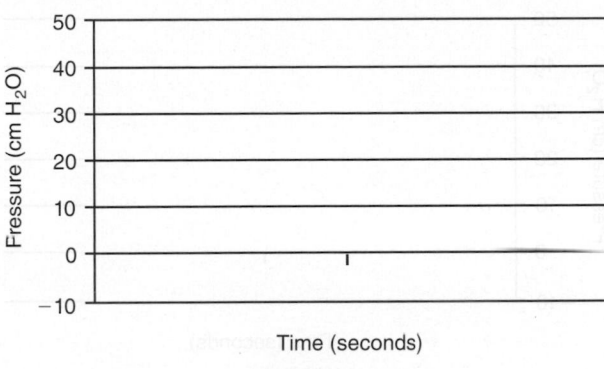

Figure 22-1

b. What changes occurred on the pressure time graphic at the baseline at the beginning of inspiration when a patient-triggered breath was simulated that did not occur with machine breaths? Draw it on Figure 22-2.

_____

_____

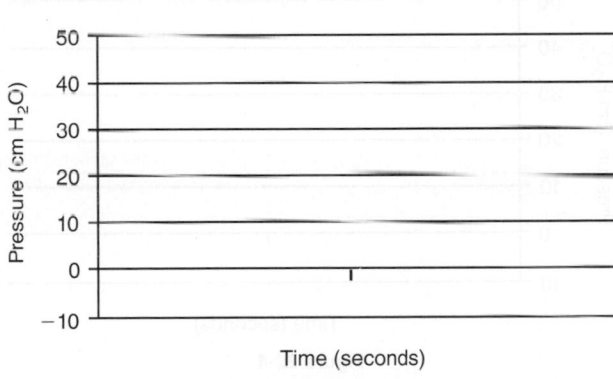

Figure 22-2

c. Change the pressure sensitivity to flow at a setting of 2 L/min. It is easier or harder to trigger?

_____

_____

12. Now change sensitivity to –3 cmH$_2$O. Gently lift or squeeze the test lung to initiate a ventilator breath to attain a total respiratory rate of 18 to 20 breaths/min.

a. What did the pressure-time graphic look like at the baseline at the beginning of inspiration with machine breaths? Draw it on Figure 22-3.

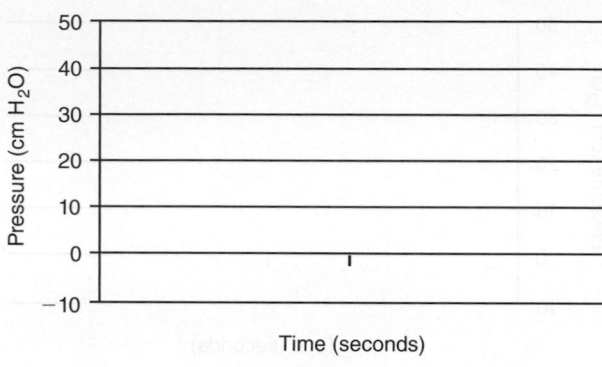

Figure 22-3

b. What changes occurred on the pressure-time graphic at the baseline at the beginning of inspiration when a patient-triggered breath was simulated that did not occur with machine breaths? Draw it on Figure 22-4.

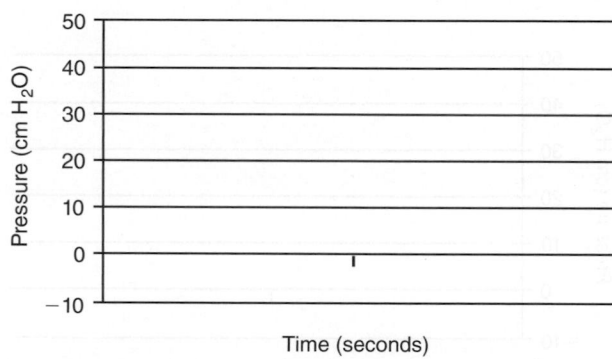

Figure 22-4

13. Now change sensitivity to −5 cmH$_2$O. Gently lift or squeeze the test lung to initiate a ventilator breath to attain a total respiratory rate of 18 to 20 breaths/min.

   a. What did the pressure-time graphic look like at the baseline at the beginning of inspiration with machine breaths? Draw it on Figure 22-5.

   _____

   _____

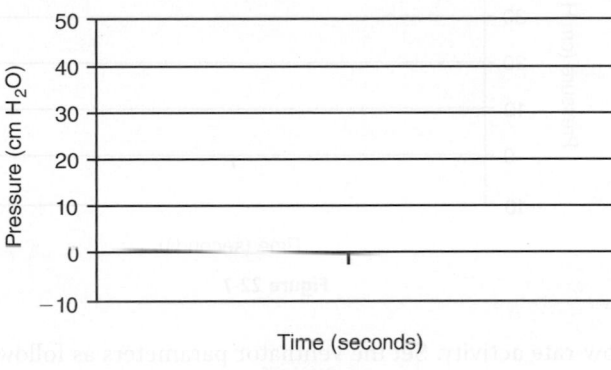

Figure 22-5

   b. What changes occurred on the pressure and time graphic at the baseline at the beginning of inspiration when a patient triggered breath was simulated that did not occur with machine breaths? Draw it on Figure 22-6.

   _____

   _____

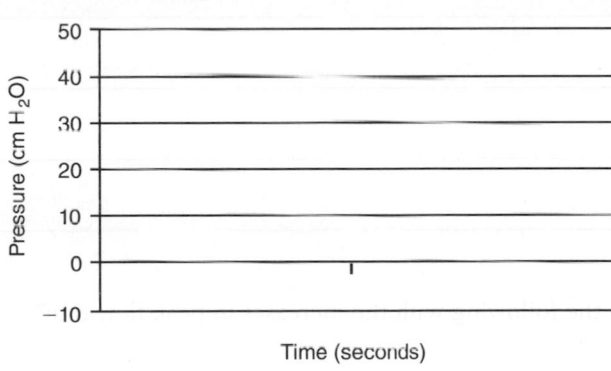

Figure 22-6

c. Illustrate the difference in negative pressure required to initiate a machine breath between the sensitivity settings of –3 and –5 cmH$_2$O. Draw it on Figure 22-7.

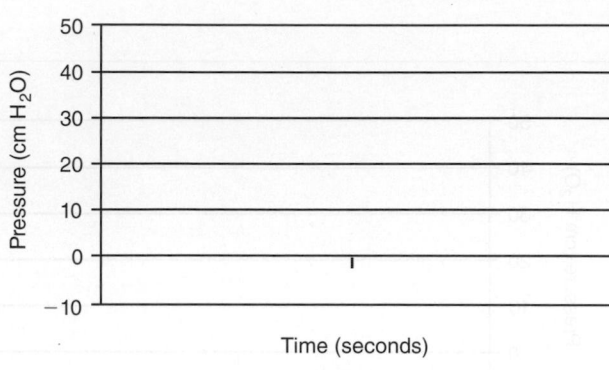

Figure 22-7

14. This is a wave form and flow rate activity. Set the ventilator parameters as follows:
- Mode: AC/VC
- V$_T$ 0.50 L
- Frequency: 12/min
- PEEP: 0 cmH$_2$O
- Sensitivity: –1 cmH$_2$O

a. Record the following with a peak flow rate set at 40, 60, and 80 L/min and a square wave form pattern.

Parameter	40 L/min	60 L/min	80 L/min
PIP (cmH$_2$O)			
Exhaled V$_T$ (mL)			
I : E ratio			

b. What changes occurred to the following with the increases in peak flow rate?

Flow rate wave form:

Pressure wave form:

I : E ratio:

_____

_____

Exhaled V_T

_____

_____

c. Record the following with a peak flow rate set at 40, 60, and 80 L/min and a decreasing wave form pattern.

Parameter	40 L/min	60 L/min	80 L/min
PIP (cmH$_2$O)			
Exhaled V_T (mL)			
I : E ratio			

d. What changes occurred to the following with the increases in peak flow rate?

Flow rate wave form:

_____

_____

Pressure wave form:

_____

_____

I : E ratio:

_____

_____

Exhaled tidal volume:

_____

_____

15. This is a PEEP activity as well as a wave form activity. Set the ventilator parameters as follows, and note the pressure wave form shape:
    - Mode: AC/VC
    - V_T 0.50 L
    - Frequency: 12/min
    - PEEP: 0 cmH$_2$O
    - Sensitivity: –1 cmH$_2$O
    - Square wave form pattern
    - Flow rate: 30 L/min

    a. Now, adjust the PEEP to read 5 cmH$_2$O. What change occurred on the pressure wave form shape?

    _____

    _____

    b. Was there any change in the flow wave form pattern?

    _____

    _____

    c. Now, adjust the PEEP to read 10 cmH$_2$O. What change occurred on the pressure wave form shape?

    _____

    _____

    d. Was there any change in the flow wave form pattern?

    _____

    _____

16. Set the ventilator parameters as follows, and note the pressure wave form shape:
    - Mode: AC/VC
    - V_T 0.50 L
    - Frequency: 12/min
    - PEEP: 0 cmH$_2$O
    - Sensitivity: –1 cmH$_2$O
    - Decreasing wave form pattern
    - Flow rate: 55 L/min

    a. Now, adjust the PEEP to read 5 cmH$_2$O. What change occurred on the pressure wave form shape?

    _____

    _____

    b. Was there any change in the flow wave form pattern?

    _____

    _____

c. Now, adjust the PEEP to read 10 cmH$_2$O. What change occurred on the pressure wave form shape?

_____

_____

d. Was there any change in the flow wave form pattern?

_____

_____

17. This is a plateau pressure activity. Set the ventilator parameters as follows:
- Mode: AC/VC
- V$_T$ 0.50 L
- Frequency: 12/min
- PEEP: 0 cmH$_2$O
- Sensitivity: −1 cmH$_2$O
- Square wave form pattern
- Flow rate: 30 L/min

Screen should display pressure-time graphic and the volume-time graphic.

a. What is a plateau pressure (P$_{plateau}$)?

_____

_____

b. Is P$_{plateau}$ attained during inspiration or expiration?

_____

_____

c. Obtain a P$_{plateau}$ Draw it on Figures 22-8 and 22-9.

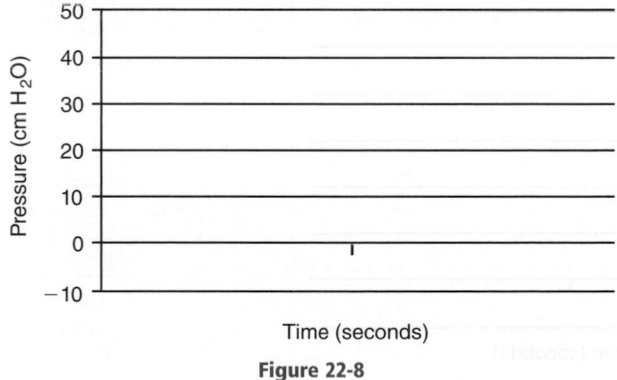

Figure 22-8

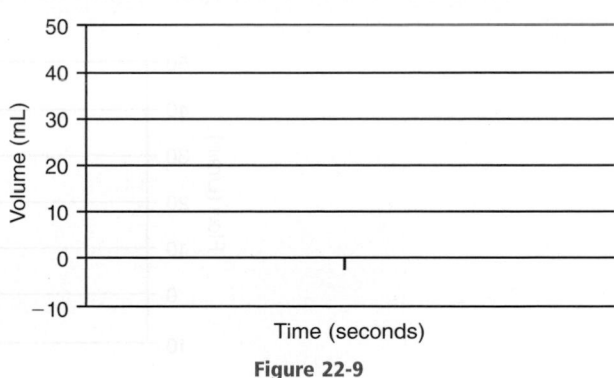

Figure 22-9

d. What are some causes of increasing plateau pressures?

_____

_____

18. This is an airway resistance activity. This activity uses resistance devices added either to the airway portion of the circuit or by turning a resistance knob. Set the ventilator parameters as follows:
- Mode: AC/VC
- V_T 0.50 L
- Frequency: 12/min
- PEEP: 2 cmH$_2$O
- Sensitivity: −1 cmH$_2$O
- Square wave form pattern
- Flow rate: 30 L/min

a. Use the resistances of 20, and 50, or turn the resistance knob once, twice, and three times. Record the following information:

Parameter	5 or One Turn	20 or Two Turns	50 or Three Turns
PIP (cmH$_2$O)			
P$_{plateau}$ (cmH$_2$O)			
PIP-P$_{plateau}$ (cmH$_2$O)			

b. What could cause an increasing PIP in a mechanically ventilated patient?

c. Why did the PIP rise and plateau pressures stay approximately the same with changes in the resistance?

d. While using the Resistance of 5 (one turn) and the Resistance of 20 (two turns), observe the flow-time graphic. Draw them on the same graphic (Figure 22-10) to compare.

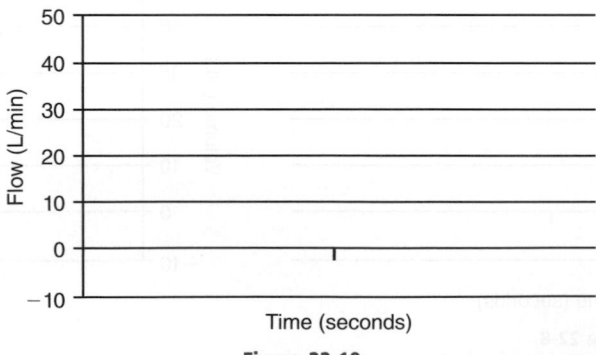

Figure 22-10

e. Why did the inspiratory portion of the flow rate wave form stay the same and the expiratory wave form change?

f. What lung condition may cause this change in the expiratory flow rate?

g. As an RT, is there any treatment or medication you could give to correct this?

19. What is the formula for airway resistance?

20. This is a compliance activity. Set the ventilator parameters as follows:
- Mode: AC/VC
- V_T 0.50 L
- Frequency: 12/min
- PEEP: 0 cmH$_2$O
- Sensitivity: 1 cmH$_2$O
- Square wave form pattern
- Flow rate: 30 L/min

Return the resistance knob to 5 (one turn), and set your test lung to the compliance settings in the chart below. If you do not have this ability, use rubber bands around the test lung. Fill in the chart, and calculate the dynamic and static lung compliances.

Parameter	0.04 L/cmH$_2$O No Rubber Band	0.03 L/cmH$_2$O 1 Rubber Band	0.025 L/cmH$_2$O 2 Rubber Bands	0.02 L/cmH$_2$O 3 Rubber Bands
PIP (cmH$_2$O)				
Exhaled V_T (mL)				
P$_{plateau}$ (cmH$_2$O)				
C$_D$ (mL/cm H$_2$O)				
C$_S$ (mL/cmH$_2$O)				

21. This is a PEEP and compliance activity. Set the ventilator parameters as follows:
- Mode: AC/VC
- V_T 0.50 L
- Frequency: 12/min
- PEEP: 5 cmH$_2$O
- Sensitivity: –1 cmH$_2$O
- Square waveform pattern
- Flow rate: 30 L/min
- Place the compliance at 0.2 (3 rubber bands)
- Resistance 5 or one turn

Fill in the chart below:

Parameter	PEEP + 5	PEEP + 10	PEEP + 12
PIP (cmH$_2$O)			
Exhaled tidal volume (mL)			
P$_{plateau}$ (cmH$_2$O)			
C$_D$ calculation (mL/cmH$_2$O)			
C$_S$ calculation (mL/cm H$_2$O)			

22. This is an alarm activity. Fill in the chart below about alarm and backup ventilation settings of initial ventilator setup for the adult patient:

Alarm	Suggested Setting
Low pressure	
Low PEEP/CPAP	
High pressure limit	
Low exhaled tidal volume	
Low exhaled minute ventilation	
High minute ventilation	
FiO_2	
Temperature	
Apnea delay	
Apnea values	

23. This is a pressure control activity. Set the ventilator parameters as follows:
- Mode: AC/PC. If not using the PB 840 Equivalent mode name: _____
- Inspiratory pressure: 10 cmH_2O
- Frequency: 12/min
- Inspiratory time: 1 second
- PEEP: 0 cmH_2O
- Sensitivity: −2 cmH_2O

Using a test lung, record the following with the inspiratory pressure changes indicated in the chart below:

Parameter	Set Inspiratory Pressure		
	10 cmH_2O	15 cmH_2O	20 cmH_2O
PIP (cmH_2O)			
Exhaled V_T (mL)			
I:E ratio			
ΔP			

b. What did the pressure-time graphics and the flow-time graphics look like for each set inspiratory pressure? Draw the three different pressures on Figures 22-11 through 22-13, and compare them.

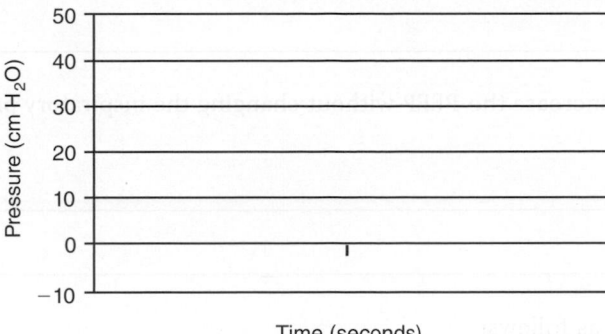

Figure 22-11

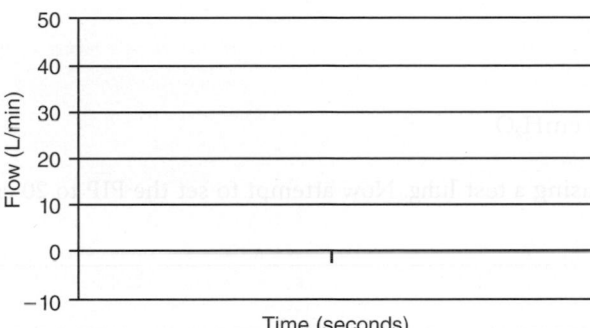

Figure 22-12

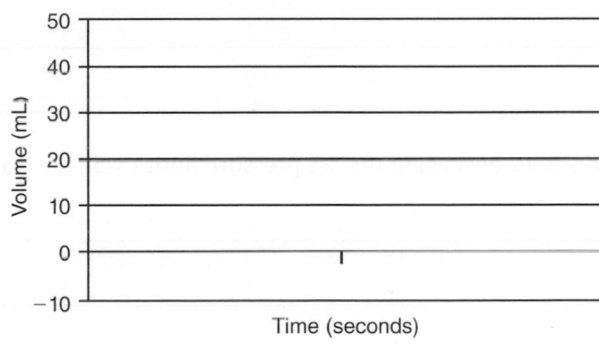

Figure 22-13

c. As the inspiratory pressure increased, what happened to the tidal volume?

_____

_____

d. As the inspiratory pressure increased, what happened to the I:E ratio?

_____

_____

e. As the inspiratory pressure increased, what happened to the ΔP value?

_____

_____

f. On your ventilator, if you increase the PEEP without changing the inspiratory pressure setting, what happens to the PIP? ΔP?

_____

_____

24. Set the ventilator parameters as follows:
    - Mode: AC/PC
    - Inspiratory pressure: 10 cmH$_2$O
    - Frequency: 12/min
    - Inspiratory time: 1 second
    - PEEP: 10 cmH$_2$O
    - Sensitivity: –2 cmH$_2$O
    - Set the pressure limit to 25 cmH$_2$O

a. Initiate the above settings using a test lung. Now attempt to set the PIP to 20 cmH$_2$O. What happens?

_____

_____

b. By definition, do limits cycle a breath?

_____

_____

c. On your particular ventilator, does exceeding the set pressure limit cycle the breath?

_____

_____

25. This is a SIMV-VC and AC/VC comparison activity. Using two ventilators and a lung simulator that are set exactly the same, set the following parameters:

Parameter	Ventilator 1	Ventilator 2
Mode	AC/VC	SIMV-VC
If not using the PB 840, equivalent mode name		
V_T	500 mL	500 mL
Frequency	15 breaths/min	15 breaths/min
Peak flow	40 L/min	40 L/min
Flow pattern	square	square
PEEP	5 cmH$_2$O	5 cmH$_2$O
Sensitivity	−2 cmH$_2$O	−2 cmH$_2$O

Attach each ventilator to a test lung. Assume that all patient lung characteristics are the same and that the patient is apneic. Observe the pressure-time and flow-time graphics on each ventilator.

a. What do you see? Draw them both in Figures 22-14 and 22-15 below. Now simulate patient triggering of breaths to a rate of 20 to 22 breaths/min.

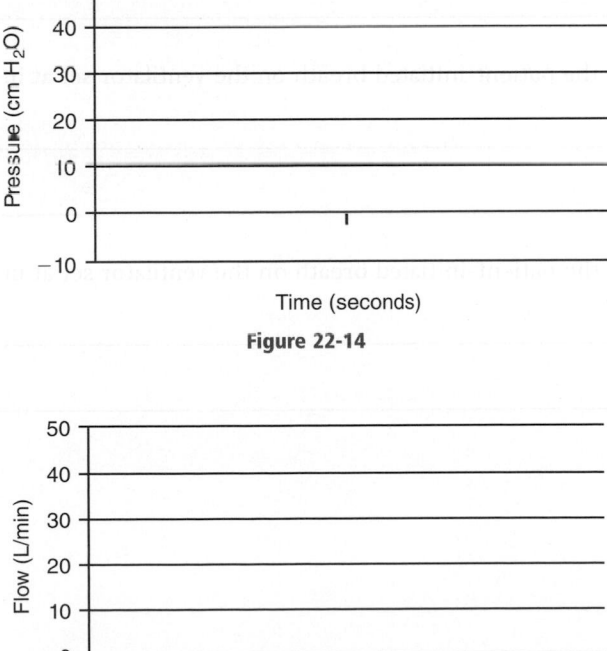

Figure 22-14

Figure 22-15

b. What do you see? Draw them both in Figures 22-16 and 22-17 below.

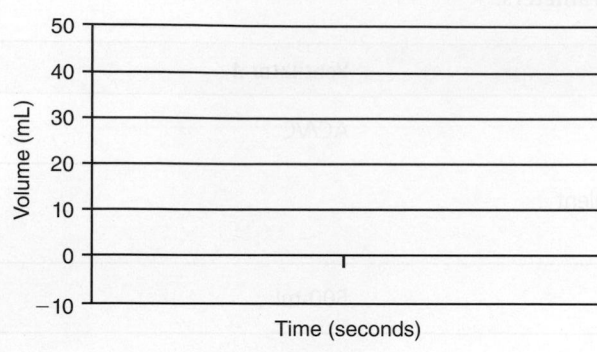

Figure 22-16

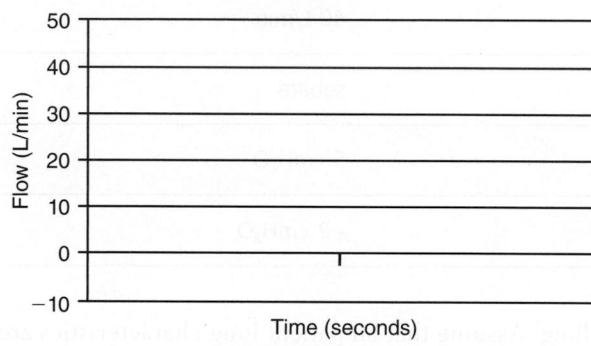

Figure 22-17

c. How is the SIMV-VC patient-initiated breath cycled?

_____

_____

d. What is the exhaled V_T of the patient-initiated breath on the ventilator set at in AC/VC?

_____

_____

e. What is the exhaled V_T of the patient-initiated breath on the ventilator set at in SIMV-VC?

_____

_____

26. Fill in the following chart with equivalent modes of ventilation terminology using the PB 840 as a baseline. Use laboratory ventilators and textbooks to get as many different types as you can.

> ✳ **Tip** It may help if you transfer these data onto 3 × 5 inch index cards. Put the cards in your pocket so that they can aid you in the clinical setting with getting to know the terminology of different ventilators.

Ventilator Name: PB 840	Ventilator Name:	Ventilator Name:	Ventilator Name:	Ventilator Name:	Ventilator Name:
AC/VC					
AC/VC +					
AC/PC					
Bilevel					
SIMV-VC					
SIMV-PC					
PAV+					

Self-Assessment Questions

1. During volume control ventilation, what happens to the delivered tidal volume when the patient's compliance worsens?
   A. Increases
   B. Decreases
   C. Stays the same
   D. It may increase or decrease

2. During pressure control ventilation, what happens to the delivered tidal volume when the patient's compliance worsens?
   A. Increases
   B. Decreases
   C. Stays the same
   D. It may increase or decrease

3. During pressure control ventilation, how is the delivered tidal volume increased?
   A. Increase the V_T being delivered
   B. Decrease the inspiratory pressure being delivered
   C. Increase the inspiratory pressure being delivered
   D. Increase the inspiratory flow being delivered

4. In volume control ventilation, what effect will changing from a square wave form pattern to a decreasing wave form pattern have on the inspiratory time?
   A. An increase in the inspiratory time
   B. A decrease in the inspiratory time
   C. It will stay the same
   D. It may increase or decrease

5. Typical parameters a respiratory therapist will set in volume control ventilation include:
   1. Inspiratory pressure
   2. V_T
   3. PEEP
   4. Inspiratory flow

   A. 1 and 4 only
   B. 1, 2, and 4 only
   C. 2, 3, and 4 only
   D. 1, 2, 3, and 4

Use the following information to answer questions 6 and 7.

During a patient-ventilator system assessment the following values are obtained:

Time	Exhaled V_T (mL)	PIP (cmH$_2$O)	P$_{plateau}$ (cmH$_2$O)
0800	600	22	18
1200	600	28	24
1600	600	36	31

6. What mode of ventilation is the patient in?
   A. Volume control
   B. Pressure control
   C. Noninvasive ventilation (NIV)
   D. Unable to determine with the information provided

7. Which of the following statements is correct?
   A. The patient's P$_{plateau}$ demonstrate improving pulmonary status.
   B. A leak exists in the patient-ventilator system.
   C. The patient's static compliance is deteriorating.
   D. The patient is likely biting on the endotracheal tube.

8. A patient who is currently intubated and mechanically ventilated following an acute asthma exacerbation is in the volume control mode. Two hours following initiation of mechanical ventilation, the high pressure alarms are going off. What is the most likely cause?
   A. Alarms were set inappropriately.
   B. The patient needs to be switched from volume control mode to pressure control mode.
   C. The cuff of the endotracheal tube has a leak.
   D. Bronchospasm has occurred.

9. A male patient is 6 feet tall and weighs 210 pounds. What is his IBW?
   A. 140 pounds
   B. 210 pounds
   C. 76 kilograms
   D. 95 kilograms

10. Complications of invasive mechanical ventilation include all of the following except:
    A. Oxygen toxicity
    B. Ventilator-induced lung injury
    C. Nosocomial pneumonia
    D. Community-acquired pneumonia

CASE STUDY 22-1

A 62-year-old man with a history of chronic obstructive pulmonary disease (COPD) presents to the emergency department (ED) with a chief complaint of worsening shortness of breath (SOB) over a 2-day history; the SOB came on following a recent upper respiratory infection. In the ED, his oxygen saturation is 86% on room air. He is complaining of severe dyspnea, is only speaking in short sentences, and appears very fatigued. His vital signs are as follows:

RR: 28 breaths/min
HR: 132 beats/min
BP: 152/94 mm Hg
Lung sounds: Diffuse wheezes and a prolonged expiratory
   phase
Arterial blood gas (ABG): Done on room air and shows a pH
   7.11; $PaCO_2$ 77 mm Hg; (HCO_3^-) 33 mEq/L; and PaO_2
   61 mm Hg.

1. What are the indications for initiation of mechanical ventilation?

_____

_____

2. The physician asks for suggestions to correct this patient's current respiratory distress. What would you suggest?

_____

_____

3. What do you think about the possibility of using noninvasive ventilation (NIV) for this patient?

_____

_____

CASE STUDY 22-2

You are called to the bedside of a patient because the nurse is concerned that the ventilator's high pressure alarm has gone off. The female patient was admitted for COPD exacerbation and was intubated earlier in the day when she failed a trial of BiPAP. You review the patient's chart and note that 30 minutes earlier, the peak pressure was 45 cmH_2O and the $P_{plateau}$ was 25 cmH_2O. At the time the nurse calls you, the peak pressure has risen to 60 cmH_2O, and the $P_{plateau}$ is now 40 cmH_2O. Her heart rate has increased from 90 beats/min to 110 beats/min, BP has fallen from 110/85 mm Hg to 90/70 mm Hg. The physical examination reveals diminished breath sounds on the left side of the chest.

1. What do $P_{plateau}$ represent?

_____

_____

2. How do you obtain a $P_{plateau}$?

_____

_____

3. What do peak pressures represent?

_____

_____

4. What do you think the problem is with this particular patient?

_____

_____

5. What should you do at this point?

_____

_____

> **CASE STUDY 22-3**

A 45-year-old, 6-foot-tall man presented to the emergency department with a 2-day history of fever and productive cough with copious amounts of brown sputum. He was hemodynamically stable with a blood pressure of 130/87 mm Hg. His chest radiograph showed a right middle lobe infiltrate, and his room air arterial blood gas (ABG) is as follows: pH 7.32; $PaCO_2$ 32 mm Hg; (HCO_3-) 18 mEq/L; (mEq/L), and PaO_2 78 mm Hg. He was started on antibiotics and admitted to the floor. Four hours later, the nurse calls you because she is concerned that he is doing worse. On your arrival at his room, his BP is 85/60 mm Hg, his pulse is 120 beats/min and his oxygen saturation, which had been 97% on 2L of oxygen via nasal cannula, is now 78% on a nonrebreather mask. The patient is displaying labored breathing with accessory muscle use and is less responsive than he was on admission. He is diaphoretic and is not able to talk. Lung examination reveals that he has crackles bilaterally in the bases posteriorly. You obtain a chest radiograph, which shows increasing bilateral, diffuse lung opacities. An ABG is done while he is on the nonrebreather mask, and it shows: pH 7.17; $PaCO_2$ 45 mm Hg; HCO_3- 14 mEq/L; and PaO_2 58 mm Hg.

1. What should you do? Is there a role for CPAP or BiPAP in his management?

_____

_____

2. What information regarding *initial* ventilator settings would you need to communicate to the physician?

_____

_____

3. How does this mode work?

_____

_____

4. How do you choose the tidal volume?

_____

_____

5. On the basis of the information above, fill in the chart below:

Setting	Suggested Starting Value
V_T	
Frequency	
Flow pattern	
FiO_2	
PEEP	

6. In volume control:

a. What would happen to the inspiratory time if you increased the flow rate?

_____

_____

b. What would happen to the inspiratory time if you switched from a square wave flow pattern to a decreasing wave flow pattern?

_____

_____

c. If you increased the patient's inspiratory time, what would happen to the mean airway pressure?

_____

_____

Monitoring and Management of the ICU Patient

■ OBJECTIVES

Upon the completion of the chapter activities and content review topics, the student should be able to:

1. Perform a complete recruitment maneuver.
2. Determine a patient's optimal positive end-expiratory pressure (PEEP) through determination of the PEEP of best compliance during a recruitment maneuver.
3. Perform calculations needed to monitor a patient's oxygenation status.
4. Perform calculations needed to monitor a patient's ventilation status.
5. Assist with chest tube placement.
6. Identify the indications for chest tube placement.
7. Perform monitoring techniques for the patient with a chest tube.

■ KEY TERMS

- Alveolar and arterial oxygen tension difference
- Dead space/tidal volume (V_D/V_T) ratio
- Intensive care unit (ICU)
- Mean airway pressure (MAP)
- Oxygen consumption
- $PaO_2:FIO_2$ (P/F) ratio
- Physiologic shunt

■ CONTENT REVIEW TOPICS

- Factitious events
- Lung protective therapy
- Monitoring cuff pressure
- Murray lung injury score

- Patient-ventilator system assessment
- Pleurodesis
- Systematic errors

■ PROCEDURAL ASSESSMENTS

- 23-1 Monitoring Oxygenation
- 23-2 Monitoring Ventilation
- 23-3 Recruitment Maneuver
- 23-4 Assisting in Chest Tube Placement
- 23-5 Patient Monitoring and Chest Tube Care

■ EQUIPMENT

- Adult ventilators
- Calculator
- Chest drainage system
- Chest tube insertion trays
- Chest tubes
- Disposable gloves
- Intubated human patient simulator, if available
- Lung simulator
- Mannequin
- Sterile draping
- Sterile gloves
- Vacuum regulator

Monitoring and management of a patient in the intensive care unit (ICU) requires the integration of all your respiratory care knowledge to successfully care for the patient. You will be measuring physiologic values, analyzing and interpreting these values, and then using the findings to manage your patient appropriately on the basis of all the information you gathered.

→ **Reality Check** Care of a patient in the ICU requires a team approach. Effective communication is imperative.

Patient monitoring and management should not be exclusively derived from technology, tests, or diagnostic procedures. Rather, it more often should involve the bedside assessments and interactions you have with your patients. As your skill set and experience grow, you will be performing and assisting with

more advanced procedures. A systematic approach to all your patients will help ensure that nothing is overlooked. Start by reviewing the charts for new notes, getting report from the off-going respiratory therapist (RT), and keeping in touch with the nurse caring for your patient. You should also check for new laboratory, culture, and chest radiography results. You can then formulate your patient care plan for the day. Changes may be required on the basis of patient assessment results or changes in the patient's condition. This chapter will cover common activities during care of patients in the ICU, along with oxygenation and ventilation monitoring indices.

≫ SKILL CHECK LISTS

23-1 Monitoring Oxygenation

Measuring a patient's oxygen saturation (SpO_2) using pulse oximetry is a handy, noninvasive way to get an idea of a patient's oxygenation status. However, in a critical care setting, a more precise measurement is often required. The ratio of partial pressure of arterial oxygen to fractional inspired oxygen (PaO_2:FiO_2 ratio or P/F ratio) and the ratio of PaO_2 to (PaO_2:PAO_2) are simple indices that can be calculated at the bedside upon obtaining arterial blood gas (ABG) values. These indices are most useful when a ventilation–perfusion ($\dot{V}/\dot{Q}$) mismatch is the primary cause of hypoxemia. The ratio's reliability decreases as hypoventilation becomes the primary cause of hypoxemia.

The P/F ratio measures the portion of the oxygen getting from the alveoli, across the alveolar–capillary membrane, to blood. The P/F ratio is normally at least 0.9 (90%). As cardiac output decreases, the ratio may become less reliable because blood passes through the capillaries at a slower rate, which can substantially decrease oxygen tension in mixed venous blood. A comparison between the pressure in the alveoli and the artery is referred to as the *alveolar-arterial pressure gradient* ($P[A\text{-}a]O_2$). When a patient is breathing room air, the $P(A\text{-}a)$ O_2 should be between 0 and 20 mm Hg.

Another index more frequently used in neonatal patients, but applicable in the pediatric and adult patient populations, is the oxygen index (OI). It is used to measure oxygenation while taking the FiO_2 and mean airway pressure into account. An OI of less than 5 is considered very good, with increasing OI values usually indicating increasing risk of mortality. An OI greater that 25 is considered very poor.

Every cell in the body requires oxygen for metabolic activity. A patient's oxygen consumption reveals information about how well the tissues are receiving, or not receiving, the oxygen that is transported by arterial blood. Because oxygen is delivered at the capillary level, comparing the blood oxygen content before and after a specific capillary describes how much oxygen is required by the tissue that is oxygenated by that capillary. Measuring oxygen consumption at this level is rather impractical; however, the average oxygen consumption for the whole body provides valuable information (Box 23-1). Information about the hemoglobin (Hb) level, mixed venous oxygen tension ($P_{\bar{V}}O_2$), and mixed venous oxygen saturation (SvO_2) enables you to calculate venous oxygen content. Comparing this to the oxygen content of blood before the tissues (CaO_2) and after the tissues ($C_{\bar{V}}O_2$) multiplied by the cardiac output allows the determination of the tissue oxygen consumption ($\dot{V}O_2$).

Nevertheless, the most accurate oxygenation measurement is the direct computation of the physiologic shunt ($\dot{Q}_s/\dot{Q}_t$). Both arterial and mixed venous blood samples are needed for measurement of physiologic shunt. Using the available data on oxygenation, understanding and interpreting the results, and knowing how to apply the findings to make decisions are all crucial in the care of the patient in the ICU. The following is the step-by-step process for monitoring oxygenation.

BOX 23-1	Measures of Decreasing Blood Oxygenation or Lung Injury

↓ SpO_2	↓ PaO_2/PAO_2
↓ PaO_2	↑ Shunt/venous admixture
↑ $P(A\text{-}a)O_2$	↑ Murray lung injury score
↓ P/F ratio	

Procedural Preparation

1. Review the patient's chart.
2. Verify the physician's order or the facility's protocol for standard of care.
3. Obtain, clean, and inspect the appropriate equipment prior to entering the patient's room.
4. Follow personal protective equipment (PPE) requirements, and observe standard precautions for any transmission-based isolation procedure.
5. Identify the patient using two patient identifiers.
6. Introduce yourself to the patient and to the family.
7. Explain the procedure to the patient and to the family, and acknowledge the patient's understanding.
8. Perform proper hand hygiene, and put on gloves, mask, and protective eyewear, as appropriate for procedure.

Implementation

1. Assess vital signs.
2. Observe for signs and symptoms of inadequate oxygenation.
3. Calculate oxygen consumption ($\dot{V}O_2$):

$$\dot{V}O_2 = \text{cardiac output} \times (CaO_2 - C_{\bar{V}}O_2)$$

$$CaO_2 = [SaO_2 \times (Hb \times 1.34)] + (PaO_2 \times 0.003 \text{ mL/dL})$$

$$C_{\bar{V}}O_2 = [S_{\bar{V}}O_2 \times (Hb \times 1.34)] + (P_{\bar{V}}O_2 \times 0.003 \text{ mL/dL})$$

$C_{\bar{V}}O_2$, O_2 content of venous blood
$P_{\bar{V}}O_2$, partial pressure of 02 in venous blood

4. Calculate the ($P[A\text{-}a]O_2$):

$$P(A\text{-}a)O_2 = P_AO_2 - P_aO_2$$

$$P_AO_2 = P_IO_2 - (PaCO_2 \times 1.25)$$

5. Calculate the P/F ratio. $\dfrac{PaO_2}{FiO_2}$

6. Calculate oxygenation index (OI):

$$\dfrac{FiO_2 \times 100 \times Mean\ airway\ pressure\ (MAP)}{PaO_2}$$

7. Remove the supplies from the patient's room, and clean the area, as needed.
8. Remove PPE, and perform proper hand hygiene prior to leaving the patient's room.

Evaluation of Procedure

1. Establish a baseline, or compare with previous measurements.
2. Observe the trends in oxygenation indices.
3. Develop an appropriate respiratory care plan based on assessment data.
4. Identify any unexpected outcomes.
5. Lower the FiO_2, when indicated.

Documentation and Reporting

1. Record your findings in the patient's chart.
2. Report any abnormal findings to the appropriate health care provider.

23-2 Monitoring Ventilation

Proper ventilation is central to the health of your patient. If your patient is not ventilating adequately, hypercapnia or hypocapnia could result. In either case, acid–base balance, and hemoglobin's ability to transport oxygen are affected. As dead space volume increases, the amount of ventilation that a patient can perform decreases. Because dead space volume cannot be directly measured, it has to be indirectly measured by utilizing the $PaCO_2$ measurement from the ABG and the partial pressure of expired carbon-dioxide ($PeCO_2$) measurement from an end-tidal CO_2 monitor. Other methods of monitoring adequate ventilation exist (Box 23-2). The dead space to tidal volume (V_D/V_T) ratio is a useful tool for monitoring ventilation and for determining how much tidal volume is participating in gas exchange. The $V_D:V_T$ ratio is equivalent to the ratio of the gradient between the $PaCO_2$ and $PeCO_2$ to the $PaCO_2$ as shown below:

$$V_D/V_T = \frac{P_aCO_2 - P_ECO_2}{P_aCO_2}$$

The ratio also provides useful information for determining the effectiveness of ventilation. By substituting normal values for $PaCO_2$ (40 mm Hg) and $PeCO_2$ (28 mm Hg) into the equation, we can see that the V_D/V_T ratio is 1:3, or 30%, in a healthy patient. In other words, one third of the air you breathe does not participate in gas exchange. The normally accepted range is 0.2 to 0.4.

As shown in Table 23-1, as the tidal volume decreases, the patient's rate increases, and minute ventilation is maintained at 6000 mL/min. Because a lower boundary of 150 mL exists on the sample patient's physiologic dead space, when the tidal volume decreases and respiratory rate increases, the physiologic dead space stays the same, resulting in the V_D/V_T ratio increasing to 0.60.

As dead space increases as a result of increased alveolar dead space, the V_D/V_T ratio increases. To maintain a normal level of lung–blood gas exchange (normal alveolar ventilation), the patient takes deeper breaths. The following is the step-by-step process for monitoring ventilation.

Procedural Preparation

1. Review the patient's chart.
2. Verify the physician's order or the facility's protocol for standard of care.
3. Obtain, clean, and inspect the appropriate equipment prior to entering the patient's room.
4. Follow PPE requirements, and observe standard precautions for any transmission-based isolation procedure.
5. Identify the patient using two patient identifiers.
6. Introduce yourself to the patient and to the family.
7. Explain the procedure to the patient and to the family, and acknowledge the patient's understanding.
8. Perform proper hand hygiene, and put on gloves, mask, and protective eyewear, as appropriate for procedure.

Implementation

1. Assess vital signs.
2. Observe for signs and symptoms of inadequate ventilation.
3. Calculate the dead space/tidal volume ratio (V_D/V_T):

$$V_D/V_T = \frac{PaCO_2 - P_ECO_2}{PaCO_2}$$

4. Calculate the minute ventilation:
   a. For patient receiving controlled mechanical ventilation (CMV):

   $$\dot{V}_E = V_T \times f$$

   b. For patient receiving synchronized intermittent mandatory ventilation (SIMV):

   $$\dot{V}_{ETOT} = (V_{Tmach})(f_{mach}) + (V_{Tpatient})(f_{patient})$$

5. Compare the inspired versus expired tidal volumes.
6. Remove the supplies from the patient's room, and clean the area, as needed.
7. Remove PPE, and perform proper hand hygiene prior to leaving the patient's room.

Evaluation of Procedure

1. Establish a baseline, or compare with previous measurements.
2. Observe trends in ventilation adequacies.

BOX 23-2   Monitoring the Adequacy of Ventilation

Respiratory volume and rate
$PaCO_2$
V_D/V_T ratio
Capnometry

TABLE 23-1 Changes in Alveolar Ventilation (mL) Associated With Changes in Rate, Volume, and Physiological Dead Space

Ventilatory Pattern	Respiratory Rate (Breaths./min)	Physiological Dead Space (mL)	Tidal Volume (mL)	V_D/V_T Ratio	Minute Ventilation (mL/min)	Dead Space Ventilation (mL/min)	Alveolar Ventilation (mL/min)
Normal	12	150	500	0.30	6,000	1,800	4,200
High rate, low volume	24	150	250	0.60	6,000	3,600	2,400
Low rate, high volume	6	150	1,000	0.15	6,000	900	5,100
Increased dead space	12	300	500	0.60	6,000	3,600	2,400
Compensation for increased dead space	12	300	650	0.46	7,800	3,600	4,200

Modified from Kacmarek RM, Stoller JK, Heuer AJ: *Egan's fundamentals of respiratory care*, ed 10, St. Louis, MO, 2013, Mosby.

3. Develop an appropriate respiratory care plan based on assessment data.
4. Identify any unexpected outcomes.
5. Lower the FIO_2 when indicated.

Documentation and Reporting

1. Record your findings in the patient's chart.
2. Report any abnormal findings to the appropriate health care provider.

23-3 Recruitment Maneuver

Recruitment maneuvers (RMs) are transient increases in distending ventilatory pressures intended to open derecruited or collapsed alveoli. These maneuvers have been shown to be safe and well tolerated in both adult and pediatric patients and with patients following cardiac surgery. RMs may improve a number of physiologic parameters, including pulmonary compliance and oxygenation. RMs have been shown to improve patient outcomes in some studies, but other studies have shown no benefit. Because of the lack of outcome data supporting their use and because of some concerns in discrete patient populations regarding safety (e.g., patients with increased intracranial pressure), their use is not universal by any means.

However, RMs are gaining wider acceptance in all areas of critical care, including pediatrics, and knowledge of their proper performance is critical for an RT. The procedure outlined below is for a step-wise increase in PEEP, sometimes referred to as a "PEEP-walk." Other forms of RMs exist, including sustained inflations at high inspiratory pressures, but the one outlined below is the most commonly referenced procedure. We also describe the PEEP determined to be the "best" for the patient as that just above the closing pressure. We define this PEEP as "optimal," with the understanding that many definitions of "optimal" PEEP exist in the literature. Our intent is to place the patient's PEEP as close to the PEEP of best compliance (using dynamic compliance) as possible. The following is the step-by-step process for recruitment maneuver.*

> ***Tip** A thorough reading of the literature on the subject of recruitment maneuvers and optimal PEEP is recommended.

Procedural Preparation

1. Review the patient's chart.
2. Identify the possible factors that preclude the use of an RM (e.g., increased intracranial pressure, significant air leak, etc.), and discuss clinical situation with the appropriate supervising health care provider.
3. Verify the physician's order or the facility's protocol for standard of care.
4. Follow PPE requirements, and observe standard precautions for any transmission-based isolation procedure.
5. Identify the patient using two patient identifiers.
6. Introduce yourself to the patient and to the family.
7. Explain the procedure to the patient and to the family, and acknowledge the patient's understanding.
8. Perform proper hand hygiene, and put on gloves, mask, and protective eyewear, as appropriate for the procedure.

Implementation

1. Position the patient.
2. Inform the bedside nurse that the RM is about to begin.
3. Assess vital signs.
4. Ensure that the patient is relaxed and comfortable, allowing ventilator-delivered control breaths.
5. Document baseline vital signs, SpO_2, end-tidal carbon dioxide concentration E_TCO_2, if available.
6. Change ventilator mode to "Pressure Control."
7. Ensure that tidal volumes are similar to baseline and adequate.
8. Review available documentation for recording changes in compliance, tidal volume, and ventilatory pressures during the maneuver.
9. Record baseline compliance, exhaled tidal volume, and ventilator pressures.
10. While maintaining a consistent delta P (ΔP), increase PEEP by 2 cmH_2O
11. After 1 minute, record compliance, tidal volume, and ventilator pressures.
12. Ensure that patient comfort, hemodynamics, and oxygenation are acceptable.
13. If increase in PEEP results in tidal volumes greater than 10 mL/kg, reduce ΔP by 2 cmH_2O.
14. If a discrete increase in PEEP results in a large improvement in compliance or tidal volume, record the pressure at which this occurs as the "opening pressure."
15. Repeat PEEP increase every minute until compliance does not increase or decrease.
16. Record this PEEP level as the PEEP where "full recruitment" is achieved.
17. Decrease PEEP by 2 cmH_2O every minute until "derecruitment" occurs.
    a. Derecruitment will be noted by a significant drop in dynamic compliance or tidal volume.
18. Record the pressure at which the drop occurred as the "closing pressure."
19. Increase PEEP again by 2 cmH_2O every minute up to full recruitment pressure, and then drop by 2 cmH_2O every minute to a PEEP of 2 cmH_2O above closing pressure.
20. Record this pressure as "optimal PEEP."
21. Reassess vital signs.
22. Remove the supplies from the patient's room, and clean the area, as needed.
23. Remove PPE, and perform proper hand hygiene prior to leaving the patient's room.

Evaluation of Procedure

1. Establish a baseline, or compare with previous measurements.
2. Develop an appropriate respiratory care plan based on assessment data.
3. Identify any unexpected outcomes.
4. Correlate your findings with changes in the patient's oxygenation, ventilation, and other vital signs.

Documentation and Reporting

1. Record final ventilator settings, PEEP level, patient vital signs, dynamic compliance (C_D), SpO_2, and E_TCO_2, if available.
2. Report any abnormal findings to the appropriate health care provider.

23-4 Assisting in Chest Tube Placement

Chest tube placement is performed to remove or drain air or blood and other fluids from the mediastinal or intrapleural spaces. Mediastinal chest tubes are typically present in a patient who has recently undergone a thoracotomy. Indications for placement are given in Box 23-3. Normally, the thoracic cavity is a closed air space. Any disturbance of the negative pressure within the intrapleural space may cause serious problems for your patients. Whether inserted following trauma or because of an underlying pulmonary pathology, the RT must be able to monitor and care for patients with chest tubes. The following is the step-by-step process for assisting with chest tube placement.

Procedural Preparation

1. Review the patient's chart.
2. Verify the physician's order or the facility's protocol for standard of care.
3. Obtain, clean, and inspect the appropriate equipment prior to entering the patient's room.
4. Follow PPE requirements, and observe standard precautions for any transmission-based isolation procedure.

BOX 23-3	Indications for Chest Tube Placement
Pneumothorax	Empyema
Hemothorax	Chylothorax
Hemopneumothorax	Hydrothorax
Tension pneumothorax	Pleural effusion
Thoracotomy	

5. Identify the patient using two patient identifiers.
6. Introduce yourself to the patient and to the family.
7. Explain the procedure to the patient and to the family, and acknowledge the patient's understanding.
8. Perform proper hand hygiene, and put on gloves, mask, and protective eyewear, as appropriate for procedure.

Implementation

1. Place the patient in a comfortable position, and instruct him or her to breathe normally.
2. Assess vital signs continuously throughout procedure, and reassure the patient, as necessary.
3. Open the chest tube insertion tray using sterile technique.
4. Assist with the preparation of the equipment and the insertion site.
5. Following insertion, connect the chest tube to the closed chest drainage system (CDS) (Figure 23-1).
6. Check the CDS for the rise and fall of the water column, and apply the ordered amount of suction.
7. Assist with suturing, and apply occlusive dressing.
8. Secure all the connection points to the drainage system.
9. Secure the tube below the dressing to the patient's skin.
10. Reassess vital signs.
11. Remove the supplies from the patient's room, and clean the area, as needed.
12. Remove PPE, and perform proper hand hygiene prior to leaving the patient's room.

Evaluation of Procedure

1. Ensure that chest radiography is ordered to confirm tube placement.

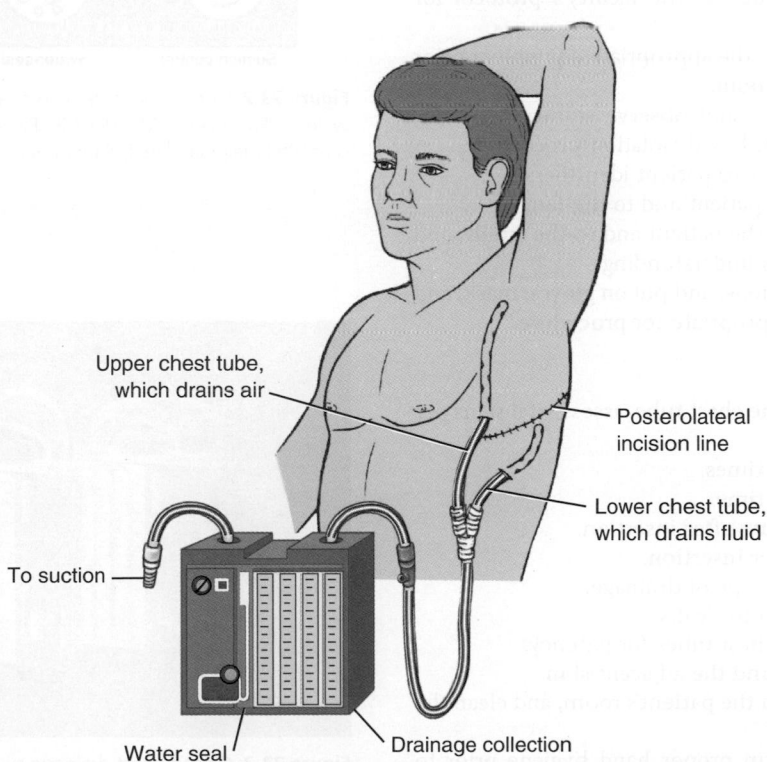

Upper chest tube, which drains air

Posterolateral incision line

Lower chest tube, which drains fluid

To suction

Water seal

Drainage collection

Figure 23-1 Closed chest drainage system. (From Evolve REACH Comprehensive Review for the NCLEX-PN Examination, St. Louis, 2009, Elsevier.)

2. Assess the patient for pain at the insertion site.
3. Ensure that vital signs are assessed every 1 to 4 hours or per your facility's protocols.
4. Develop an appropriate respiratory care plan based on assessment data.
5. Identify any unexpected outcomes.

Documentation and Reporting

1. Record vital signs during and after the procedure in the patient's chart.
2. Report any abnormal findings to the appropriate health care provider.

23-5 Patient Monitoring and Chest Tube Care

Monitoring patients with chest tubes should include cardiopulmonary and vital sign assessments. In addition, you must be aware of the situation that dictated chest tube insertion in the first place. Recurrence of that condition may require further interventions or more frequent patient assessment. Drainage type and amount should be evaluated along with the chest tube system itself. Different types of chest tube drainage systems are shown in Figures 23-2 and 23-3. Thorough knowledge of the system utilized at your facility is vital. Placement of the system should be secure and out of the way so that no one trips over it and it does not get dislodged. The following is the step-by-step process for patient monitoring and chest tube care.

Procedural Preparation

1. Review the patient's chart.
2. Verify the physician's order or the facility's protocol for standard of care.
3. Obtain, clean, and inspect the appropriate equipment prior to entering the patient's room.
4. Follow PPE requirements, and observe standard precautions for any transmission-based isolation procedure.
5. Identify the patient using two patient identifiers.
6. Introduce yourself to the patient and to the family.
7. Explain the procedure to the patient and to the family, and acknowledge the patient's understanding.
8. Perform proper hand hygiene, and put on gloves, mask, and protective eyewear, as appropriate for procedure.

Implementation

1. Following placement of the chest tube, assess vital signs per protocol or:
   a. Every 15 minutes two times.
   b. Every 30 minutes one time.
   c. Every 1 hour for 4 hours after insertion.
   d. Every 2 to 4 hours after insertion.
2. Monitor the amount and type of drainage.
3. Assess patient and system for leaks
4. Maintain and check the chest tubes for patency.
5. Assess the insertion site and the adjacent skin.
6. Remove the supplies from the patient's room, and clean the area, as needed.
7. Remove PPE, and perform proper hand hygiene prior to leaving the patient's room.

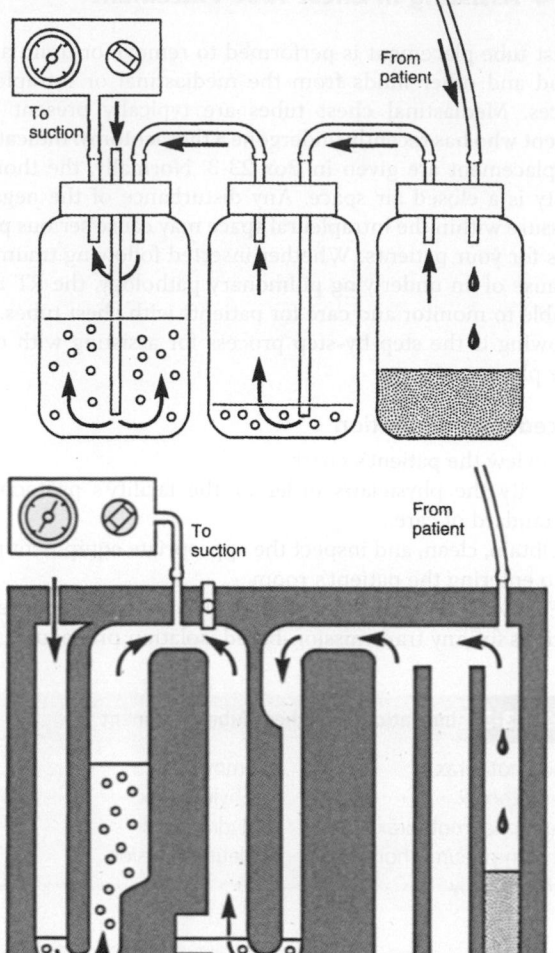

Figure 23-2 Disposable system correlating with a three-bottle system. (From Luce JM, Tyler ML, Pierson DJ: *Intensive respiratory care*, Philadelphia, 1984, Saunders.)

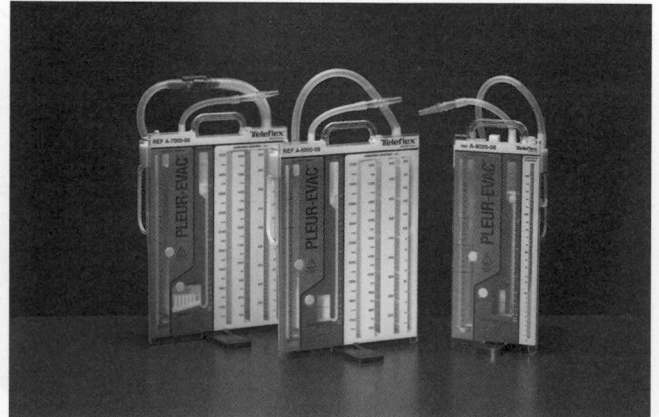

Figure 23-3 Closed chest drainage systems. (Pleur-Evac is a registered brand of Teleflex Medical, Research Triangle Park, NC.)

Evaluation of Procedure

1. Establish a baseline, or compare with previous measurements.
2. Develop an appropriate respiratory care plan based on assessment data.
3. Identify any unexpected outcomes.

Documentation and Reporting

1. Record your findings in the patient's chart.
2. Report any abnormal findings to the appropriate health care provider.

Bibliography

American Association of Colleges of Nursing: *AACN procedure manual for critical care*, ed 6, St. Louis, MO, 2011, Saunders.

Cairo JM: *Pilbeam's mechanical ventilation*, ed 5, St. Louis, MO, 2012, Mosby.

Kacmarek RM, Stoller JK, Heuer AJ: *Egan's fundamentals of respiratory care*, ed 10, St. Louis, MO, 2013, Mosby.

Hess DR, Bigatello LM: Lung recruitment: the role of recruitment maneuvers, *Am J Respirat Crit Care Med* 47(3):296, 2002: http://ajrccm.atsjournals.org/cgi/content/abstract/172/2/206. Accessed 2012.

*Dr. Brigham Willis provided content for Recruitment Maneuvers.

1. Label the images in Figure 23-4.

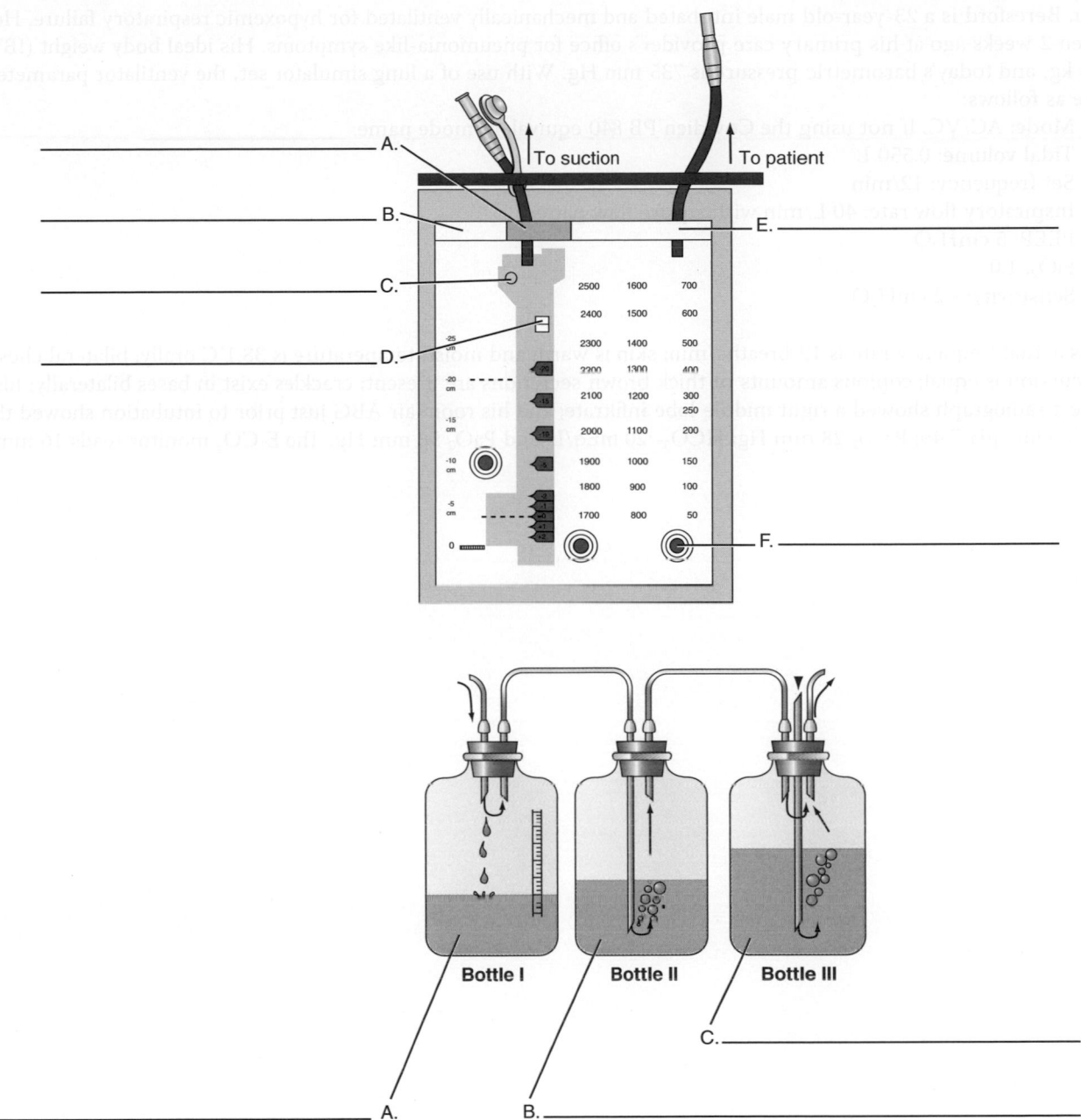

Figure 23-4

*The following exercises will use the terminology from the Covidien PB 840. You can use **any ventilator** to complete the exercise.*

Use the following scenario for questions 2 through 8.

Mr. Beresford is a 23-year-old male intubated and mechanically ventilated for hypoxemic respiratory failure. He was seen 2 weeks ago at his primary care provider's office for pneumonia-like symptoms. His ideal body weight (IBW) is 75 kg, and today's barometric pressure is 735 mm Hg. With use of a lung simulator set, the ventilator parameters are as follows:

- Mode: AC/VC. If not using the Covidien PB 840 equivalent mode name: _____
- Tidal volume: 0.550 L
- Set frequency: 12/min
- Inspiratory flow rate: 40 L/min with square flow pattern
- PEEP: 5 cmH$_2$O
- F$_I$O$_2$: 1.0
- Sensitivity: −2 cmH$_2$O

His actual frequency rate is 12 breaths/min; skin is warm and moist; temperature is 38.1°C orally; bilateral chest excursion is equal; copious amounts of thick brown secretions are present; crackles exist in bases bilaterally; his chest radiograph showed a right middle lobe infiltrate; and his room air ABG just prior to intubation showed the following: pH 7.49; Pa$_{CO_2}$ 28 mm Hg; HCO$_3$- 20 mEq/L; and PaO$_2$ 58 mm Hg. The E$_T$CO$_2$ monitor reads 16 mm Hg.

2. Fill in the following ventilator flow sheet as completely as you can (Figure 23-5).

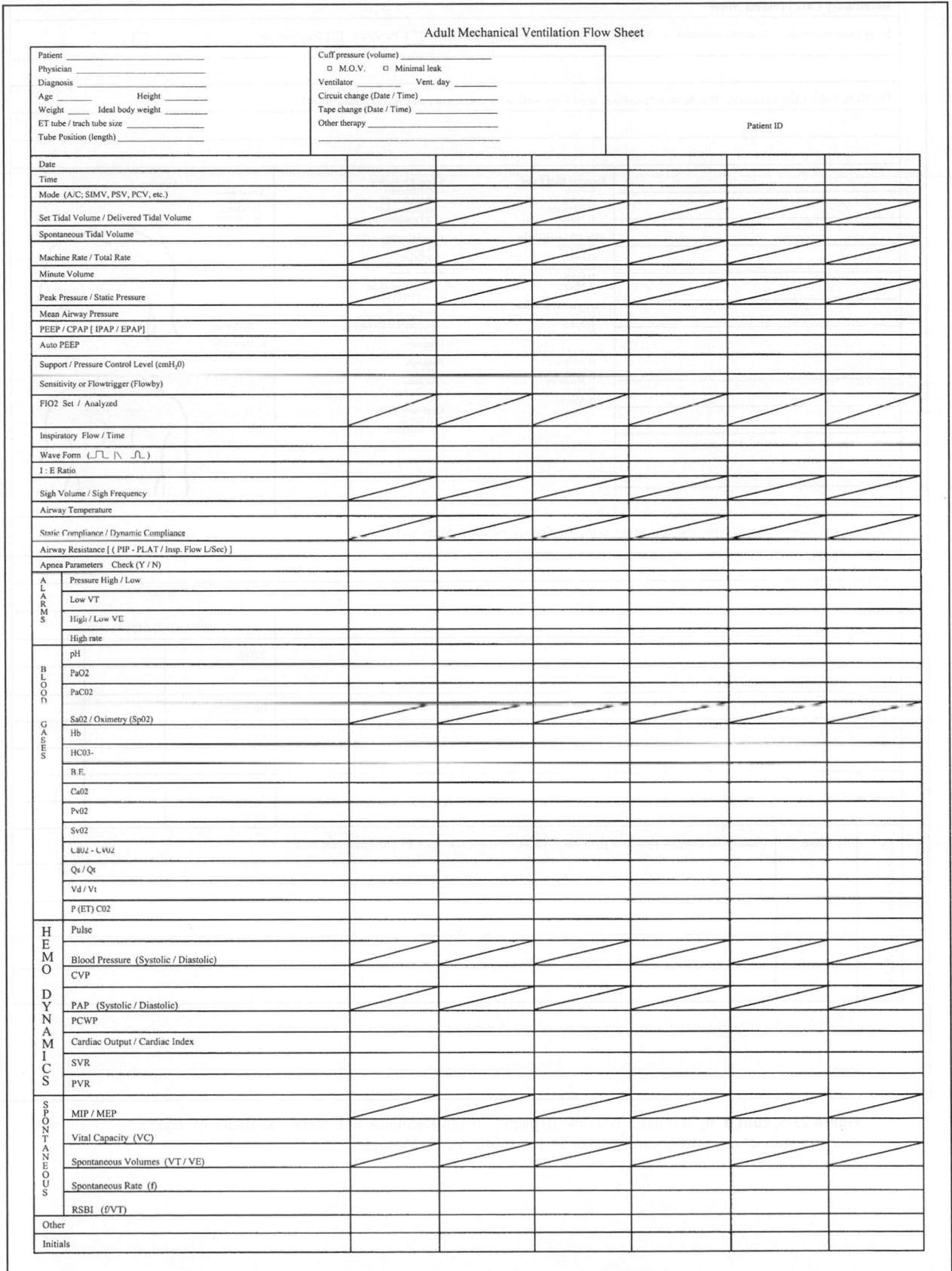

Figure 23-5 A, Ventilator flow sheet, page 1.

Continued

Adult Mechanical Ventilation Flow Sheet

Respiratory Care Progress Notes

S: (pt Awareness, response, sedations / paralytics) Responds ☐ Non-responsive ☐ Sedated ☐ Paralytics ☐ See comment ☐ ☐

O: (WOB, Color, Chest Expansion, BBS, Sputum Production, latest x-ray, pertinent pt assessment concerns, lab values, fluids)

General Skin Color
☐ Pink
☐ Ashy
☐ Cyanotic
☐ Jaundice

Skin Characteristics
☐ Warm
☐ Dry
☐ Diaphoretic
☐ Cool
☐ Moist

Mucous Membranes
☐ Pink
☐ Ashy
☐ Cyanotic

Work of Breathing
☐ Normal
☐ Mild
☐ Moderate
☐ High
☐ Absent

Chest Excursion
☐ Bilateral
☐ Unilateral
☐ Diminished
☐ Paradoxical/Flail

Chest Configuration
☐ Normal
☐ Other_____

☐ Subcutaneous
   Emphysema

☐ Tactile Fremitus
☐ Tracheal Deviation
☐ Abdominal
Distention

Nailbeds
☐ Pink
☐ Ashy
☐ Cyanotic

Capillary Refill
☐ Rapid
☐ Sluggish

Anterior

Auscultation
1) Clear
2) Wheeze
3) Crackles
4) Rhonchi

Posterior
A. Good Aeration
B. Diminished
C. Absent

A: (Pt history, Admit dx. & date, events leading to intubation/trach/ventilation, significant problems, etc.)

P: (Care plan , standing orders, treatments)

WEANING MECHANICS		
TIME		
VC		
I/E FORCES		
VT		
RR		
VE		
f/VT		

Pt. EVENTS/ CHANGES	Time	(Reasons for changes, significant pt. events, CT Scan, chest tube placement, BP problems, codes, etc.)

Signature _____   Initials _____

_____   _____

_____   _____

B

Figure 23-5, cont'd B, Ventilator flow sheet, page 2. (From Kacmarek RM, Stoller JK, Heuer AJ: *Egan's fundamentals of respiratory care*, ed 10, St. Louis, MO, 2013, Mosby.)

3. What type of humidification device would you choose? Why?

_____

_____

4. Interpret the patient's ABG results: _____

5. Assuming normal adult hemoglobin, what do you expect the pulse-oximeter reading to be?

_____

6. Calculate all of the following and determine if the value is normal, high, or low:

V_E: _____

Total cycle time (TCT): _____

Inspiratory time (I-time): _____

PAO_2: _____

$P(A-a)O_2$: _____

P/F: _____

PaO_2/ PAO_2: _____

C_D: _____

C_S: _____

Resistance: _____

V_D: _____

7. Calculate the oxygen index (OI) using a mean airway pressure of 14 cmH_2O

_____

_____

8. Which ventilator parameter would you adjust, if any? _____

9. Working with a lab partner, perform a complete recruitment maneuver (RM) with proper documentation of opening pressure, closing pressure, full recruitment pressure, and "optimal PEEP" using a pig lung or the equivalent. Obtain a signature from your instructor once the maneuver has been successfully completed.

Signature:_____

Self-Assessment Questions

1. Tissue oxygenation depends on:

   1. FIO_2
   2. PAO_2
   3. CaO_2
   4. $PaCO_2$

   A. 1 and 3 only
   B. 1, 2, and 4 only
   C. 1 only
   D. 1, 2, and 3 only

2. A healthy person breathing room air has a $P(A-a)O_2$ of approximately:
   A. 5 to 15 mm Hg
   B. 20 to 30 mm Hg
   C. 60 to 80 mm Hg
   D. 80 to 100 mm Hg

Use the following information to answer questions 3 through 7.
- Mode of ventilation: AC/VC
- Set frequency: 12 breaths/min
- Actual frequency: 20 breaths/min
- Set V_T: 500 mL
- FIO_2: 0.6
- Mean airway pressure: 11 cmH$_2$O
- $PaCO_2$: 58 mm Hg
- PaO_2: 62 mm Hg

3. What is the oxygenation index?
   A. 1.06
   B. 10.6
   C. 106
   D. Unattainable based on presented data

4. What is the P/F ratio?
   A. 1.03
   B. 103
   C. 37
   D. Unattainable based on presented data

5. According to the available information, the patient has normal oxygenation.
   A. True
   B. False

6. What is the minute ventilation?
   A. 10 L/min
   B. 6 L/min
   C. 3 L/min
   D. Unattainable based on presented data

7. Your patient experiences severe pain during placement of a chest tube and becomes tachypneic with a total frequency of 34 breaths/min. What acid–base abnormality is most likely?
   A. Respiratory acidosis
   B. Respiratory alkalosis
   C. Metabolic acidosis
   D. Metabolic alkalosis

8. Chest tube placement is indicated in:
   A. Myocardial infarction
   B. Pneumothorax
   C. Acute respiratory distress syndrome (ARDS)
   D. Acute cardiogenic pulmonary edema

9. Monitoring ventilation includes measurement of:

   1. Tidal volume
   2. Frequency
   3. PaO_2
   4. $PaCO_2$

   A. 3 and 4 only
   B. 1 and 4 only
   C. 1, 2, and 3 only
   D. 1, 2, and 4 only

10. When a patient is receiving mechanical ventilation, only the inspired tidal volume is important.
    A. True
    B. False

CASE STUDY 23-1

A 47-year-old male patient with an ideal body weight (IBW) of 75 kg is intubated and receiving mechanical ventilation in the volume-control mode following exacerbation of his asthma.

Settings:
Rate: 16 breaths/min
Tidal volume: 600 mL
PEEP: 8 cmH$_2$O
F$_I$O$_2$: 0.5

1. After using a lung simulator and an adult ventilator, fill out the ventilator flow sheet (Figure 23-6).

_____

_____

2. All of a sudden, the peak airway pressure alarm goes off. What are some likely causes?

_____

_____

3. How can these causes be corrected?

_____

_____

4. If you were having a difficult time managing the patient's peak airway pressure, what other mode of ventilation would you consider?

_____

_____

5. Can you figure out what peak inspiratory pressure you would need to use to keep a tidal volume of 6 mL/kg?

_____

_____

6. Using the same flow sheet (see Figure 23-6), initiate a change to pressure control. Chart your settings.

_____

_____

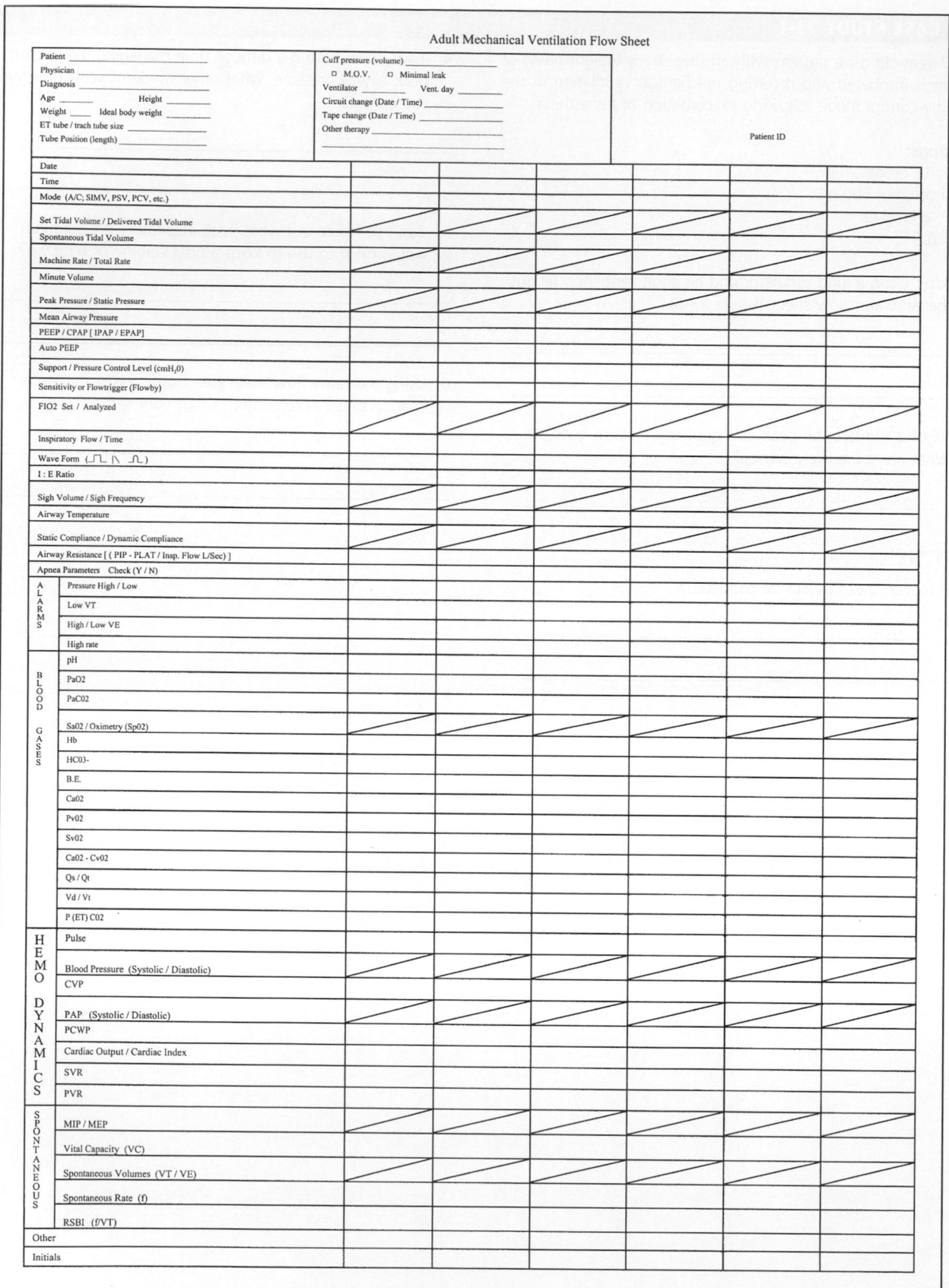

Figure 23-6 A, Ventilator flow sheet, page 1.

Adult Mechanical Ventilation Flow Sheet

Respiratory Care Progress Notes

S: (pt Awareness, response, sedations / paralytics)   Responds ☐   Non-responsive ☐   Sedated ☐   Paralytics ☐   See comment ☐   ☐

O: (WOB, Color, Chest Expansion, BBS, Sputum Production, latest x-ray, pertinent pt assessment concerns, lab values, fluids)

General Skin Color
☐ Pink
☐ Ashy
☐ Cyanotic
☐ Jaundice

Skin Characteristics
☐ Warm
☐ Dry
☐ Diaphoretic
☐ Cool
☐ Moist

Mucous Membranes
☐ Pink
☐ Ashy
☐ Cyanotic

Work of Breathing
☐ Normal
☐ Mild
☐ Moderate
☐ High
☐ Absent

Chest Excursion
☐ Bilateral
☐ Unilateral
☐ Diminished
☐ Paradoxical/Flail

Chest Configuration
☐ Normal
☐ Other____

☐ Subcutaneous
   Emphysema

☐ Tactile Fremitus
☐ Tracheal Deviation
☐ Abdominal
Distention

Nailbeds
☐ Pink
☐ Ashy
☐ Cyanotic

Capillary Refill
☐ Rapid
☐ Sluggish

Anterior

Auscultation
1) Clear
2) Wheeze
3) Crackles
4) Rhonchi

Posterior
A. Good Aeration
B. Diminished
C. Absent

A: (Pt history, Admit dx. & date, events leading to intubation/trach/ventilation, significant problems, etc.)

P: (Care plan , standing orders, treatments)

WEANING MECHANICS		
TIME		
VC		
I/E FORCES		
VT		
RR		
VE		
f/VT		

Pt. EVENTS / CHANGES	Time	(Reasons for changes, significant pt. events, CT Scan, chest tube placement, BP problems, codes, etc.)

Signature _____   Initials _____

_____   _____

_____   _____

B

Figure 23-6, cont'd B, Ventilator flow sheet, page 2. (From Kacmarek RM, Stoller JK, Heuer AJ: *Egan's fundamentals of respiratory care*, ed 10, St. Louis, MO, 2013, Mosby.)

Venous Access

▪ OBJECTIVES

Upon the completion of the chapter activities and content review topics, the student should be able to:

1. Identify basic complete blood cell count and basic metabolic panel values.
2. Perform venipuncture with a butterfly collection needle and Vacutainer.
3. Interpret basic laboratory values.
4. Identify complications associated with venous access.
5. Perform initiation of intravenous therapy.
6. Perform discontinuation of intravenous therapy.
7. Perform peripherally inserted central catheter line placement.

▪ KEY TERMS

- Basic metabolic panel (BMP)
- Complete blood cell count (CBC)
- Comprehensive metabolic panel (CMP)
- Erythrocytes
- Hematology
- Hematoma
- Keep vein open (KVO)
- Leukocytes
- Modified Seldinger technique
- Over-the-needle IV catheter (ONC)
- Peripherally Inserted Central Catheter (PICC)
- Thrombocytes
- Venipuncture

▪ CONTENT REVIEW TOPICS

- Central line bundles
- Critical test value
- National Committee for Clinical Laboratory Standards
- Vascular access specialist
- Radiograph interpretation

▪ PROCEDURAL ASSESSMENTS

24-1   Venipuncture
24-2   Interpreting Basic Laboratory Values
24-3   Initiating Intravenous Access
24-4   Discontinuing Intravenous Access
24-5   Placing a Peripherally Inserted Central Catheter Line

▪ EQUIPMENT

- 2 × 2 or 4 × 4 Sterile gauze pads
- Alcohol preps
- Catheter stabilization device
- Disposable gloves, face shield, goggles
- IV catheters or over-the-needle IV catheter (ONC) safety device needle
- IV infusion fluid
- IV pole
- IV tube
- Mannequin or artificial phlebotomy practice arm
- Needle or butterfly needle
- PICC line kit
- Saline lock
- Sharps container
- Sterile drapes
- Sterile gloves
- Syringe
- Tape
- Tegaderms or transparent dressing
- Tourniquets
- Vacutainer

The respiratory therapist (RT) is mainly a "lung specialist" whose focus and area of expertise is the pulmonary care of patients. However, in this high-tech era of medicine, the focus is on patient care teams that include multiple disciplines and specialties, hospital workforce restructuring, and therapist-driven protocols, and the responsibilities of RTs have expanded. Many responsibilities that used to belong to hospital staff specialists other than RTs are shifting to the respiratory care department. Venipuncture, venous access, and peripherally inserted central catheter (PICC) line placement are skills that can be acquired by the RT with proper procedural education and clinical practice. As a student, you should be familiar with the standards and safety procedures at your clinical facility relating to needle safety and methods to report an accidental needle stick.

> → **Reality Check** Venous access is becoming a procedure that is done under ultrasound guidance to ensure the best outcomes for patients.

In addition to the skills needed to perform various types of venous access, the RT must possess a practical understanding of lab and diagnostic tests. The RT must understand values for the complete blood cell count (CBC), basic metabolic panel (BMP), and coagulation studies. A CBC provides a description of the number of circulating leukocytes (white blood cells [WBCs]), erythrocytes (red blood cells [RBCs]), and thrombocytes (platelets), whereas a BMP includes the predominant electrolytes and glucose values (see "Normal Values" in Appendix A). This chapter will cover the skills needed to perform various aspects of venous access, including blood draws, initiating venous access, and discontinuing venous access, along with basic interpretation of laboratory values.

≫ SKILL CHECK LISTS

24-1 Venipuncture

The RT is frequently called on to draw venous blood specimens that will be used for a variety of laboratory tests. Specimens are then sent to the laboratory to aid in the diagnosis of conditions such as electrolyte imbalances as well as to monitor the effects of treatments and medications. Hematology is the branch of medicine involved in the study of blood morphology, physiology, and pathology. Although obtaining blood specimens is a fairly routine procedure, precautions must be taken because it is a hazardous procedure if not carefully performed.

RTs must follow universal precautions and all facility policies and procedures with regard to venipuncture. Figures 24-1 illustrates the steps for applying a tourniquet and cleansing the puncture site.

Although venous access is reasonably safe for a patient, he or she may experience complications as a result of the procedure. A few that may occur are hematoma (localized collection of blood outside the blood vessels) formation, excessive bleeding, and syncope (fainting) during the procedure. Common access sites are shown in Figure 24-2.

The following is the step-by-step process for venipuncture using two different methods.

Procedural Preparation

1. Review the patient's chart.
2. Verify the physician's order or the facility's protocol for standard of care.
3. Obtain, clean, and inspect the appropriate equipment prior to entering the patient's room.
4. Follow personal protective equipment (PPE) requirements, and observe standard precautions for any transmission-based isolation procedure.
5. Identify the patient using two patient identifiers.
6. Introduce yourself to the patient and to the family.
7. Explain the procedure to the patient and to the family, and acknowledge the patient's understanding.
8. Perform proper hand hygiene, and put on gloves, mask, and protective eyewear, as appropriate for the procedure.

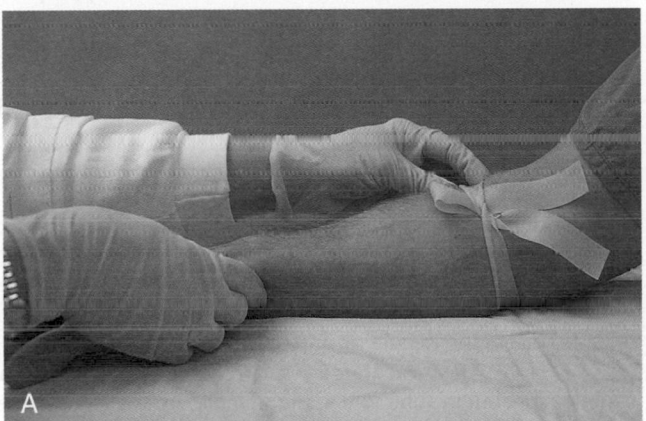
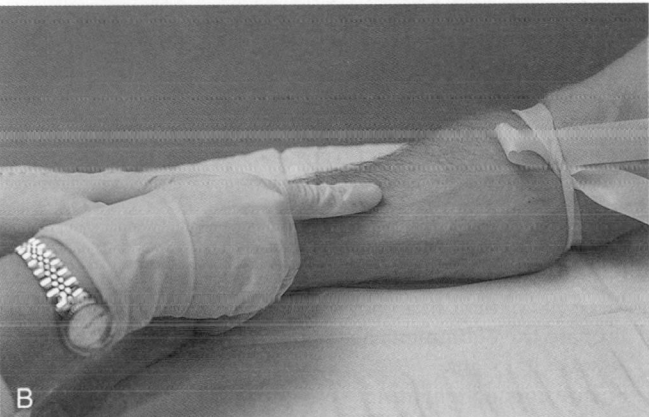
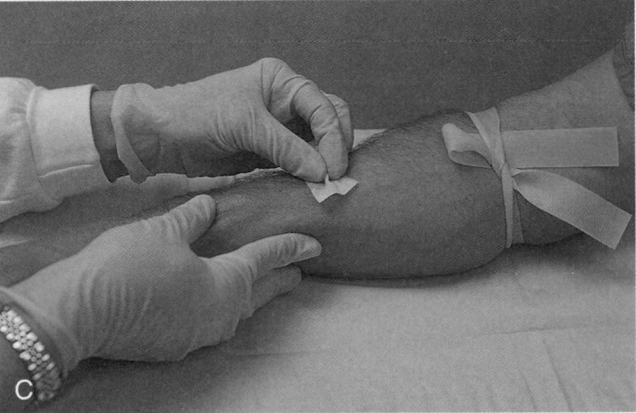

Figure 24-1 A, Apply the tourniquet. **B,** Locate the site. **C,** Cleanse the site. (From Elkin MK, et al: *Nursing interventions and clinical skills,* ed 4, St. Louis, MO, 2008, Mosby.)

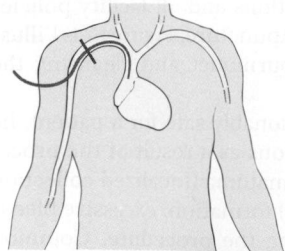

Subclavian catheter site

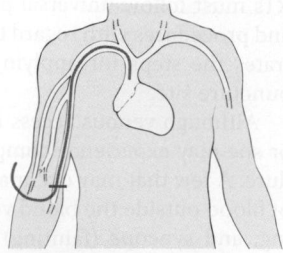

Peripherally inserted
central catheter (PICC)

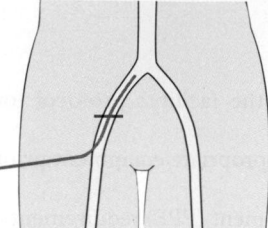

Femoral catheter site

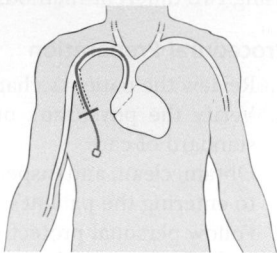

Hickman catheter site

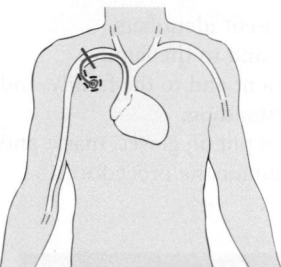

Subclavian catheter
with implantable
vascular access port

Figure 24-2 Sites of central venous access. (From Fuhrman MP: Management of complications of parenteral nutrition. In Matarese LE, Gottschlich MM, eds: *Contemporary nutrition support practice: a clinical guide,* Philadelphia, 1998, WB Saunders.)

Implementation

1. Place the patient in a comfortable position.
2. Prepare the equipment needed at the bedside.
3. Assess vital signs.
4. Ensure adequate lighting.
5. Choose the appropriate site for the venipuncture.
6. Apply a tourniquet above the selected site (about 3–4 inches) and gently palpate the vein with your finger (see Figure 24-1).
7. Instruct the patient to clench his or her fist.
   Syringe with Needle or Butterfly Method
   a. Prepare a syringe with the needle or butterfly securely attached.
   b. Cleanse the site (see Figure 24-1).
   c. Remove the needle or butterfly cover.
   d. Pull the patient's skin taut with your thumb or forefinger about 1 inch below the site.
   e. Hold the syringe and needle or butterfly at a 15-degree to 30-degree angle (Figure 24-3).
   f. Insert the needle or butterfly slowly into the vein.
   g. Hold the syringe securely, and pull back on the plunger while watching for blood return.
   h. Obtain the desired amount of blood.

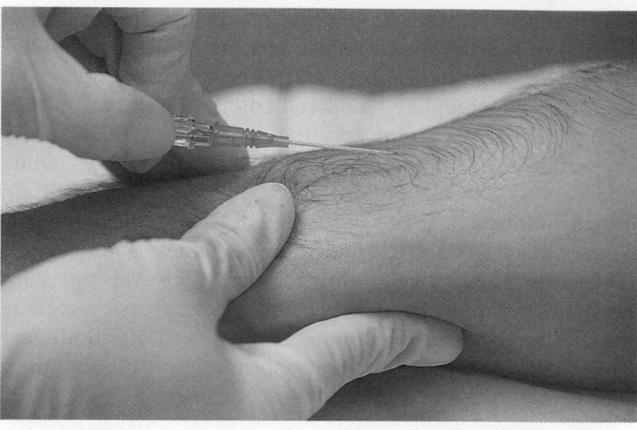

Figure 24-3 Pull the patient's skin taut with your thumb, and hold the syringe and needle at a 15-degree or 30-degree angle. (From Elkin MK, et al: *Nursing interventions and clinical skills,* ed 4, St. Louis, MO, 2008, Mosby.)

   i. Release the tourniquet after the specimen is obtained.
   j. Apply pressure with a 2 × 2 inch gauze, and withdraw the needle or butterfly from the vein.
   k. Dispose of the used sharps in the proper container.
   l. Follow all the recommended Occupational Safety and Health Administration (OSHA) practice standards.
   m. Fill the blood tubes, if needed, and invert them if additives are present.
   Vacutainer Method
   a. Attach a double-ended needle to the appropriate vacuum tube.
   b. Place the blood specimen tube in the Vacutainer without puncturing the rubber stopper.
   c. Prepare a syringe with the needle or butterfly securely attached.
   d. Cleanse the site.
   e. Remove the needle or butterfly cover.
   f. Pull the patient's skin taut with your thumb or forefinger about 1 inch below the site.
   g. Hold the syringe and needle or butterfly at a 15-degree to 30-degree angle.
   h. Insert the needle or butterfly slowly into the vein.
   i. Hold the Vacutainer securely, and advance the specimen tube onto the needle in the Vacutainer (Figure 24-4).
   j. Observe the blood flow.
   k. Remove the specimen tube after it is filled, and if necessary, insert additional tubes.
   l. Release the tourniquet after the last sample is obtained.
   m. Apply pressure with a 2 × 2 inch gauze, and withdraw the needle or butterfly from the vein.
   n. Dispose of the used sharps in the proper container.
   o. Follow all the recommended OSHA practice standards.
8. Apply gauze with tape to the puncture site.
9. Check the tubes, and wipe with alcohol, if necessary.
10. Assist the patient to a comfortable position, if previously moved.
11. Label every tube with the patient's information, date and time the specimen was collected, and the initials of the person who collected it.
12. Dispose of all the used supplies and soiled equipment.

13. Remove the unused supplies from the patient's room, and clean the area, as needed.
14. Remove PPE, and perform proper hand hygiene prior to leaving the patient's room.
15. Bag and transport the tube to the laboratory according to your facility's protocols.

Evaluation of Procedure

1. Reassess the venipuncture site.
2. Establish a baseline, or review laboratory data.
3. Develop an appropriate respiratory care plan based on laboratory data.
4. Identify any unexpected outcomes.

Documentation and Reporting

1. Record data related to the venipuncture sampling in the patient's chart.
2. Report any "stat" critical values to the appropriate health care provider.

24-2 Interpreting Clinical Lab Data

Most often, the physician orders specific tests, depending on the patient's clinical presentation, to confirm a differential diagnosis or to obtain information regarding the patient's response to therapy. Other reasons for laboratory and diagnostic tests include, but are not limited to, screening, evaluating the severity of a patient's disease, or assessing current management of the care the patient is receiving. By themselves, laboratory data offer a snap-shot of your patient's illness; and they should not be looked at independently to determine a respiratory care plan but should be considered in conjunction with the patient's chief complaint, history of present illness, and past medical history.

> ✳ **Tip** Lab values will vary from hospital to hospital. Make sure that you know the reference ranges used at your facility.

Before you can understand laboratory data and how abnormalities or deviations in the data relate to a patient's condition, you must know what the normal values are and how to obtain them correctly (see "Normal Values" in Appendix A, which lists the values of typical laboratory values common in respiratory care). Physicians commonly utilize a diagram, called a *fishbone diagram*, to list the most common parts of the CBC and BMP. This diagram is provided in Figure 24-5. This chapter will use a case study approach to help the RT student interpret basic clinical laboratory data as they relate to the pulmonary status of their patients. The following is the step-by-step process for interpreting basic laboratory values.

Procedural Preparation

1. Review the patient's chart.
2. Identify the laboratory values that relate to the respiratory status of the patient, for interpretation.

Implementation

1. Evaluate the CBC:
   a. WBC count
   b. WBC differential:
      i. Segmented neutrophils
      ii. Bands
      iii. Eosinophils
      iv. Basophils
      v. Lymphocytes
      vi. Monocytes
   c. Platelet count
   d. RBC count
   e. Hemoglobin
   f. Hematocrit
2. Evaluate the BMP or the comprehensive metabolic panel:
   a. Electrolyte levels:
      i. Sodium
      ii. Potassium
      iii. Chloride
      iv. Total carbon dioxide
      v. Magnesium
      vi. Phosphorus
      vii. Calcium
      viii. Ionized calcium
      ix. Creatinine
      x. Blood urea nitrogen (BUN)

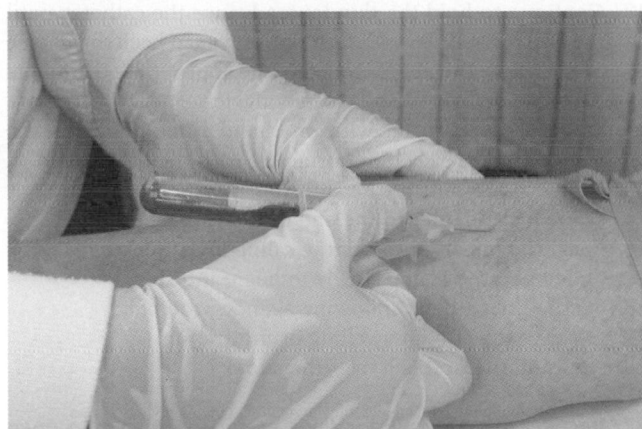

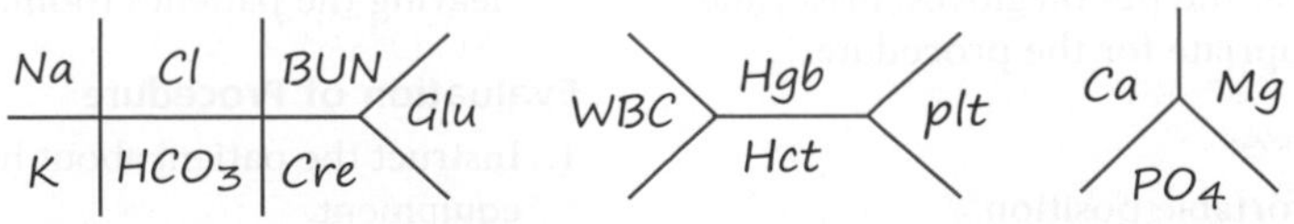

Figure 24-4 Hold the Vacutainer tightly, and let the blood collect in the container. (From Elkin MK, et al: *Nursing interventions and clinical skills,* ed 4, St. Louis, MO, 2008, Mosby.)

Figure 24-5 The "fishbone" diagram. A short-hand method used when writing down laboratory values by hand.

xi. Lactate

xii. Osmolarity

b. Glucose level

3. Evaluate enzyme tests

a. Liver enzymes

i. Alanine aminotransferase (ALT)

ii. Aspartate aminotransferase (AST)

iii. Alkaline phosphatase (ALK)

iv. Total bilirubin (T Bil)

b. Pancreatic enzymes:

i. Lipase

ii. Amylase

c. Muscle enzymes:

i. Creatine phosphokinase (CPK)

ii. Lactate dehydrogenase (LDH)

d. Cardiac enzymes protein tests:

i. Troponin

ii. B-type natriuretic peptide (BNP)

4. Evaluate coagulation studies:

a. Prothrombin time (PT)

b. Partial thromboplastin time (PTT)

c. International normalized ratio (INR)

Evaluation of Procedure

1. Identify any critical test values (Table 24-1).
2. Develop an appropriate respiratory care plan based on laboratory data.

Documentation and Reporting

1. Report any critical test values immediately to the appropriate health care provider.

24-3 Initiating Intravenous Access

Patients in the emergency room, on the general floors, and in the intensive care units may all require intravenous (IV) access at some point during their hospital stay. The RT may be summoned on an urgent basis to initiate IV therapy. Fluids, medications, and blood products may be delivered through IV access. The following is the step-by-step process for initiating IV access.

Procedural Preparation

1. Review the patient's chart.
2. Verify the physician's order or the facility's protocol for standard of care.
3. Obtain, clean, and inspect the appropriate equipment prior to entering the patient's room.
4. Follow PPE requirements, and observe standard precautions for any transmission-based isolation procedure.
5. Identify the patient using two patient identifiers.
6. Introduce yourself to the patient and to the family.
7. Explain the procedure to the patient and to the family, and acknowledge the patient's understanding.
8. Perform proper hand hygiene, and put on gloves, mask, and protective eyewear, as appropriate for the procedure.

Implementation

1. Place the patient in a comfortable position.
2. Assess vital signs.
3. Ensure adequate lighting.

4. Organize the equipment on the bedside table.
5. Prepare IV infusion tube for the solution:
   a. Verify that the IV solution has been correctly prepared and labeled, and check the expiration date.
   b. Open and place the roller clamp about 2 to 5 cm below the drip chamber in the "off" position.
   c. Remove the protective sheath over the IV tube port on the IV solution bag.
   d. Insert the infusion spike into the fluid bag.
   e. Prime the infusion tube by compressing drip chamber and filling to one third to one half full.
   f. Remove protector cap on the end of the tube (if applicable), release roller clamp, and allow the fluid to fill the tube.
   g. Remove air bubbles, and replace the protector cap on the end of the infusion tube.
6. Prepare a heparin or normal saline lock for infusion.
7. Put on face shield and mask, if indicated.
8. Identify the accessible vein, and apply a tourniquet over the gown sleeve 3 to 4 inches above the proposed insertion site.
9. Select an appropriate, well-dilated vein for IV insertion.
10. Cleanse the site with an appropriate antiseptic in a circular pattern.
11. Perform venipuncture:
    a. Anchor the vein by placing your thumb over the vein and stretching the skin distal to the selected site.
    b. Advise the patient to remain still, and warn him or her of a quick, sharp stick.
    c. Insert an over-the-needle IV catheter (ONC) safety device needle with the bevel up at a 10- to 30-degree angle slightly distal to the actual site in the direction of the vein.
12. Observe the flash of blood, lower the needle until almost flush with the patient's skin, and advance the catheter approximately one eighth to one fourth of an inch.
13. Continue to hold the skin taut, advance the catheter until the hub rests at the insertion site, and snap back the needle or withdraw the needle by using the appropriate technique for the specific ONC's IV safety device.
14. Stabilize the catheter with one hand while removing the needle, and release the tourniquet with the other hand.
15. Connect the end of the infusion tube set of heparin or saline lock adapter to the end of the catheter.
16. Flush the injection cap of the saline lock, if needed.
17. Slide open the clamp slowly to begin infusion.
18. Secure the catheter following agency protocol.
19. Observe the site for swelling or infiltration.
20. Apply sterile dressing over the site.
21. Secure the tube.
22. Recheck the IV tube for flow, or set to "keep vein open (KVO)."
23. Dispose of the sharps in the appropriate container.
24. Remove the supplies from the patient's room, and clean the area, as needed.
25. Remove PPE, and perform proper hand hygiene prior to leaving the patient's room.

Evaluation of Procedure

1. Instruct the patient about how to move around with the IV equipment.
2. Observe the patient's response to IV therapy.
3. Identify any unexpected outcomes.

TABLE 24-1 Sample Critical Test Results Reflecting Abnormalities in Electrolyte and Other Common Laboratory Tests.*

Test	Sample Critical Test Result*	Common Pathologic Conditions Associated with Abnormally High Levels	Common Pathologic Conditions Associated with Abnormally Low Levels
Sodium (Na+)	>155 mmol/L <125 mmol/L	**Hypernatremia:** Dehydration from excessive water loss or fluid restriction Excessive administration of saline fluids or diuretics (usually ≥180 mmol)	**Hyponatremia:** Over hydration or abnormal secretion of antidiuretic hormone Severe vomiting or diarrhea Congestive heart failure Renal or hepatic failure Addison disease
Potassium (K+)	>6.0 mmol/L <3.0 mmol/L	**Hyperkalemia:** Acute or chronic kidney disease Addison disease Severe alcoholism Rhabdomyolysis values ≥6 mmol are life-threatening	**Hypokalemia:** Severe vomiting or diarrhea Chronic renal disease High-dose β-agonist therapy
Chloride (Cl⁻)	>120 mmol/L <70 mmol/L	*Hyperchloremia:* Excessive chloride administration (usually saline resuscitation during shock) Metabolic acidosis Diabetes insipidus	*Hypochloremia:* Severe vomiting or diarrhea Metabolic alkalosis Adrenal insufficiency Severe burns Excessive IV dextrose administration
Total carbon dioxide	>40 mmol/L <15 mmol/L	Ventilatory failure	Metabolic acidosis Hyperventilation syndrome Severe diarrhea
Calcium (Ca)	>13.5 mmol/L <6.5 mmol/L	*Hypercalcemia:* Hyperparathyroidism Lithium or thiazide diuretic therapy Metastatic cancer Multiple myeloma	*Hypocalcemia:* Hypoparathyroidism Blood transfusions Acute pancreatitis Vitamin D deficiency
Ionized calcium (Ca⁺⁺)	>1.5 mmol/L <0.8 mmol/L		
Glucose (GLU)	>500 mg/dL <50 mg/dL	*Hyperglycemia:* Diabetes mellitus Severe sepsis	*Hypoglycemia:* Excessive insulin administration Inadequate dietary intake of carbohydrates
Creatinine (Cr)	>10 mg/dL	Acute kidney injury Chronic renal failure	Protein starvation Liver disease
Blood urea nitrogen (BUN)	>100 mg/dL	Acute kidney injury Chronic renal failure Dehydration	Liver disease Malnutrition
Magnesium (Mg⁺⁺)	>4.5 mg/dL <1.0 mg/dL	*Hypermagnesemia:* Chronic renal failure Addison's disease Diabetic ketoacidosis Dehydration	*Hypomagnesemia:* Cirrhosis Pancreatitis Severe alcoholism Hemodialysis Toxemia of pregnancy Ulcerative colitis
Phosphorus (PO₄⁻)	<1.0 mg/dL	*Hyperphosphatemia:* Commonly found in patients with renal failure, hepatic failure, bone metastasis, hypocalcemia, or hypoparathyroidism	*Hypophosphatemia:* Most often seen in chronic hyperventilation syndrome Also caused by hypercalcemia, hyperparathyroidism, and malnutrition
Lactate	>4.0 mmol /L		Primarily caused by anaerobic metabolism Frequently found in patients with hemorrhagic or septic shock May also be due to reduced hepatic clearance, dehydration, or trauma
Osmolarity	>320 mOsm/kg <240 mOsm/kg		

*Values for reference ranges and critical test results are from the University of California, San Francisco Moffit-Long Hospital, and San Francisco General Hospital: http://pathology.ucsf.edu/labmanual/mftlng-mtzn/test/test-index.html and http://pathology.ucsf.edu/sfghlab/test/ReferenceRanges.html: Accessed 9 January, 2011.

mg/dL, Milligrams per deciliter; *mmol/L*, millimoles per liter; *mOsm/kg*, milliosmoles per kilogram.

(From in Kacmarek RM, Stoller JK, Heuer AJ: *Egan's fundamentals of respiratory care*, ed 10, St. Louis, MO, 2013, Mosby.)

Documentation and Reporting

1. Record all the information about the insertion site and the infusion.
2. Document if ultrasonography was used during placement.
3. Report any abnormal findings to the appropriate health care provider.

24-4 Discontinuing Intravenous Access

As a member of the health care team, the RT may be called upon to discontinue IV access because it is no longer needed for patient care, it has become infected or nonfunctional, or the patient is being discharged. Care must be taken to dispose of all objects used for IV access in the proper medical waste container. The following is the step-by-step process for discontinuing IV access.

Procedural Preparation

1. Review the patient's chart.
2. Verify the physician's order or the facility's protocol for standard of care.
3. Obtain, clean, and inspect the appropriate equipment prior to entering the patient's room.
4. Follow PPE requirements, and observe standard precautions for any transmission-based isolation procedure.
5. Identify the patient using two patient identifiers.
6. Introduce yourself to the patient and to the family.
7. Explain the procedure to the patient and to the family, and acknowledge the patient's understanding.
8. Perform proper hand hygiene, and put on gloves, mask, and protective eyewear, as appropriate for the procedure.

Implementation

1. Place the patient in a comfortable position.
2. Turn the IV tube roller clamp to the "off" position.
3. Remove the dressing on the IV site and the tape securing catheter carefully and gently.
4. Cleanse the site with an appropriate antiseptic, and allow the area to dry.
5. Place sterile gauze over the site, and withdraw the catheter completely.
6. Apply pressure to the site for 2 to 3 minutes, according to the patient's medical or medication history.
7. Inspect the catheter for intactness and the tip for integrity.
8. Apply clean, folded gauze dressing over the site, and secure it with tape.
9. Discard the used IV catheter and the used IV supplies in the appropriate container.
10. Remove the supplies from the patient's room, and clean the area, as needed.
11. Remove PPE, and perform proper hand hygiene prior to leaving the patient's room.

Evaluation of Procedure

1. Observe the site for any evidence of bleeding, redness, pain, drainage, or swelling.
2. Identify any unexpected outcomes.

Documentation and Reporting

1. Record your findings in the patient's chart.
2. Report any abnormal findings to the appropriate health care provider.

24-5 Placing a Peripherally Inserted Central Catheter Line

The responsibilities and scope of practice of an RT are growing, and our profession itself is advancing. A new task that the RT is taking on is that of peripherally inserted central catheter (PICC) placement. Placed into a large vein, a PICC line is a soft, thin plastic line, similar to an intravenous (IV) line (Figure 24-6), which allows for administration of fluids, blood, blood products, and medications to the patient. It is indicated for long-term venous access needs (longer than 7 days to several months). PICC lines have a wider range of use compared with short-term venous access lines. For patient comfort, to ensure patency before venous puncture, and for the best procedural results, utilization of ultrasonography during the procedure should be the standard of care. The following is the step-by-step process for PICC line placement.

> → **Reality Check** PICC line placement is a relatively new responsibility for the RT. In the past, it was a procedure performed almost exclusively by nurses.

Procedural Preparation

1. Review the patient's chart.
2. Verify the physician's order or the facility's protocol for standard of care.
3. Check the chart for the consent form.
4. Obtain, clean, and inspect the appropriate equipment prior to entering the patient's room.
5. Follow PPE requirements, and observe standard precautions for any transmission-based isolation procedure.
6. Identify the patient using two patient identifiers.
7. Introduce yourself to the patient and to the family.

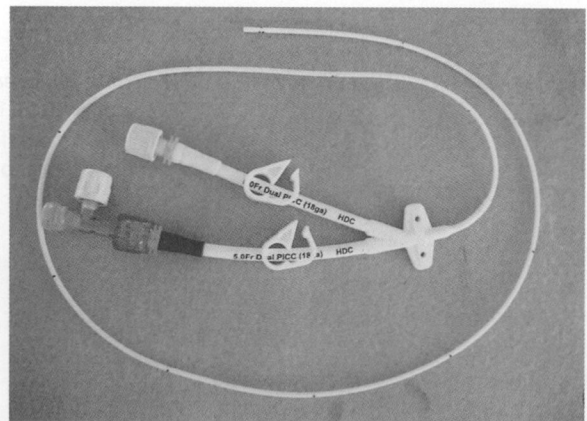

Figure 24-6 Peripherally inserted central catheter (PICC) line. (From Roberts J and Hedges J: Clinical procedures in emergency medicine, ed 5, Philadelphia, 2010, Saunders)

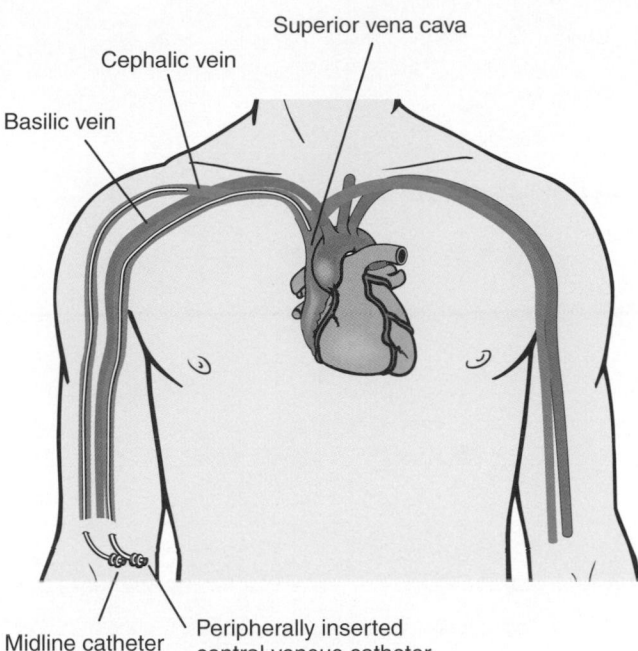

Cephalic vein

Basilic vein

Superior vena cava

Midline catheter

Peripherally inserted
central venous catheter

Figure 24-7 Peripherally inserted central catheter (PICC) line
placement. (From ENA: *Sheehy's emergency nursing*, ed 6,
St. Louis, MO, 2009, Mosby.)

BOX 24-1 Steps of a Modified Seldinger Technique

1. Insert a peripheral intravenous (IV) catheter, and observe for blood return in the flashback chamber.
2. Remove the stylet, and advance the guidewire 5 to 10 centimeters (cm) through the IV catheter.
3. Remove the IV catheter, and insert the dilator or introducer over the guidewire.
4. Gently advance the dilator or introducer until the tip is well within the vein.
5. Remove the dilator and guidewire, leaving the introducer in place.
6. Insert the catheter approximately 15 to 20 cm into the vein.

---

8. Explain the procedure to the patient and to the family, and acknowledge the patient's understanding.
9. Perform proper hand hygiene, and put on gloves, mask, and protective eyewear, as appropriate for the procedure.

Implementation

1. Place the patient in a comfortable position.
2. Assess vital signs, and check for pacers, filters, and tunneled catheters.
3. Perform vein assessment, and choose a site (Figure 24-7).
4. Wash the insertion area with soap and water, discard the used supplies, and remove your gloves.
5. Measure and make note of the required catheter length.
6. Position the tourniquet high on the patient's arm, but do not constrict blood flow.
7. Open the PICC line insertion kit, and place it onto a sterile field.
8. Put on sterile gown and gloves.
9. Fill a 10-mL syringe with normal saline.
10. Add the injection port to the extension tube, and prime it with normal saline, leaving the syringe attached.
11. Use ultrasonography to identify the correct vessel.
12. Prepare the site with 2% chlorhexidine.
13. Remove and discard your gloves.
14. Apply the tourniquet.
15. Put on a new pair of sterile gloves.
16. Place the patient in a 15- to 25-degree Trendelenburg position (if not contraindicated)

17. Place sterile drapes over the prepped area.
18. Use ultrasonography to identify landmarks, and administer local anesthesia (1% lidocaine without epinephrine), as indicated.
19. Advance the insertion needle into the vein.
20. Perform the modified Seldinger technique (Box 24-1).
21. Release the tourniquet, and instruct the patient to drop the chin to the chest.
22. Advance the remainder of the catheter while monitoring the patient's heart rate and rhythm.
23. Instruct the patient to turn the head away from the insertion site.
24. Pull the introducer from the insertion site, and remove it.
25. Apply the pressure cap, secure the line, and apply antimicrobial patch and dressing.
26. Reassess vital signs.
27. Remove the supplies from the patient's room, and clean the area, as needed.
28. Remove PPE, and perform proper hand hygiene prior to leaving the patient's room.

Evaluation of Procedure

1. Order a postinsertion radiograph to confirm placement.
2. Monitor the patient for complications, hematoma, pain, and poor or no blood return.
3. Identify any unexpected outcomes.

Documentation and Reporting

1. Record your findings in the patient's chart.
2. Report any abnormal findings to the appropriate health care provider.

Bibliography

American Association of Colleges of Nursing: *AACN procedure manual for critical care*, ed 6, St. Louis, MO, 2010, Saunders.

Kacmarek RM, Stoller JK, Heuer AJ: *Egan's fundamentals of respiratory care*, ed 10, St. Louis, MO, 2013, Mosby.

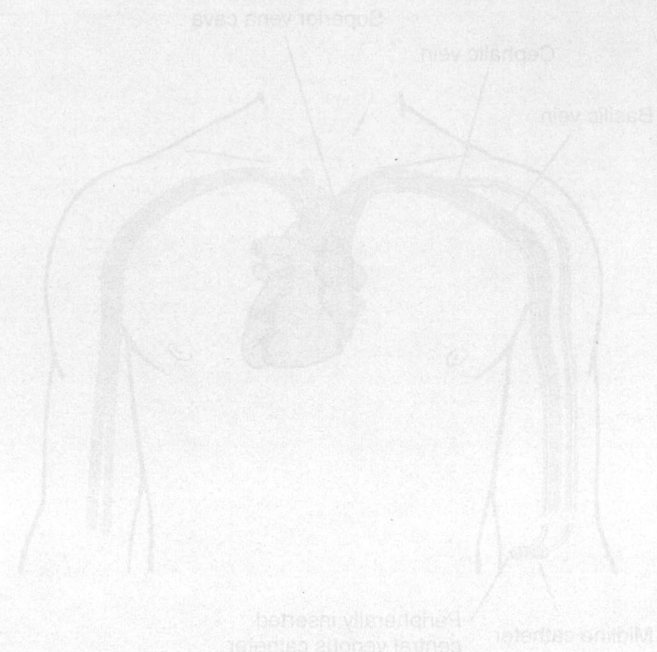

Superior vena cava

Cephalic vein

Basilic vein

Midline catheter

Peripherally inserted central venous catheter

Figure 24-7 Peripherally inserted central catheter (PICC) line placement. (From RNA, Sheehy's emergency nursing, ed 6, St. Louis, MO, 2008, Mosby.)

8. Explain the procedure to the patient and to the family and acknowledge the patient's understanding.

9. Perform proper hand hygiene, and put on gloves, mask, and protective eyewear, as appropriate for the procedure.

Implementation

1. Place the patient in a comfortable position.
2. Assess vital signs, and check for patency, filters, and unneeded catheters.
3. Perform vein assessment and choose a site (Figure 24-7).
4. Wash the insertion area with soap and water, discard the used supplies, and remove your gloves.
5. Measure and make note of the required catheter length.
6. Position the tourniquet high on the patient's arm, but do not constrict blood flow.
7. Open the PICC line insertion kit, and place it onto a sterile field.
8. Put on sterile gown and gloves.
9. Fill a 10 mL syringe with normal saline.
10. Add the injection port to the extension tube, and prime it with normal saline, leaving the syringe attached.
11. Use ultrasonography to identify the correct vessel.
12. Prepare the site with 2% chlorhexidine.
13. Remove and discard your gloves.
14. Apply the tourniquet.
15. Put on a new pair of sterile gloves.
16. Place the patient in a 15- to 25-degree Trendelenburg position (if not contraindicated).

17. Place sterile drapes over the prepped area.
18. Use ultrasonography to identify landmarks, and administer local anesthetic (1% lidocaine without epinephrine), as indicated.
19. Advance the insertion needle into the vein.
20. Perform the modified Seldinger technique (Box 24-1).
21. Release the tourniquet, and instruct the patient to drop the chin to the chest.
22. Advance the remainder of the catheter while monitoring the patient's heart rate and rhythm.
23. Instruct the patient to turn the head away from the insertion site.
24. Pull the introducer from the insertion site, and remove it.
25. Apply the pressure cap, secure the line, and apply antimicrobial patch and dressing.
26. Reassess vital signs.
27. Remove the supplies from the patient's room, and clean the area, as needed.
28. Remove PPE, and perform proper hand hygiene prior to leaving the patient's room.

Evaluation of Procedure

1. Order a postinsertion radiograph to confirm placement.
2. Monitor the patient for complications, hematoma, pain, and poor or no blood return.
3. Identify any unexpected outcomes.

Documentation and Reporting

1. Record your findings in the patient's chart.
2. Report any abnormal findings to the appropriate health care provider.

Bibliography

American Association of Colleges of Nursing: *PICC procedure manual for critical care*, ed 6, St. Louis, MO, 2010, Saunders.

Rosenzweig RA, Shelby DC: *Heart & lung: fundamentals of respiratory care*, ed 10, St. Louis, MO, 2014, Mosby.

Lab Activities

1. What is thrombocytopenia?

_____

_____

2. Name the three complications a patient with thrombocytopenia may have following a venous access procedure.

a. _____

b. _____

c. _____

3. Fill in the following chart:

Common Conditions Associated with Electrolyte Abnormalities

Test	Common Pathologic Condition Associated with Abnormally High Levels	Common Pathologic Condition Associated with Abnormally Low Levels
Sodium (Na⁺)	Critical test result value: _____ Term used to describe: _____ Common pathologic condition associated with abnormally high levels:	Critical test result value: _____ Term used to describe: _____ Common pathologic condition associated with abnormally low levels:
Potassium (K⁺)	Critical test result value: _____ Term used to describe: _____ Common pathologic condition associated with abnormally high levels:	Critical test result value: _____ Term used to describe: _____ Common pathologic condition associated with abnormally low levels:
Chloride (Cl⁻)	Critical test result value: _____ Term used to describe: _____ Common pathologic condition associated with abnormally high levels:	Critical test result value: _____ Term used to describe: _____ Common pathologic condition associated with abnormally low levels:

Continued

Test	Common Pathologic Condition Associated with Abnormally High Levels	Common Pathologic Condition Associated with Abnormally Low Levels
Total carbon dioxide (CO_2)	Critical test result value: _____ Common pathologic condition associated with abnormally high levels: _____	Critical test result value: _____ Common pathologic condition associated with abnormally low levels: _____

Obtain a mannequin or an artificial phlebotomy practice arm to use for activities 4–6.

4. Obtain all the appropriate equipment needed for venipuncture.

   Perform four successful venipunctures using both the butterfly or needle method and the Vacutainer. Have your lab partner sign off to confirm proper technique used throughout the procedures.

   Butterfly/Needle Method   **Vacutainer**

   Signature:_____   Signature:_____

   Signature:_____   Signature:_____

   Signature:_____   Signature:_____

   Signature:_____   Signature:_____

5. Obtain all the appropriate equipment needed for initiation and discontinuation of intravenous (IV) access.

   Perform four successful initiations of IV access followed by properly discontinuing of the IV access. Have your lab partner sign off to confirm proper technique used throughout the procedures.

   Initiation   **Discontinuation**

   Signature:_____   Signature:_____

   Signature:_____   Signature:_____

   Signature:_____   Signature:_____

   Signature:_____   Signature:_____

6. Obtain all the appropriate equipment needed for PICC line placement.

Perform four successful PICC line placements (or as many as you can, given the lab supplies available). Have your lab partner sign off to confirm proper technique used throughout the procedures.

PICC line placement:

Signature: _____

Signature: _____

Signature: _____

Signature: _____

7. Locate the sharps container in your lab. Dispose of all the used sharps appropriately.

8. Define the abnormal laboratory value for each of the conditions listed below, and list a clinical situation that could result in the value.

a. Leukocytosis _____

b. Leukopenia _____

c. Neutropenia _____

d. Anemia _____

e. Polycythemia _____

f. Thrombocytopenia _____

g. Thrombocytosis _____

Self-Assessment Questions

1. Which of the following is an indication for PICC line placement?
   A. Four-hour medication drip
   B. Blood draw for pregnancy test
   C. Frequent arterial blood gas testing
   D. Course of 10-day IV antibiotic administration

2. What lab test would indicate a patient at risk for excessive bleeding following venipuncture?
   A. PvO_2 value of 82 mm Hg
   B. Platelet count of 88×10^3
   C. White blood cell count of $5.9 \times 10^3/\mu L$
   D. Red blood cell value of $4.0 \times 10^6/\mu L$

3. Complications associated with venipuncture include:

   1. Hematoma formation
   2. Excessive bleeding
   3. Syncope
   4. Polycythemia

   A. 1 and 2 only
   B. 1 and 4 only
   C. 1, 2, and 3 only
   D. 1, 2, 3, and 4

4. Which of the following orders may be needed following PICC line placement to rule out complications?
   A. Radiography
   B. Magnetic resonance imaging
   C. Arterial blood draw from PICC line for blood gas analysis
   D. Complete blood cell count

5. During PICC line placement, ultrasonography should be used:
   A. Only after Administration confirms that the patient has valid medical insurance
   B. Only if the patient requests it
   C. As a standard of care for every patient
   D. If the physician is performing the procedure

6. How long is the application of pressure needed to control excessive bleeding following venipuncture on a patient receiving warfarin?
   A. About 5 seconds
   B. About 10 seconds
   C. About 15 seconds
   D. Until the bleeding has stopped

7. How many inches above the venipuncture site should the tourniquet be placed?
   A. 1–2
   B. 3–4
   C. 5–6
   D. 7–8

8. Used IV catheters or over-the-needle catheter (ONC) safety device needles do not need to be placed in a sharps container if blood is not visible in the catheter.
   A. True
   B. False

9. Sterile gloves are needed during venipuncture of a patient with human immunodeficiency virus (HIV) infection.
   A. True
   B. False

10. Consent is not needed for PICC line placement if a patient needs long-term venous access.
    A. True
    B. False

›› CASE STUDY 24-1

Miss Robert walks into her pulmonologist's office with complaints of tiredness and cough. The physician orders a complete blood cell count (CBC) and a basic metabolic panel (BMP).

1. Is initiation of intravenous (IV) access necessary?

_____

_____

2. What technique can be used to obtain the blood samples?

_____

_____

3. Miss Robert's current medication history includes albuterol 2 puffs via a metered-dose inhaler (MDI), as needed (PRN), Combivent 2 puffs via an MDI twice daily, and warfarin 2 mg orally (PO) daily. Will any of these medications influence the ability of her blood to clot following a blood draw procedure?

_____

_____

›› CASE STUDY 24-2

You are the RT working the night shift in the intensive care unit when you are called by a nurse to evaluate the respiratory status of a patient. The patient is a 52-year-old male recently admitted to the unit following a farm accident in which his left arm was severely lacerated by a piece of farm equipment. The patient has no significant pulmonary history and is complaining of shortness of breath. His lung sounds are clear and equal, his respiratory rate is 24 breaths/min, HR 100 beats/min, with weak radial pulses bilaterally. He has no other complaints. His hematocrit is 21%, and his hemoglobin is 7 g/dL.

1. Are these lab values normal?

_____

_____

2. On the basis of his history and his present condition, what is a likely cause of his shortness of breath?

_____

_____

3. As the RT, what can you do for him?

_____

_____

Discontinuing Ventilatory Support

▪ OBJECTIVES

Upon the completion of the chapter activities and content review topics, the student should be able to:

1. Evaluate a patient for readiness for a spontaneous breathing trial.
2. Perform a spontaneous breathing trial procedure.
3. Describe the guidelines for extubation.
4. List the acceptable weaning indices used to predict a patient's readiness for discontinuation of ventilatory support.
5. Determine an appropriate weaning mode for a patient.
6. Perform the weaning procedure.
7. Describe factors that may lead to ventilator dependence.
8. Perform a terminal weaning procedure.

▪ KEY TERMS

- Spontaneous breathing trial (SBT)
- Terminal weaning
- Ventilator-associated pneumonia (VAP)
- Ventilator dependence
- Weaning

▪ CONTENT REVIEW TOPICS

- Adaptive support ventilation
- Computer-based weaning
- Noninvasive ventilation (NIV) during weaning

▪ PROCEDURAL ASSESSMENTS

25-1 Implementing a Spontaneous Breathing Trial
25-2 Weaning Process
25-3 Terminal Weaning

▪ EQUIPMENT

- 50-psi air source
- 50-psi oxygen source
- Adult circuits for ventilators
- Intubated human patient simulator, if available
- Mechanical ventilators
- Test lungs or lung simulator

R emoving a patient from ventilatory support may range from a routine procedure that takes minutes to the need for a systematic approach that takes days to weeks. However rapid or time consuming the undertaking, discontinuation of ventilatory support requires the evaluation of a patient's physiologic and psychological status and, at times, even requires ethical considerations. Physiologic parameters for weaning and extubation are provided in Table 25-1.

> ✳ **Tip** Be familiar with ventilator "lingo" at your facility. A *spontaneous breathing trial* (SBT) and *weaning* are not the same thing. Be succinct with your wording, and keep with department terminology.

Many terms such as *gradual withdrawal, liberation, slow wean,* and *discontinuations* are used when discussing the concept of discontinuing a patient from a mechanical ventilator. It is relatively easy with some patients. All it takes is simply testing their ability to breathe on their own, disconnecting the ventilator, and extubating them. However, weaning, the reduction of ventilatory support for a patient, is a process. Timing is everything when discontinuing ventilatory support or weaning. If the ventilatory support is stopped and the patient is extubated too soon, the risks are reintubation and the adverse effects associated with it. However, the potential for

ventilator-associated pneumonia (VAP), a lower respiratory tract infection that develops more than 48 to 72 hours after endotracheal (ET) intubation, or even death must be considered as adverse effects of leaving a patient on the ventilator too long. This chapter will discuss the aspects of discontinuing ventilatory support.

≫ SKILL CHECK LISTS

25-1 Implementing a Spontaneous Breathing Trial

Supporting a patient during an exacerbation of a chronic pulmonary condition or an acute pulmonary illness at times requires mechanical ventilation. It is not, however, without consequences. These could range from airway damage such as tracheal stenosis to ventilator dependence, defined as the need for ventilatory support for lengthy periods, usually longer than 2 weeks. Discontinuing ventilatory support is a complex issue. Both premature discontinuation and delayed discontinuation of ventilatory support are associated with adverse patient outcomes. A way to test a patient's readiness for successful discontinuation of mechanical ventilatory support is a SBT. Extubation should be considered but not integrated into the SBT process. Guidelines for extubation are provided in Box 25-1. The following is the step-by-step process for a spontaneous breathing trial.

TABLE 25-1 Physiologic Parameters for Weaning and Extubation of Adults

Parameter	Acceptable Value
VENTILATORY PERFORMANCE AND MUSCLE STRENGTH	
VC	>15 mL/kg (IBW)
V_E	<10–15 L/min
V_T	>4–6 mL/kg (IBW)
f	<35 breaths/min
f/V_T	<60–105 breaths/min/L (spontaneously breathing patient)
Ventilatory pattern	Synchronous and stable
PImax (up to 20-s measurement from RV)	<−20 to −30 cm H_2O
MEASUREMENT OF DRIVE TO BREATHE	
$P_{0.1}$	>−6 cm H_2O
MEASUREMENT AND ESTIMATION OF WOB	
WOB*	<0.8 J/L
Oxygen cost of breathing*	<15% of total $\dot{V}O_2$
Dynamic compliance (C_D)	>25 mL/cm H_2O
V_D/V_T	<0.6
CROP index	>13 mL/breaths/min
MEASUREMENT OF ADEQUACY OF OXYGENATION	
PaO_2	≥60 mm Hg (FiO_2 <0.4)
PEEP	≤5–8 cm H_2O
PaO_2/FiO_2	>250 mm Hg (consider at 150–200 mm Hg)
PaO_2/P_AO_2	>0.47
$P(A-a)O_2$	<350 mm Hg (FiO_2 =1)
% $\dot{Q}_S/\dot{Q}_T$	<20% to 30%

*Actual measure of work of breathing (WOB).
%Q_S/Q_T, Percent shunt; *CROP*, compliance, respiratory rate, oxygenation, and inspiratory pressure; *f*, respiratory rate; *f/V$_T$*, rapid shallow breathing index; *FiO$_2$*, fractional inspired O$_2$; *IBW*, ideal body weight; *P(A-a)O$_2$*, alveolar-to-arterial partial pressure of O$_2$; *P$_{0.1}$*, pressure on inspiration measured at 100 milliseconds (ms); *PaO$_2$*, partial pressure of O$_2$ in the arteries; *PaO$_2$/FiO$_2$ (P/F)*, ratio of partial pressure of O$_2$ (PO$_2$) in the arteries to FiO$_2$; *PaO$_2$/P$_A$O$_2$*, ratio of arterial PO$_2$ to alveolar PO$_2$; *PEEP*, positive end expiratory pressure; *PImax*, maximum inspiratory pressure; *RV*, residual volume; *VC*, vital capacity; *V$_D$/V$_T$*, ratio of dead space to tidal volume; *V$_E$*, minute ventilation; *VO$_2$*, oxygen (O$_2$) consumption per minute; *V$_T$*, tidal volume.

(From Cairo JM: *Pilbeam's mechanical ventilation*, ed 5, St. Louis, 2011, MO, Mosby.)

Procedural Preparation

1. Review the patient's chart.
2. Verify the physician's order or the facility's protocol for standard of care.
3. Obtain, clean, and inspect the appropriate equipment prior to entering the patient's room.
4. Follow personal protective equipment (PPE) requirements, and observe standard precautions for any transmission-based isolation procedure.
5. Identify the patient using two patient identifiers.
6. Introduce yourself to the patient and to the family.
7. Explain the procedure to the patient and to the family, and acknowledge the patient's understanding.
8. Perform proper hand hygiene, and put on gloves, mask, and protective eyewear, as appropriate for the procedure.

BOX 25-1 Practical Guidelines for Extubation

- No immediate need for mechanical ventilation or intubation exists.
- The medical course does not suggest impending respiratory failure or other indications for mechanical ventilation.
- Procedures necessitating intubation and general anesthesia are not immediately planned.
- Adequate oxygenation and ventilation with spontaneous ventilation have been achieved.
- The patient's FiO$_2$ requirement can be achieved with a mask or nasal cannula.
- The patient no longer needs mechanical ventilatory assistance.
- Weaning is successful.
- Minimal risk of upper airway obstruction exists.
- The patient has minimal edema or mass encroachment of the oropharynx and upper airway; oral and upper airway anatomy is otherwise normal.
- The result of a "cuff-leak" test is positive.
- Airway protection is adequate, and risk of aspiration is minimal.
- Level of consciousness and neuromuscular function allow gag reflex and adequate cough.
- Gastric contents are minimized by discontinuation of tube feedings for 4 to 6 hours before extubation.
- Clearance of pulmonary secretions is adequate.
- Level of consciousness and muscular strength allow effective coughing.
- Secretion volume and thickness are not worsening.

From Kacmarek RM, Stoller JK, Heuer AJ: *Egan's fundamentals of respiratory care*, ed 10, St. Louis, MO, 2013, Mosby.

Implementation

1. Place the patient in a comfortable position.
2. Assess vital signs.
3. Assess the patient for SBT readiness, including the following:
   a. Correction of reversible causes for mechanical ventilation
   b. Adequacy of oxygenation
   c. Adequacy of ventilation
   d. Presence of airway leak
   e. Laboratory values
   f. Chest radiography
   g. Hemodynamic stability
   h. Current sedation medications
   i. Patient's ability to generate an inspiratory effort
4. Record the patient's baseline values:
   a. General appearance
   b. Breath sounds
   c. Blood pressure
   d. Heart rate and rhythm
   e. SpO$_2$
5. Advise the patient when the SBT will commence.
6. Change the ventilator to a spontaneous mode with zero pressure support ventilation (PSV) and zero continuous positive airway pressure (CPAP):
   a. Minimal CPAP settings may be used, per facility protocols.

b. Minimal PSV settings may be used, per facility protocols.
7. Maintain the fractional inspired oxygen (FiO_2) that the patient was receiving on mechanical ventilation.
8. Monitor and record the SBT start data, including the following:
   a. Ventilator mode and settings
   b. Patient's general appearance
   c. Pulse oximetry
   d. Blood pressure
   e. Cardiac monitoring
   f. Use the ventilator to monitor the following:
      i. Respiratory rate and tidal volume
      ii. Minute ventilation
      iii. Rapid-shallow-breathing index (RSBI)

> ✳ **Tip** RSBI has less predictive value for patients older than 70 years or those who have required mechanical ventilation for longer than 8 days.

9. Consider extubation if the patient tolerated the SBT for 30 to 120 minutes.

> → **Reality Check** Discontinuing mechanical ventilation does not equal extubation. Some patients are ready to come "off the vent" but should be considered for a tracheostomy if they are not able to maintain their secretions or airway patency.

10. Identify the SBT failing criteria, and reestablish previous ventilator settings.
11. Reassess vital signs at the end of the SBT.
12. Remove the supplies from the patient's room, and clean the area, as needed.
13. Remove PPE, and perform proper hand hygiene prior to leaving the patient's room.

Evaluation of Procedure

1. Establish a baseline, or compare with previous SBT attempts.
2. Develop an appropriate respiratory care plan based on SBT data.
3. Repeat the SBT over multiple days, as needed or per protocol.
4. Identify any unexpected outcomes.

Documentation and Reporting

1. Record your findings in the patient's chart
2. Notify the physician of the SBT results.
3. Report any abnormal findings to the appropriate health care provider.

25-2 Weaning Process

The key to patient readiness to be weaned from ventilatory support is the resolution or improvement of the cause of mechanical ventilation in the first place. *Ventilator dependency* is the term used to describe the patient who needs ventilatory support for lengthy periods (more than 2 weeks). Evaluation

and patient assessment prior to the decision to wean includes length of mechanical ventilation and both respiratory and nonrespiratory factors that may lead to ventilator dependence. Box 25-2 lists some respiratory and nonrespiratory factors. Good oxygenation, ventilation, and cardiovascular status are also important when considering readiness to wean.

> ✳ **Tip** Try to time SBTs or weaning processes such that they do not conflict with patient transport for radiography, magnetic resonance imaging (MRI), or an invasive procedure.

No "perfect" mode to wean a patient exists. An example of a weaning protocol is given in Figure 25-1. The choice of mode is dependent on the clinical experience and judgment of the physician and the respiratory therapist (RT). The patient's response to a mode should also play a role in the process. A probability of successful weaning curve using different methods is provided in Figure 25-2. The following is the step-by-step process for the weaning process.

> ✳ **Tip** Weaning indices include the RSBI, airway occlusion pressure, and measures of WOB. It is important to be familiar with the capabilities of your specific ventilator along with facility protocols.

Procedural Preparation

1. Review the patient's chart.
2. Verify the physician's order or the facility's protocol for standard of care.
3. Obtain, clean, and inspect the appropriate equipment prior to entering the patient's room.
4. Follow PPE requirements, and observe standard precautions for any transmission-based isolation procedure.

BOX 25-2	Factors That Contribute to Ventilator Dependence

Respiratory Factors
- Ventilator workload exceeds capacity
- ↓ Lung or chest wall compliance
- ↑ Airway resistance
- ↑ Dead space
- Ventilatory muscle weakness or fatigue
- Oxygenation problems

Nonrespiratory Factors
- Cardiovascular factors
- Myocardial ischemia
- Heart failure
- Hemodynamic instability
- Neurologic factors
- ↑ or ↓ Central drive to breathe
- Multisystem organ failure
- ↓ Peripheral nerve transmission
- Fear and anxiety
- Stress
- Altered mental status
- Depression
- Poor nutrition
- Equipment shortcomings

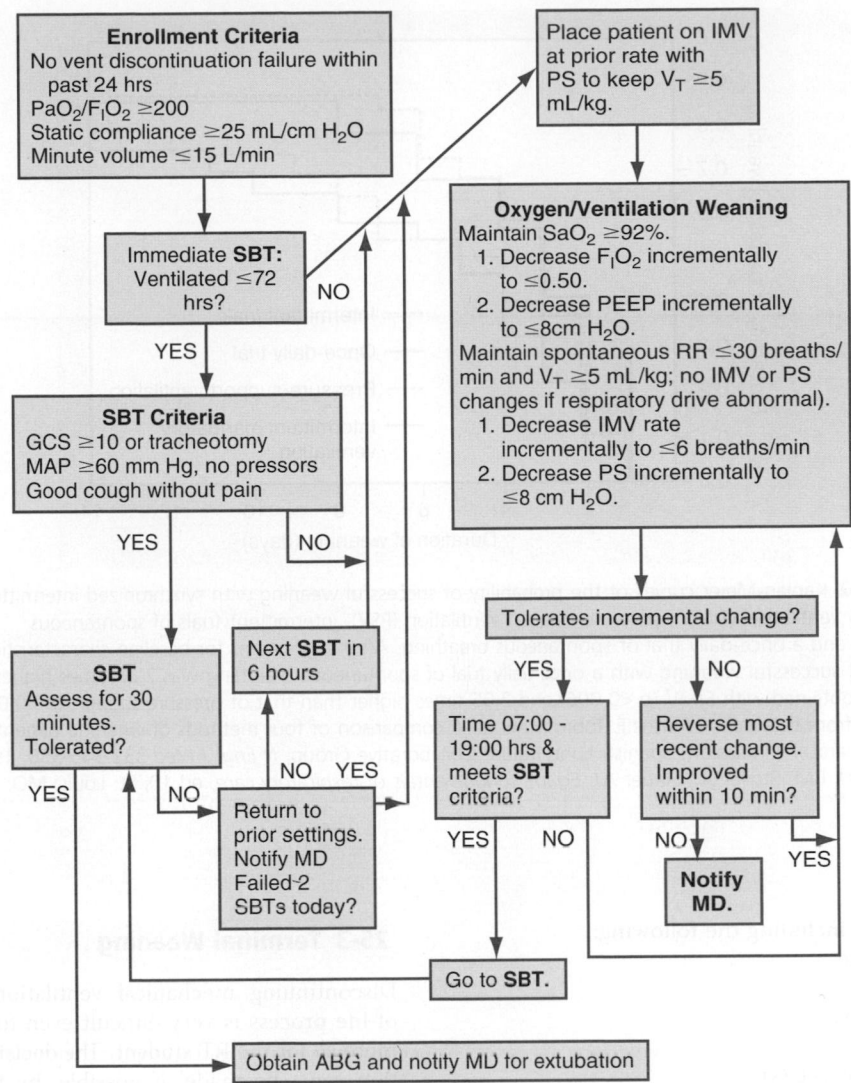

Figure 25-1 Example of a weaning protocol. (Redrawn from Marelich GP, Murin S, Batistella FF, et al: Protocol weaning of mechanical ventilation in medical and surgical patients by respiratory care practitioners and nurses: effect of weaning time and incidence of ventilator-associated pneumonia. Reproduced with permission from the American College of Chest Physicians. *Chest* 118:459, 2000.)

5. Identify the patient using two patient identifiers.
6. Introduce yourself to the patient and to the family.
7. Explain the procedure to the patient and to the family, and acknowledge the patient's understanding.
8. Perform proper hand hygiene, and put on gloves, mask, and protective eyewear, as appropriate for the procedure.

Implementation

1. Place the patient in a comfortable position.
2. Assess vital signs.
3. Inform the patient that the trial will feel different from how they felt on full support, and instruct the patient to breathe normally.
4. Determine the weaning process mode:
   a. Gradually lengthening SBTs via the mechanical ventilator or with a T-piece alternating with mechanical ventilatory support:
      i. Connect the patient to a heated aerosol via T-piece.
      ii. Carefully monitor the patient in the absence of ventilator alarms.
   b. Pressure support method:
      i. Start the patient at a PSV level to achieve a tidal volume of 6 to 10 mL/kg IBW.
      ii. Decrease PSV by 2 to 4 cmH_2O, according to protocol or as the patient tolerates.
   c. Synchronized intermittent mandatory ventilation (SIMV) method:
      i. Place the patient in the SIMV mode.
      ii. Set the tidal volume or inspiratory pressures and rate equivalent to those settings in controlled mechanical ventilation.
      iii. Gradually and progressively lower the SIMV rate.
      iv. Consider PSV if WOB increases.

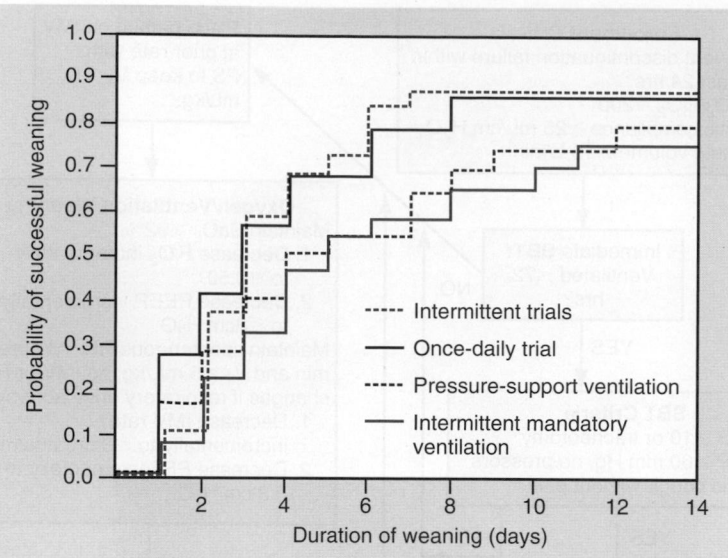

Figure 25-2 Kaplan-Meier curves of the probability of successful weaning with synchronized intermittent mandatory ventilation (SIMV), pressure support ventilation (PSV), intermittent trials of spontaneous breathing, and a once-daily trial of spontaneous breathing. After adjustment for baseline characteristics, the rate of successful weaning with a once-daily trial of spontaneous breathing was 2.83 times higher than that obtained with SIMV ($p < 0.006$) and 2.05 times higher than that of pressure support ($p < 0.04$). (Modified from Esteban A, Frutos F, Tobin M, et al: A comparison of four methods of weaning patients from mechanical ventilation. Spanish Lung Failure Collaborative Group, *N Engl J Med* 332:345-350, 1995, in Kacmarek RM, Stoller JK, Heuer AJ: *Egan's fundamentals of respiratory care*, ed 10, St. Louis, MO, 2013, Mosby.)

5. Monitor patient data, including the following:
   a. General appearance
   b. RR
   c. Respiratory pattern
   d. HR
   e. Electrocardiography (ECG)
   f. SpO_2
   g. Ventilator graphics
6. Place the patient back on stable, nonfatiguing ventilator settings at either of the following times:
   a. After predetermined time
   b. When signs of intolerance to weaning emerge
7. Perform a patient–ventilator system assessment following the weaning process.
8. Remove supplies from the patient's room, and clean the area, as needed.
9. Remove the PPE, and perform proper hand hygiene prior to leaving the patient's room.

Evaluation of Procedure

1. Establish a baseline, or compare with previous weaning attempts.
2. Develop an appropriate respiratory diagnosis based on assessment data.
3. Identify any unexpected outcomes.

Documentation and Reporting

1. Record the procedure in the patient's chart.
2. Notify the physician of the results of weaning.
3. Report any abnormal findings to the appropriate health care provider.

25-3 Terminal Weaning

Discontinuing mechanical ventilation as part of the end-of-life process is very difficult even for the seasoned RT and more so for the RT student. The decision to withdraw ventilation must be made, if possible, by the patient and by the family. However, the entire health care team plays an integral role in this process. Acute care hospitals, as well as long-term acute care facilities, may have an ethics committee to decide on cases in which it is difficult for the family to make a decision regarding end-of-life issues, including terminal weaning. The following is the step-by-step process for terminal weaning.

Procedural Preparation

1. Review the patient's chart.
2. Verify the physician's order or the facility's protocol for standard of care.
3. Obtain, clean, and inspect the appropriate equipment prior to entering the patient's room.
4. Follow PPE requirements, and observe standard precautions for any transmission-based isolation procedure.
5. Identify the patient using two patient identifiers.
6. Introduce yourself to the patient and to the family.
7. Explain the procedure to the patient and to the family, and acknowledge the patient's understanding.
8. Perform proper hand hygiene, and put on gloves, mask, and protective eyewear, as appropriate for the procedure.

Implementation

1. Place the patient in a comfortable position.
2. Assess vital signs.
3. Ensure that all key health care team members are present.
4. Ensure that all key family members are present.
5. Prepare the patient and family for what to expect:
   a. Changes in ventilatory pattern
   b. Noisy breathing
6. Turn off all of the ventilator alarms.
7. Withdraw the ventilatory support.
8. Provide oxygen therapy, as ordered or per protocol.
9. Reassess vital signs only as necessary to ensure patient comfort.
10. Provide time for the patient and the family to be alone, if indicated.
11. Remove the supplies from the patient's room, and clean the area, as needed.
12. Remove PPE, and perform proper hand hygiene prior to leaving the patient's room.

Evaluation of Procedure

1. Note any use of oxygen therapy.
2. Identify any unexpected outcomes.
3. Ensure patient comfort.

Documentation and Reporting

1. Record the procedure in the patient's chart.
2. Report any abnormal findings to the appropriate health care provider.

Bibliography

Cairo JM: *Pilbeam's mechanical ventilation Physiological and clinical applications*, ed 5, St. Louis, MO, 2011, Mosby.

Kacmarek RM, Stoller JK, Heuer AJ: *Egan's fundamentals of respiratory care*, ed 10, St. Louis, MO, 2013, Mosby.

MacIntyre N: Discontinuing mechanical ventilatory support, *Chest* 132(3):1049-1056, 2007.

Multifactor Clinical Score and Outcome of Mechanical Ventilation Weaning Trials: Burns Wean Assessment Program, *Am J Crit Care* 19(5): 2010.

Prendergast TJ, Puntillo KA: Withdrawal of life support: intensive caring at the end of life, *JAMA* 288:2732-2740, 2002.

Lab Activities

1. Fill in the following chart comparing available weaning methods:

Method	Advantages	Disadvantages
SBT		
SIMV		
PSV		

2. Fill in the following chart pertaining to factors that may increase the ventilatory workload:

Situation	Factors
Increased ventilatory demand	
Decreased compliance	
Increased resistance	

3. Fill in the criteria portion of the following chart pertaining to indices that are used to predict successful weaning and mechanical ventilator discontinuation:

Measurement	Criteria
OXYGENATION	
a. FIO_2	
b. PEEP (cm H_2O)	
c. PaO_2 (mm Hg)	
d. SaO_2 (%)	
e. SvO_2 (%)	
f. $PaO_2 : FIO_2$ ratio	
g. P/F ratio	
h. $P(A\text{-}a)O_2$ (mm Hg)	

Continued

Measurement	Criteria
VENTILATION	
a. $PaCO_2$ (mm Hg)	
b. pH (mm Hg)	
VENTILATORY MECHANICS	
a. Respiratory rate (f) (breath/min)	
b. V_T (mL/kg)	
c. VC (mL/kg)	
d. C_S (mL/cm H_2O)	
e. f/V_T	
RESPIRATORY MUSCLE STRENGTH	
MIF (cm H_2O)	
VENTILATORY DRIVE	
a. Minute ventilation $\dot{V}_E$ for normal $PaCO_2$ (L/min)	
b. V_{DS}/V_T	
c. $P_{0.1}$ (cm H_2O)	
d. $P_{0.1}/MIP$	
WORK OF BREATHING (WOB)	
Spontaneous WOB	
Pressure-time index	
VENTILATORY RESERVE	
MVV (L/min)	

4. On the basis of the presented data, calculate the rapid shallow breathing index (RSBI), and fill in the chart:

Frequency (breaths/min)	Tidal volume (L)	RSBI
22	0.5	
22	0.25	
15	0.5	

Frequency (breaths/min)	Tidal volume (L)	RSBI
15	0.25	
32	0.5	
32	0.25	

5. In what time frame must the RSBI be calculated?

_____

6. List the nonrespiratory factors that affect weaning:

_____

_____

_____

_____

_____

_____

_____

_____

_____

_____

_____

_____

_____

_____

_____

_____

_____

_____

_____

7. What are the criteria for confirming cardiovascular stability?

_____

_____

_____

Use a lung simulator for the following exercise. Set it up to match the scenario presented.

Miss Wall is a 23-year-old female intubated and mechanically ventilated for apnea 2 days ago following an overdose of oxycontin and heroin. Her current ventilator settings are as follows:
- Ventilator: PB 840
- Mode: AC/VC
- V_T: 450 mL
- PIP: 22 cmH$_2$O
- Set frequency: 12 breaths/min
- Actual frequency: 18 breaths/min
- PEEP: 5 cmH$_2$O
- FiO$_2$: 0.3
- P$_{plateau}$: 14 cmH$_2$O

Physical assessment and vital signs are as follows:
- Patient is alert and follows simple commands with sedation medications discontinued
- Airway patent with 7.5 mm endotracheal tube 23 cm at teeth, scant secretions
- Breath sounds clear with good aeration in the apices and bases anteriorly
- BP: 118/74 mm Hg
- HR: 78 beats/min regular sinus rhythm on the monitor
- SpO$_2$: 98%
- Temperature: 37°C via Foley
- No arterial blood gas test today

8. On the basis of the above data, do you feel an SBT is appropriate at this time? Why, or why not?

9. Set up for a spontaneous breathing trial on the ventilator you are using. Have a partner simulate breathing at a rate of 12 to 20 breaths/min on your lung simulator. Fill out the ventilator flow sheet (Figure 25-3, *A* and *B*) with the new data.

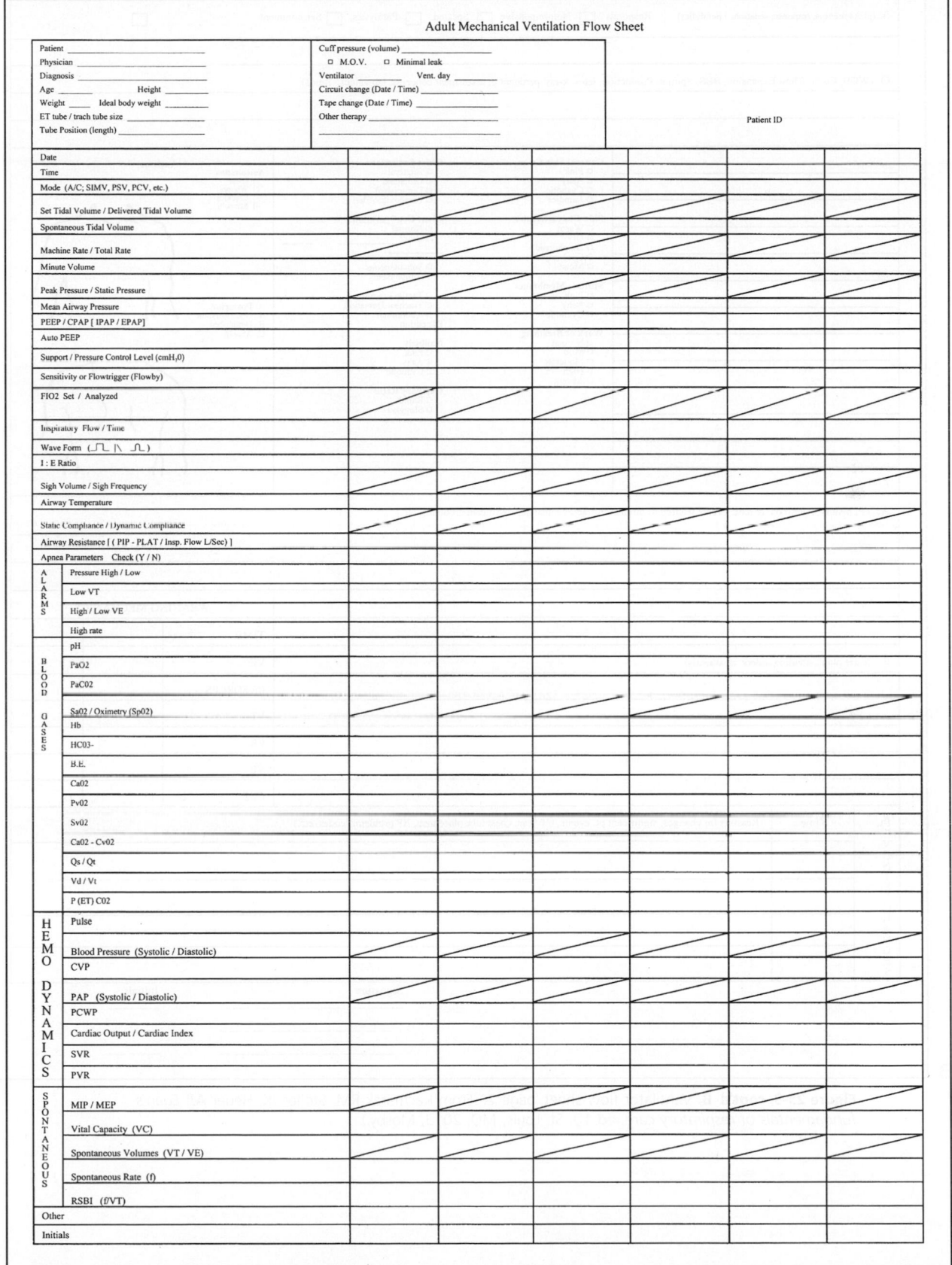

Adult Mechanical Ventilation Flow Sheet

Patient _____
Physician _____
Diagnosis _____
Age _____ Height _____
Weight _____ Ideal body weight _____
ET tube / trach tube size _____
Tube Position (length) _____

Cuff pressure (volume) _____
☐ M.O.V. ☐ Minimal leak
Ventilator _____ Vent. day _____
Circuit change (Date / Time) _____
Tape change (Date / Time) _____
Other therapy _____

Patient ID

Date						
Time						
Mode (A/C; SIMV, PSV, PCV, etc.)						
Set Tidal Volume / Delivered Tidal Volume						
Spontaneous Tidal Volume						
Machine Rate / Total Rate						
Minute Volume						
Peak Pressure / Static Pressure						
Mean Airway Pressure						
PEEP / CPAP [IPAP / EPAP]						
Auto PEEP						
Support / Pressure Control Level (cmH$_2$0)						
Sensitivity or Flowtrigger (Flowby)						
FIO2 Set / Analyzed						
Inspiratory Flow / Time						
Wave Form (⎍ ⃒\ ⎍)						
I : E Ratio						
Sigh Volume / Sigh Frequency						
Airway Temperature						
Static Compliance / Dynamic Compliance						
Airway Resistance [(PIP - PLAT / Insp. Flow L/Sec)]						
Apnea Parameters Check (Y / N)						
ALARMS Pressure High / Low						
Low VT						
High / Low VE						
High rate						
BLOOD GASES pH						
PaO2						
PaCO2						
SaO2 / Oximetry (SpO2)						
Hb						
HCO3-						
B.E.						
CaO2						
PvO2						
SvO2						
CaO2 - CvO2						
Qs / Qt						
Vd / Vt						
P (ET) CO2						
HEMODYNAMICS Pulse						
Blood Pressure (Systolic / Diastolic)						
CVP						
PAP (Systolic / Diastolic)						
PCWP						
Cardiac Output / Cardiac Index						
SVR						
PVR						
SPONTANEOUS MIP / MEP						
Vital Capacity (VC)						
Spontaneous Volumes (VT / VE)						
Spontaneous Rate (f)						
RSBI (f/VT)						
Other						
Initials						

A

Figure 25-3 A, Ventilator flow sheet, page 1.

Continued

Adult Mechanical Ventilation Flow Sheet

Respiratory Care Progress Notes

S: (pt Awareness, response, sedations / paralytics)   Responds ☐   Non-responsive ☐   Sedated ☐   Paralytics ☐   See comment ☐   ☐

O: (WOB, Color, Chest Expansion, BBS, Sputum Production, latest x-ray, pertinent pt assessment concerns, lab values, fluids)

General Skin Color
☐ Pink
☐ Ashy
☐ Cyanotic
☐ Jaundice

Skin Characteristics
☐ Warm
☐ Dry
☐ Diaphoretic
☐ Cool
☐ Moist

Mucous Membranes
☐ Pink
☐ Ashy
☐ Cyanotic

Work of Breathing
☐ Normal
☐ Mild
☐ Moderate
☐ High
☐ Absent

Chest Excursion
☐ Bilateral
☐ Unilateral
☐ Diminished
☐ Paradoxical/Flail

Chest Configuration
☐ Normal
☐ Other_____

☐ Subcutaneous
   Emphysema

☐ Tactile Fremitus
☐ Tracheal Deviation
☐ Abdominal
Distention

Nailbeds
☐ Pink
☐ Ashy
☐ Cyanotic

Capillary Refill
☐ Rapid
☐ Sluggish

Anterior

Auscultation
1) Clear
2) Wheeze
3) Crackles
4) Rhonchi

Posterior
A. Good Aeration
B. Diminished
C. Absent

A: (Pt history, Admit dx. & date, events leading to intubation/trach/ventilation, significant problems, etc.)

P: (Care plan, standing orders, treatments)

WEANING MECHANICS		
TIME		
VC		
I/E FORCES		
VT		
RR		
VE		
f/VT		

Pt. EVENTS / CHANGES	Time	(Reasons for changes, significant pt. events, CT Scan, chest tube placement, BP problems, codes, etc.)

Signature   Initials
_____   _____
_____   _____
_____   _____

B

Figure 25-3, cont'd B, Ventilator flow sheet, page 2. (From Kacmarek RM, Stoller JK, Heuer AJ: *Egan's fundamentals of respiratory care*, ed 10, St. Louis, MO, 2013, Mosby.)

Self-Assessment Questions

1. Methods for discontinuing ventilatory support include:

   1. CPAP
   2. Airway pressure release ventilation
   3. SIMV
   4. PSV

   A. 1 only
   B. 1 and 3 only
   C. 1, 2, and 4 only
   D. 1, 3, and 4 only

2. The long-term need for ventilatory support, usually longer than 2 weeks, is termed:
   A. Terminal mechanical ventilation
   B. Ventilator dependence
   C. Increased ventilatory workload
   D. Weaning indices

3. Successful discontinuation of ventilatory support includes improvement and monitoring of:

   1. Oxygenation status
   2. Cardiovascular function
   3. Ventilatory workload versus capacity
   4. Normalcy of arterial blood gases

   A. 1 and 2 only
   B. 1 and 4 only
   C. 1, 2, and 3 only
   D. 1, 2, 3, and 4

4. The most important criterion to consider when evaluating for ventilator discontinuation or weaning is:
   A. Arterial blood gas values
   B. Weaning mode
   C. Therapist-driven protocols
   D. Alleviation or reversal of condition that necessitated initiation of mechanical ventilation

5. The rapid shallow breathing index is:
   A. Frequency/tidal volume (f/V_T)
   B. $P_{0.1}$
   C. Work of breathing (WOB)
   D. $P_{0.1}/MIP$

6. What percentage of patients removed from ventilatory support experience severe respiratory distress that necessitates the reinstitution of mechanical ventilation?
   A. 2%
   B. 5%
   C. 15%
   D. 25%

7. Following disconnection from the ventilator and extubation, your patient begins experiencing shortness of breath and stridor. What medication is appropriate at this time?
   A. Albuterol
   B. Nebulized racemic epinephrine
   C. Atrovent
   D. Tobramycin (TOBI)

8. Terminal weaning is a decision made exclusively by the treating pulmonologist.
   A. True
   B. False

9. An important element in managing respiratory muscle fatigue is properly nourishing the patient and replacing depleted electrolytes.
   A. True
   B. False

10. All SBTs must be performed for a minimum of 2 hours.
    A. True
    B. False

▶▶ CASE STUDY 25-1

Mr. T is a 79-year-old man with congestive heart failure, chronic obstructive pulmonary disease (COPD), and end-stage renal failure, which requires hemodialysis. He had lived on an Indian reservation in upstate New York before moving to Phoenix, Arizona, for relief from the cold weather. He lives with his daughter. At the time he was admitted to the hospital, he had been planning to meet with an oncologist that his pulmonologist referred him to following an abnormal chest x-ray. His shortness of breath has been worsening over the last month, and he has been hospitalized two times in the last 5 weeks for exacerbation of his COPD. While eating breakfast with a friend, he developed severe dyspnea, and the paramedics were called. He was brought to the emergency room, where he was found to be unresponsive. He was intubated and admitted to the intensive care unit (ICU). Despite optimal mechanical ventilation over the last 10 days, he remains unable to breathe without a ventilator and requires medications to maintain his blood pressure. He is not responsive to his daughter's voice or any simple commands.

1. Define the term *terminal weaning*.

_____

_____

2. What are some determinants of the decision to withdraw ventilation?

_____

_____

■ OBJECTIVES

Upon the completion of the chapter activities and content review topics, the student should be able to:

1. Identify indications for continuous positive airway pressure.
2. Initiate and assess neonatal and pediatric noninvasive positive pressure ventilation.
3. Identify indications for invasive mechanical ventilation.
4. Describe the complications associated with intubation.
5. Initiate and assess neonatal and pediatric invasive mechanical ventilation.
6. Initiate and assess high-frequency positive pressure ventilation, both high-frequency jet ventilation and high-frequency oscillatory ventilation.

■ KEY TERMS

- Bilevel positive airway pressure (BiPAP)
- Continuous positive airway pressure (CPAP)
- High-frequency oscillatory ventilation (HFOV)
- High-frequency jet ventilation (HFJV)
- Positive end-expiratory pressure (PEEP)

■ CONTENT REVIEW TOPICS

- Administration of surfactant
- Closing pressure
- Lung recruitment
- Neonatal and pediatric resuscitation and ventilation
- Opening pressure
- Pulmonary compliance

■ PROCEDURAL ASSESSMENTS

26-1 Initiating Neonatal and Pediatric Noninvasive Positive Pressure Ventilation

26-2 Assessing the Neonatal and Pediatric Noninvasive Positive Pressure Ventilation System

26-3 Initiating Neonatal and Pediatric Mechanical Ventilation

26-4 Assessing the Neonatal and Pediatric Ventilator System

26-5 Initiating High-Frequency Ventilation

■ EQUIPMENT

- Circuits
- Compressed air source
- Compressed oxygen source
- CPAP or BiPAP ventilator
- Disposable gloves
- Interfaces
- Intubated human patient simulator, if available
- Test lungs or lung simulator
- Neonatal and pediatric mechanical ventilator(s)

The use of mechanical ventilation is one of the most significant advances in the history of medicine, enabling therapies, procedures, and interventions in an incredibly wide array of otherwise unrelated subspecialties. Nearly all of the critical care and surgical interventions we currently provide would be impossible or prohibitively difficult without the use of mechanical ventilation. Many thousands, even millions, of lives have likely been saved because of this technology. However, the use of mechanical ventilation also brings with it a host of associated problems and complications. Referencing the delicate nature of the appropriate use of mechanical ventilation, and obviously indulging in a bit of hyperbole, a respected mentor of the author of this chapter once referred to the mechanical ventilator as "the single deadliest instrument ever placed in the hands of physicians" (and respiratory therapists [RTs]). As such, the appropriate selection of patients for, management of, and ultimate timely liberation from mechanical ventilation can dramatically affect patient outcomes.

→ **Reality Check** Implementing and managing mechanical ventilation in neonates and children may be even more difficult than in adults.

The history of pediatric mechanical ventilation is rich, originating, for the most part, in the early twentieth century. Alexander Graham Bell in 1889 described his design for a neonatal ventilator. Recognizing the need for assisted ventilation in neonates with surfactant deficiency, he said, "Many children, especially those prematurely born, die from inability to expand their lungs sufficiently when they take their first breath. I have no doubt that in many of those cases, lives could be saved by starting the respiration artificially by means of apparatus operating in the manner described above." The history of mechanical ventilator use in the 1920s during the polio epidemic is generally well known. Subsequently, many advances in mechanical ventilation have come from pediatric and neonatal applications, including some of the first uses of continuous positive airway pressure (CPAP) and high-frequency ventilation (HFV).

The broad range of patient sizes, diagnoses, and unique anatomies leads to added levels of complexity when initiating or managing mechanical ventilation in a neonate, infant, or child. Pediatric respiratory care is truly a specialty in and of itself. This chapter intends to outline the basics of a number of neonatal and pediatric respiratory procedures and competencies. It is hoped that understanding of the procedures in this chapter will provide a fundamental knowledge for the RT caring for children needing mechanical ventilation. It is also expected that this understanding will result in safer, higher-quality care for children and will transform the ventilator from a ventilatory device to a safe, reliable tool in the hands of a skilled RT.

>> SKILL CHECK LISTS

26-1 Initiation of Neonatal and Pediatric Noninvasive Positive Pressure Ventilation

Noninvasive positive pressure ventilation is a life-saving intervention in neonatal and pediatric care. The ability to non-invasively provide respiratory support, improve upper and lower airway patency, and improve lung recruitment has proven invaluable. Noninvasive support can be utilized simply as CPAP or as bilevel positive airway pressure (BiPAP), with additional inspiratory pressure added to spontaneous or controlled breaths. Widespread use of nasal CPAP has reduced intubation times, intubation rates, pulmonary morbidity, and bronchopulmonary dysplasia rates dramatically in neonates. Pediatric applications of both CPAP and BiPAP, including those in acute lung injury, asthma, and postoperative conditions, have also resulted in significant improvements in care. Indications for CPAP in children are listed in Box 26-1.

Noninvasive positive pressure ventilation is positive pressure applied to the upper oropharynx through a noninvasive interface, providing improved pulmonary mechanics and modest lung recruitment. Interfaces are varied but include nasal prongs, nasal masks, nasal–oral masks, full-face masks, and helmets. Images of these interfaces are given in Figure 26-1. The effort required to adequately set up a CPAP interface is well worth it, as avoiding intubation and its attendant complications is a worthy goal. A respiratory therapist skilled in the application of noninvasive ventilator interventions is invaluable in a pediatric or neonatal unit. The following is the step-by-step process for initiating neonatal and pediatric noninvasive positive pressure ventilation.

> → **Reality Check** CPAP is generally well tolerated, but achieving an adequate seal of the mask may be tricky. Convincing a toddler that strapping a mask over the mouth and nose is a good idea can be, in a word, difficult.

Procedural Preparation

1. Review the patient's chart.
2. Verify the physician's order or the facility's protocol for standard of care.
3. Obtain, clean, inspect, and test the appropriate equipment prior to entering the patient's room.
4. Follow personal protective equipment (PPE) requirements, and observe standard precautions for any transmission-based isolation procedure.
5. Identify the patient using two patient identifiers.
6. Introduce yourself to the patient and to the family.
7. Explain the procedure to the patient and to the family, and acknowledge the patient's understanding.
8. Perform proper hand hygiene, and put on gloves, mask, and protective eyewear, as appropriate for the procedure.

Implementation

1. Place the patient in a comfortable position.
2. Assess vital signs.
3. Assess the upper airway for abnormalities.
4. Obtain the interface and the securing devices.
5. Establish and implement the appropriate settings or execute the physician's orders:
   a. CPAP level
   b. Inspiratory positive airway pressure (IPAP) and expiratory positive airway pressure (EPAP) levels (if ordered)
   c. Rate (if ordered)
   d. Fractional inspired oxygen (FIO_2)
6. Apply and secure the device to the patient.
7. Ensure suitable fit and minimal leak.
8. Ensure patient comfort.
9. Reassess vital signs.
10. Set the alarms appropriately.
11. Set up the noninvasive monitors.
12. Remove the supplies from the patient's room, and clean the area, as needed.
13. Remove PPE, and perform proper hand hygiene prior to leaving the patient's room.

Evaluation of Procedure

1. Establish a baseline, or compare with previous measurements.

BOX 26-1	Indications for Continuous Positive Airway Pressure in Children

Respiratory Distress
- Tachypnea
- Retractions or accessory muscle use
- Grunting
- Nasal flaring
- Head bobbing

Abnormal Breathing Patterns
- Apnea of prematurity
- Obstructive sleep apnea

Lung Disease
- Decreased lung volumes on chest radiography
- Pneumonia
- Tracheomalacia
- Pulmonary edema
- PaO_2 <50 mm Hg, with FIO_2 ≥0.60

Other
- Postextubation failure

From Kacmarek RM, Stoller JK, Heuer AJ: *Egan's fundamentals of respiratory care*, ed 10, St. Louis, MO, 2013, Mosby-Elsevier.

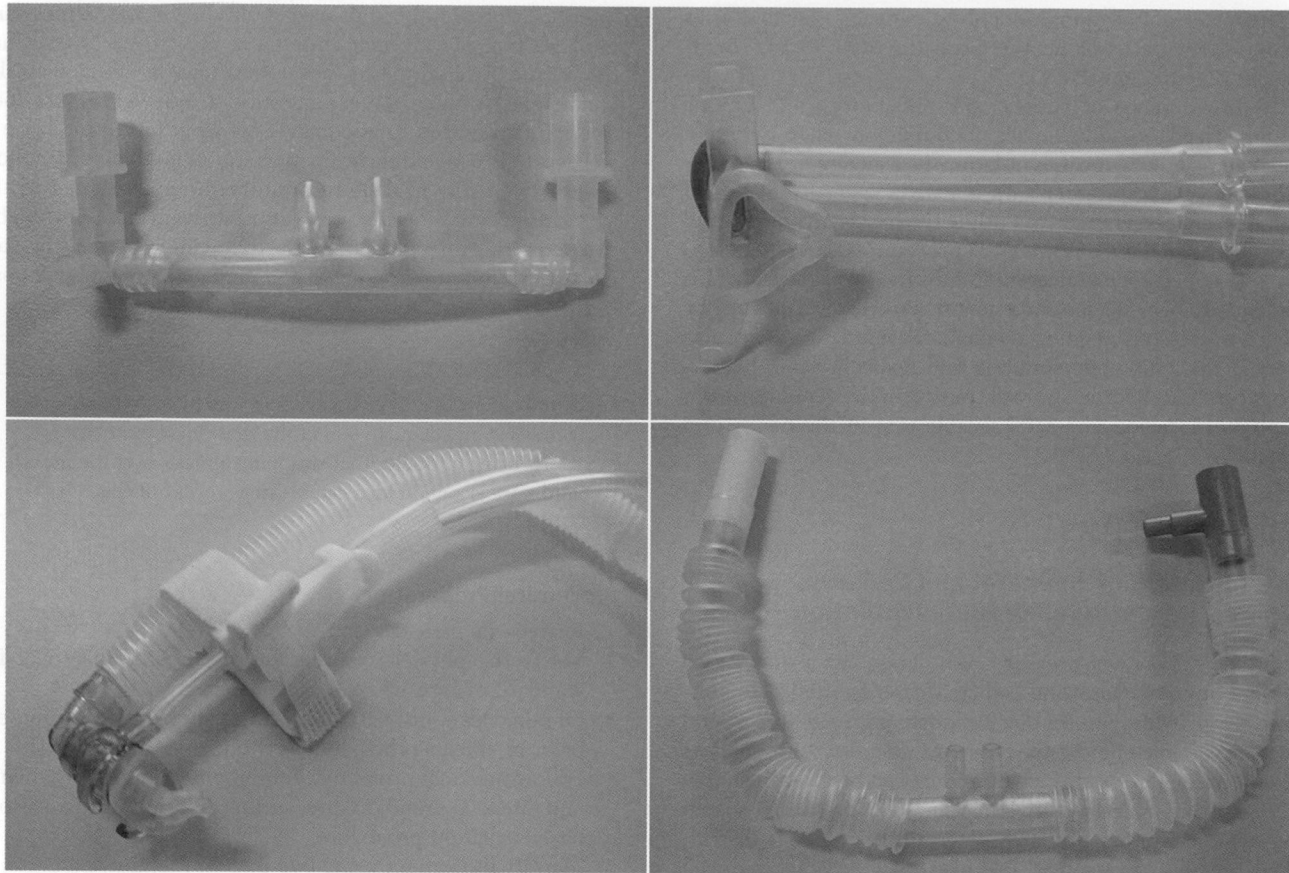

Figure 26-1 Patient interfaces for CPAP and NPPV. (From Kacmarek RM, Stoller JK, Heuer AJ: *Egan's fundamentals of respiratory care*, ed 10, St. Louis, MO, 2013, Mosby-Elsevier.)

2. Develop an appropriate respiratory care plan based on assessment data.
3. Identify any unexpected outcomes.

Documentation and Reporting

1. Record your findings in the patient's chart.
2. Report any abnormal findings to the appropriate health care provider.

26-2 Assessing the Neonatal and Pediatric Noninvasive Positive Pressure Ventilation System

Appropriate monitoring of the adequacy of therapy is important for any respiratory intervention, but for noninvasive respiratory support, it is even more critical. The odds of a child of any age being continuously compliant with a therapy that involves blowing liters of air up the nose every minute are extremely slim. Added to this difficulty is the fact that most masks are not well designed for children, which creates extremely challenging problems with leak management. Considering all these factors together, the astute RT needs to pay frequent attention to the adequacy of therapy when a noninvasive positive pressure system is utilized on any pediatric patient. Constant communication between the RT, the bedside nurse, and the ordering physician is critical to the continued success of the management of noninvasive respiratory support in children. The following is the step-by-step process for

assessing the neonatal and pediatric noninvasive positive pressure ventilation system.

> → **Reality Check** A perfectly functioning system may go awry in seconds because of a child rolling over, pulling the mask off, or crying and fighting the delivery of the support.

Procedural Preparation

1. Review the patient's chart for the patient's current vital signs and NIV settings.
2. Review the patient's most recent arterial blood gas (ABG) or SpO$_2$ values.
3. Review the most recent chest radiograph.
4. Identify the current sedation medications.
5. Verify the physician's order or the facility's protocol for standard of care.
6. Obtain, clean, and inspect the appropriate equipment prior to entering the patient's room.
7. Follow PPE requirements, and observe standard precautions for any transmission-based isolation procedure.
8. Identify the patient using two patient identifiers.
9. Introduce yourself to the patient and to the family.
10. Explain the procedure to the patient and to the family, and acknowledge the patient's understanding.
11. Perform proper hand hygiene, and put on gloves, mask, and protective eyewear, as appropriate for the procedure.

Implementation

1. Approach the patient before you approach the CPAP generator.
2. Assess the patient:
   a. Overall appearance and comfort
   b. Nasal prong or mask position
   c. Skin integrity at all contact points
   d. Breath sounds; suction, if indicated
   e. Chest-rise
   f. Peripheral pulses
   g. Indwelling catheter(s)
   h. Chest tubes
   i. Need for oral care
3. Assess the NIV generator function and settings:
   a. Security of circuit connections
   b. Heat and humidification device and airway temperature
   c. Adequacy of seal
   d. Adequacy of delivery of tidal volume
   e. Pressure level(s), depending on mode:
      i. CPAP level
      ii. IPAP and EPAP levels
   f. Set frequency
   g. Spontaneous frequency
   h. Flow rate
   i. Set F_{IO_2}
   j. Analyzed F_{IO_2}
   k. Monitoring of alarms
4. Ensure that the manual ventilation device and the suction equipment are available at the patient's bedside.
5. Remove the supplies from the patient's room, and clean the area, as needed.
6. Remove PPE, and perform proper hand hygiene prior to leaving the patient's room.

Evaluation of Procedure

1. Establish a baseline, or compare with previous measurements.
2. Develop an appropriate respiratory care plan based on assessment data.
3. Identify any unexpected outcomes.

Documentation and Reporting

1. Record your findings in the patient's chart.
2. Report any abnormal findings to the appropriate health care provider.

26-3 Initiating Neonatal and Pediatric Mechanical Ventilation

The initiation of neonatal or pediatric mechanical ventilation begins with the decision to intubate or not intubate a patient. Clinical indications for mechanical ventilation and initial ventilator settings are given in Boxes 26-2 and 26-3. This decision is difficult and has many implications, as intubating too early or too late may both result in increased patient morbidity. Complications and hazards of endotracheal intubation in infants and children are listed in Box 26-4. In general, it is a well-tolerated and safe procedure when done with care and attention to detail. The RT plays a key role in the proper

initiation of pediatric mechanical ventilation, and the establishment of age-appropriate and disease-appropriate therapeutic goals at the outset of therapy.

The actual procedure for the initiation of pediatric and neonatal ventilation is, in a number of ways, more complex than the same procedure in adults. A number of complicating factors include wide variations in patient size, the question regarding the need to utilize a cuffed endotracheal tube (ETT), less "wiggle room" in the placement of the ETT, difficulty with tube placement because of the small size of the oropharyngeal opening, and many others. In addition, age-related factors may be critical to understanding and properly managing pediatric mechanical ventilation. Table 26-1 illustrates ETT sizes based on weight, along with formulas to estimate size (Box 26-5). For example, for premature infants or children with congenital heart disease, oxygenation goals may be set at a significantly lower level than that for an adult. Consideration for the patient's developmental and physical maturational state, as well as physiologic status and attendant pathophysiology, is essential. The following is the step-by-step process for initiating neonatal and pediatric mechanical ventilation.

Procedural Preparation

1. Review the patient's chart.
2. Verify the physician's order or the facility's protocol for standard of care.
3. Obtain, clean, and inspect the appropriate equipment prior to entering the patient's room.
4. Follow PPE requirements, and observe standard precautions for any transmission-based isolation procedure.
5. Identify the patient using two patient identifiers.
6. Introduce yourself to the patient and to the family.
7. Explain the procedure to the patient and to the family, and acknowledge the patient's understanding.
8. Perform proper hand hygiene, and put on gloves, mask, and protective eyewear, as appropriate for the procedure.

Implementation

1. Place the patient in a comfortable position.
2. Assess vital signs.
3. Establish an airway:
   a. Ensure or consult on the proper tube size for the procedure.
   b. Ensure proper depth of tube placement.
   c. Assist with or perform the tube securing procedure.
4. Establish and implement the appropriate settings or execute the physician's orders:
   a. Mode
   b. Tidal volume or inspiratory pressure
   c. Frequency
   d. Inspiratory time
   e. Inspiratory rise time
   f. Flow pattern
   g. PEEP level
   h. F_{IO_2}
   i. Pressure support
   j. Inspiratory cycle off % or ventilator specific equivalent
   k. Trigger
5. Reassess vital signs.
6. Set the alarms appropriately.
7. Remove the supplies from the patient's room, and clean the area, as needed.

BOX 26-2 Clinical Indications for (But Not Limited to) Mechanical Ventilation

Pulmonary Disorders

Restrictive Process

- Respiratory distress syndrome
- Acute respiratory distress syndrome
- Pulmonary hemorrhage
- Pulmonary hypoplasia or agenesis
- Congenital pneumonia
- Pneumothorax or air leaks
- Pleural effusion or chylothorax
- Aspiration syndromes (blood, amniotic fluid)
- Flail chest
- Bronchopleural fistula
- Abdominal distension
- Diaphragmatic hernia
- Congenital lung cysts; tumors
- Rib cage anomalies
- Extrinsic masses

Obstructive Process

- Meconium aspiration
- Congenital lobar emphysema
- Asthma
- Bronchiolitis
- Cystic fibrosis
- Bronchopulmonary dysplasia

Airway

- Laryngomalacia
- Tracheomalacia
- Choanal atresia
- Pierre Robin syndrome
- Micrognathia
- Nasopharyngeal tumor
- Subglottic stenosis

Extrapulmonary Disorders

Neurologic and Muscular Disorders

- Myasthenia gravis
- Muscular dystrophy
- Guillain-Barré syndrome
- Cerebral edema
- Cerebral hemorrhage
- Spinal cord injury or disease
- Phrenic nerve damage

Hypoventilation

- Sleep apnea
- Overdose or poisoning
- Postoperative recovery

Increased Intracranial Pressure

- Infection
- Head trauma
- Near-drowning
- Reye's syndrome

Cardiovascular Dysfunction

- Cardiac shunting
- Cyanotic heart disease
- Circulatory collapse
- Hypovolemia
- Anemia
- Polycythemia
- Congestive heart failure
- Postoperative cardiac surgery
- Persistent pulmonary hypertension

Metabolic

- Acidosis
- Hypoglycemia
- Hypothermia
- Hyperthermia

From Walsh BK, Czervinske MP, DiBlasi RM: *Perinatal and pediatric respiratory care*, ed 3, St. Louis, MO, 2010, Saunders.

BOX 26-3 Calculation of Effective Tidal Volume

$$V_{Teff} = V_{Tset} - [(Pstatic* - PEEP) \times Circuit]$$

Determination of Compliance Factor of Circuit

1. With the circuit assembled and connected to the ventilator, the connection of the patient to the circuit is occluded.
2. A known volume of gas is delivered into the circuit through the ventilator, and the resulting peak inspiratory pressure is noted.
3. The resulting pressure is divided by the delivered volume to obtain the compliance factor of the circuit. This is generally 1 mL/cm H_2O for infant circuits and 2 to 3 mL/cm H_2O for larger circuits.

*If static or plateau pressure measurement cannot be obtained because of airway leaks, the peak inspiratory pressure may be used as an approximation. *Circuit*, Compliance or compression factor of circuit; *PEEP*, positive end-expiratory pressure set on ventilator; P_{static}, static (plateau) pressure measured during inflation; V_{Teff}, effective tidal volume; V_{Tset}, tidal volume set on ventilator. (From Walsh BK, Czervinske MP, DiBlasi RM: *Perinatal and pediatric respiratory care*, ed 3, St. Louis, MO, 2010, Saunders.)

BOX 26-4 Complications and Hazards of Endotracheal Intubation in Infants and Children

Palatal grooving (neonates)
Incisal enamel hypoplasia
Accidental extubation
Tube blockage
Tracheal stenosis
Esophageal perforation
Tracheal perforation

BOX 26-5 Estimating Catheter Sizes

Estimating Formula for Tube Internal Diameter (ID) in Minutes:

Tube ID = (Age + 16) ÷ 4
Tube ID = Height (cm) ÷ 20

Estimating Formula for Tube Length in Centimeters:

Oral: 12 + (Age ÷ 2)
Nasal: 15 + (Age ÷ 2)

TABLE 26-1 Endotracheal Tube and Suction Catheter Sizes for Infants and Children

Age or Weight	ETT Internal Diameter (mm)	Tube Length (cm) Oral	Tube Length (cm) Nasal	Suction Catheter (F)
NEWBORN				
<1000 g	2.5	9–11	11–12	6
1000–2000 g	3	9–11	11–12	6
2000–3000 g	3.5	10–12	12–14	6
>3000 g	4	11–12	13–14	8
CHILDREN				
6 months	3–4	11–12	12–14	6–8
18 months	3.5–4.5	11–13	13–15	8
2 years	4–5	12–14	14–16	8–10
3–5 years	4.5–5.5	12–15	14–17	8–10
6 years	5.5–6	14–16	16–18	10
8 years	6–6.5	15–17	17–19	10–12
12 years	6–7	17–19	19–21	10–12
16 years	6.5–7.5	19–21	21–23	10–12

From Kacmarek RM, Stoller JK, Heuer AJ: *Egan's fundamentals of respiratory care*, ed 10, St. Louis, MO, 2013, Mosby.

8. Remove PPE, and perform proper hand hygiene prior to leaving the patient's room.

Evaluation of Procedure

1. Establish a baseline, or compare with previous measurements.
2. Develop an appropriate respiratory care plan based on assessment data.
3. Identify any unexpected outcomes.

Documentation and Reporting

1. Record your findings in the patient's chart.
2. Report any abnormal findings to the appropriate health care provider.

26-4 Assessing the Neonatal and Pediatric Ventilator System

The status of neonatal and pediatric patients can change dramatically within a very short period. Neonates with surfactant deficiency, once provided with exogenous surfactant, can have dramatic changes in pulmonary compliance very quickly. In the postoperative period, pediatric patients with cardiac disease may have rapid changes in pulmonary blood flow and intrathoracic volume and pressure. Pediatric patients with asthma can have rapid and dramatic responses to treatment or worsening of disease. Many other examples exist, but they all point to the critical need for the bedside RT to closely and frequently scrutinize all aspects of a patient's mechanical ventilator therapies. In addition, patient–ventilator synchrony is extremely difficult to achieve in children, given their inability to participate voluntarily with many interventions as well as their relatively small flow rates and patient-generated pressure changes.

> ✳ **Tip** Timely weaning and liberation from mechanical ventilation should be a goal at the forefront of every RTs mind when caring for infants and children. The faster the children can be safely extubated, the better off they will be.

Time spent on a mechanical ventilator is the single biggest determinant of length of stay in the intensive care unit (ICU); pulmonary morbidities, including ventilator-associated pneumonia; and ICU morbidities, including catheter-related bloodstream infections. As such, every pediatric and neonatal patient requires frequent and thoughtful reevaluation and assessment of his or her current ventilator needs. Dr. Thomas Petty once said, "Intermittent mandatory cerebration (IMC) is the preferred method of mechanical ventilation. Even better, continuous mandatory contemplation (CMC) must emerge as the preferred method used in all forms of respiratory care." To the bedside practitioner, what this means is that at every assessment, we must ask ourselves if the current therapy is appropriate, whether the current therapy can be more optimally configured for the patient, and whether the patient can be weaned from or taken off the ventilator. Significantly, the bedside RT is in the unique position to do the most in these situations. Physicians generally are pulled in too many directions to adequately assess and thoughtfully adjust ventilator settings on a real-time basis, and bedside nurses, at least in the United States, often do not pay specific attention to the details of the ventilator. It is up to the RT to advocate for the mechanically ventilated patient. The following is the step-by-step process for assessing the neonatal and pediatric ventilator system.

Procedural Preparation

1. Review the patient's chart for the patient's current vital signs and ventilator settings.
2. Review the patient's most recent ABG or SpO$_2$ values.
3. Review the patient's most recent chest radiograph.
4. Identify the current sedation medications.
5. Verify the physician's order or the facility's protocol for standard of care.
6. Obtain, clean, and inspect the appropriate equipment prior to entering the patient's room.
7. Follow PPE requirements, and observe standard precautions for any transmission-based isolation procedure.
8. Identify the patient using two patient identifiers.

9. Introduce self to the patient and to the family.
10. Explain the procedure to the patient and to the family, and acknowledge the patient's understanding.
11. Perform proper hand hygiene, and put on gloves, mask, and protective eyewear, as appropriate for the procedure.

Implementation

1. Approach and assess the patient before assessing ventilator functions and settings.
2. Assess the patient:
   a. Overall appearance, comfort, and ventilator synchrony
   b. Airway position, patency, and security
   c. Breath sounds; suction, if indicated
   d. Chest-rise
   e. Peripheral pulses
   f. Indwelling catheter(s)
   g. Chest tubes
   h. Head of bed elevated by at least 30 degrees
   i. Need for oral care
3. Assess the ventilator function and settings:
   a. Security of circuit connections
   b. Heat and humidification device; airway temperature
   c. Mode
   d. V_T or inspiratory pressure
   e. Exhaled tidal volume
   f. Set frequency
   g. Spontaneous frequency
   h. Inspiratory time
   i. Flow rate
   j. Flow pattern
   k. Mean airway pressure (MAP)
   l. PEEP level
   m. Set FIO_2
   n. Analyzed FIO_2
   o. Pressure support
   p. Trigger
   q. Monitoring of alarms
   r. Static compliance (C_S) calculation
4. Ensure that the manual ventilation device and the suction equipment are available at the patient's bedside.
5. Ensure that replacement tracheostomy tubes are available at the patient's bedside.
6. Remove the supplies from the patient's room, and clean the area, as needed.
7. Remove PPE, and perform proper hand hygiene prior to leaving the patient's room.

Evaluation of Procedure

1. Establish a baseline, or compare with previous measurements.
2. Develop an appropriate respiratory care plan based on assessment data.
3. Ensure that lung protective therapy is in place.
4. Consider discontinuation of mechanical ventilation or weaning.
5. Identify any unexpected outcomes.

Documentation and Reporting

1. Record your findings in the patient's chart.
2. Report any abnormal findings to appropriate health care provider.

26-5 Initiating High-Frequency Ventilation

HFV is one of a number of respiratory care techniques pioneered largely in the pediatric realm. Today, HFV has emerged as a common tool in respiratory care and truly is the ultimate application of a low-tidal volume, adequate recruitment ventilator strategy. It allows for high mean airway pressures without high alveolar peak pressures, theoretically minimizing the deleterious effects of mechanical ventilation. Effective tidal volumes in HFV are significantly smaller than the anatomic dead space. Ventilation is achieved through effective gas admixture throughout the respiratory tree because of the high velocities of injected gas bursts, resulting in continuous gas exchange, rather than tidal gas exchange as normally occurs during mechanical ventilation. Combined with a constant mean airway pressure for lung recruitment, HFV is extremely effective in a variety of clinical situations. Although definitive evidence of the therapeutic superiority of HFV over low-tidal volume strategies is lacking, many investigations show that HFV may be equally effective and safe compared with conventional strategies.

> → **Reality Check** The history of the development of HFV is fascinating, with the original concept coming from observations of the effectiveness of canine panting. It was developed because of the need for a form of mechanical ventilation that did not affect a subject's hemodynamics. Stereo speakers were used in its first implementation!

A number of forms of HFV exist, but we are focusing on the two most common: (1) jet ventilation and (2) oscillatory ventilation. High-frequency jet ventilation (HFJV) utilizes injection of a high-velocity stream of gas from an in-line jet. The jet is usually placed in the ventilator circuit just proximal to the patient's ETT, through use of a specialized ETT connector (Figure 26-2). Jet parameters, including rate, peak

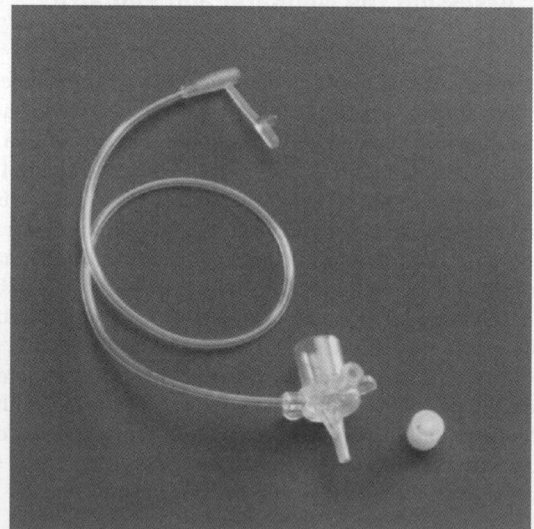

Figure 26-2 LifePort endotracheal tube (ETT) adapter. Jet pulses are delivered through the side lumen of the ETT. Connection to a conventional ventilator is provided at the proximal ETT opening. This ETT adaptor made specifically for this device now makes reintubation optional. (Courtesy of Bunnell Inc., Salt Lake City, UT.)

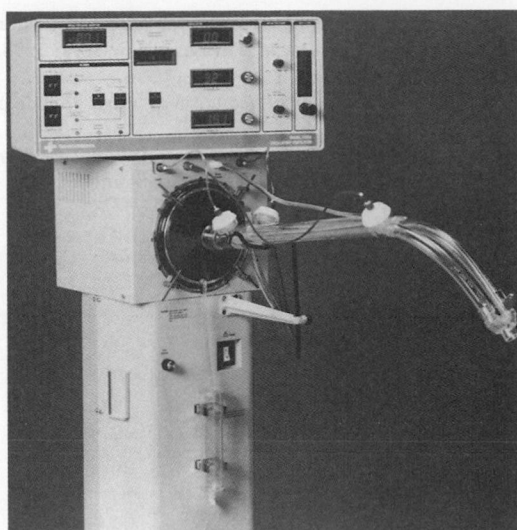

Figure 26-3 A high-frequency oscillatory ventilator (SensorMedics 3100A). (From Walsh BK, Czervinske MP, DiBlasi RM. *Perinatal and pediatric respiratory care*, ed 3, St. Louis, MO, 2010, Saunders.)

inspiratory pressure (PIP), and inspiratory time (I-time), are set on the jet ventilator, and a conventional ventilator is used to provide PEEP and "sigh" breaths, if desired. The MAP is determined from a combination of the PEEP and the injected jet PIP and is displayed on the jet ventilator. Of note, jet ventilation can also be of use in emergency situations when an airway cannot be achieved, through a needle or catheter in the cricothyroid membrane or through a small-bore tube exchanger. Generally, HFJV is thought to be useful in patients with severely compromised lung compliance, air leak syndrome, or both. Of note, current widely available HFJV technology does not allow for effective use in patients weighing over 15 to 20 kg.

High-frequency oscillatory ventilation (HFOV) is the most widely used HFV in children and adults (Figure 26-3). In HFOV, injected air flow is achieved through the use of an oscillating pump or diaphragm, connected just proximal to the ETT, with continuous bias flow and a low-pass downstream filter. Oscillation of the diaphragm in the ventilator results in a sinusoidal wave of gas, with an active expiration phase. Gas is essentially "pushed" and "pulled" in and out of the patient, at usual rates of 240 breaths/min; 4 Hz in larger patients to 840 breaths/min (14 Hz) in neonates. No conventional ventilator is necessary, and the MAP and PIP are set on the oscillatory ventilator. The I-time is usually left at 33%. HFOV is most often used in situations similar to those in which HFJV is used, namely, severely compromised pulmonary compliance as well as air leak syndrome. Significantly, however, HFOV is the HFV mode of choice for larger children and adults, as there is no size restriction on its use. The following is the step-by-step process for HFV.

Procedural Preparation

1. Review the patient's chart.
2. Verify the physician's order or the facility's protocol for standard of care.
3. Obtain, clean, and inspect the appropriate equipment prior to entering the patient's room.

4. Follow PPE requirements, and observe standard precautions for any transmission-based isolation procedure.
5. Identify the patient using two patient identifiers.
6. Introduce yourself to the patient and to the family.
7. Explain the procedure to the patient and to the family, and acknowledge the patient's understanding.
8. Perform proper hand hygiene, and put on gloves, mask, and protective eyewear, as appropriate for the procedure.

Implementation

1. Place the patient in a comfortable position.
2. Assess baseline data:
   a. Ventilatory status
   b. Oxygenation status
   c. Circulatory status
3. Ensure patency of the ETT.
4. Suction the patient, if needed.
5. Perform a recruitment maneuver of 35 to 40 centimeters of water (cmH$_2$O) for 30 to 40 seconds.
6. Establish and implement the appropriate settings or execute the physician's orders.
   For oscillation:
   a. Mean airway pressure
   b. Frequency:
      i. 9 to 14 Hz in neonates
      ii. 6 to 8 Hz in children
      iii. 4 to 6 Hz in older patients
   c. FIO$_2$
   d. Amplitude (delta P [ΔP])
   e. Inspiratory time %
   f. Bias flow
   For jet ventilation:
   a. Mean airway pressure and PEEP
   b. Rate of jet ventilator
      i. 420 breaths/min (7 Hz) in neonates
      ii. 300 breaths/min (5 Hz) in children
   c. HFV on-time: Typically 0.02 seconds
   d. HFV PIP
   e. Rate of conventional ventilator
   f. Settings for conventional mechanical ventilator breaths
   g. FIO$_2$
   h. Servo pressure and MAP
7. Reassess vital signs.
8. Set the alarms appropriately.
9. Remove the supplies from the patient's room, and clean the area, as needed.
10. Remove PPE, and perform proper hand hygiene prior to leaving the patient's room.

Evaluation of Procedure

1. Establish a baseline, or compare with previous measurements.
2. Develop an appropriate respiratory care plan based on assessment data.
3. Consider addition of inhaled pulmonary vasodilator therapy.
4. Identify any unexpected outcomes.

Documentation and Reporting

1. Record your findings in the patient's chart.
2. Report any abnormal findings to the appropriate health care provider.

Bibliography

Fuhrman BP: *Pediatric critical care*, ed 4, St. Louis, MO, 2011, Saunders.

Kacmarek RM, Stoller JK, Heuer AJ: *Egan's fundamentals of respiratory care*, ed 10, St. Louis, MO, 2013, Mosby.

Lumb AB: *Nunn's applied respiratory physiology*, ed 7, London, UK, 2010, Churchill Livingstone.

Marini JJ: Physiological basis of ventilatory support. In Lenfant C, editor: *Lung biology in health and disease*, New York, 1998, Marcel Dekker.

Rennie JM: *Roberton's textbook of neonatology*, ed 4, Philadelphia, PA, 2005, Elsevier.

Walsh BK, Czervinske MP, DiBlasi RM: *Perinatal and pediatric respiratory care*, ed 3, St. Louis, MO, 2010, Saunders.

Lab Activities

1. Using a lung simulator and an infant CPAP device, initiate CPAP for a variety of patient sizes—neonatal, infant, toddler, and child. Have your instructor sign off once you complete the setup.

   a. Settings: _____

   Signature for 3-kg neonate with apnea of prematurity: _____

   b. Settings: _____

   Signature for 10-kg infant with tracheomalacia: _____

   c. Settings: _____

   Signature for 20-kg toddler with pulmonary edema: _____

   d. Settings: _____

   Signature for 30-kg child with postextubation failure: _____

2. Using a lung simulator and a neonatal or pediatric ventilator, initiate conventional mechanical ventilation for a variety of patient sizes—neonatal, infant, toddler, and child—selecting an appropriately sized airway.

   a. Weight in grams: _____

   Tube size: _____

   Settings:

   RR (breaths/min): _____

   V_T (mL/kg): _____

   Inspiratory time (seconds): _____

   PEEP (cmH$_2$O): _____

   F$_I$O$_2$: _____

   Signature for 2-kg neonate born at 27 weeks' gestation: _____

   b. Tube size: _____

   Settings:

   RR (breaths/min): _____

   V_T (mL/kg): _____

   Inspiratory time (seconds): _____

   PEEP (cmH$_2$O): _____

   F$_I$O$_2$: _____

   Signature for 10-kg toddler with pneumonia: _____

   c. Tube size: _____

     Settings:

     RR (breaths/min): _____

     V_T (mL/kg): _____

     Inspiratory time (seconds): _____

     PEEP (cmH_2O): _____

     FiO_2: _____

     Signature for 20-kg small child, following cardiac valve repair:_____

   d. Tube size: _____

     Settings:

     RR (breaths/min): _____

     V_T (mL/kg): _____

     Inspiratory time (seconds): _____

     PEEP (cmH_2O): _____

     FiO_2: _____

     Signature for 30-kg child, following an accidental drug overdose:_____

  Fill out a ventilator flow sheet (Figure 26-4) for this patient.

3. Imagine the patient represented in lab activity 2b failed to respond to conventional mechanical ventilation. Initiate HFOV. Use the same ventilator flow sheet in Figure 26-4 to document your settings. Have your instructor sign off on your flow sheet once you complete the setup. Work with a lab partner.

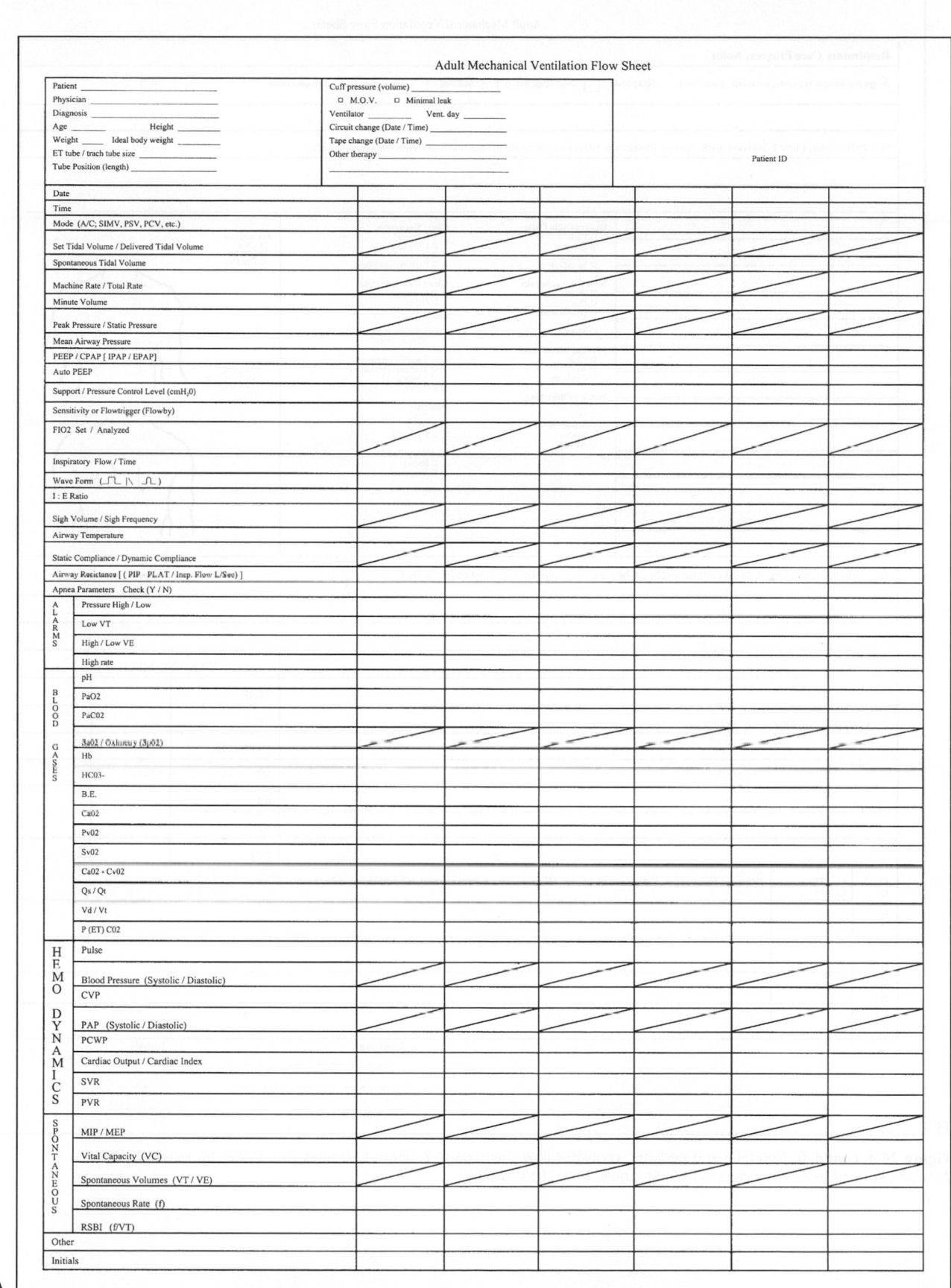

Figure 26-4 A, Neonatal and pediatric ventilator flow sheet, page 1.

Continued

Adult Mechanical Ventilation Flow Sheet

Respiratory Care Progress Notes

S: (pt Awareness, response, sedations / paralytics) Responds ☐ Non-responsive ☐ Sedated ☐ Paralytics ☐ See comment ☐

O: (WOB, Color, Chest Expansion, BBS, Sputum Production, latest x-ray, pertinent pt assessment concerns, lab values, fluids)

General Skin Color
☐ Pink
☐ Ashy
☐ Cyanotic
☐ Jaundice

Skin Characteristics
☐ Warm
☐ Dry
☐ Diaphoretic
☐ Cool
☐ Moist

Mucous Membranes
☐ Pink
☐ Ashy
☐ Cyanotic

Work of Breathing
☐ Normal
☐ Mild
☐ Moderate
☐ High
☐ Absent

Chest Excursion
☐ Bilateral
☐ Unilateral
☐ Diminished
☐ Paradoxical/Flail

Chest Configuration
☐ Normal
☐ Other_____

☐ Subcutaneous Emphysema

☐ Tactile Fremitus
☐ Tracheal Deviation
☐ Abdominal Distention

Nailbeds
☐ Pink
☐ Ashy
☐ Cyanotic

Capillary Refill
☐ Rapid
☐ Sluggish

Auscultation   Anterior
1) Clear
2) Wheeze
3) Crackles
4) Rhonchi

Posterior
A. Good Aeration
B. Diminished
C. Absent

A: (Pt history, Admit dx. & date, events leading to intubation/trach/ventilation, significant problems, etc.)

P: (Care plan , standing orders, treatments)

WEANING MECHANICS		
TIME		
VC		
I/E FORCES		
VT		
RR		
VE		
f/VT		

Pt. EVENTS/CHANGES	Time	(Reasons for changes, significant pt. events, CT Scan, chest tube placement, BP problems, codes, etc.)

Signature _____ Initials _____

_____ _____

_____ _____

B

Figure 26-4, cont'd B, Neonatal and pediatric ventilator flow sheet, page 2. (From Kacmarek RM, Stoller JK, Heuer AJ: *Egan's fundamentals of respiratory care*, ed 10, St. Louis, MO, 2013, Mosby.)

Self-Assessment Questions

1. Indications for CPAP in children include:

   1. Tachypnea
   2. Retractions or accessory muscle use
   3. pH of 7.11
   4. Frequent apneic episodes followed by bradycardia

   A. 1 and 2 only
   B. 1 and 3 only
   C. 1, 2, and 3 only
   D. 1, 2, 3, and 4

2. The following conditions are thought to be responsive to CPAP except:
   A. Atelectasis
   B. Apnea of prematurity
   C. Untreated diaphragmatic hernia
   D. Pulmonary edema

3. Lung disease processes that are indications for CPAP include:

   1. Pneumonia
   2. Tracheomalacia
   3. Pneumothorax
   4. Pulmonary edema

   A. 1 and 4 only
   B. 1, 2, and 4 only
   C. 2 and 3 only
   D. 1, 2, 3, and 4

4. CPAP is indicated when:
   A. The infant is apneic
   B. The $PaCO_2$ level is less than 7.10 mm Hg
   C. The arterial oxygenation is inadequate despite elevated FIO_2
   D. All of the above

5. Weaning and discontinuation of CPAP should be considered when FIO_2 is less than:
   A. 0.7
   B. 0.6
   C. 0.5
   D. 0.4

6. Indications for mechanical ventilation include:

   1. PaO_2 <50 mm Hg
   2. $PaCO_2$ >65 mm Hg
   3. Persistent pulmonary hypertension of the newborn (PPHN)
   4. Congenital diaphragmatic hernia

   A. 1 and 2 only
   B. 3 and 4 only
   C. 1, 2, and 3 only
   D. 1, 2, 3, and 4 only

7. What tidal volume is generally considered safe for neonatal and pediatric patients?
   A. 2–3 mL/kg
   B. 3–4 mL/kg
   C. 6–8 mL/kg
   D. 10–12 mL/kg

8. What inspiratory time is usually set for the neonatal patient receiving mechanical ventilation?
   A. 0.2–0.4 seconds
   B. 0.4–0.6 seconds
   C. 0.6–0.8 seconds
   D. 0.8–1.0 seconds

9. Types of high-frequency ventilation (HFV) include:

   1. High-frequency oscillatory ventilation (HFOV)
   2. High-frequency jet ventilation (HFJV)
   3. Airway pressure release ventilation (APRV)
   4. Pressure regulated volume control (PRVC)

   A. 1 and 3 only
   B. 1, 2, and 3 only
   C. 1 and 2 only
   D. 1, 2, 3, and 4

10. Considerations for extubation in neonatal and pediatric patients includes:

    1. FIO_2 requirements <0.4
    2. Normal vital signs
    3. Ability to protect airway
    4. Spontaneous tidal volumes <4–5 mL/kg

    A. 1, 2, and 3 only
    B. 1 and 2 only
    C. 2, 3, and 4 only
    D. 1, 2, 3, and 4 only

CASE STUDY 26-1

A 4-year-old toddler in the pediatric intensive care unit (PICU) has been receiving continuous nebulization of albuterol for her asthma. Her condition has not improved, and the decision has been made to intubate and mechanically ventilate her. Using a pediatric mechanical ventilator and a lung simulator, answer the following questions:

1. What size ETT would you choose?

_____

_____

2. What mode of ventilation would you choose?

_____

_____

3. Would you initially use PEEP? Why, or why not?

_____

_____

Pulmonary Rehabilitation

Kathryn Patterson

▪ OBJECTIVES

Upon the completion of the chapter activities and content review topics, the student should be able to:

1. Identify pertinent interview information that would guide the initial exercise program and the progression of exercise.
2. Perform a 6-minute-walk test (6MWT).
3. Calculate a patient's target heart rate (THR).
4. Explain and use the dyspnea scale.
5. Explain and use the Borg scale.
6. Instruct a patient on the proper method for pursed-lip breathing (PLB).
7. Instruct a patient on the proper method for diaphragmatic breathing (DB).
8. Instruct a patient on the proper method for active cycle of breathing technique (ACBT).
9. Instruct a patient on the proper method for autogenic drainage (AD).
10. Instruct a patient with a weak diaphragm on the proper method for the use of an inspiratory muscle trainer (IMT).
11. Identify appropriate topics for education.

▪ KEY TERMS

- Active cycle breathing technique (ACBT)
- Autogenic drainage
- Borg scale
- Comorbidities
- Diaphragmatic breathing (DB)
- Forced expiratory technique (FET)
- Inspiratory muscle trainer (IMT)
- Pursed-lip breathing (PLB)
- Reconditioning
- 6-minute-walk test (6MWT)
- Target heart rate (THR)

▪ CONTENT REVIEW TOPICS

- AARC pulmonary rehabilitation toolkit
- Better breathers clubs
- Bronchial hygiene
- COPD
- Dyspnea
- GOLD guidelines
- Maximum inspiratory pressure (MIP)
- Metabolic equivalent (MET) level
- National Home Oxygen Patients Association (NHOPA)
- Negative inspirawtory force (NIF)
- Smoking cessation

▪ PROCEDURAL ASSESSMENTS

27-1 Performing a 6-Minute-Walk Test
27-2 Teaching Pursed-Lip Breathing
27-3 Teaching Diaphragmatic Breathing
27-4 Teaching the Use of an Inspiratory Muscle Trainer
27-5 Teaching the Active Cycle Breathing Technique
27-6 Autogenic Drainage

▪ EQUIPMENT

- A chair that can be easily moved along the walking course
- A source of oxygen
- Automated electronic defibrillator
- Borg scales (level of perceived exertion, modified dyspnea)
- Countdown timer (or stopwatch)
- Nose clip
- Portable oxygen device
- Small straw
- Sphygmomanometer
- Two small cones to mark the turnaround points
- Worksheets on a clipboard

Pulmonary rehabilitation is an integral part of keeping a patient healthy at his or her home. The respiratory therapist (RT), who strives to keep a discharged patient strong and focuses on helping him or her function at home, must understand the importance of patient education regarding pulmonary rehabilitation. When patients understand the importance of the techniques and activities that will help them get and stay fit, they will successfully return to a functional strength and to a status where activities of daily living (ADLs) are attainable.

Patient goals are developed with the help of the RT. They must be realistic and agreeable to the patient. Some common educational topics discussed in pulmonary rehabilitation are listed in Box 27-1. A clear understanding of these goals and a discussion of progress toward them should involve the patient's family as well. Examples of goals may be resuming a leisure activity that the patient once enjoyed, returning to work, or participating more in family responsibilities. Teaching patients to recognize how they feel, preparing them to use the tools that help cope with shortness of breath (SOB), and facilitating in rebuilding their strength and endurance are ways that pulmonary rehabilitation can decrease hospitalizations and prevent readmissions. The most common cause of intensive care unit (ICU) readmission is a pulmonary problem. Boxes 27-2 and 27-3 list patient characteristics and risk factors associated with ICU readmissions.

Common Educational Topics in Pulmonary Rehabilitation

- Anatomy and physiology of the lung
- Pathophysiology of lung disease
- Airway management
- Breathing retraining strategies
- Energy conservation and work simplification techniques
- Medications
- Self-management skills
- Benefits of exercise and safety guidelines
- Exercise modifications
- Oxygen therapy
- Environmental irritant avoidance
- Respiratory and chest therapy techniques
- Symptom management
- Psychological factors: Coping, anxiety, depression, panic control
- Stress management
- End-of-life planning
- Smoking cessation
- Travel, leisure, sexuality
- Nutrition

From Hodgkin JE, Celli BR, Connors GL: *Pulmonary rehabilitation: guidelines for success,* ed 4, St. Louis, 2009, Mosby.

BOX 27-2 **Patient Characteristics that Can Increase ICU Readmissions**

Patient characteristics include:
- Advanced age
- Having chronic health conditions
- Receiving dialysis
- ICU admission was from a step-down unit
- After emergency surgery
- Has a nonoperative diagnosis
- Has a higher acute physiology score at time of discharge

BOX 27-3 **Risk Factors Associated with Higher ICU Readmission Rates**

- Location before intensive care unit admission
- Age
- Comorbid conditions
- Diagnosis
- ICU length of stay
- Physiologic abnormalities at time of ICU discharge
- Discharge to a step-down unit

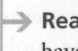 **Reality Check** Many pulmonary rehabilitation facilities have licensed counselors to help patients cope with social adjustment disorders, depression, or both.

This is important not only for the individual but also for the hospital financially, since Medicare now has a 30-day readmission criterion for reimbursement. Common goals for a pulmonary rehabilitation program are listed in Box 27-4.

BOX 27-4 **Common Goals for Pulmonary Rehabilitation Programs**

- Control of respiratory infections
- Basic airway management
- Improvement in ventilation and cardiac status
- Improvement in ambulation and types of physical activity
- Reduction in overall medical costs
- Reduction in hospitalizations
- Psychosocial support
- Occupational retraining and placement (when and where)
- Family education, counseling, and support
- Patient education, counseling, and support
- Control of respiratory infections

From Kacmarek RM, Stoller JK, Heuer AJ: *Egan's fundamentals of respiratory care,* ed 10, St. Louis, MO, 2013, Mosby.

Reality Check Reimbursement issues are a hot topic in pulmonary rehabilitation. It is a service covered by Centers for Medicare and Medicaid Services, but conditions and outcomes must be met. The 30-day readmission criterion may cause refusal of payment on a readmission within 30 days of discharge if the admission diagnosis is related to the previous admission.

In the case of chronic obstructive pulmonary disease (COPD) as well as other obstructive disorders, pulmonary rehabilitation is an integral part of efforts to decrease repeated admissions and save both patient health and medical costs.

This chapter will cover educational topics such as evaluation tools, breathing techniques, and the use of equipment aids in pulmonary rehabilitation.

Patient Interviewing: Review

When beginning to structure a pulmonary rehabilitation program, you should first determine the patient's chief complaint related to his or her diagnosis and the duration of this symptom. Even though the patient's medical history may be provided by the referring physician's office, interviewing the patient and his or her significant other may enhance your evaluation. Symptoms such as dyspnea, fatigue, cough, sputum production, sleep disturbance, pain, and swelling contribute to the overall picture. Orthopedic concerns, comorbidities, hospitalizations, smoking history, exposure to second-hand smoke, and occupational exposure to noxious substances need to be explored. Outcomes, from the start of the program to the finish, can be measured by providing surveys at the beginning and again at the end of the program. These may include a depression questionnaire and an SOB questionnaire. Outcome may also be estimated "before and after" the 6-minute-walk test (6MWT). These beginning parameters are obtained as part of the intake or interview session.

Reality Check Immobility during recent hospitalization may lead to decreased muscle mass caused by decreased protein synthesis and muscle catabolism. This may result in lower extremity weakness.

TABLE 27-1 Occupational Therapy Multidimensional Functional Assessment*

Dimensions of Function	Measurement of Dimension and Assessment Goals	Evaluation Methods and Tools
Participation	Determine impact of health conditions and of social and physical environment on everyday lifestyle, particularly social and productive activities	Interview Canadian Occupational Performance Measure School Function Assessment Functional Status Questionnaire
	Identify important activities for performance-based assessment	Activity configuration Activity checklist Environmental assessment
Activity	Determine ability to perform specific activities relative to difficulty, assistance needed, duration limits, and outlook on activity	Activity analysis Metabolic equivalent table Rate of perceived dyspnea Rate of perceived exertion
	Determine areas of strength that enable performance Determine which impairments should be evaluated in depth	Functional Independence Measure (FIM) Wee-FIM Assessment of Motor and Process Skills
Body functions and structure	Determine degree of severity, location, or duration of impairments that impede activities and social participation	Endurance: 6- or 12-minute-walk test Strength: manual muscle test, grip strength
	Determine whether the impairment can be remediated or whether it should be compensated for	Range of motion: goniometry Oxygen saturation: pulse oximetry
	Determine areas of strength	Visual perception, cognitive performance, and motor control tools

*Organized according to International Classification of Functioning and Disability (ICF) Dimensions of Function: Participation, Activity, and Body Functions and Structure Data from International Classification of Functioning, Disability and Health (ICF): http://www.who.int/classifications/icf/en/. Accessed January 2008. (In Hodgkin JE, Celli BR, Connors GL, editors: *Pulmonary rehabilitation: guidelines for success*, ed 4, St. Louis, MO, 2009, Mosby.)

Diagnostic and laboratory tests such as pulmonary function test, electrocardiography (ECG), and arterial blood gas (ABG) analysis are helpful in establishing a patient's baseline status and ruling out any contraindications. The Global Initiative for Chronic Obstructive Lung Disease (GOLD) guidelines for assessing stages of COPD are available on the Internet. They have been updated and published in the *Annals of Internal Medicine* (see 155:179-191, 2011).

> **Reality Check** Stage III is commonly associated with referral into Pulmonary Rehabilitation; however, this guideline suggests more study of referral during stage II to improve quality of life and decrease readmissions.

The patient's medication regimen, oxygen saturation at rest, nutrition, and fluid status must also be evaluated before starting any exercise. Functional status is often assessed using activities of daily living (ADLs). See Tables 27-1 and 27-2 for examples of this assessment. Vaccines are important to protect patients from common infections. If patients are vaccinated, they are less likely to be readmitted with an exacerbation of their underlying pulmonary condition. If their vaccination status is not up to date, provide instructions on how and where to get vaccinated.

Information regarding respiratory support groups should be offered to your patients. These groups allow patients to share their feelings about their pulmonary problems and their concerns with others and gather useful information that will help them cope with their situation. The Lung Association is a useful resource for finding these groups in the patient's area. The respiratory support group may provide the patient with

long-term support. Better Breathers Clubs (BBCs) are affiliated with the Lung Association, but stand-alone support groups exist as well.

> **Reality check** Adult education is a complex issue. Most adults are self-directed, rely on past experiences, and learn what they need to know only for real life situations that they can apply immediately. Patient backgrounds are diverse, and the educator needs to be aware of this to provide successful patient and family education.

>> SKILLS CHECK LIST

27-1 Performing the 6-Minute-Walk Test

As an RT, you will interview patients entering pulmonary rehabilitation. Information you gather will allow you to structure a program to meet your patient's specific needs. Performance of the 6MWT may provide a baseline for exercise prescription. Initially, pulmonary rehabilitation may be done in the hospital setting. However, it is typically done on an out-patient basis. Indications and contraindications for the 6MWT are given in Table 27-3. The Borg scale is commonly used to assess dyspnea, perceived level of exertion, and pain. An adaptation of this scale is given in Table 27-4.

The Borg scale is part of the 6MWT, but other dyspnea scales may also be used. Dyspnea scales and the patient's target heart rate (THR) will allow you to establish a baseline and safely progress through your patient's pulmonary rehabilitation plan.

TABLE 27-2 Metabolic Equivalent Values for Some Occupational Performance Areas

MET Levels (Oxygen Consumed) [Level of Activity]	Self-Care Activities	Work and Productive Activities	Play and Leisure Activities
1.5–2.0 METS (4–7 mL/kg/min) [Very light/minimal]	Eating	Desk work	Playing cards
	Shaving, grooming	Typing	Sewing
	Getting in and out of bed	Writing	Knitting
	Standing		
2–3 METS (7–11 mL/kg/min) [Light]	Showering in warm water	Ironing	Level bicycling (8 km or 5 mph)
	Level walking (3.25 km or 2 mph)	Light woodworking	Billiards
		Riding lawn mower	Bowling
			Golfing with power cart
3–4 METS (11–14 mL/kg/min) [Moderate]	Dressing, undressing	Cleaning windows	Bicycling (10 km or 6 mph)
	Walking (5 km or 3 mph)	Making beds	Fly-fishing (standing in waders)
		Mopping floors	Horseshoe pitching
		Vacuuming	
		Bricklaying	
		Machine assembly	
4–5 METS (14–18 mL/kg/min) [Heavy]	Showering in hot water	Scrubbing floors	Bicycling (13 km or 8 mph)
	Walking (5.5 km or 3.5 mph)	Hoeing	Table tennis
		Raking leaves	Tennis (doubles)
		Light carpentry	
5–6 METS (18–21 mL/kg/min) [Heavy]	Walking (6.5 km or 4 mph)	Digging in garden	Bicycling (16 km or 10 mph)
		Shoveling light earth	Canoeing (6.5 km or 4 mph)
			Ice-skating or roller-skating (15 km or 9 mph)
6–7 METS (21–25 mL/kg/min) [Very heavy]	Walking (8 km or 5 mph)	Snow shoveling	Bicycling (17.5 km or 11 mph)
		Splitting wood	Light downhill skiing
			Ski touring (4 km or 2.5 mph)

MEQ, Metabolic equivalents; *mL/kg/min*, milliliters of oxygen consumed per kilogram body weight per minute; *km*, kilometer; *mph*, miles per hour.
Schell BA, Scaffa M, Gillen G and Cohn ES: *Willard & Spackman's Occupational therapy*, ed 12, Philadelphia, 2013, Lippincott, Williams and Wilkins, Inc.

> ✳ **Tip** Blood glucose should be monitored in the patient with diabetes before the 6MWT. If cardiac comorbidities exist, the electrocardiography (ECG) monitoring may be required.

The following is the step-by-step process for performing the 6MWT. A protocol is detailed in Box 27-5.

Procedural Preparation

1. Review the patient's chart.
2. Verify the physician's order or the facility's protocol for standard of care.
3. Obtain, clean, and inspect the appropriate equipment.
4. Follow personal protective equipment (PPE) requirements, and observe standard precautions for any transmission-based isolation procedure.
5. Identify the patient using two patient identifiers.
6. Introduce yourself to the patient and to the family.
7. Explain the procedure to the patient and to the family, and acknowledge the patient's understanding.
8. Perform proper hand hygiene, and put on gloves.
9. Confirm that the patient is wearing comfortable clothing and appropriate shoes for walking.
10. Advise the patient to use the usual walking aids during the test.
11. Confirm that the padtient has not exercised vigorously within 2 hours of beginning the test.

12. Ensure that the patient has been resting in a chair located near the starting position for at least 10 minutes prior to the test.

Implementation

1. Place the patient in a comfortable position at the start line, and instruct patient to breathe normally.
2. Apply the pulse oximeter on the patient's finger, and use a carry strap for device.
3. Adjust the pulse oximeter to "continuously read."
4. Prepare the clipboard with the documentation.
5. Assess 0 minute stats:
   a. Oxygen use in L/min
   b. FIO_2
   c. SpO_2
   d. HR
   e. BORG
   f. Pain
   g. RR
   h. Blood pressure
   i. Breath sounds
6. Set the timer to 6 minutes.
7. Place the cone at the starting point, and prepare a cone to mark the point where the patient completes the test.
8. Show and explain the Borg scale and pain level scale to the patient before the test.
9. Explain the objective of the test to the patient.

TABLE 27-3 Indications and Contraindications for a 6MWT

Indications	Dyspnea during rest or exertion
	Hypoxemia or hypercapnia
	Reduced exercise tolerance
	Unexpected deterioration or worsening of symptoms against a background of chronic dyspnea and reduced but stable exercise tolerance
	Need for surgical intervention
	Chronic respiratory failure
	Ventilator dependence
	Increasing need for acute care intervention
Absolute contraindications	Unstable angina during the previous month
	Myocardial infarction during the previous month
Relative contraindications	Resting heart rate greater than 120 beats/min
	Resting systolic blood pressure >180 mm Hg
	Resting diastolic blood pressure >100 mm Hg
	Resting systolic blood pressure <80 mm Hg
	Resting diastolic blood pressure <50 mm Hg
	Angina
	Resting Borg scale >6
	Dizziness
	Nausea
	Resting SpO_2 <80% with breathing oxygen or room air

6MWT, 6-minute-walk test; *beats/min*, beats per minute; *SpO_2*, saturation of peripheral oxygen.

10. Demonstrate the test by walking one lap of the track or a distance premeasured for the patient.
11. Instruct the patient on how to perform the test, and explain that he or she will:
    a. Walk around the track as many times as he or she can in 6 minutes.
    b. Be exerting himself or herself and may feel out of breath.
    c. Be permitted to slow down, stop, sit down, and rest, if needed.
    d. Be asked to use the Borg scale and pain level readings at 3 and 6 minutes.
12. Instruct the patient to begin the test.
13. Update the patient after the first minute and every minute thereafter.
14. Assess the 3-minute stats:
    a. Oxygen use in L/min
    b. FiO_2
    c. SpO_2
    d. HR
    e. BORG
    f. Pain
    g. RR
    h. Blood pressure
    i. Breath sounds

15. Instruct patient to sit in chair and assess 6 minute stats
    a. Oxygen use in L/min
    b. FiO_2
    c. SpO_2
    d. HR
    e. BORG
    f. Pain
    g. RR
    h. Blood pressure
    i. Breath sounds
16. Remove the supplies from the area and clean the area, as needed.
17. Remove PPE, and perform proper hand hygiene.

Evaluation of Procedure

1. Establish a baseline, and compare with the 0-, 3- and 6-minute measurements.
2. Develop an appropriate respiratory care plan based on assessment data.
3. Identify any unexpected outcomes.
4. Trend the test over several pulmonary rehabilitation sessions.

Documentation and Reporting

1. Record your findings in the patient's chart.
2. Record the number of laps the patient completed.
3. Report any abnormal findings to the appropriate health care provider.

27-2 Teaching Pursed-Lip Breathing

Breathing techniques help patients gain awareness of their breathing and make it possible for them to reduce dyspnea during activities. Pursed-lip breathing (PLB) facilitates the elimination of trapped air, thus enabling better diaphragmatic excursion. The following is the step-by-step process for teaching the pursed-lip breathing technique.

Procedural Preparation

1. Review the patient's chart.
2. Verify the physician's order or the facility's protocol for standard of care.
3. Follow PPE requirements, and observe standard precautions for any transmission-based isolation procedure.
4. Identify the patient using two patient identifiers.
5. Introduce yourself to the patient and to the family.
6. Explain the procedure to the patient and to the family, and acknowledge the patient's understanding.
7. Perform proper hand hygiene, and put on gloves.

Implementation

1. Place the patient in a comfortable position, and instruct him or her to breathe normally.
2. Assess vital signs.
3. Instruct the patient to close the mouth and inhale slowly and deeply through the nose.
4. Instruct the patient to exhale though pursed lips, as in whistling.
5. Instruct the patient to prolong exhalation to twice the length of inspiration.

6. Instruct the patient to practice pursed lip breathing during an activity.
7. Instruct the patient to practice exhaling during the most strenuous part of a task.

Evaluation of Procedure

1. Develop an appropriate respiratory care plan based on assessment data.
2. Note any use of oxygen therapy.
3. Evaluate the patient's ability to demonstrate the procedure.
4. Identify any unexpected outcomes.

Documentation and Reporting

1. Record your findings in the patient's chart.
2. Report any abnormal findings to the appropriate health care provider.

27-3 Teaching Diaphragmatic Breathing Techniques

Many individuals need to learn breathing techniques that will help them maximize their lung function. Often the diaphragm is weak and needs strengthening. Patients need to be conscious of proper diaphragmatic breathing (DB). It can be used along with the PLB technigue to aid in the patient's ease of breathing. The following is the step-by-step process for teaching DB techniques.

Procedural Preparation

1. Review the patient's chart.
2. Verify the physician's order or the facility's protocol for standard of care.
3. Follow PPE requirements, and observe standard precautions for any transmission-based isolation procedure.
4. Identify the patient using two patient identifiers.
5. Introduce yourself to the patient and to the family.
6. Explain the procedure to the patient and to the family, and acknowledge the patient's understanding.
7. Perform proper hand hygiene, and put on gloves.

Implementation

1. Place the patient in a comfortable position, and instructs patient to breathe normally
2. Assess vital signs, and obtain a baseline pulse oximetry reading.
3. Instruct the patient to place one hand on the abdomen just below the rib cage and the other hand on the chest.
4. Instruct the patient to observe the rise and fall of the abdominal wall during inspiration and expiration.
5. Explain the relationship between the abdominal wall and the diaphragm.
6. Instruct the patient to perform DB in conjunction with PLB.
7. Coach the patient to keep the upper chest movement to the minimum.

TABLE 27-4 Instructions for Evaluating Perceived Dyspnea and Perceived Exertion

1. The patient identifies an activity that is important and problematic and then performs that activity.
2. The patient is shown the following 10-point scales and asked to rate perceptions of dyspnea and exertion.
3. Descriptive terms in the scales serve as verbal anchors to assist the patient in rating.
4. To evaluate outcomes, retest using the same activity, rating scales, and instructions.

Note: If assessing for change in activity performance, the patient uses newly acquired energy conservation and breathing strategies in the retest session. If assessing for impairment of endurance, the original activity is replicated.

Perceived Dyspnea Scale		Perceived Exertion Scale	
Instructions: "How would you rate your shortness of breath during the activity? On a scale of 0 to 10, with 0 being no shortness of breath and 10 being shortness of breath so severe that you must stop and rest, what number best indicates your experience of shortness of breath?"		*Instructions:* "Rate how hard you were working (or the amount of physical effort) during the activity. On a scale of 0 to 10, with 0 being no effort and 10 being your maximum possible effort, what number best indicates your level of effort?"	
My shortness of breath is:		My level of effort is:	
0	None	0	None
0.5	Very slight, just noticeable	0.5	Very slight
1		1	Slight
2	Mild	2	Mild
3	Moderate	3	Moderate
4	Somewhat heavy	4	Somewhat strong
5	Strong, heavy	5	Strong, heavy
6		6	
7	Severe	7	Very strong
8		8	
9		9	
10	Very, very severe; I must stop and rest	10	Very, very strong, almost the maximum possible

Adapted with permission from Borg G: Psychophysical bases of perceived exertion, *Med Sci Sports Exerc* 14:377, 1982. In Hodgkin JE, Celli BR, Connors GL: *Pulmonary rehabilitation: guidelines for success,* ed 4, St. Louis, MO, 2009, Mosby.

8. If diaphragmatic movement is not satisfactory, gently push in on the abdomen during exhalation to get the desired response.
9. Remove PPE, and perform proper hand hygiene prior to leaving the patient's room.

Evaluation of Procedure

1. Develop an appropriate respiratory care plan based on assessment data.
2. Note any use of oxygen therapy.
3. Identify any unexpected outcomes.
4. Correct any paradoxical movement.

Documentation and Reporting

1. Record your findings in the patient's chart.
2. Report any abnormal findings to the appropriate health care provider.

27-4 Teaching the Use of an Inspiratory Muscle Trainer

It has been shown that patients with COPD experience muscle weakness as a result of air trapping, not utilizing the diaphragm through its normal range of motion, and poor nutrition. The inspiratory muscle trainer (IMT) allows the respiratory muscles to be exercised. It should be used in conjunction with both PLB and DB techniques.

> **✳ Tip** Think of inspiratory muscle trainer (IMT) use as weight training for the diaphragm.

The following is the step-by-step process for teaching the use of an IMT.

Procedural Preparation

1. Review the patient's chart.
2. Verify the physician's order or the facility's protocol for standard of care.
3. Obtain, clean, and inspect the appropriate equipment.
4. Follow PPE requirements, and observe standard precautions for any transmission-based isolation procedure.
5. Identify the patient using two patient identifiers.
6. Introduce yourself to the patient and to the family.
7. Explain the procedure to the patient and to the family, and acknowledge the patient's understanding.
8. Perform proper hand hygiene, and put on gloves.

Implementation

1. Place the patient in a comfortable position, and instruct him or her to breathe normally.
2. Assess vital signs.
3. Bring the negative inspiratory force (NIF) meter and the IMT to the patient.
4. Using the NIF meter, instruct the patient to generate the strongest negative pressure possible with one breath and then repeat two more times making the best effort.
5. Calculate one third of the best effort.
6. Set the IMT device to generate a slightly greater effort than one third of the best effort.

7. Explain to the patient that he or she will feel resistance to breathing only on inspiration.
8. Inform the patient that 30 minutes per session per day for at least 5 days per week is the goal.
9. If patient is unable to complete 30 minutes, advise him or her to break the effort into two 15-minute sessions.
10. Instruct the patient to cough.
11. Reassess vital signs.
12. Remove the supplies used, and clean the area, as needed.
13. Remove PPE, and perform proper hand hygiene.

Evaluation of Procedure

1. Establish a baseline, or compare with previous measurements.
2. Develop an appropriate respiratory care plan based on assessment data.
3. Note any use of oxygen therapy.
4. Identify any unexpected outcomes.

Documentation and Reporting

1. Record your findings in the patient's chart.
2. Document the NIF value and the starting IMT setting.
3. Document the patient's ability to perform therapy and any coaching needed.
4. Report any abnormal findings to the appropriate health care provider.

27-5 Teaching the Active Cycle Breathing Technique

As the RT caring for the patient in pulmonary rehabilitation, the patient's breathing will be your priority. Patients must constantly be reminded of the diaphragm and its importance to valuable breathing techniques such as the active cycle breathing technique (ACBT). The forced expiratory technique (FET), known as the *huff cough*, is only effective if patients are coached to control their breathing prior to initiating the cough. This combination includes controlled DB with periodic thoracic expansion to loosen mucus and the FET to move secretions centrally for removal. The following is the step-by-step procedure for teaching the ACBT.

Procedural Preparation

1. Review the patient's chart.
2. Verify the physician's order or the facility's protocol for standard of care.
3. Follow PPE requirements, and observe standard precautions for any transmission-based isolation procedure.
4. Identify the patient using two patient identifiers.
5. Introduce yourself to the patient and to the family.
6. Explain the procedure to the patient and to the family, and acknowledge the patient's understanding.
7. Perform proper hand hygiene, and put on gloves.

Implementation

1. Place the patient in a comfortable position, and instruct him or her to breathe normally.
2. Assess vital signs.
3. Instruct the patient to relax and control the breathing by using DB.

BOX 27-5 | 6-Minute-Walk Policy

Purpose

To provide a protocol for all pulmonary rehabilitation staff to follow when performing evaluation of the 6-minute-walk test (6MWT). This protocol will allow maximum patient safety and consistency among team members and avoid variances in technique. The 6MWT better reflects activities of daily living than other walk tests. It helps measure the functional status of the patient.

Absolute Contraindications

- Unstable angina during the previous month
- Myocardial infarction during the previous month

Relative Contraindications

- Resting heart rate >120 beats per minute (beats/min)
- Resting systolic blood pressure of >180 mm Hg
- Resting diastolic blood pressure of >100 mm Hg
- Resting systolic blood pressure of <80 mm Hg
- Resting diastolic blood pressure of <50 mm Hg
- Asymptomatic (i.e., primary pulmonary hypertension [PPH]), as directed by referring physician for 6MWT
- Angina
- Resting BORG scale >6
- Dizziness
- Nausea
- Resting oxygen saturation level <80% on oxygen or room air

Other Safety Issues

- If available, results from a resting electrocardiogram done during the previous 6 months should also be reviewed before testing.
- Stable exertional angina is *not* an absolute contraindication, but a patient with these symptoms should perform the test *after using* his or her antiangina medication (verify that the patient has taken the antiangina medication), and the patient should have rescue nitrate medication readily available.

Required Equipment

- Countdown timer (or stopwatch)
- Mechanical lap counter
- Two small orange cones to mark the start and stop points of the patient's walk
- Chairs set up strategically around the walk track for the patient to sit on, if needed
- 6MWT documentation form on a clipboard
- Source of oxygen with nasal cannula ready for emergency or if patient uses oxygen for activity or walking, as prescribed by physician
- Sphygmomanometer
- Stethoscope
- Cutaneous pulse oximeter, with finger or forehead probe
- Quick-acting β_2-albuterol metered-dose inhaler (MDI) for emergency use
- Rescue nitrate medication, NTG 0.4 sublingual every 5 min ×3; then call to emergency room (ER) for transport
- Aspirin
- Distance marker to determine last lap distance
- BORG scale 0–10 point
- Walker with wheels, if indicated
- Staff performing the test should know the emergency response system if the patient falls or has a cardiac arrest
- Know the location of the CRASH cart in pulmonary diagnostics

- Wheel chair, if the patient needs assistance during or after the test

Patient Preparation

- Instruct the patient to wear comfortable clothing.
- Instruct the patient to wear appropriate shoes for walking.
- Patients should use their usual walking assistive devices during the test as they use at home (i.e., cane, walker, etc.).
- Light meal is acceptable before the test.
- Patients should not have exercised vigorously within 2 hours of beginning test.
- The patient's usual medical regimen should be followed the day of the test (i.e., medications, inhalers, breathing treatments, etc.).

Policy (not facility specific)

1. If the patient arrives without oxygen, *but* has it prescribed at a certain liter per minute (L/min), place the patient on oxygen system, and have him or her use oxygen per the physician's order for L/min.
2. If the patient's resting oxygen saturation is 88% or greater and he or she does *not* use oxygen at home, have the patient perform the 6MWT without supplemental oxygen.
3. If the patient's resting oxygen saturation is less than 88% on room air, perform the 6MWT with the patient on continuous oxygen at 2 L/min via nasal cannula.
4. *Wait* for 10 minutes after any change in oxygen delivery to start the walk test.
5. *Do not* use pulsed oxygen for the 6MWT. (An oxygen prescription walk test will be done to titrate oxygen or to verify adequacy of the pulsed oxygen system the patient is using at home; this is a separate test from our pre- or post-6MWT.)
6. *Do not titrate oxygen during the walk test*; leave it at the prescribed liter flow from the referring doctor or the 2 L/min patient started on per protocol.
7. *Do not walk with the patient or behind him or her.*
8. *No* warm-up should be performed before the test.
9. Only one patient should be testing for a 6MWT at a time.
10. Abnormal results: Inform the referring physician about adverse symptoms documented on the 6MWT, and ask for advice.

Reasons for Stopping 6MWT

- Chest pain
- Intolerable dyspnea, (i.e., BORG scale > or equal to 7)
- Leg cramps
- Staggering
- Diaphoresis
- Pale or ashen appearance

If a test is stopped for any of the above reasons or the patient just cannot continue, have the patient sit. A careful assessment *must* be performed, with documentation of the vital signs as noted on the 6MWT documentation form.

Patient Instructions

"The object of this test is to walk as far as possible for 6 minutes. You will walk around the track. Six minutes is a long time to walk. You will be exerting yourself. You may get out of breath or become exhausted. You are permitted to slow down, to stop, and to rest, as necessary. You may use any of the chairs placed around the track to sit and rest if you have to, *but* resume walking as soon as you are able. I will be asking you to perform

Continued

| BOX 27-5 | 6-Minute-Walk Policy—cont'd |

your BORG and pain scale exercises at the 3- and 6-minute marks. I will also be looking at the oximeter to get the oxygen saturation reading and heart rate. You are not to try to read the oximeter while walking. That is our job. Do not talk to anyone during the test, but tell us if you have any sudden symptoms, and when we ask you about your BORG and pain scale levels.

You will be walking the track as many times as you can. Now I'm going to show you."

Demonstrate by walking one lap yourself.

"I am going to use this counter to keep track of the number of laps you complete. I will click it each time you return to this starting point. *Remember* that the object is to walk *as far as possible* for 6 minutes, but don't run or jog."

If you have all the 0 data points, then you can proceed.

"Are you ready for the 6MWT?"

1. Position the patient at the starting line. You should also stand near the starting line during the entire test, unless the patient needs your help. **Do not walk with the patient**. When you tell the patient to *start*, start the timer, and carefully observe your patient as he or she walks, looking for symptoms, gait issues, and so on.

2. The staff performing the test should not talk to anyone during the walk. Use an even tone of voice when using the standard phrases of encouragement. Watch the patient. Do not get distracted and lose count of the laps. Each time the patient returns to the starting line, click the lap counter once. *Let the participant see you do it; exaggerate the click by using body language, like using a stop watch at a race.*

3. What you tell the patient during the test:
   After the first minute, tell the patient (in even tones):
   "You are doing well. You have 5 minutes to go."
   When the timer shows 4 minutes remaining, tell the patient:
   "Keep up the good work. You have 4 minutes to go."
   When the timer show 3 minutes remaining, tell the patient:
   "You are doing well. You are halfway done."
   When the timer shows 1 minutes remaining, tell the patient:

   "Keep up the good work. You have only 2 minutes left."
   When the timer shows 1 minute remaining, tell the patient:
   "You are doing well. You have only 1 minute to go."
   When the timer is 15 seconds from completion of the test, tell the patient:
   "In a moment I'm going to tell you to stop. When I do, just stop right where you are, and I will come to you."
   When the timer rings (or buzzes), tell the patient:
   "STOP!"

4. Walk over to the patient. Consider providing the wheel chair if he or she looks exhausted. Mark the spot where the patient stopped, by placing an orange cone on the floor.

5. Record the 6-minute data.

6. Congratulate the patient on his or her good effort, and offer a drink of water when you are waiting for your recovery times.
   Do not use other words of encouragement.
   If the patient stops walking during the test and needs a rest, tell the patient:
   "You can sit and rest if you like. Continue walking whenever you feel able."

7. Do not stop the timer. If the patient stops before the 6 minutes are up and refuses to continue (or you decide the patient should not continue), take the wheel chair for the patient to sit on, discontinue the walk, and note on the worksheet the distance, the time stopped, and the reason for stopping prematurely. Gather the ending data points.

8. Have the patient proceed to the nearest chair. Proceed with data collection on blood pressure and recovery.

9. Record the number of laps as shown by the counter, and use the distance marker to determine the last lap distance. Record this information.

10. When the patient has returned to resting parameters and has no new symptoms, he or she may leave. At this time, do your calculation on the 6MWT form.

Modified from Hodgkin JE, Celli BR, Connors GL: Pulmonary rehabilitation: guidelines for success, ed 4, St. Louis, MO, 2009, Mosby.

4. Instruct the patient to perform three or four thoracic expansion exercises:
   a. Instruct the patient to perform deep inhalation and relaxed exhalation.
   b. Inform the patient that this may be accompanied by percussion, vibration, or compression.

5. Instruct the patient to, again, perform three or four thoracic expansion exercises.

6. Instruct the patient to perform one or two exercises using the FET.

7. Instruct the patient to again perform three or four thoracic expansion exercises.

8. Remove PPE, and perform proper hand hygiene.

Evaluation of Procedure

1. Develop an appropriate respiratory care plan based on assessment data.

2. Evaluate the color, consistency, volume, and odor of sputum.

3. Note any use of oxygen therapy.

4. Identify any unexpected outcomes.

Documentation and Reporting

1. Record your findings in the patient's chart.

2. Report any abnormal findings to the appropriate health care provider.

27-6 Autogenic Drainage

The RT must be skilled in teaching patients to manipulate the tidal volume breath below the usual levels and into the functional residual capacity (FRC). This will help loosen secretions. If the patient becomes sensitive and feels the urge to cough, he or she is instructed to do DB at normal lung volumes until the urge passes. At this point, the patient can attempt to move back into the lower lung volume to work on mucus loosening. The patient is then instructed to move into middle lung volume with the hopes the mucus will move more into the central airway. After mucus is moved centrally, the patient is encouraged to breathe larger volumes to facilitate expulsion with an FET. The following is the step-by-step process for autogenic drainage (AD).

Procedural Preparation

1. Review the patient's chart.
2. Verify the physician's order or the facility's protocol for standard of care.
3. Follow PPE requirements, and observe standard precautions for any transmission-based isolation procedure.
4. Identify the patient using two patient identifiers.
5. Introduce yourself to the patient and to the family.
6. Explain the procedure to the patient and to the family, and acknowledge the patient's understanding.
7. Perform proper hand hygiene, and put on gloves, mask, and protective eyewear, as appropriate for the procedure.

Implementation

1. Place the patient in a comfortable position, and instruct him or her to breathe normally.
2. Assess vital signs.
3. Instruct the patient to use DB during the three phases of AD:
   a. Full inspiratory capacity maneuver, followed by low lung volume breathing
   b. Breathing at low to middle lung volumes
   c. Breathing at increasing lung volumes in preparation for expulsion of mucus

4. Instruct the patient to perform forced expiratory technique once all the three phases are complete.
5. Repeat steps 3 and 4 until all mucous is removed.
6. Remove PPE, and perform proper hand hygiene.

Evaluation of Procedure

1. Develop an appropriate respiratory care plan based on assessment data.
2. Evaluate the color, consistency, volume, and odor of sputum.
3. Note any use of oxygen therapy.
4. Identify any unexpected outcomes.

Documentation and Reporting

1. Record your findings in the patient's chart.
2. Report any abnormal findings to the appropriate health care provider.

Bibliography

Fan E: Critical illness neuromyopathy and the role of PT and rehabilitation in critically ill patients, *RC J* 57(6):933, 2012.

Hodgkin JE, Celli BR, Connors GL: *Pulmonary rehabilitation, guidelines for success*, ed 4, St. Louis, MO, 2009, Mosby.

Kacmarek RM, Stoller JK, Heuer AJ: *Egan's fundamentals of respiratory care*, ed 10, St. Louis, MO, 2013, Mosby.

Kramer AA, Higgins TL, Zimmerman JE: Intensive care unit readmissions in US hospitals: patient characteristics, risk factors, and outcomes. *Crit Care Med*, 40(1):3-10, 2012.

Rosenberg AL, Watts C: Patients readmitted to ICUs: A systematic review of risk factors and outcomes. *Chest*, 118: 492-502, 2000.

1. List the eight indications for pulmonary rehabilitation.

a. _____

b. _____

c. _____

d. _____

e. _____

f. _____

g. _____

h. _____

2. List the 10 contraindications for pulmonary rehabilitation.

a. _____

b. _____

c. _____

d. _____

e. _____

f. _____

g. _____

h. _____

i. _____

j. _____

3. Have a lab partner perform a 6-minute-walk test (6MWT) while breathing through a small straw. Fill in the form (Figure 27-1) provided.

Pulmonary Rehabilitation Assessment
Timed Distance Walk Test - 6 Minutes

Date: _____ Age: _____

Appropriate shoes? **Y / N**

Recent medication changes? **Y / N**
(ie., Prednisone dose, on antibiotics?)

_____

_____

Bronchodilator:

Not prescribed _____

Not used today _____

Used, time _____

Name _____

6 minute type walk:

Initial _____

Discharge _____

Maintenance _____

Other _____

Pre-walk symptoms:

Cough _____   Sputum _____   Wheezing _____

Leg cramps _____   Fatigue _____   Other _____

Chest pain _____   Chest pressure _____   _____

Orthopedic issues:

_____

_____

O_2 Walk System? Y / N

O_2 Delivery Device:

Cannula ____

Oxymizer ____

Non-rebreather ____

Venti Mask ___% ____

Other _____

How O_2 transported?

Pushed ____

Pulled ____

Carried ____

Staff carried ____

Other _____

O_2 Flow Type:

Cont flow ____

Cyclinder ____

Pulsed ____

Liquid ____

Peripheral Circulation:

Good ____

Poor ____

Raynaud's ____

Scleraderma ____

Other ____

_____

MMRC Dyspnea Scale:

Grade 0 ____

Grade 1 ____

Grade 2 ____

Grade 3 ____

Grade 4 ____

Oximeter Probe Site:

Finger ____

Forehead ____

Other ____

Fall risk? Y / N   Why:

Neuropathy _____

Gait _____

Balance _____

Other _____

_____

Borg Scale: 0 (no problem) 10 (ER time)   Pain Scale: 0 (no problem) 10 (ER pain)

0 min.	3 min.	6 min.	Post	Recovery
F_IO_2 _____	F_IO_2 _____	F_IO_2 _____	F_IO_2 _____	F_IO_2 _____
O_2 lpm _____	O_2 lpm _____	O_2 lpm _____	O_2 lpm _____	O_2 lpm _____
SpO_2 % _____	SpO_2 % _____	SpO_2 % _____	SpO_2 % _____	SpO_2 % _____
HR _____	HR _____	HR _____	HR _____	HR _____
BORG _____	BORG _____	BORG _____	BORG _____	BORG _____
Pain _____	Pain _____	Pain _____	Pain _____	Pain _____
RR _____	RR _____	RR _____	RR _____	RR _____
BP _____	BP _____	BP _____	BP _____	BP _____
Lung sounds _____	Lung sounds _____	Lung sounds _____	Lung sounds _____	Lung sounds _____

#1 Rest Time: _____   #2 Rest Time: _____   #3 Rest Time: _____   **Total Rest Time:** _____

Figure 27-1 6-minute-walk test form. (From Hodgkin JE, Celli BR, Connors GL: *Pulmonary rehabilitation: guidelines for success*, ed 4, St. Louis, MO, 2009, Mosby.)

Pulmonary Rehabilitation Assessment
Timed Distance Walk Test - 6 Minutes

Ht. _____ Wt. _____ IBW_____ BMI_____

IBW MALE LBS = [50 +(2.3 (ht. in inches - 60)] 2.2

IBW FEMALE LBS = [45.5 +(2.3 (ht. in inches - 60)] 2.2

Actual Total Distance (ft):_____ = _____ laps (114 ft) + _____ ft.

Predicted distance: _____ ft   % Predicted: _____

Men 6MWD Reference equations in healthy male adults:

    [3,740 ft. - (5.61 x BMI) - (6.94 x age)] - 501 ft. for the lower limit of normal

Women 6MWD Reference equations in healthy female adults:

    [3,337 ft. - (6.24 x BMI) - (5.83 x age)] - 456 ft. for the lower limit of normal

MPH _____ = {ft. walked (10)} / 5280

METS_____ = [(MPH) (26.83 meters/min) (0.1 mL/kg/min) + 3.5 mL/kg/min] / 3.5mL/kg/min

MMRC_____

BODE Index _____ Restrictive Diag. BODE not applicable

THR Range _____

Check formula used:

_____ Standard formula: THR = (220 - age) X (70 - 75%)

_____ Karvonen's formula: THR Low End = HRR X .70 + RHR

                              THR High End = HRR X .75 + RHR

_____ Other, % _____

Calculations:

220 - age = Max Perceived Heart Rate (MPHR)

THR High End = HRR X .75 + RHR

MPHR - Resting HR = Heart Rate Reserve (HRR)

DURING walk symptoms:

Cough _____   Sputum _____   Wheezing _____

Leg cramps _____   Fatigue _____   Other _____

Chest pain _____   Chest pressure _____   _____

Supportive devices used during walk:

Cane _____

Walker with wheels _____

Walker with no wheels _____

Other _____

Other comments:

_____

_____

Staff Signature: _____

Figure 27-1, cont'd

a. Did he or she maintain appropriate oxygen levels?

b. Consider the dyspnea reported by your lab partner. Generally, it should be 0. With limitation of breathing through a straw, what level did he or she report on the dyspnea scale?

c. Did he or she complain of any symptoms?

d. Did you notice any changes in your lab partner's vital signs during the 6MWT?

e. Generally, with exercise, we expect systolic blood pressure and heart rate (HR) to increase. Did you see this?

> → **Reality check** A target HR is calculated to keep the patient in a safe range during exercise. This HR range will safeguard against excess work of the heart and possible complications. The Karvonen formula is used for the calculation.

4. Calculate your lab partner's target HR by using the Karvonen equation, and record it below.

✳ **Tip** To set a target heart rate (THR) for patient exercise, use the *Karvonen formula*:

$$THR = [MHR - RHR] \times [50\% - 70\%] + RHR$$

where MHR = maximum heart rate at limit of exercise tolerance, and RHR = resting heart rate. A good THR for a patient with chronic obstructive pulmonary disease (COPD), with MHR of 150 beats per minute (beats/min) and RHR of 90 beats/min, would be [{150 – 90} × 0.60] + 90 = 126 beats/min.

From Kacmarek RM, Stoller JK, Heuer AJ: *Egan's fundamentals of respiratory care*, ed 10, St. Louis, MO, 2013, Mosby.

Target heart rate (THR): _____

5. How do you calculate the average speed in a 6MWT?

_____

_____

_____

6. Match the educational topic to the point that would be covered during that lecture. Some items may overlap. You could choose more than one for a particular educational topic.

1. ___ Anatomy and physiology of the lung		a.	When to call the doctor
2. ___ Pathophysiology of the lung		b.	Nicotine replacement therapy
3. ___ Breathing retraining		c.	Showering
4. ___ Energy conservation		d.	Adhering to medical regimen
5. ___ Medications		e.	Location of the diaphragm
6. ___ Self-management		f.	Improved walk distance
7. ___ Benefits of exercise		g.	Relaxation techniques
8. ___ Oxygen therapy		h.	Prearrangement with airline
9. ___ Environment		i.	Definition of COPD
10. ___ Symptom management		j.	Inhaler technique
11. ___ Psychosocial issues		k.	Portable oxygen concentrator
12. ___ Stress management		l.	Eating six small meals daily
13. ___ Smoking cessation		m.	Pursed-lip breathing
14. ___ Travel		n.	Allergies
15. ___ Nutrition		o.	Depression

Self-Assessment Questions

1. One method for calculating target heart rate (THR) is called the _____ equation.
   a. Borg
   b. Karvonen
   c. Dyspnea
   d. Exertion

2. All of the following would be appropriate to gather during patient evaluation and assessment except:
   a. Pulmonary function tests (PFTs)
   b. Medications
   c. Sexual orientation
   d. Vaccines

3. Functional status may be obtained from:
   a. Chief complaint
   b. Nutrition
   c. 6MWT
   d. Smoking history

4. Necessary equipment for the 6MWT includes all of the following except:
   a. Arterial blood gas syringe
   b. Stethoscope
   c. Oximeter
   d. Blood pressure cuff

5. For the purpose of releasing trapped air, the patient is instructed to perform:
   a. Diaphragmatic breathing
   b. Pursed-lip breathing
   c. Use the inspiratory muscle trainer
   d. Segmental

6. An example of a reasonable goal that a patient may want to achieve might be:
   a. Go jogging
   b. Reverse disease
   c. Return to golfing
   d. Climb mountains

7. Therapy to improve the strength of the diaphragm using a threshold resistor is:
   a. Using the IMT
   b. Performing activities of daily living
   c. PLB
   d. Metabolic equivalent

8. Pulmonary rehabilitation reconditioning that would benefit the patient include all of the following except:
   a. Upper extremity
   b. Lower extremity
   c. Respiratory muscles
   d. Brain

9. Appropriate topics of education include all of the following except:
   a. Medications
   b. ABG values interpretation
   c. Symptom management
   d. Nutrition

10. Most commonly patients with chronic obstructive pulmonary disease (COPD) are referred to pulmonary rehabilitation when they are at stage_____.
    a. I
    b. II
    c. III
    d. IV

▶▶ CASE STUDY 27-1

A 60-year-old patient has been referred to your pulmonary rehabilitation program. He has been hospitalized three times in the past 3 months with exacerbation of chronic obstructive pulmonary disease (COPD). He is on inhalers and oxygen and states that he has not been educated in any way about his condition. He no longer smokes. He is complaining of dyspnea and fatigue and says that he sits around all day.

1. List three other questions that you would like to ask him during his interview process.

   _____

   _____

2. Give three education topics that you would like to teach him.

   a. _____

   b. _____

   c. _____

3. Would he benefit from breathing retraining? If so, what techniques would you like to teach?

   _____

   _____

Polysomnography Technology

Wendi M. Nugent and Susan Townsley

■ OBJECTIVES

Upon the completion of the chapter activities and content review topics, the student should be able to:

1. Describe the process of patient setup and data acquisition.
2. Identify the various types of polysomnographic testing protocols and their respective uses.
3. Identify polysomnographic monitoring devices.
4. Identify polysomnographic signals, including classification of sleep-related breathing disorders.
5. Describe patient preparation tips for polysomnographic testing.

■ KEY TERMS

- Arousal
- Biopotentials
- Central Sleep Apnea Syndrome (CSA)
- Cheyne-Stokes Respirations (CSR)
- Claustrophobia
- Comorbidity
- Complex Sleep Apnea Syndrome
- Electrooculogram
- Montage
- Narcolepsy
- Obesity Hypoventilation Syndrome
- Obstructive Sleep Apnea Syndrome (OSA)
- Parasomnia
- Periodic Limb Movement Disorder (in sleep) (PLMD)
- Polysomnogram
- Polysomnographic technologist
- Polysomnography (PSG)
- Primary Snoring
- REM Behavior Disorder (RBD)
- Sleep Terrors
- Somnambulism
- Upper Airway Resistance Syndrome

■ CONTENT REVIEW TOPICS

- Cardiac dysrhythmias
- Chronic obstructive pulmonary disease
- Einthoven's Triangle
- Normal vital signs
- Patient assessment

- Pulse oximetry
- Respiratory patterns

■ PROCEDURAL ASSESSMENTS

28-1 Assessing the Polysomnography Patient
28-2 Educating the Polysomnography Patient
28-3 Introducing and Fitting for Positive Airway Pressure Interface
28-4 Applying Monitoring Devices for the Polysomnography
28-5 Acquiring Polysomnographic Data
28-6 Manually Scoring of the Polysomnogram

■ EQUIPMENT

- Abrasive Skin Prep
- Airflow Thermistor or Thermocouple, and Nasal Pressure Transducer
- Alcohol wipes
- Cotton tipped applicators
- Digital amplifier
- EEG conductive paste
- EEG gold disk electrodes with long lead wires
- Electrode input (jack) box
- Flexible cloth or paper metric measuring tape (washable or disposable)
- Gauze 2 × 2 cm gauze squares
- Hair clips
- Hypoallergenic medical tape
- Nontoxic China marker
- PAP delivery unit with heated humidifier
- Remote operation and digital readout at PSG acquisition device screen
- PAP interfaces (nasal mask, nasal pillows, full face mask, chin support strap)
- Polysomnographic acquisition device
- Pulse oximeter with probe (typically a module within the acquisition device)
- Respiratory effort sensors, thoracic and abdominal belts
- Snap-on long lead wires
- Snoring microphone
- Stick-on surface electrodes (pregelled ECG electrodes)
- Supplemental oxygen (when indicated)

This chapter provides an overview of polysomnographic technology and the duties of the polysomnographic technologist. It is not intended to be an in-depth and comprehensive tool for learning about the technical responsibilities and sleep disorders that are encountered in a sleep lab.

Polysomnography (*poly*—many, *somno*—sleep, *graphy*—tracing) (PSG) is the acquisition of various physiologic signals transmitted to a recording device for interpretation. To acquire and record the physiologic signals, sleep laboratories use computerized technology to digitalize and amplify the acquired signals. A series of electrodes and transducers are attached to the patient to record brainwaves (electroencephalography [EEG]) (Figure 28-1), cardiac wave forms (electrocardiography [ECG]), respiratory events (effort, air flow, saturation of peripheral oxygen [SpO$_2$]), limb movements, snoring, and other parameters during sleep. The data are then available for detailed review to assist qualified physicians in the diagnosis and treatment of sleep disorders. Respiratory therapists (RTs) who have been trained in polysomnographic testing play an integral role in the diagnosis and treatment of sleep-related breathing disorders. Examples of the most common sleep disorders

and some frequently performed sleep studies are listed in Boxes 28-1 and 28-2. Of the over 90 identified sleep disorders, 14 are related to sleep-disordered breathing. The most common sleep disorder diagnosed in the sleep lab is obstructive sleep apnea. The goal of the trained respiratory therapist is to help normalize disordered breathing during the overnight procedure. Normalizing breathing through the elimination of sleep apnea helps to restore neurologic sleep patterns and to provide the patient with restorative sleep, decreasing or eliminating the symptoms of snoring and excessive daytime sleepiness. This

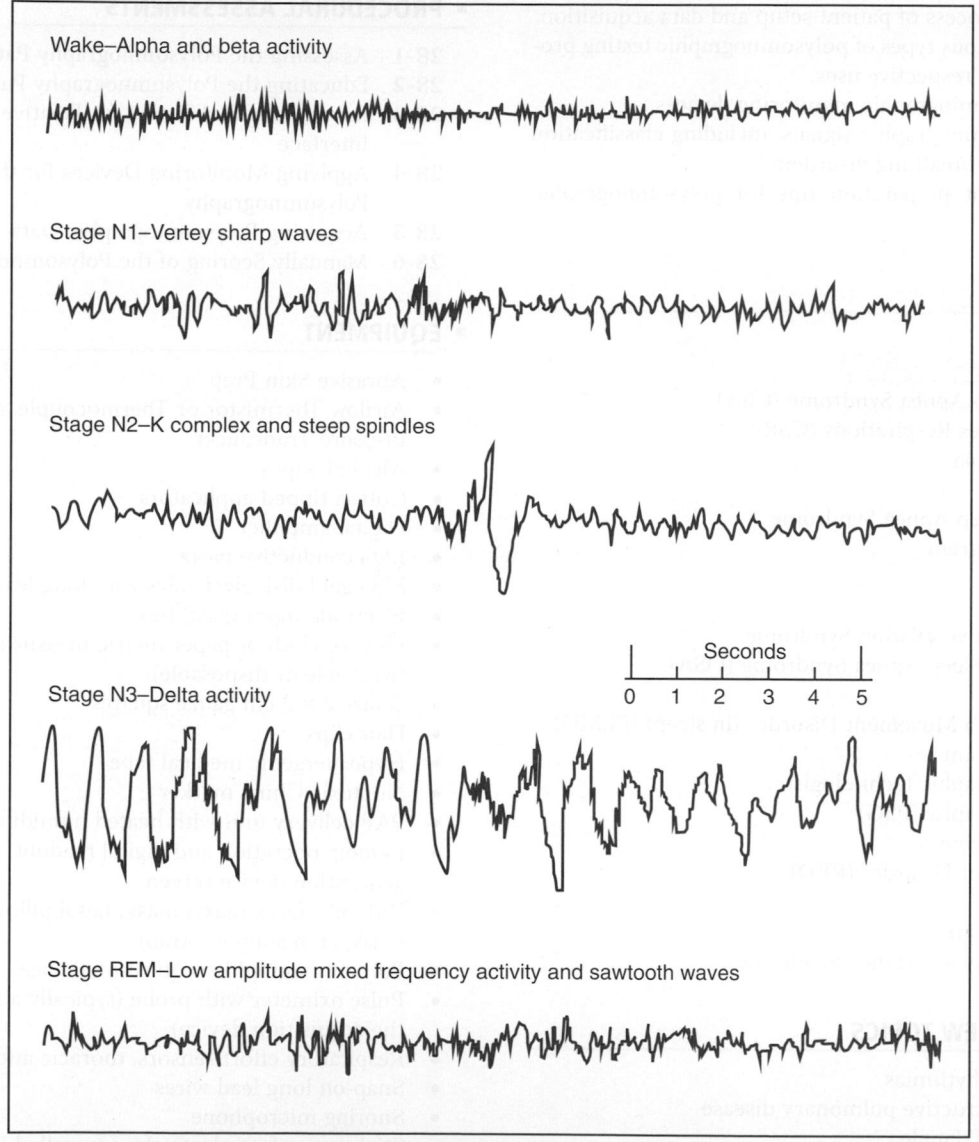

Figure 28-1 EEG of Human Sleep Stages. Wakefulness (Stage W) is identified by posterior alpha activity (patient relaxed with eyes closed) and anterior beta activity, active chin EMG and eye blinks. Slow rolling eye movements, theta activity and vertex sharp waves help to determine Stage N1 sleep. Stage N2 sleep is characterized by sleep spindles and K complexes. High amplitude (75μv) slow waves (delta activity) for 20% or more of the epoch are scored as Stage N3. Stage N3 is also referred to as slow wave sleep (SWS) or delta sleep. The EEG of REM sleep consists of low amplitude mixed frequency EEG- and REM-specific sawtooth waves. Eye movements (EOG) and chin EMG are used for the scoring of REM sleep. Sharp rapid eye movements of REM can resemble reading eye movements of wakefulness, however, the chin EMG will be greatly reduced from baseline levels, indicating the relative muscle paralysis of REM sleep, helping to differentiate from Stage W. (Source: Iber C, Ancolo-Israel S, Chesson A, Quan S: *The AASM Manual for the Scoring of Sleep and Associated Events, Rules, and Terminology and Technical Specifications.* © 2007 American Acacemy of Sleep Medicine).

BOX 28-1 Common Sleep Disorders

- Sleep-disordered breathing:
  - Obstructive sleep apnea syndrome (OSA)
  - Central sleep apnea syndrome (CSA)
  - Cheyne-Stokes respiration (CSR)
  - Obesity hypoventilation syndrome (Pickwickian Syndrome)
  - Complex sleep apnea syndrome
  - Upper airway resistance syndrome
  - Primary snoring
- Insomnia
- Narcolepsy
- Parasomnias:
  - Somnambulism—sleep walking
  - Sleep terrors
  - REM behavior disorder (RBD)
- Periodic limb movement disorder in sleep (PLMD)

BOX 28-2 Frequently Performed Sleep Studies

- **Nocturnal polysomnogram (NPSG):** a standard overnight diagnostic sleep study used to assess sleep disorders, including sleep apnea, narcolepsy, parasomnias, periodic limb movement disorders, 24 hour sleep–wake cycle disruptions, and so on. PSG monitoring includes physiological measurements such as respiratory effort and airflow, EEG (brain waves), EOG (eye movements), ECG (heart rhythms), chin and limb EMG (muscle movement), oxygen saturation (SpO$_2$), and snoring. These parameters are standard on every attended sleep lab–based overnight PSG both diagnostic and therapeutic.
- **PAP titration study:** In lab PSG for the therapeutic PAP treatment of previously diagnosed sleep apnea
- **Split-night polysomnography:** In lab sleep study that encompasses both the diagnosis and the therapeutic CPAP treatment of sleep apnea
- **Multiple Sleep Latency Testing (MSLT):** a series of daytime nap PSG studies that measure how long it takes a patient to fall asleep after a full night's sleep documented by in lab NPSG and to document the presence of REM sleep during the naps. Used for differential diagnosis for excessive daytime sleepiness and narcolepsy. Only EEG, EOG, ECG, and chin EMG are monitored.
- **Maintenance of wakefulness testing (MWT):** a series of daytime PSG studies developed to provide an objective measure of a patient's ability to remain awake under standardized conditions for a defined period of time after a full night's sleep documented by NPSG. Only EEG, EOG, ECG, and chin EMG are monitored. This procedure is often used post PAP or narcolepsy treatment in an attempt to determine treatment efficacy.

ECG, Electrocardiography; *EEG,* electroencephalography; *EMG,* electromyography; *EOG,* electrooculography; *REM,* rapid eye movement; *S$_P$O$_2$,* saturation of peripheral oxygen.

chapter will cover the indications, methodology, and interpretation of polysomnographic testing for the respiratory therapist (RT).

→ **Reality Check** Pediatric polysomnography has age-specific parameters for patient hookup and sleep stage scoring and is not included in this chapter.

✳ **Tip** The National Board for Respiratory Care (NBRC) offers an examination for the sleep technologist that is a subspecialty for current respiratory care practitioners (RCPs). The examination allows for credentialing as a Certified Respiratory Technician-Sleep Disorder Specialist (CRT-SDS) or a Registered Respiratory Therapist-Sleep Disorder Specialist (RRT-SDS). The Board of Registered Polysomnographic Technologists (BRPT) offers the Registered Polysomnographic Technologist (RPSGT) credentialing examination. The American Association of Sleep Medicine (AASM) offers the Registered Sleep Technologist (RST) examination.

>> SKILL CHECK LISTS

28-1 Assessing the Polysomnography Patient

Patient safety is the primary concern for the RT during diagnostic and positive airway pressure (PAP) titration sleep study procedures. Medical history taking and physical assessment of the patient are the first steps in preparing a patient for polysomnography. It is preferable to obtain a baseline set of vital signs, including blood pressure, prior to testing for all patients. Additionally, any special needs should be addressed prior to initiating patient preparation procedures. Patient-specific accommodations may include a bedside commode or easy access to handicapped bathroom facilities. Padded bedrails may be needed if seizures are suspected. Other assessments include factors complicating communication between the technologist and the patient, for example, the inability to follow simple verbal instructions because of language barriers, neurologic status, anxiety, or hearing loss. The sleep lab should also be prepared to provide supplemental oxygen when it is prescribed. The patient should be queried about medication or tape allergies. Use of medical tapes and adhesive surface electrodes during patient preparation may cause some patients to experience skin irritation. The technologist should also determine if the patient has issues with claustrophobia, before presenting the patient with options for PAP interfaces (masks).

✳ **Tip** All patients should have vital signs measured prior to the start of the PSG study. If the patient has complaints of chest discomfort, shortness of breath, or pain, vital signs should be obtained again; if the values are outside normal limits, contact the sleep lab medical director or the physician on call.

→ **Reality Check** Sleep labs require a detailed medical history from the referring physician as well as a sleep questionnaire completed by the patient detailing the primary sleep complaint.

Upon checking into the sleep lab, the patient is asked to complete a presleep questionnaire, which includes information about their activities the night before and the day of testing (Figure 28-2). This questionnaire will provide an indication of the quality of sleep the night prior to testing, napping on the testing day, medications taken prior to arriving at the lab, current state of wakefulness or sleepiness, and consumption of caffeine, alcohol, or other substances that may impact sleep.

Comorbidities such as cardiac disease, hypertension, diabetes, seizures, neuromuscular abnormalities, and pulmonary disease should be identified and documented. Disorders such as seizures may alter the process for data acquisition, and interpretation of the sleep study; cardiac abnormalities may present increased risks to the apnea patient during the night; and some medications may alter the appearance of the EEG data or lead to other changes in the recording. The technologist must be

---

SLEEP DISORDERS LABORATORY—PRESLEEP QUESTIONNAIRE

Name: _____ DOB: _____ Date: _____

Sleep specialist: _____ Form completed by: _____

I. HEALTH HISTORY (Check all that apply)

☐ Arthritis
☐ Back/Hip/Knee problems
☐ Bleeding problems
☐ Blood pressure problems
☐ Breathing problems
☐ Cancer
☐ Chipped or loose teeth

☐ Diabetes
☐ Dialysis
☐ Emotional problems
☐ Heart disease
☐ Hepatitis
☐ Infections/Communicable
   disease (i.e., VRE, MRSA, HIV)

☐ Insomnia
☐ IV device (i.e., Port, PICC, etc.)
☐ Kidney disease
☐ Seizures
☐ Sensory loss
   ☐ Hearing   ☐ Vision
☐ Sleep walking

☐ Skin problems/Wounds
☐ Sleep apnea
☐ Stomach/Bowel problems
☐ Stroke/TIA
☐ Exposure to toxic substances:

_____
_____
☐ Other: _____

II. PSYCHOSOCIAL–Sleeping problems:
☐ None   ☐ Difficulty falling asleep   ☐ Difficulty staying asleep   ☐ Other _____

IV. ALLERGIES/MEDICATIONS
List allergies and describe reactions to drugs, food, tape, Betadine, iodine-containing latex and tape (i.e., latex, rubber, other).

Allergy/Reaction   *Allergy/Reaction*   *Allergy/Reaction*

Did you bring any medications from home?   ☐ Yes   ☐ No If yes, please list.

V. HOSPITALIZATIONS
Have you been hospitalized for illness or surgeries in the last 6 months?   ☐ Yes   ☐ No If yes, please list.

_____

VI. PRE-SLEEP QUESTIONS
1. Has today been an unusual day in any way?
   ☐ Yes   ☐ No If yes, please explain: _____
2. How many hours of sleep did you get last night?_____
3. Did you take a nap today?   ☐ Yes   ☐ No If yes, how many, what time, and how long: _____
4. Did you consume any alcoholic beverages today?
   ☐ Yes   ☐ No If yes, what time, and how much: _____
5. Did you consume any caffeinated food or drinks today?
   ☐ Yes   ☐ No If yes, what time, and how much: _____
6. Please list below any medications you took today:
   a._____   b._____
   c._____   d._____
7. Do you have any physical complaints right now?
   If yes, please describe: _____
8. Do you feel ready to go to sleep right now?
   If no, please describe reason: _____
9. Please circle the description number that best describes how you feel right now:
   1. Active, alert, wide awake 2. Relaxed, awake 3. Foggy, anxious to sleep 4. Sleepy, prefer to be lying down
   5. Almost asleep, can't stay awake anymore

VII. CLINICIAN OBSERVATIONS - LABORATORY USE ONLY
Arrival date _____ Arrival time _____ Mode _____ Accompanied by _____
Mental status: ☐ Calm ☐ Anxious ☐ Withdrawn ☐ Alert ☐ Arousable ☐ Disoriented ☐ Unconscious ☐ Confused ☐ Fall/Risk assessment
CLINICAL NOTES: _____

_____

Technologist Signature: _____

Figure 28-2 PreSleep Questionnaire. (Modified from St. Joseph Health Center, SSM, St. Louis, MO.)

cognizant of potential health risks to the patient during the night and any possible recording difficulties (i.e., cardiac abnormalities, excessive movements, required nocturnal medications, etc.) that may impact patient safety.

Permission must be obtained from the patient to monitor, record, and treat sleep-related breathing disorders diagnosed during the sleep study. Standard medical procedure consent forms are signed and dated by the patient as well as the technologist prior to beginning polysomnography. Patients must be made aware that they will be video recorded during the hours of the sleep study. Video recording is essential to polysomnography to document technologist–patient interactions, sleeping position, parasomnias, seizures, or other behavioral events that may occur during the night. The following is the step-by-step process for assessing the polysomnography patient.

> **✱ Tip** The sleep technologist should review the presleep questionnaire (see Figure 28-1) with the patient.

> **→ Reality Check** Video recording provides documentation of the patient during sleep and interactions with the technologist who is entering and leaving the room while the patient is sleeping.

Procedural Preparation

1. Review the patient's chart.
2. Verify the physician's order and the facility's protocol for standard of care and appropriate study type (i.e., baseline PSG only, split night-baseline and titration, titration only, Multiple Sleep Latency Test (MSLT), etc.)
3. Identify the patient using two patient identifiers.
4. Follow the facility's protocol for patient interaction, and introduce yourself to the patient and the family.

Implementation

1. Obtain the patient's history for medication and substance allergies.
2. Ask the patient to verbally describe the reason he or she has come to the sleep lab, and his or her expectations of the testing procedure and potential treatments to be accomplished during the study.
3. Determine if the patient has had issues with claustrophobia.
4. Determine if the patient has special physical needs to be addressed prior to the start of the procedure (i.e., bedside commode, supplemental oxygen, padded bedrails, etc.).
5. Instruct the patient to complete a presleep questionnaire (see Figure 28-2), which includes information about the patient's activity the day of testing, prescribed medications already taken and medications to be taken while in the sleep lab, quality of sleep the night prior to testing, time the patient awoke, and any nap(s) taken on the day of testing.
6. Review the completed presleep questionnaire with the patient to ensure accuracy.
7. Determine any comorbidities that may be of concern during the procedure (i.e., cardiovascular abnormalities, diabetes, seizures, neuromuscular disorders, pulmonary disease, etc.).
8. Obtain written permission from the patient to monitor, record, and acquire video during the procedure and to treat breathing-related sleep disorders diagnosed in the sleep lab.

Evaluation of Procedure

1. Establish rapport with the patient, and gain his or her confidence.
2. Develop an appropriate sleep-related breathing treatment plan based on assessment data.
3. Identify any unexpected testing outcomes.

Documentation and Reporting

1. Record the PSG findings in the patient's chart.
2. Report any abnormal findings to the appropriate health care provider.
3. Inform the patient about the poststudy follow-up process.

28-2 Educating the Polysomnography Patient

The technologist must be able to clearly communicate the reason for polysomnographic testing and to explain the process of ancillary monitoring device application to the patient. Discuss with the patient sleep-disordered breathing, the negative health effects sleep disorders can have, and the benefits of PAP therapy, should it be indicated. Answer all patient questions and concerns before proceeding with the test to ease patient anxieties and help him or her become more comfortable and compliant with the testing procedures. The following is the step-by-step process for educating the polysomnography patient.

> **✱ Tip** Technologist to patient PAP discussions should include the interface and PAP pressure acclimation process, equipment orientation, and discussion of potential benefits of PAP therapy.

> **→ Reality Check** Patient anxiety can be relieved with proper explanation of testing and treatment procedures.

Procedural Preparation

1. Review the patient's chart.
2. Verify the physician's order or the facility's protocol for standard of care and for appropriate study type (i.e., split-night, titration, MSLT, etc.).

Implementation

1. Clearly explain the reason for PSG testing to the patient, making sure that he or she understands.
2. Explain the process of ancillary monitoring device application.
3. Educate the patient regarding sleep-disordered breathing and PAP treatment.
4. Discuss PAP therapy, including the acclimation process, equipment orientation, and the benefits of PAP therapy (see PAP therapy).
5. Answer all the questions and concerns the patient has before proceeding with testing to ensure the patient's comfort and compliance with the procedure.

Evaluation of Procedure

1. Establish patient confidence.
2. Determine patient competence.

3. Develop an appropriate plan of action based on patient's response to education.

4. Identify any unexpected outcomes.

Documentation and Reporting

1. Record patient education in the patient's chart.

28-3 Introducing and Fitting the Positive Airway Pressure Interface

The process of fitting the PAP interface (mask) may cause anxiety in some patients (Figure 28-3). A detailed explanation of the equipment used for PAP therapy helps alleviate stress for the patient. Several interface options should be presented to the patient with an explanation of pros and cons for each device. Patient comfort is the most important factor for compliance, and sufficient time should be exercised when assisting a patient with choosing the appropriate interface. A proper fit of the interface provides an adequate seal with minimal tension of the headgear. Interface manufacturers provide a wide variety of interface sizes and styles intended to accommodate differences in facial morphology, facial hair, and style preferences. Ask the patient to choose the style of interface that appears most appropriate for him or her, keeping in mind this is a new experience for most patients and that they may have no idea about what is suitable. For example, does the patient like to read or watch TV in bed while falling asleep? Does the patient need glasses? If so, the patient may prefer a nasal pillow type interface that allows the use of glasses while the patient is wearing the interface. Is the patient a mouth breather? If so, try a full-face interface that covers the mouth.

✳ Tip The interface should be comfortable for the patient while lying in the favorite sleeping position.

→ Reality Check A full understanding of PAP interfaces (masks) is critical for the sleep technologist to better assist the patient with interface choice. Training and experience with multiple interfaces allows the technologist to guide the patient to the most appropriate interface based on the patient's likes, dislikes, and needs.

Next, the concept of how PAP works by keeping the airway open should be explained to the patient. Understanding how the PAP device will improve breathing and subsequently sleep and daytime alertness may aid in patient adoption of the PAP devices. (See Box 28-3—PAP Devices.) In the case of patients who experience claustrophobia, ask them to hold the interface in place without the headgear or PAP pressure to acclimate to the feel of the interface, as this allows for the interface to be pulled away at will. Once the patient develops some confidence and comfort with the interface, add 4 cmH$_2$O PAP pressure, and allow the patient to experience breathing with the interface held against the face. Once the patient is able to hold the interface in place without pulling it away, assist with placing the headgear and adjusting the strap tension to keep

---

BOX 28-3 **PAP Devices**

PAP devices have evolved over the years from strictly continuous positive airway pressure (CPAP) to bi-Level positive airway pressure and automated devices. The following is a brief description of each of the device types and how they are used:

- CPAP—positive pressure is set at one pressure level to keep the airway open, acting as a pneumatic splint. Some systems offer a "ramp or flex" pressure setting to allow the patient to get used to gradually increasing levels of positive pressure as they fall asleep.

- Bi-level—inspiratory and expiratory pressures are set, typically 3–4 cm/H$_2$O apart to allow the patient to inhale with a higher level of pressure to open the airway and exhale against a lower level of pressure. Bi-level is especially useful for patients who are placed on higher PAP levels, which are difficult for some patients to exhale against. Bi-level devices also offer ventilator assist with timed and spontaneous options.

- Autotitration, non-invasive ventilation bi-level devices— PAP systems that utilize back-up rates, alarms and servo ventilatory support through sophisticated algorithms to determine the amount of positive pressure required to keep the patient's airway open on a breath-by-breath basis. These devices are used for treating patients with complex sleep apnea; sleep stage dependent apnea; and patients who may be going through significant physical changes such as weight loss, respiratory diseases such as COPD, restrictive thoracic diseases, complex sleep apnea, Cheyne-Stokes respiration, and neuromuscular diseases.

---

the interface in proper position. With the interface in place and the PAP unit turned on to the lowest pressure (4 cmH$_2$O), coach the patient to do easy, relaxed breathing through the nose. Often the patient will open the mouth to exhale when first trialing PAP, so encouragement to keep his or her mouth closed may be necessary. Extreme caution should be taken to avoid overtightening the headgear. Overtightening the straps will reduce the cushioning properties of the interface seal and create more leaks. Each interface manufacturer has a predetermined intentional leak for their interface products, and a proper fit will reflect a leak value within the manufacturers' guidelines.

→ Reality Check The idea of "strapping" a device on the face may be frightening for patients with claustrophobia. Providing these patients with training and allowing them to control interface placement on the face will help the patient to better tolerate PAP therapy.

PAP acclimation in the sleep lab is very time consuming but should not be skipped or shortened to save time. A patient who fully understands PAP therapy and has experienced the device and developed confidence in the therapy will experience a more successful titration process during the night.

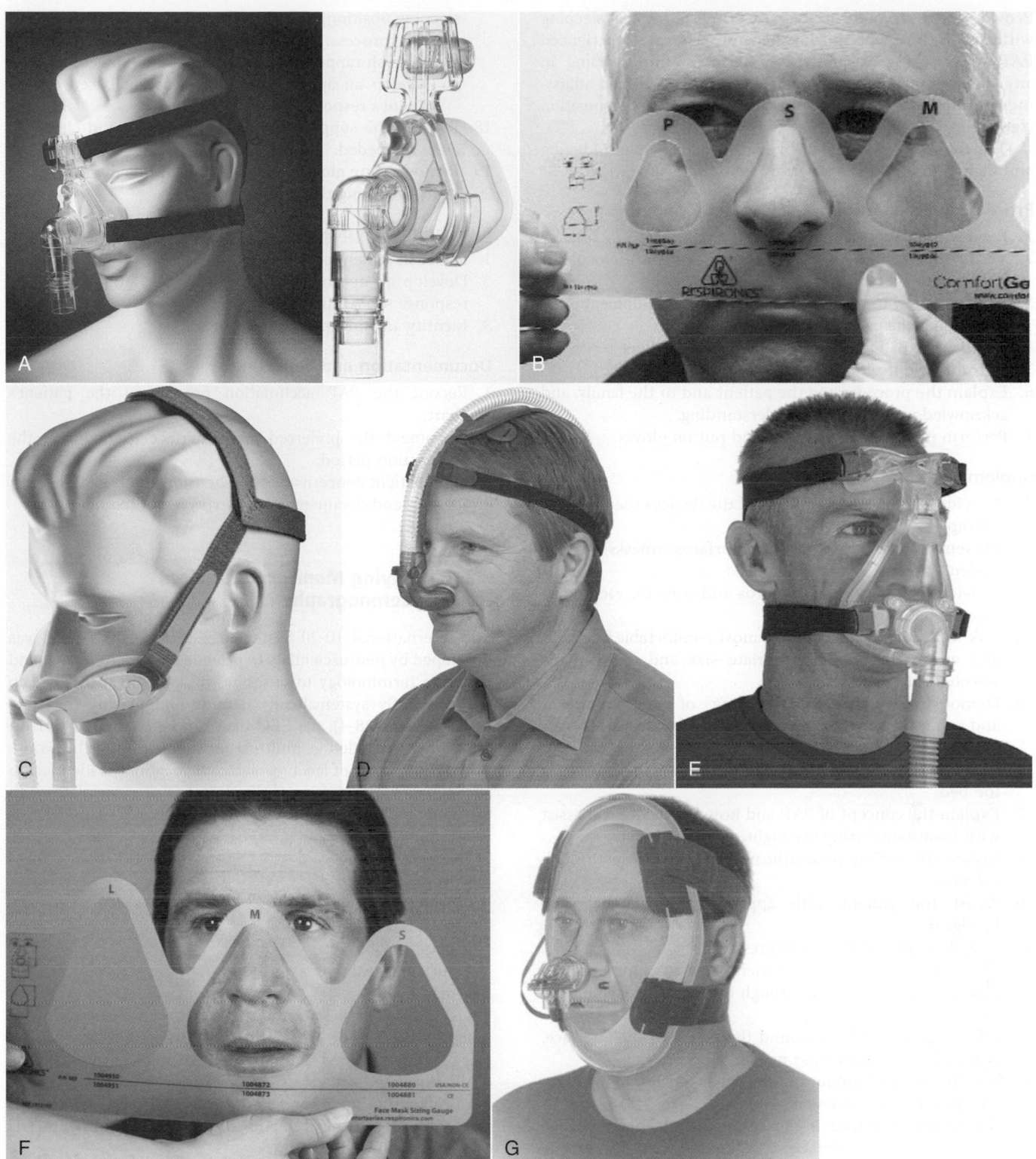

Figure 28-3 PAP Interface Examples. **A,** Nasal mask and headgear. **B,** A fitting gauge is used to ensure correct fitting of nasal mask. **C,** Nasal mini-mask and headgear. **D,** Nasal pillows and headgear. **E,** Full-face mask or oronasal mask. **F,** Sizing gauge used to determine proper size of full-face mask. **G,** Total face mask. (**A and C, F, and G,** Courtesy of Philips Respironics, Murrysville, PA. **D,** Image used with permission. Nellcor Puritan-Bennett, LLC, Boulder, CO, doing business as Covidien. **E,** Courtesy of ResMed, San Diego, CA.)

Provide encouragement to the patient by stating that sleeping with the device will quickly become natural. Experienced PAP users, using a variety of interfaces, find sleeping in any desired position comfortable, with only minor adjustments required, when moving to a new sleeping position (see Figure 28-3).

The following is the step-by-step process for introducing and fitting for a positive airway pressure interface.

Procedural Preparation

1. Review the patient's chart.
2. Verify the physician's order or the facility's protocol for standard of care.
3. Obtain, clean, and inspect the appropriate equipment prior to entering the patient's room.
4. Identify the patient using two patient identifiers.
5. Introduce yourself to the patient and to the family.
6. Explain the procedure to the patient and to the family, and acknowledge the patient's understanding.
7. Perform proper hand hygiene, and put on gloves.

Implementation

1. Provide a detailed explanation of the devices used for PAP therapy.
2. Present multiple options of interfaces (masks) to the patient.
3. Provide explanations of the pros and cons for each interface device.
4. Ask the patient to choose the most comfortable interface, and ensure that the appropriate size and fit has been selected for the patient.
5. Demonstrate your understanding of PAP interfaces and appropriate application for each device to the patient.
6. Instruct the patient to sit comfortably on the side of the bed.
7. Explain the concept of PAP and how the device will assist with breathing during the night.
8. Instruct the patient to breathe normally in and out through the nose.
9. Assist the patient with applying the interface and headgear.
10. Introduce PAP at 4 cmH$_2$O pressure.
11. Reassure and support the patient, and ask him or her to relax and breathe easily through the nose throughout the process.
12. Assess for any leak(s) around the edges of the interface, and make adjustments, as needed.
13. Use the minimal amount of headgear tension to maintain an adequate interface seal.
14. Adjust the interface if measured leak is unacceptable, or change the interface if adequate seal cannot be maintained.
15. Instruct the patient to lie down in the supine position:
    a. The interface may need a slight adjustment when moving into the supine position to maintain a good seal.
16. Assure the patient that PAP will be initiated only if indicated by findings on the polysomnogram.
17. Determine patient tolerance of interface and PAP pressure by allowing time to acclimate to any changes with interface or position (allow the patient to move to the preferred

sleeping position) and to ensure the patient is comfortable with the process:
    a. Establish rapport and gain patient confidence.
    b. Develop an appropriate plan of action based on the patient's response to PAP.
18. Remove the supplies from patient's room, and clean the area, as needed.
19. Remove your gloves, and perform proper hand hygiene prior to leaving the patient's room.

Evaluation of Procedure

1. Establish patient confidence.
2. Develop an appropriate care plan based on the patient's response to PAP therapy.
3. Identify any unexpected outcomes.

Documentation and Reporting

1. Record the PAP acclimation process in the patient's chart.
2. Document the preferred PAP interface used during the acclimation period.
3. Note patient concerns or apprehension about PAP therapy.
4. Identify and document any unexpected outcomes.

28-4 Applying Monitoring Devices for Polysomnography

The International 10-20 System of electrode placement was developed by neuroscientists to provide a standard format and common terminology to describe the location of EEG scalp electrodes. By systematically naming and placing the electrodes (Figure 28-4), the EEG data can be compared serially, even when recorded at multiple locations around the world. The 10-20 System of labeling electrode locations is identical in all languages. The naming of the electrode sites correlates with the cortical structures under the electrodes, for example:

T—temporal lobe
F—frontal lobe
FP—frontal polar
C—central fissure
O—occipital lobe
P—parietal lobe
A—auricular (ear)
M—mandible

The 10-20 System is so termed "10-20" because electrodes are spaced either 10% or 20% of the total distance between a given pair of predetermined landmarks such as the area at the bridge of the nose, or "nasion," or the protrusion on the back of the head called the "inion," and so on. The 10-20 System also provides uniform spacing of electrodes for accurate and symmetrical comparison of EEG data.

Nomenclature for the International 10-20 System was developed to give each electrode site a logical alphabetical abbreviation that immediately identifies it with the lobe or area of the brain to which it refers. All of the alphabetical characters refer to the area of brain over which they are located with the exception of "z" which is used for the numerical subscript zero or the midline zero reference (FPz, Fz, Cz, Pz). Refer to Figure 28-4A for descriptions of the regions covered in electrode placement. Table 28-1 lists the alphabetical abbreviations used.

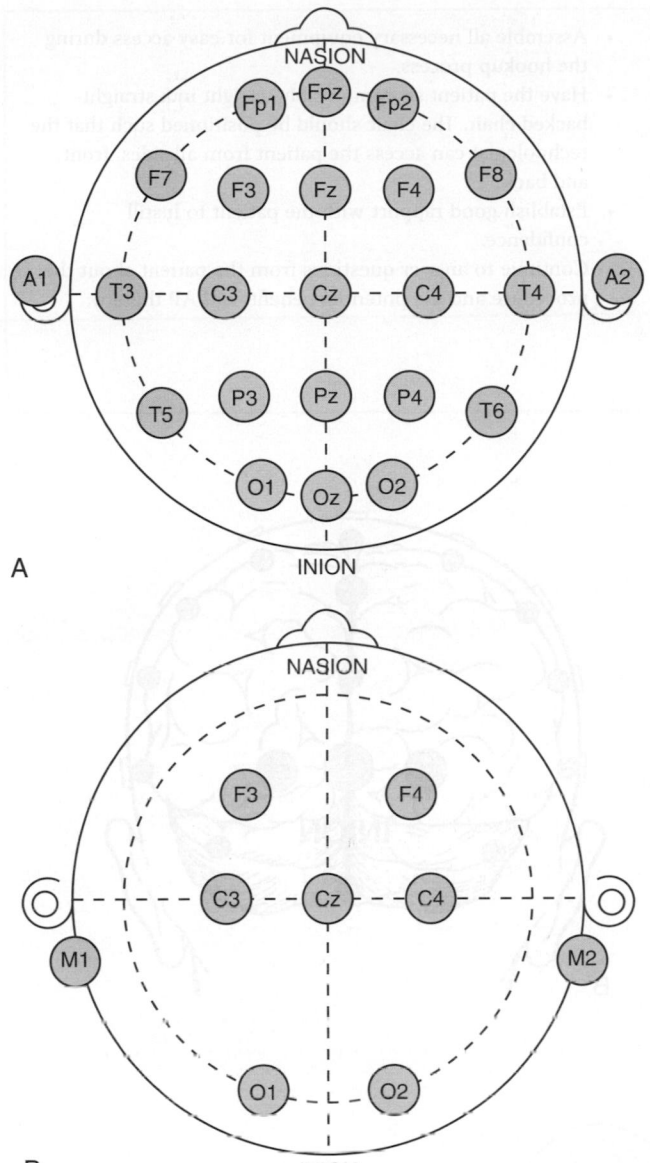

Figure 28-4 A. EEG electrode placement locations. B. EEG Electrode Placement for PSG.

TABLE 28-1 Nomenclature for the International 10-20 Electrode Placement System

C	Central	P	Parietal
F	Frontal	A	Auricular
Fp	Frontal polar	M	Mastoid
T	Temporal	Z	Midline
O	Occipital		

The numbers refer to the right or left hemisphere. All of the even subscripted numbers refer to the right hemisphere, and all the odd numbered subscripts refer to the left hemisphere of the brain. The numbered subscripts also define the electrode location in relation to the midline. For example, the smaller the subscript, the closer it is to the midline. When electrode sites

are properly measured and electrodes are applied according to the 10-20 System, the coverage of the right and left hemispheres is symmetrical.

There are four skull landmarks for the 10-20 System. Locating these landmarks is the first step in the measuring procedure. Each landmark is marked with a nontoxic skin pencil or china marker. These are not electrode positions, but reference points from which the basic measurements are derived. They are listed in Figures 28-4A and 28-5A, B and C.

The sequence of measurement in the 10-20 System is critical for accurate placement of EEG electrodes. The 10-20 System uses measurement in centimeters, rather than inches, to prevent errors in determining 10% or 20% of distances between landmarks. Electrodes are placed over the point where two lines intersect (forming a cross) from the measured distances. The sequence of measurement and measuring procedure are given in Boxes 28-4 and 28-5.

By the end of this procedure, 19 standard electrode positions should be identified on the scalp (see Figure 28-5). PSG reference electrodes M1 and M2, plus an EEG ground electrode make a full complement of 22 electrodes sites. For polysomnography, only those EEG electrode sites and signals useful for sleep staging are applied and acquired. Patients with seizures or neurologic disorders may require additional EEG electrodes and channels for a more in-depth assessment of brain activity during sleep. Standard polysomnography acquisition records the following EEG channels: F3, F4, C3, C4, O1, O1, M1 and M2, (see Figure 28-4B).

Eye movements during sleep are also recorded to aid in the determination of sleep stages. The cornea of the eye is more positive, and the retina of the eye is more negative, and as a result, eye movements create measureable biopotential wave forms called an electrooculogram (EOG). To monitor eye movement biopotentials for scoring sleep stages, electrodes are placed on the outer canthus of each eye. The American Academy of Sleep Medicine (AASM) recommends that the left eye monitoring electrode be placed 1 centimeter (cm) lateral and 1 cm below the outer canthus of the left eye; the right eye monitoring electrode is placed 1 cm lateral and 1 cm above the outer canthus of the right eye to create the biopotentials to record eye movements. Offsetting the electrodes up and down from the horizontal plane allows for detection of both vertical *and* horizontal eye movement, relevant to rapid eye movement (REM) sleep, as well as the slow, rolling eye movements seen in drowse or stage N1 sleep (Figure 28-6).

Because of a relatively paralyzed state, to prevent the physical acting out of dreams, skeletal muscles, including the facial muscles, relax and lose tone during REM sleep. To document this relative paralysis and loss of muscle tone during REM sleep, electrodes are placed on the chin or jaw to record submental electromyography (EMG). These electrodes are instrumental in the identification of REM sleep when the muscle tone and recorded EMG signal drops dramatically. The AASM guidelines recommend placing two to three electrodes for chin EMG monitoring (recording from all three simultaneously is acquisition device vendor specific, but three electrodes are usually placed, with one as a backup). One electrode is placed at the midline of the chin on the mentalis muscle and two are placed (right and left of the midline) 4 cm apart on the submentalis muscle, located 2 cm below the inferior edge of the mandible. In the case of a patient with significant facial hair or other issues, the chin EMG electrodes may also be placed on

✳ **Tips** when preparing the patient for the application of monitoring devices:
- Explain the application process of electrode location and placement and the function of recording sleep waveforms during the testing.
- Identify and explain devices needed to measure airflow, breathing effort, heart rate, and oxygen levels.
- Assure the patient that monitoring devices will be placed and secured to minimize interference with normal sleeping positions and movement during the test.
- Ask the patient to prepare for bed by changing into sleepwear and performing bedtime routines (i.e., washing face, brushing teeth, etc.).

- Assemble all necessary equipment for easy access during the hookup process.
- Have the patient sit comfortably upright in a straight-backed chair. The chair should be positioned such that the technologist can access the patient from all sides, front and back.
- Establish good rapport with the patient to instill confidence.
- Continue to answer questions from the patient about the procedure and the potential benefits of PAP therapy.

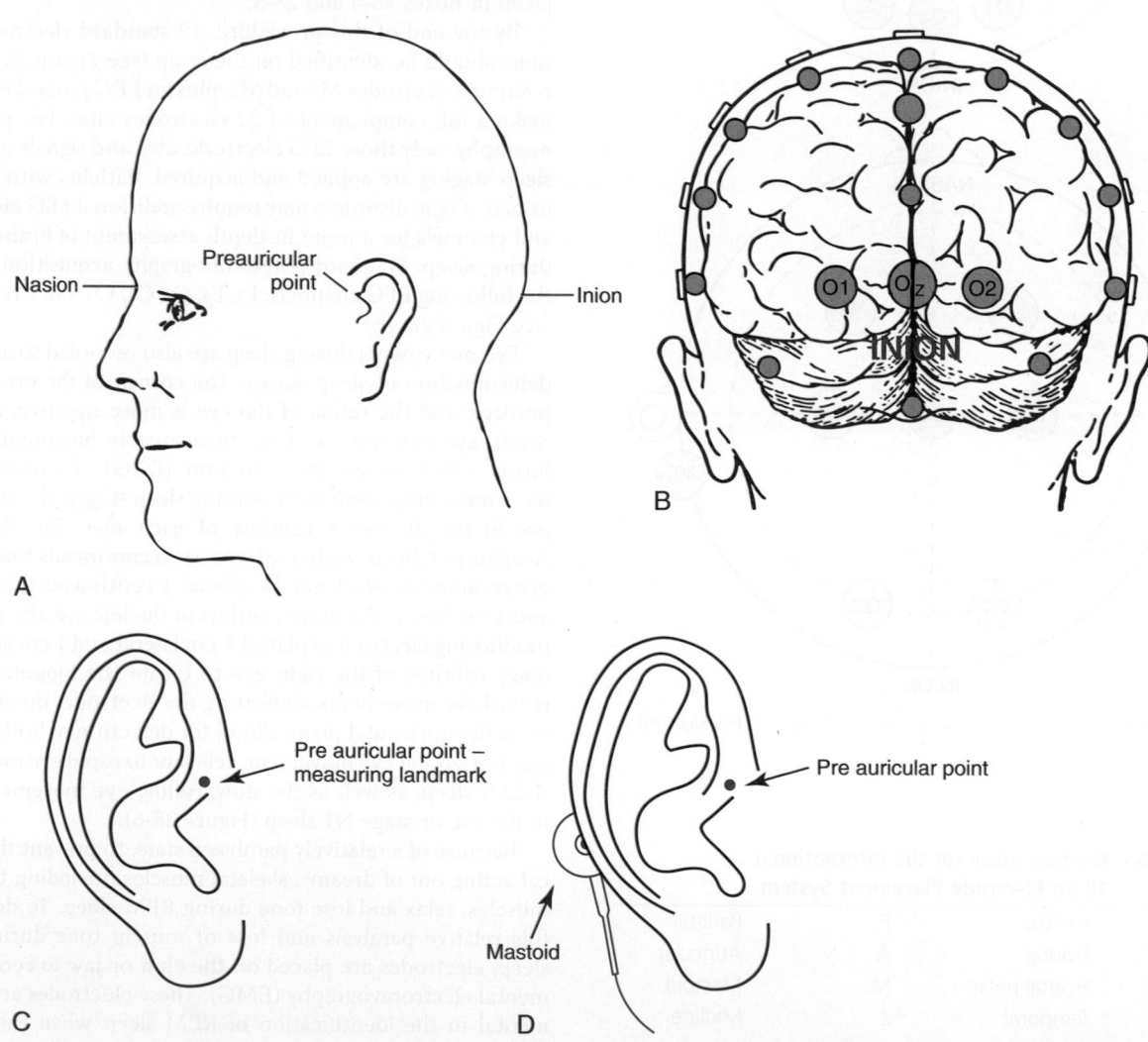

Figure 28-5 Skull Landmarks for the International 10-20 System. **A,** The nasion: The indentation between the forehead and the nose, located between the eyes. The inion is a ridge or bump that can be felt as you run your finger up the back of the neck to the skull. If the location of the inion in not obvious, ask the patient to tilt the head back while you are trying to feel the ridge. If the location of the inion is still in doubt, it should be marked as the same level as the preauricular points. The preauricular points are located at the indentations just above the cartilage (tragus) that covers the external ear opening. Preauricular points must be located at both the right and left sides. **B,** Occipital scalp electrode locations using the 10-20 System. **C,** The dot is landmark for the preauricular point. **D,** Mastoid reference electrode placement behind ear.

BOX 28-4 Measuring Procedure of the International 10-20 System

- Locate the skull landmarks:
  - Nasion
  - Inion
  - Preauricular points right and left
- Measure the distances along the midline between the nasion and the inion with the tape measure in centimeters. (See Box 28-5A)
- Determine what half (50%) of this distance is and mark Cz perpendicular to the tape.
- Determine 10% of the total nasion–inion distance and mark FPz on the forehead and mark Oz at the back of the head, both 10% up from the landmarks.
- Determine 20% of the total distance from FPz for location of Fz (Fz is halfway between FPz and Cz).
- 20% of the total distance back from Cz is Pz (Pz is halfway between Cz and Oz).
- Measure the distance between the right and left preauricular points making sure that the tape goes through Cz.
- Place the second mark for Cz, creating a cross exactly halfway between the preauricular points. This completes the two marks for the Cz position.
- Measure up 10% from the right preauricular point, and place a lateral mark perpendicular to the tape. This is the first mark for T4
- Place a lateral mark perpendicular to the tape for electrode position $C4$ halfway between $T4$ and Cz.
- Follow the same procedure for the left side of the head to locate $T3$ and $C3$.
- Measure the circumference of the head making sure that the tape goes through FPz and the occipital Oz reference points and $T3$ and $T4$.
- Divide the circumference of the head into 10 equal parts as follows:
  - Determine 10% of the total circumference of the head and mark this distance on your tape measure.
  - Position the tape measure so that it straddles the midline at the level of FPz. Make a vertical mark at 5% on each side of the midline (FPz). The right mark is $FP2$ and the left mark is $FP1$.
- Do the same process to find $O1$ and $O2$, make a vertical mark at 5% on each side of the midline (Oz). The right mark is $O2$ and the left mark is $O1$.
- Place your 10% tape measurement at $FP2$ and then make a vertical mark for $F8$ on the right. Proceed moving posteriorly along the circumference line making vertical marks for $T4$ and $T6$.
- Repeat this procedure for the left side of the head, moving posteriorly from the $FP1$ mark.
- Measure the distance from $FP1$ and $O1$ going through $C3$. At 50% of this distance make the intersecting mark that completes the cross for electrode position $C3$.
- Locate $F3$ halfway between $FP1$ and $C3$.
- $P3$ is halfway between $C3$ and $O1$.
- Repeat this procedure on the right hemisphere. At 50% of the distance between $FP2$ and $O2$ is $C4$. This completes the mark for the $C4$ position.
- Locate $F4$ halfway between $FP2$ and $C4$.
- $P4$ is halfway between $C4$ and $O2$.
- With the tape, measure the distance from $F7$ to $F8$ through Fz. Determine 50% of this distance and mark. This becomes the final mark for Fz.
- The final mark for $F3$ is placed halfway between Fz and $F7$.
- The final mark for $F4$ is halfway between $F8$ and Fz.
- Measure the distance from $T5$ to $T6$ through Pz. Mark one half of this distance. This mark completes the Pz location.
- One half of the distance from Pz to $T5$ distance is the final mark for $P3$.
- One half of the distance from Pz to $T6$ is the final mark for $P4$.
- Place the referential electrodes M1 (left) and M2 (right) on the mastoid process, which is the bony area behind the ear, just below the hairline.
  - The electrodes should be placed on the bony area just below the hairline behind the ear, to minimize ECG artifact coming from the carotid arteries.

BOX 28-5 Sequence of Measurement for the International 10-20 System

1. Measure nasion to inion followed by subdivisions for FPz, Fz, Cz, Pz, and Oz.
2. Measure preauricular point to preauricular point passing the tape measure through Cz, completing the Cz placement and locating one mark of $T3$, $C3$, $C4$, and $T4$.
3. Circumference measurement through Oz, FPz, $T3$, and $T4$, followed by the division of this total distance into 10 equal segments to locate the vertical mark for $FP1$, $F7$, $T3$, $T5$, $O1$ $FP2$, $F8$, $T4$, $T6$, $O2$, and completing $T3$ and $T4$.
4. Measure $FP1$ to $O1$ through $C3$, on the left side of the head for the location of $F3$, $C3$, and $P3$, completing the location of $C3$. Repeat for the right side of the head.
5. Measure $F7$ to $F8$ through Fz to complete electrode position for $F3$, Fz, and $F4$.
6. Measure $T5$ to $T6$ through Pz, to complete electrode position for $P3$, Pz, and $P4$.

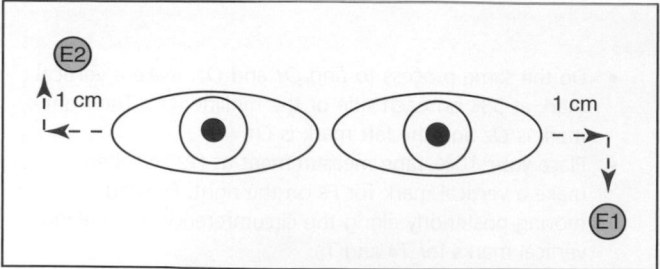

Figure 28-6 E1 is 1 cm out and 1 cm down from left outer canthus. E2 is 1 cm out and 1 cm up from the right outer canthus.

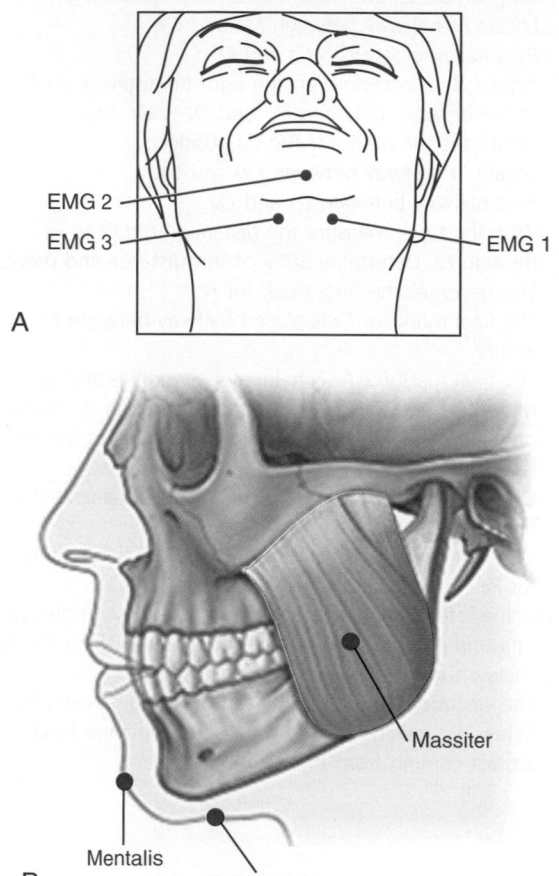

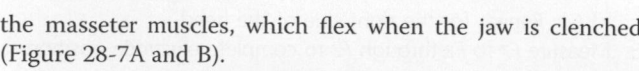

Figure 28-7 Chin EMG Lead Placement. **A,** Mentalis and submentalis muscle is primary lead placement. **B,** Masseter muscle—alternate chin EMG site.

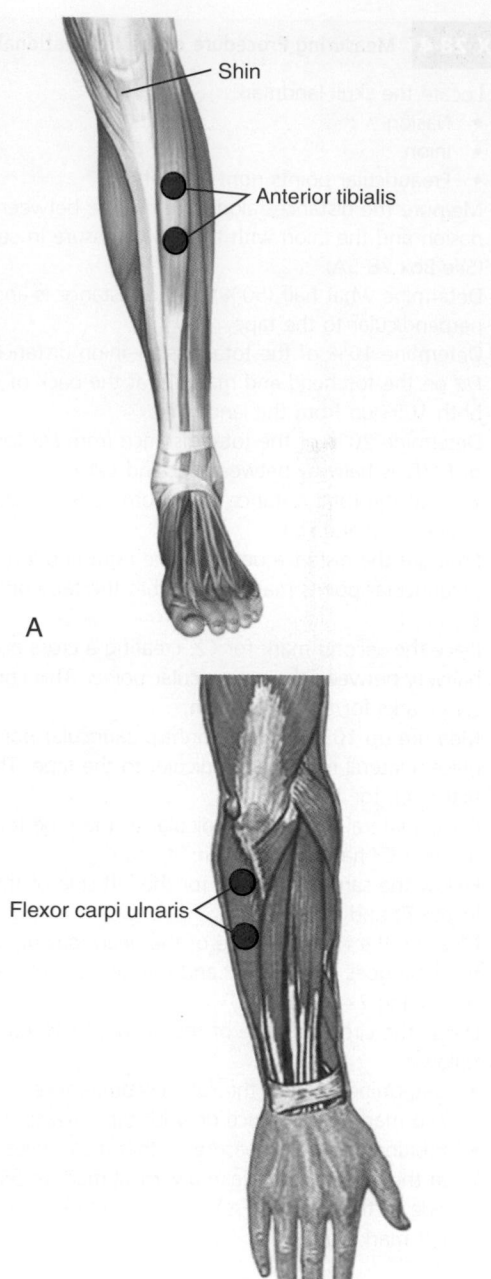

Figure 28-8 Limb EMG Lead Placement. **A,** Anterior tibialis placement. **B,** Alternate site—Flexor carpi ulnaris.

the masseter muscles, which flex when the jaw is clenched (Figure 28-7A and B).

Right-leg and left-leg EMG electrodes are placed on the anterior tibialis muscles to record leg movements. The AASM recommends placing two electrodes on each leg 2 to 3 cm apart, about 4 cm down from the knee and 1 cm from the outside of the shin bone for two channel monitoring of both legs (Figure 28-8, *A*). To find the muscle, ask the patient to flex the leg as if stepping on the gas pedal to determine maximum muscle movement. Pull the lead wires up through the leg of the pajama bottoms and up through the pajama top, with the leads exiting through the neck hole of the pajama top, to

prevent the leads from being dislodged during the night. An alternative limb monitoring site is the flexor carpi ulnaris on the forearm (see Figure 28-8, *B*).

Standard snap style ECG electrodes are used to monitor ECG activity on the polysomnogram. The AASM recommends two to three leads placed on the right shoulder and left hip or rib cage, in a modified Einthoven's Triangle; when three leads are used, the left shoulder is added (Figure 28-9).

An airflow thermistor or thermocouple and a pressure transducer (Figures 28-11, *A&B*)are placed together between the nose and upper lip, with the three prongs of the cannulas resting at the nostrils and over the mouth to detect both nasal and oral breathing. A microphone is placed on either side of the trachea to record the sounds and vibrations of snoring. To monitor respiratory effort, respiratory inductance plethysmography (RIP) belts are placed on the chest and abdomen, preferably on the outside of the patient's pajamas or t-shirt. The

chest or thoracic respiratory effort belts should be placed just below the arm pits and above the nipples encircling the thorax. The abdominal effort belt is placed below the lower rib cage and around the abdomen. It is recommended that the patient's breathing be observed to determine where the greatest excursion occurs to most accurately place the effort belts. The belts, which come in different sizes and are adjustable, should be placed tight enough to move with respiration but not so tight that they no longer have room to expand. To monitor SpO_2 levels during the study, the polysomnographic monitoring device will have a pulse oximetry module built into the recorder and a proprietary finger probe that fits their jack box (Figures 28-10 and 28-11).

Snoring sounds are also monitored to provide correlation with obstructive events. A snoring microphone is taped on either side of the trachea. To find the correct location, ask the patient to hum, paper tape should be applied (Figure 28-12).

After all of the electrodes have been applied, the lead wires are gathered together at the base of the patient's neck and bundled with a Velcro strip at two to three locations to prevent the wires from becoming entangled during the night. The following is the step-by step process for the application of monitoring devices for polysomnography.

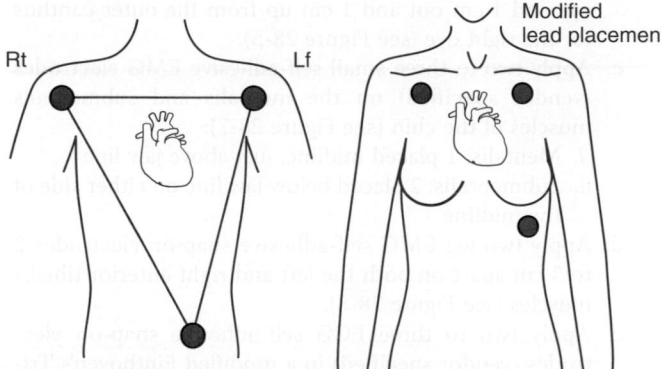

Figure 28-9 ECG Lead Placement. This shows the Einthoven's Triangle configuration for ECG lead placement. Some machines require three leads and others just two.

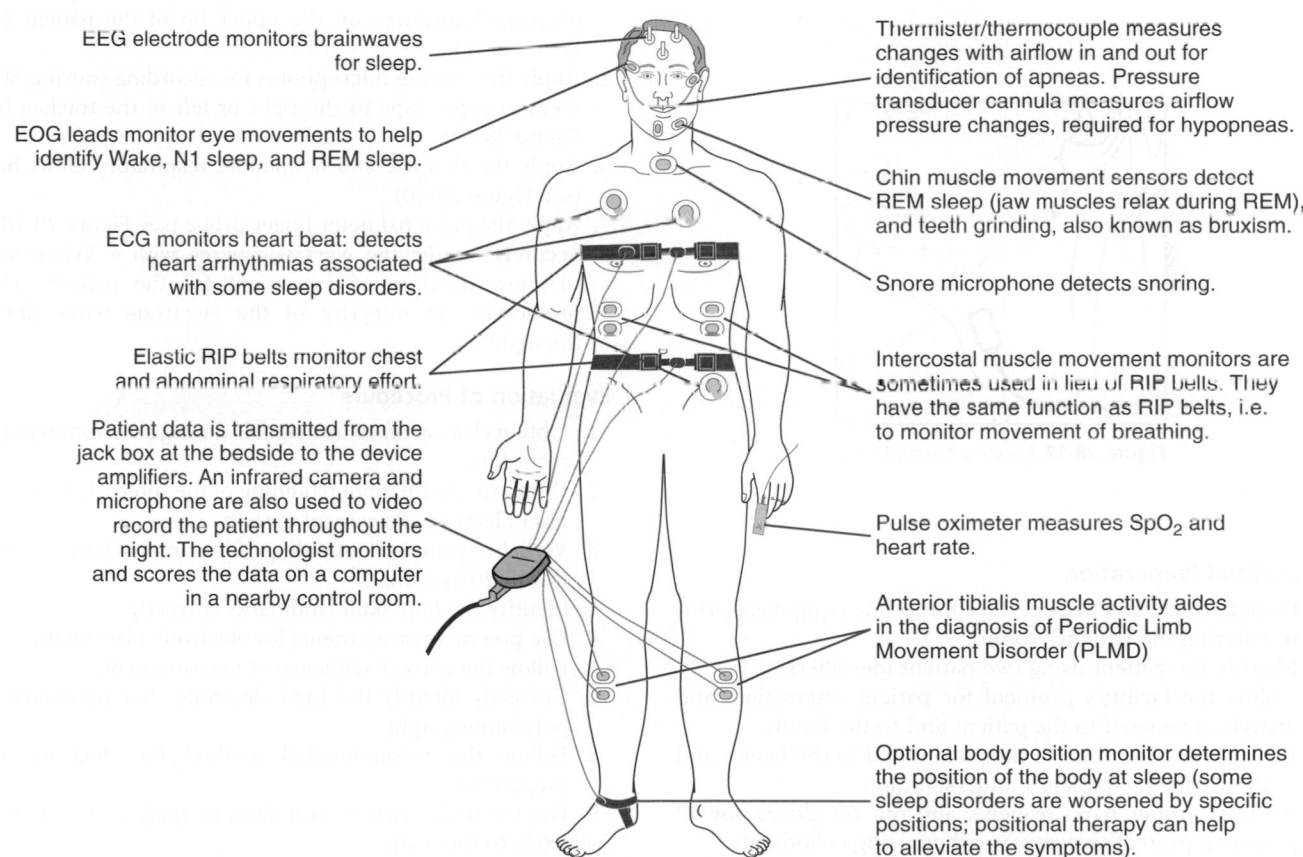

EEG electrode monitors brainwaves for sleep.

EOG leads monitor eye movements to help identify Wake, N1 sleep, and REM sleep.

ECG monitors heart beat: detects heart arrhythmias associated with some sleep disorders.

Elastic RIP belts monitor chest and abdominal respiratory effort.

Patient data is transmitted from the jack box at the bedside to the device amplifiers. An infrared camera and microphone are also used to video record the patient throughout the night. The technologist monitors and scores the data on a computer in a nearby control room.

Thermister/thermocouple measures changes with airflow in and out for identification of apneas. Pressure transducer cannula measures airflow pressure changes, required for hypopneas.

Chin muscle movement sensors detect REM sleep (jaw muscles relax during REM), and teeth grinding, also known as bruxism.

Snore microphone detects snoring.

Intercostal muscle movement monitors are sometimes used in lieu of RIP belts. They have the same function as RIP belts, i.e. to monitor movement of breathing.

Pulse oximeter measures SpO_2 and heart rate.

Anterior tibialis muscle activity aides in the diagnosis of Periodic Limb Movement Disorder (PLMD)

Optional body position monitor determines the position of the body at sleep (some sleep disorders are worsened by specific positions; positional therapy can help to alleviate the symptoms).

Figure 28-10 Patient is ready for a sleep study with RIP belts to detect thoracic and abdominal respiratory effort. ECG leads are placed. EEG leads are placed on the head. EOG electrodes are placed above and below the eyes. EMG electrodes are placed. A snoring microphone is placed on the front of the neck. A thermistor and pressure tranducer are placed to monitor airflow at the nose and mouth. A pulse oximeter is placed for measurement of SpO_2 and heart rate. Finally, electrodes are placed on the right and left anterior tibialis muscles.

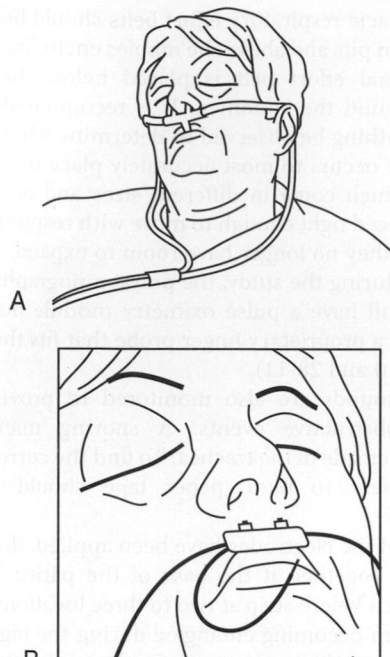

Figure 28-11 Airflow Monitoring Devices. **A,** Nasal-oral pressure transducer cannula. This detects and amplifies airflow pressure changes. **B,** Nasal-oral thermistor and thermocouple that detects temperature differences in inhaled and exhaled air.

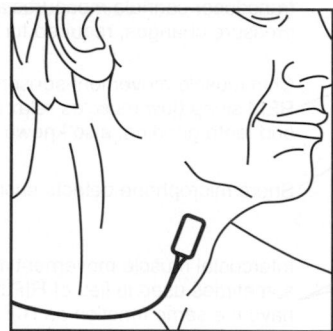

Figure 28-12 Snoring Microphone.

Procedural Preparation

1. Obtain, clean, and inspect the appropriate equipment prior to entering the patient's room.
2. Identify the patient using two patient identifiers.
3. Follow the facility's protocol for patient interaction, and introduce yourself to the patient and to the family.
4. Explain the procedure to the patient and to the family, and acknowledge the patient's understanding.
5. Perform proper hand hygiene, and put on gloves (for all patients), protective eyewear (when using collodion).

Implementation

1. Utilize accurate EEG electrode placement using the International 10-20 Electrode Placement System after correctly measuring and identifying EEG for PSG electrode sites.

2. Prepare each electrode site with a mildly abrasive gel and a cotton swab to ensure quality, artifact-free tracings.
3. Apply the appropriate electrode to the site by using electrode paste and a 1 cm × 1 cm gauze square.
   a. Some labs may attach the electrodes by using collodion and gauze with a conductive gel.
   b. Apply the EOG electrodes by using offset pattern of 1 cm lateral and 1 cm down from the outer canthus for the left eye and 1 cm out and 1 cm up from the outer canthus for the right eye (see Figure 28-5).
   c. Apply two to three small self-adhesive EMG electrodes (vendor specified) on the mentalis and submentails muscles of the chin (see Figure 28-7):
      i. Mentalis: 1 placed midline, just above jaw line
      ii. Submentalis: 2 placed below jaw line on either side of the midline
   d. Apply two leg EMG self-adhesive snap-on electrodes 2 to 3 cm apart on both the left and right anterior tibialis muscles (see Figure 28-8).
   e. Apply two to three ECG self-adhesive snap-on electrodes (vendor specified) in a modified Einthoven's Triangle, with one electrode on the right shoulder and one electrode on the left hip, and, if a third electrode is used, an additional electrode on the left shoulder (see Figure 28-9).
4. Place and secure with tape, two types of airflow monitoring devices, an oral nasal thermistor or thermocouple, *and* a pressure transducer on the upper lip of the patient (see Figure 28-11).
5. Apply the snoring microphone, for recording snoring, with medical paper tape to the right or left of the trachea (see Figure 28-12).
6. Apply the thoracic and abdominal respiratory effort belts (see Figure 28-10).
7. Apply the pulse oximeter finger probe (see Figure 28-10).
8. Securely bundle the electrode wires with a Velcro strip to allow freedom of movement for the patient, while protecting the integrity of the electrode wires during the night.

Evaluation of Procedure

1. Obtain clear, artifact-free signals during polysomnography recording.
2. Demonstrate full understanding of the International 10-20 EEG Electrode Placement System.
3. Verbalize your understanding of the nomenclature used in the 10-20 System.
4. Identify the four skull landmarks correctly.
5. Use precise measurements for electrode placement.
6. Follow the correct sequence of measurement.
7. Correctly identify the EEG electrode sites necessary for polysomnography.
8. Follow the recommended method for electrode site preparation.
9. Use electrode paste or collodion to apply each EEG electrode to the scalp.
10. Demonstrate appropriate caution when using collodian, taking into consideration patient safety with regard to room ventilation and fire precautions.

Documentation and Reporting

1. Record the PSG recording in the patient's chart.

28-5 Acquiring Polysomnographic Data

Currently, sleep diagnostics are performed using a computerized acquisition medical device to obtain and record the signals derived from the ancillary monitoring devices. The computerized system converts the analog EEG waveforms into numerical (digitized) signals. This process is known as *analog-to-digital conversion*. The digitized waveforms are displayed in real time on the computer screen. The rate at which the waveform data are sampled to convert them to a numerical format is known as the *sampling rate*. The sampling rate must be fast enough to ensure good signal quality (Figure 28-13). The sampling rate is expressed in hertz (Hz). For example, 500 Hz is 500 sample times per second. The AASM recommends the sampling rates shown in Table 28-2.

EEG signals that have been digitized and saved during the recording can be manipulated during and after acquisition, allowing changes to the montage, filters, gain, and the number of recorded seconds or minutes displayed on the screen.

The EEG activity is the basis for determining sleep staging for PSG. All of the additional acquired physiologic signals are collected and displayed simultaneously to show the relationships between events. The designated recording sites and their arrangement in the record are known as the *montage*. Standard polysomnography includes the acquisition of EEG activity, chin muscle activity, air flow and pressure, respiratory effort, ECG, leg muscle activity, and pulse oximetry. The AASM recommends acquiring EEG from electrode sites F3, F4, C3, C4, O1, O2, M1, M2. It is acceptable for the computer screen to display F4-M1, C4-M1, O2-M1 only, in an effort to save screen space. The acquisition of all of the EEG signals ensures backup in the event that a connection fails during the night. For enhanced recordings the montage can be modified to include the entire compliment of EEG electrodes for evaluation of seizure disorders. Additional muscle channels such as flexor carpi ulnaris for the arms and intercostal EMG for respiratory effort may be added to the montages for additional monitoring. The montage will display the label of each signal, including the reference source (M1, M2), where relevant.

Prior to the start of the PSG to ensure that all of the ancillary monitors have been placed correctly and are working properly, the patient is asked to perform a biocalibration procedure. The patient is asked to look left, look right, look up and down, blink and close the eyes (EOG) (EEG changes with eyes closed), grind teeth together (chin EMG), make a snoring sound (snore microphone), flex each leg (limb EMG), breath in and out through the mouth and nose separately (thermistor or thermocouple and pressure transducer), and breathe deeply to expand the RIP belts, ensuring respiratory muscle movements are captured.

The following is the step-by step process for acquiring polysomnographic data.

Procedural Preparation

1. Prepare the patient for bedtime.
2. Assist the patient to bed, and assist him or her to find a comfortable supine position.
3. Explain the process of biocalibration to the patient.
4. Select the appropriate testing protocol (i.e., split-night, titration, MSLT, MWT).

Implementation

1. Perform amplifier and montage calibration per vendor guidelines, using the appropriate filters; sensitivity and gain settings for each channel recorded confirms all signals from the amplifier are responding correctly.
2. Ask the patient to perform biocalibration immediately before the "lights out" command.
3. Ensure that the signals obtained are clear and artifact free and that all of the ancillary devices are working properly.
4. Instruct the patient to get into a comfortable position, close his or her eyes, and try to go to sleep.
5. Mark the record with the "lights out" tag to begin the procedure.
6. Document physiologic data at 30-minute intervals.
7. Document body position changes, interventions, or disruption in monitoring.
8. Document ending of the testing period with the "lights on" tag.
9. Perform montage calibrations to verify signal integrity.

Evaluation of Procedure

1. Adjust the monitoring devices, as needed, to obtain artifact-free signals.
2. Document the maneuvers performed during biocalibration.

TABLE 28-2 American Association of Sleep Medicine Recommended Sampling Rates

Modality	Desirable	Minimal
EEG, EOG, EMG, ECG	500 Hz	200 Hz
Airflow	100 Hz	25 Hz
Oximetry	25 Hz	10 Hz
Nasal pressure	100 Hz	25 Hz
Esophageal pressure	100 Hz	25 Hz
Body position	1 Hz	1 Hz
Snoring sounds	500 Hz	200 Hz
Thoracic or abdominal	100 Hz	25 Hz

ECG, Electrocardiography; *EEG,* electroencephalography; *EMG,* electromyography; *EOG,* electrooculography.
(Data from AASM: *The AASM scoring manual*: http://www.aasmnet.org/scoringmanual/default.aspx. Accessed.)

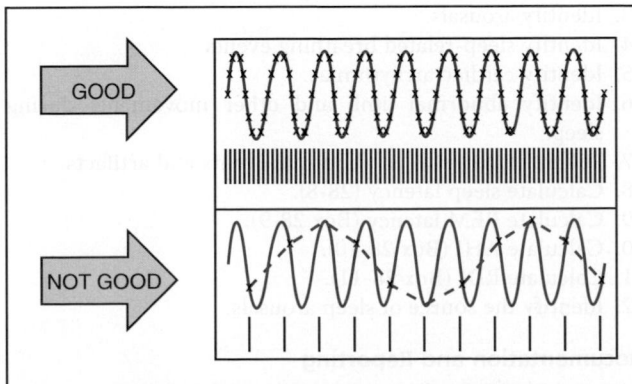

Figure 28-13 Signal Sampling Rate Chart.

3. Document the data obtained at the required intervals during the procedure.
4. Document the pertinent data, when needed, between the regular charting intervals.
5. End the recording interval with the "lights on" tag.
6. Perform amplifier calibration at the end of testing period to verify signal integrity.

Documentation and Reporting

1. Document each biocalibration maneuver in the polysomnographic record.
2. Obtain clear, artifact-free signals during polysomnography, and fix the ancillary device issues, as needed.
3. Document the data obtained at the required intervals during the procedure.
4. Ensure that the PSG event tags are present to allow for data assessment.

28-6 Manual Scoring Of The Polysomnogram

Once the polysomnographic data have been recorded, they must be analyzed in great detail to fully evaluate the night's sleep. Scoring is used to determine sleep stages, sleep architecture and arousals from sleep (EEG, EOG, chin EMG), sleep-related breathing abnormalities (SpO_2, airflow, snoring, and effort), cardiac abnormalities (ECG), and limb (anterior tibialis EMG) and other movement abnormalities. The AASM has provided well-defined rules for scoring all aspects of the polysomnographic and these rules should be consulted routinely to ensure accuracy. The polysomnographic data are reviewed multiple times in their entirety prior to compiling the data for final interpretation.

The initial pass through the data will establish sleep staging for each 30-second epoch beginning at the "lights out" tag and through to the "lights on" tag at the ending of the testing procedure. Sleep stages include W (wake), N1, N2, N3, and R (REM). *Sleep onset* is defined as the time it takes a patient to have the first epoch other than W after "lights out." Typically, but not always, the first stage is N1. N1 is defined by slow, rolling eye movements, attenuation of alpha activity (8–13 Hz sinusoidal wave forms seen in wake), low amplitude mixed frequency (LAMF) EEG activity in the 4- to 7-Hz range, and the occurrence of vertex sharp waves over the central electrodes. N1 is followed by N2. N2 is determined by the onset of sleep spindles (fast sinusoidal wave forms greater than 14 Hz) and K-complexes (high amplitude wave forms with sleep spindles) not associated with arousals. N3, or slow wave sleep, typically follows N2 and is defined by slow delta wave forms (0.5–2 Hz) with an amplitude of 75 microvolts (μV) or greater, comprising 20% or more of the epoch. REM sleep, which typically appears about 90 minutes after sleep onset, is determined by the presence of rapid eye movements and a flattening of the muscle activity in the chin EMG electrodes (typically the lowest amplitude in the study) and the presence of sawtooth waves (2–6 Hz). Brainwave activity is low amplitude mixed frequency (LAMF) EEG, and it may look similar to wake.

Once sleep staging is complete, the next pass through will identify respiratory events, evaluating each event for type of event, duration, associated sleep arousals, and oxygen desaturations. Apneas and hypopneas are measured from the lowest point of the last normal breath to the beginning of the first normal breath after the apnea or hypopnea. Respiratory events are described in Box 28-6.

Following the respiratory scoring, the polysomnogram is reviewed for cardiac arrhythmias that may or may not be related to respiratory events. Another pass through the record will document limb or other movements and associated arousals that are independent of respiratory events previously noted. The scorer must determine which events have caused the arousal and the impact on the overall sleep patterns. Depending on the amount of sleep disturbance found in the polysomnogram, more passes through the record may be needed to score all of the events. Scoring a single polysomnogram recording may take several hours when the patient has had a very disturbed sleep or significant respiratory and limb movements or other sleep pathologies. Most technologists will score the recording a few hours at a time throughout the night so that most of the scoring is completed by morning. Scoring sections of the data throughout the night is also required for split-night PAP studies because the criteria for the introduction of PAP therapy must be met and documented.

Once the record scoring is complete, the calculations for sleep efficiency, sleep latencies, and respiratory and movement indexes may be calculated by the acquisition device computer, providing a detailed analysis and report of the technologist scored data (see Box 28-7 for sleep stage scoring rules). The following is the step-by-step process for manual scoring of the polysomnogram.

Procedural Preparation

1. Review the patient's chart.

Implementation

1. Perform an initial pass through the record to score sleep stages, according to the AASM guidelines.
2. Perform a second pass through the record to score sleep-related breathing events, according to the AASM guidelines.
3. Perform additional passes through the record, as needed, for cardiac events, limb movements, and other event-related arousals, according to the AASM guidelines.
4. Demonstrate understanding of sleep architecture.

Evaluation of Procedure

1. Identify sleep onset.
2. Identify changes in sleep stages.
3. Identify arousals.
4. Identify sleep-related breathing events.
5. Identify cardiac arrhythmias.
6. Identify abnormal limb and other movements during sleep.
7. Differentiate between abnormal events and artifacts.
8. Calculate sleep latency (28-8).
9. Calculate REM latency (Box 28-9).
10. Calculate AHI (Box 28-10).
11. Calculate RDI (Box 28-11).
12. Identify the source of sleep arousals.

Documentation and Reporting

1. Record patient information in the patient's chart.

BOX 28-6	Respiratory Events

1. **Obstructive sleep apnea (OSA)**—continued inspiratory effort associated with a ≥ 90% decrease in airflow from the peak signal excursion of the thermal sensor of pre-event baseline (diagnostic study), or PAP device flow (titration study), for ≥ 10 seconds. Typically associated with an EEG arousal and oxygen desaturation

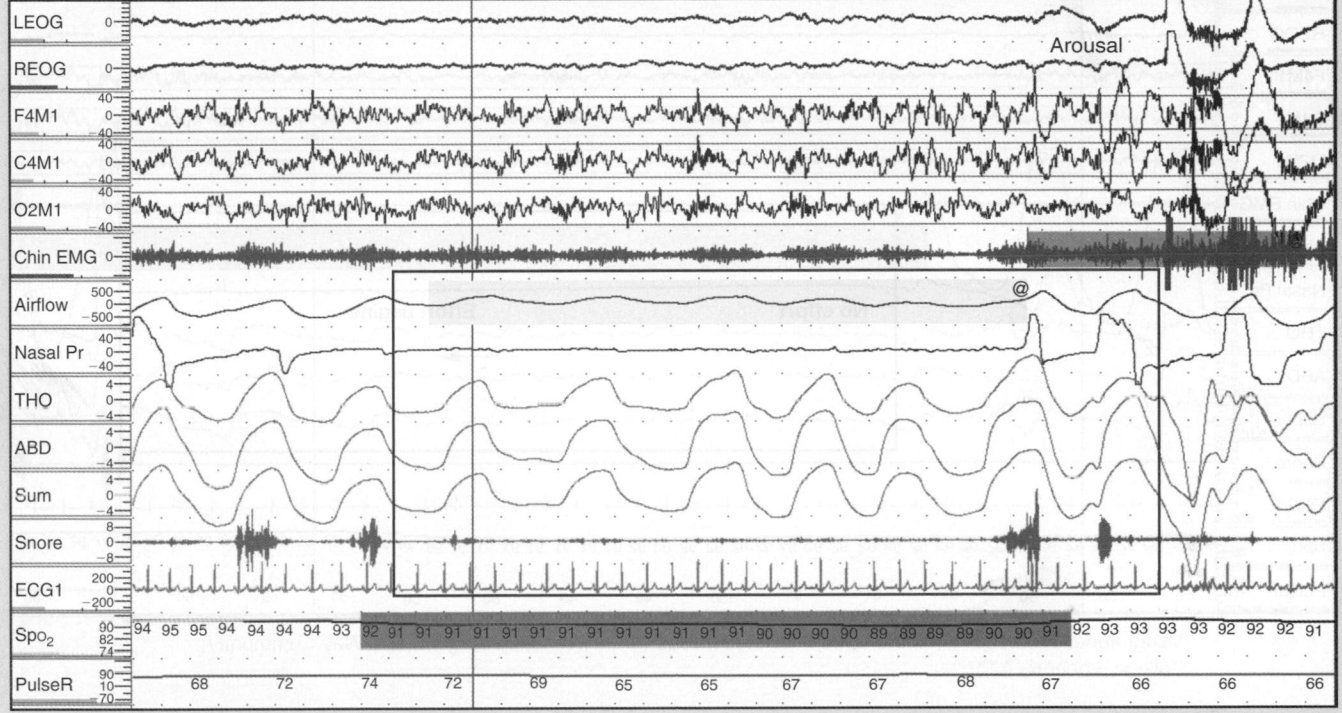

Obstructive sleep apnea (OSA) in N2 sleep, 1-minute screen. (With permission from Wendi M. Nugent, GateWay Community College, Phoenix, AZ.)

2. **Central sleep apnea (CSA)**—no inspiratory effort or airflow for ≥ 10 seconds. Typically associated with an EEG arousal and oxygen desaturation

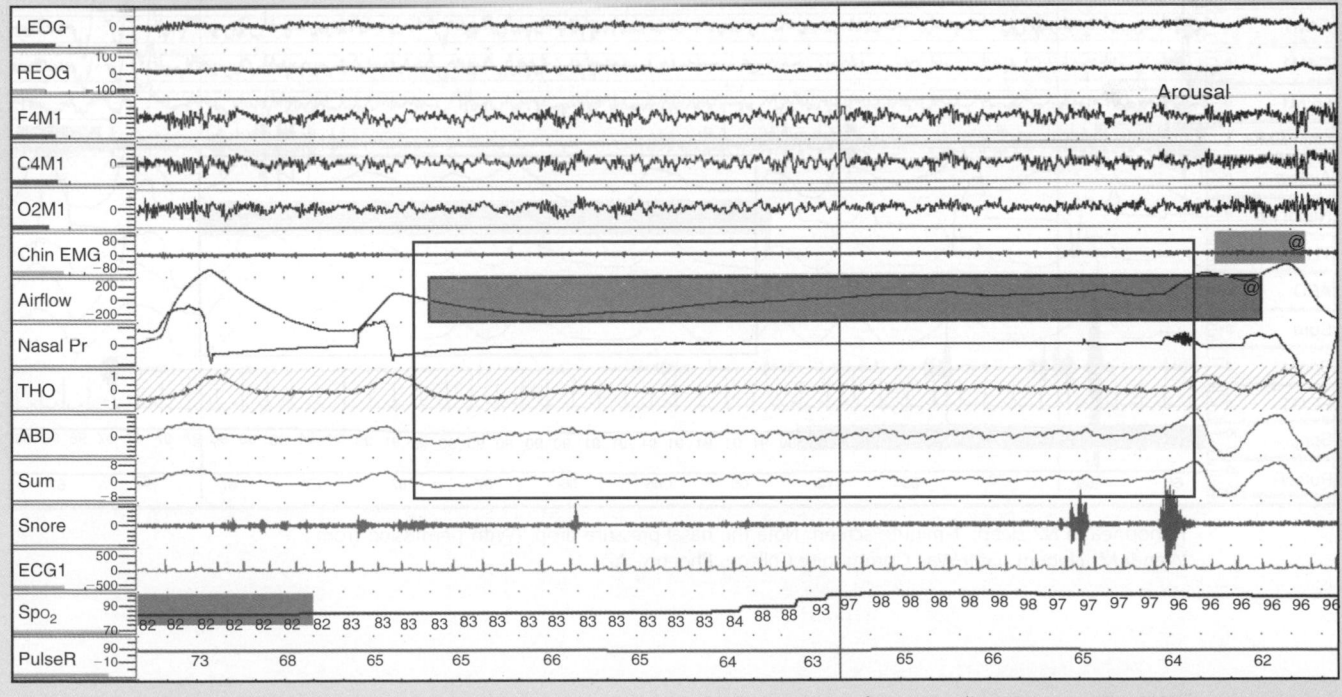

Central sleep apnea (CSA) in REM Sleep, 1-minute screen. (With permission from Wendi M. Nugent, GateWay Community College, Phoenix, AZ.)

Continued

BOX 28-6   Respiratory Events—cont'd

3. **Mixed apnea**—initially onset of central apnea with no effort or airflow, followed by resumption of inspiratory effort and no airflow, for ≥ 10 seconds

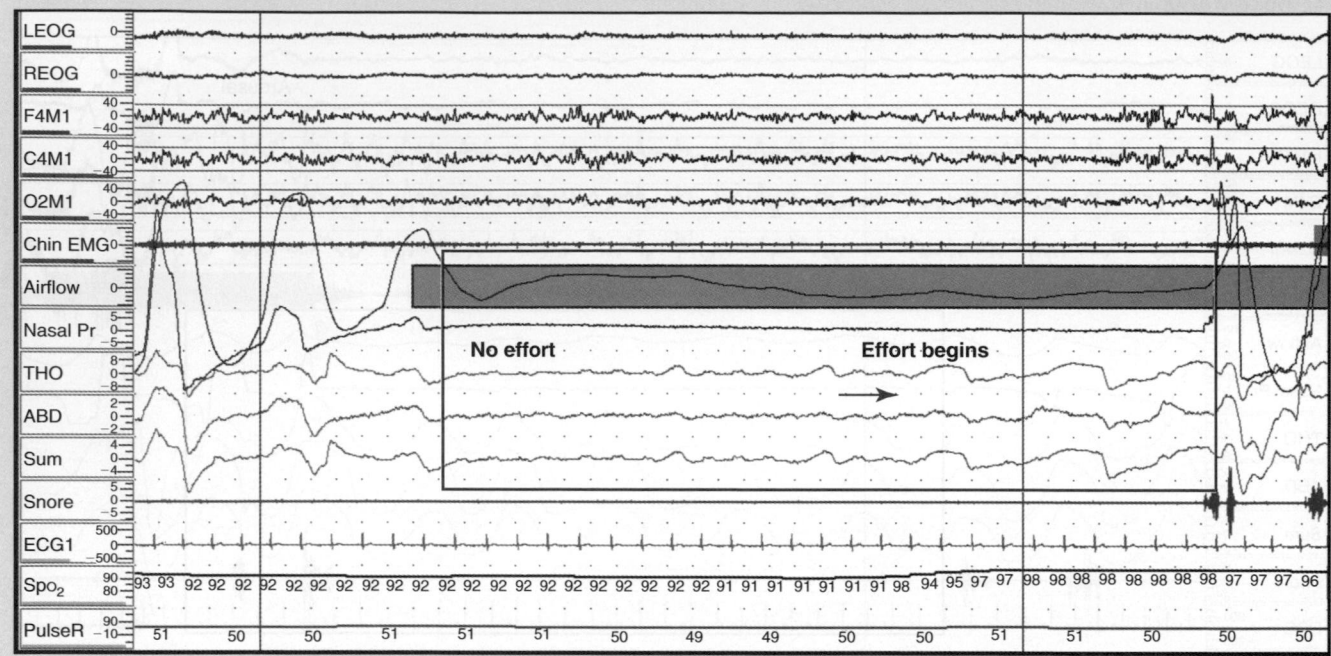

Mixed apnea N2 sleep, 1-minute screen. (With permission from Wendi M. Nugent, GateWay Community College, Phoenix, AZ.)

4. **Hypopnea**—scored when the peak signal excursions drop by ≥ 30% of pre-event baseline using nasal pressure (diagnostic study), PAP flow measurement (titration study), for ≥ 10 seconds associated with either ≥ 3% arterial oxygen desaturation or an arousal.

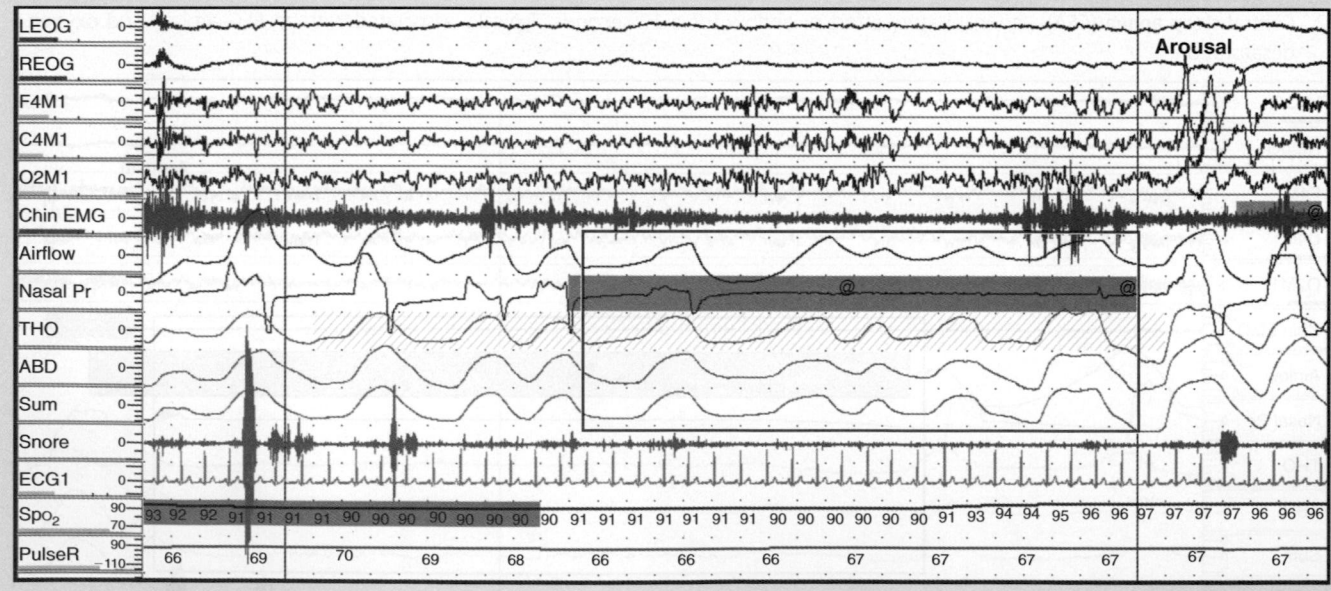

Hypopnea in N2 sleep, 1-minute screen. Note the nasal pressure drop. (With permission from Wendi M. Nugent, GateWay Community College, Phoenix, AZ.)

BOX 28-6   **Respiratory Events—cont'd**

5. **Respiratory effort related arousal (RERA)**—when an apparent respiratory event does not meet criteria for an apnea or a hypopnea, score a RERA.

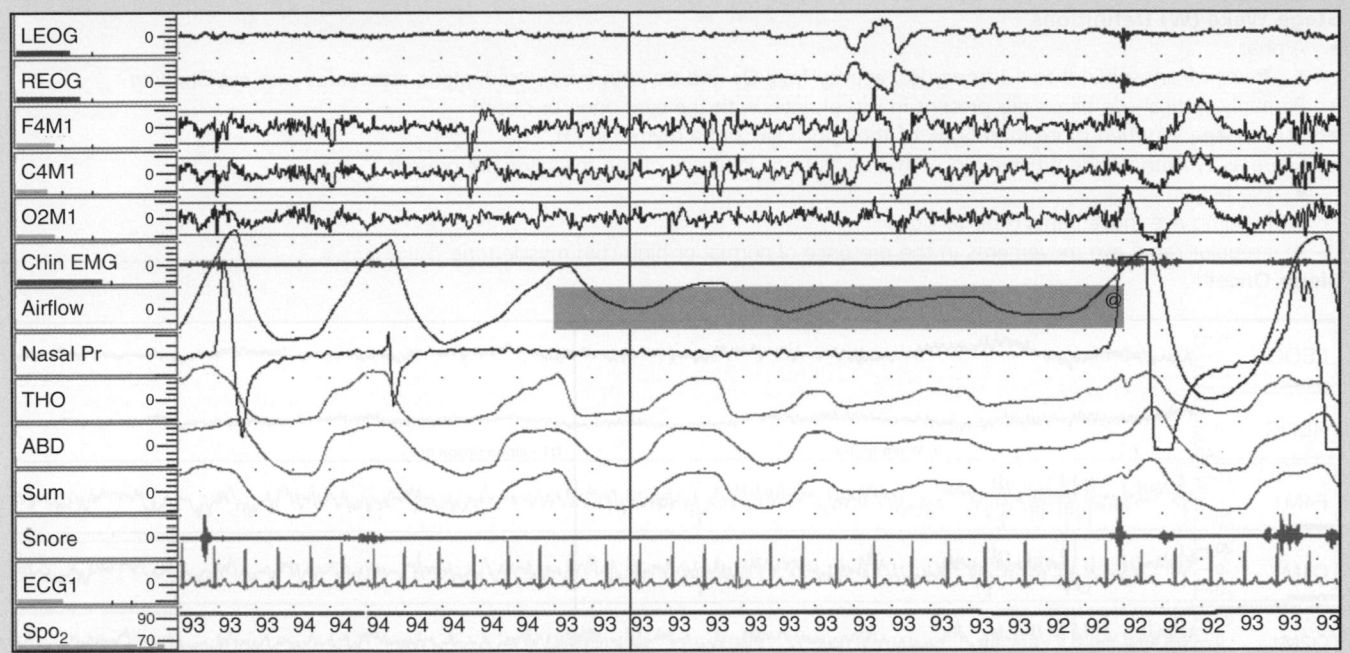

Respiratory event related arousals (RERAs) during REM sleep, 30-second screen. (With permission from Wendi M. Nugent, GateWay Community College, Phoenix, AZ.)

  a. RERA is a sequence of respiratory events lasting ≥ 10 seconds, which display increasing respiratory effort or flattening of the nasal pressure wave forms leading to arousal.

6. **Hypoventilation**—using an end tidal or transcutaneous CO_2 monitoring device, score hypoventilation if there is a ≥ 10 mm Hg increase in $PaCO_2$ during sleep in comparison to an awake supine value

7. **Cheyne-Stokes Breathing (CSB)**—score CSB if there are at least three consecutive cycles of crescendo/decrescendo changes in breathing amplitude, associated with at least one of the following:

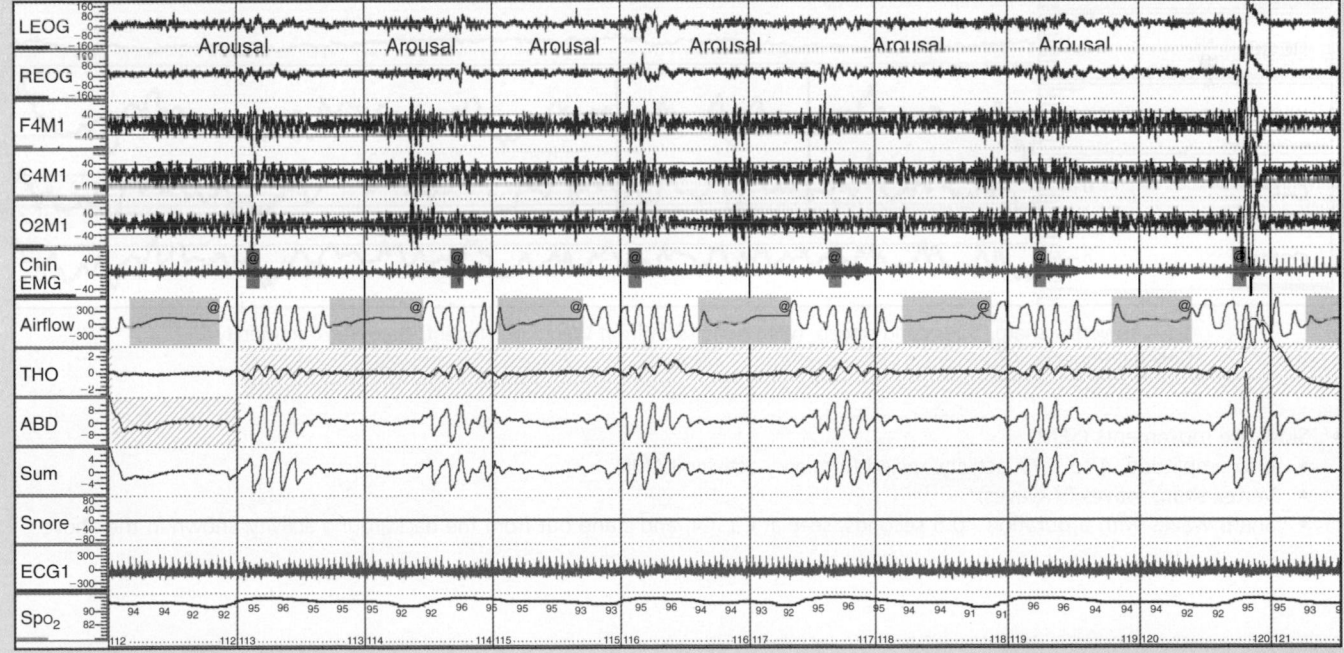

Cheyne-Stokes respiration, N2 sleep, 5-minute screen. Note arousals displayed in the chin and EEG channels occur in the middle of the respiration cycle. (With permission from Wendi M. Nugent, GateWay Community College, Phoenix, AZ.)

  a. Five or more central apneas or hypopneas per hour of sleep

  b. Cyclic crescendo/decrescendo change in breathing amplitude has a duration of ≥ 10 seconds

Note: Use the thermal sensor (thermistor or thermocouple) to score apneas and the pressure transducer to score hypopneas.

BOX 28-7	Sleep Stage Scoring Rules

Stage Wake (W) Definitions

- Alpha:
  - Trains of sinusoidal 8 to 13 hertz (Hz) activity from O1 and O2 with eyes closed, alpha attenuates with eye opening
- Primarily vertical eye blinks are present in wakefulness with the eyes open or closed
- Score stage W when more than 50% of the epoch has alpha rhythm in O1, O2
- Score as W without identifiable alpha rhythm as stage W if any of the following are present:
  - Eye blinks
  - Reading eye movements (side to side)
  - Irregular rapid eye movements in the presence of normal or high chin muscle tone

Sleep Onset

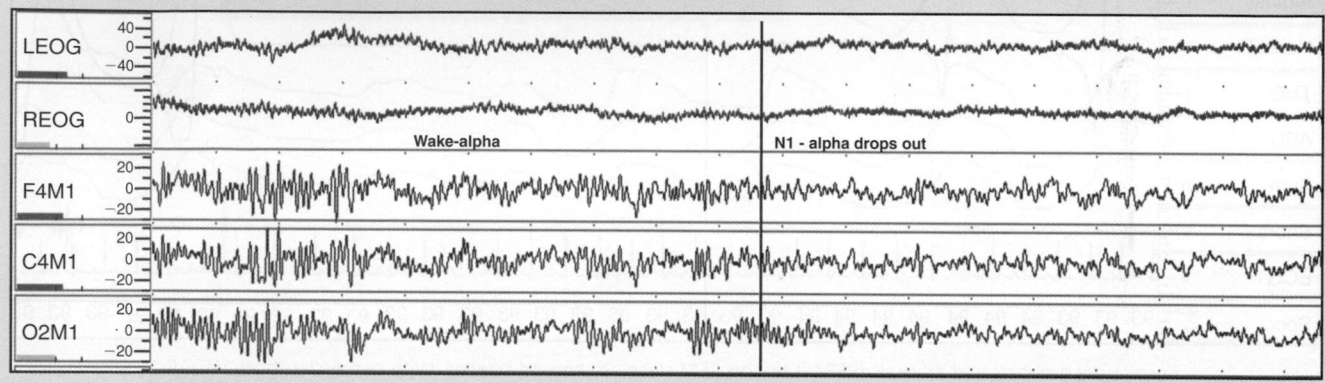

Sleep onset, 30-second screen. (With permission from Wendi M. Nugent, GateWay Community College, Phoenix, AZ.)

- The first epoch scored as any stage other than stage W, is typically stage N1

Stage N1 Definitions

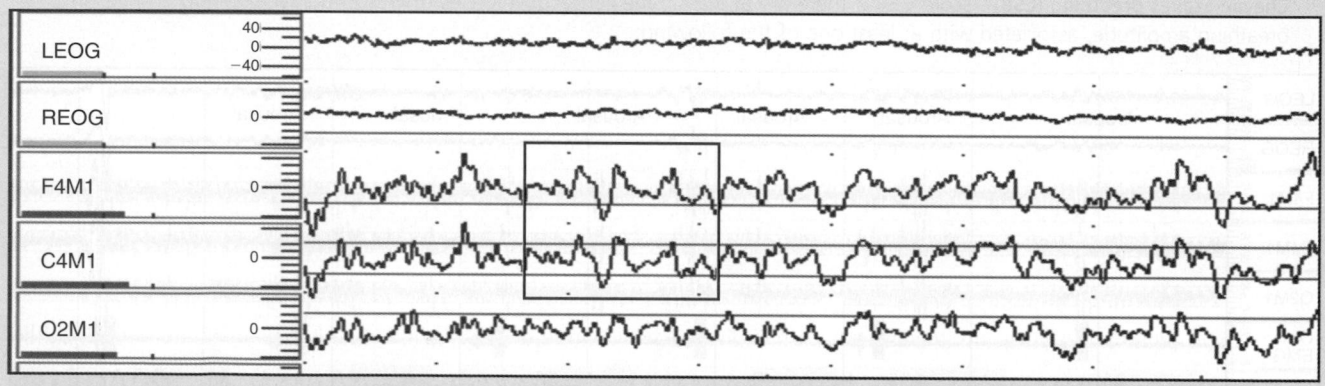

N1 with vertex sharp, 30-second screen. (With permission from Wendi M. Nugent, GateWay Community College, Phoenix, AZ.)

- Slow eye movements (SEM):
  - Low amplitude, 4 to 7 Hz activity, mixed frequency activity (LAMF):
  - Vertex sharp waves (V waves):
  - Sharp waves with a duration <0.5 seconds, seen at C3, C4, and stand out from the background activity, shown in the above.

BOX 28-7	Sleep Stage Scoring Rules—cont'd

Stage N2 Definitions

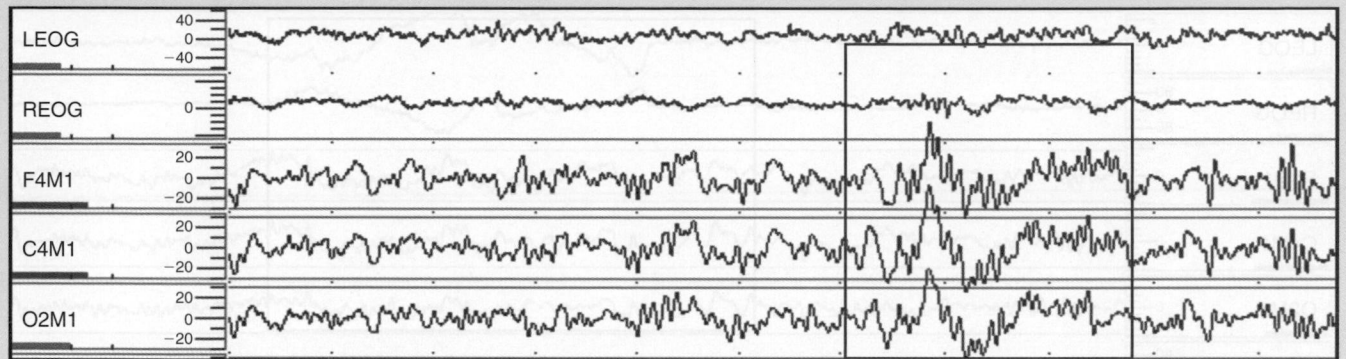

N2 with K-complex and sleep spindles, 30-second screen. (With permission from Wendi M. Nugent, GateWay Community College, Phoenix, AZ.)

- Score stage N2 if one or both of the following occur during the first half of the epoch or if occurred in the last half of the previous epoch:
  - K-complexes not associated with arousals (blue box)
  - Trains of sleep spindles

Stage N3 Definitions

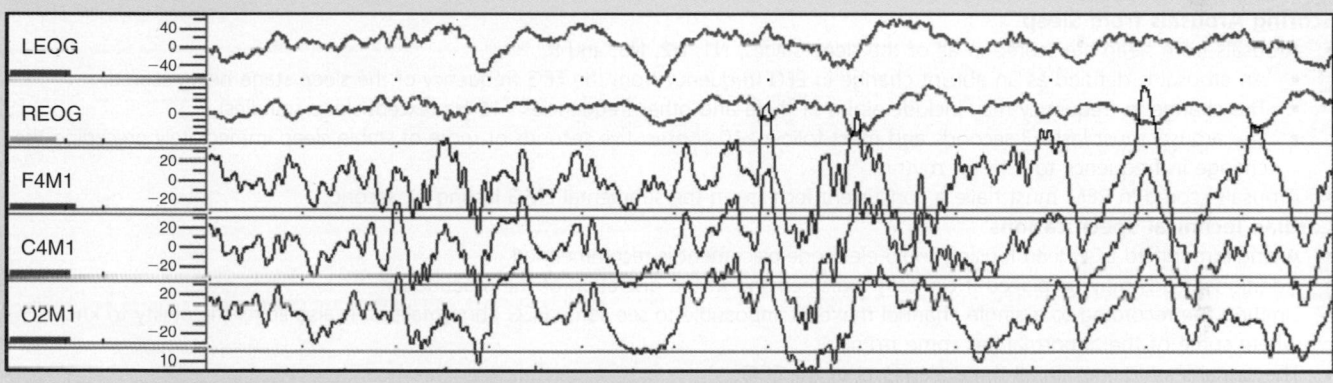

N3 with high amplitude delta, 30-second screen. (With permission from Wendi M. Nugent, GateWay Community College, Phoenix, AZ.)

- Score stage N3 when 20% or more of an epoch consists of:
  - Slow waves at 0.5 to 2 Hz
  - Peak to peak amplitude of ≥ to 75 microvolts (µV)
  - Slow waves are seen at the highest amplitude over F3 and F4

Continued

BOX 28-7	Sleep Stage Scoring Rules—cont'd

Stage REM (R) Definitions

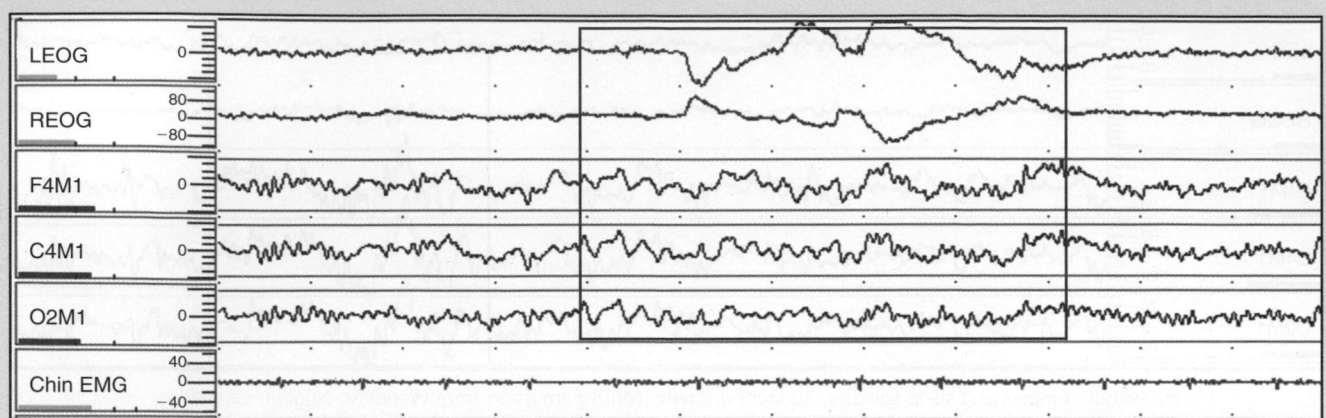

REM sleep with rapid eye movements and sawtooth waves, 30-second screen. (With permission from Wendi M. Nugent, GateWay Community College, Phoenix, AZ.)

- Score stage REM sleep in epochs when *all* of the following attributes are present:
  - Low amplitude, mixed frequency EEG (LAMF)
  - Low chin EMG tone
  - Rapid Eye Movements

Scoring Arousals from Sleep

- Arousals from sleep are scored in all of the sleep stages, N1, N2, N3, and R.
  - An arousal is defined as an abrupt change in EEG frequency from the EEG frequency of the sleep stage being scored.
  - The change in frequency may include alpha or theta and other frequencies >16 Hz (except sleep spindles).
  - The arousal must last ≥3 seconds and must follow ≥10 consecutive seconds or more of stable sleep immediately preceding the change in frequency to a faster rhythm.
- Arousals scored in REM must have a concurrent increase in the submental EMG lasting ≥1 second.

Cardiac Technical Specifications

- A single modified ECG lead II using torso electrode placement is recommended.
- Additional leads may be placed if clinically indicated and at the discretion of the practitioner.
- Limiting the recording to a single channel makes it impossible to see some ECG abnormalities. It also limits the ability to know where some of the abnormalities come from.
- The signal should contain all three elements of the ECG:
  - P wave
  - QRS complex
  - T wave

Definitions

- Tachycardia: Heart rate that is faster than normal:
  - Score sinus tachycardia during sleep for a sustained sinus heart rate of greater than 90 beats per minute (beats/min) for adults.
  - Score wide complex tachycardia (WCT):
    - For a rhythm lasting a minimum of three consecutive beats
    - At a rate greater than 100 beats/min
    - With QRS duration of ≥ 120 milliseconds (msec)
  - Score narrow complex tachycardia:
    - For a rhythm lasting a minimum of three consecutive beats
    - At a rate of greater than 100 beats/min
    - With QRS duration of less than 120 msec

BOX 28-7 Sleep Stage Scoring Rules—cont'd

- Bradycardia: Heart rate that is slower than normal:
  - Score bradycardia during sleep for a sustained heart rate of less than 40 beats/min for ages 6 years though adulthood:
    - Sustained is defined as more than 30 seconds of a stable rhythm to distinguish it from transient responses associated with SDB events or arousals.
- Asystole: Period of time with no heart beat:
  - Score asystole events when cardiac pauses are > 3 seconds in duration.
- Fibrillation: Fast oscillations and fluttering of the heart:
  - Score atrial fibrillation events in the presence of an:
    - Irregular ventricular rhythm with variable rapid oscillations replacing consistent P waves
- Arrhythmias such as heart block should be reported if the recorded quality of the ECG is sufficiently accurate:
  - If a clear P wave is not followed by a QRS complex, score as heart block.
- Ectopic beats that are deemed clinically significant should be reported:
  - Ectopic or premature beats, such as premature ventricular contractions (PVCs) may occur during sleep; if they occur frequently, they should be reported.

Scoring Movements during Sleep

Scoring Periodic Limb Movements

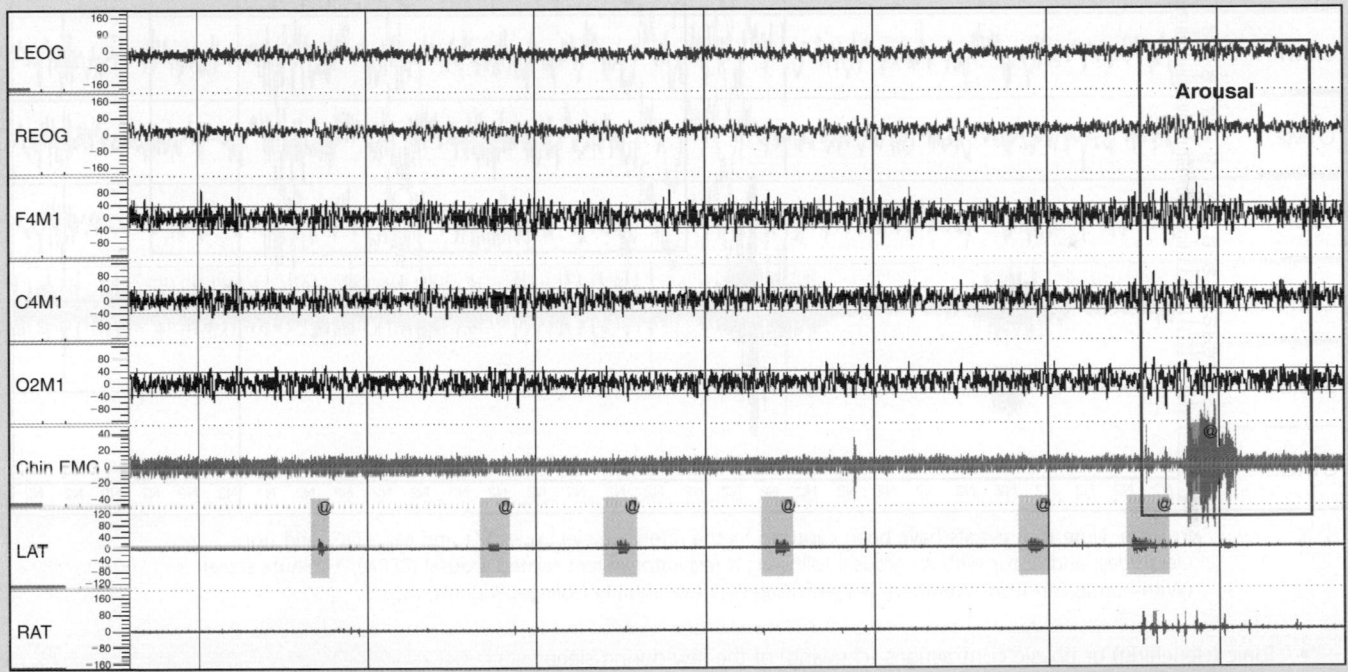

Periodic limb movements N2 sleep with arousal, 5-minute screen (With permission from Wendi M. Nugent, GateWay Community College, Phoenix, AZ.)

- Periodic limb movement (PLM) event:
  - 8 µV increase in EMG voltage above resting EMG, not associated with apneas or other arousal events
- PLM Series
  - Four consecutive leg movement events or more within a 90-second period
- Alternating leg muscle activation (ALMA):
  - Alternating leg movements, much like peddling a bicycle
  - Both legs must be monitored independently to score ALMAs

Continued

BOX 28-7	Sleep Stage Scoring Rules—cont'd

Other Movements during Sleep That Can Be Scored

- Bruxism

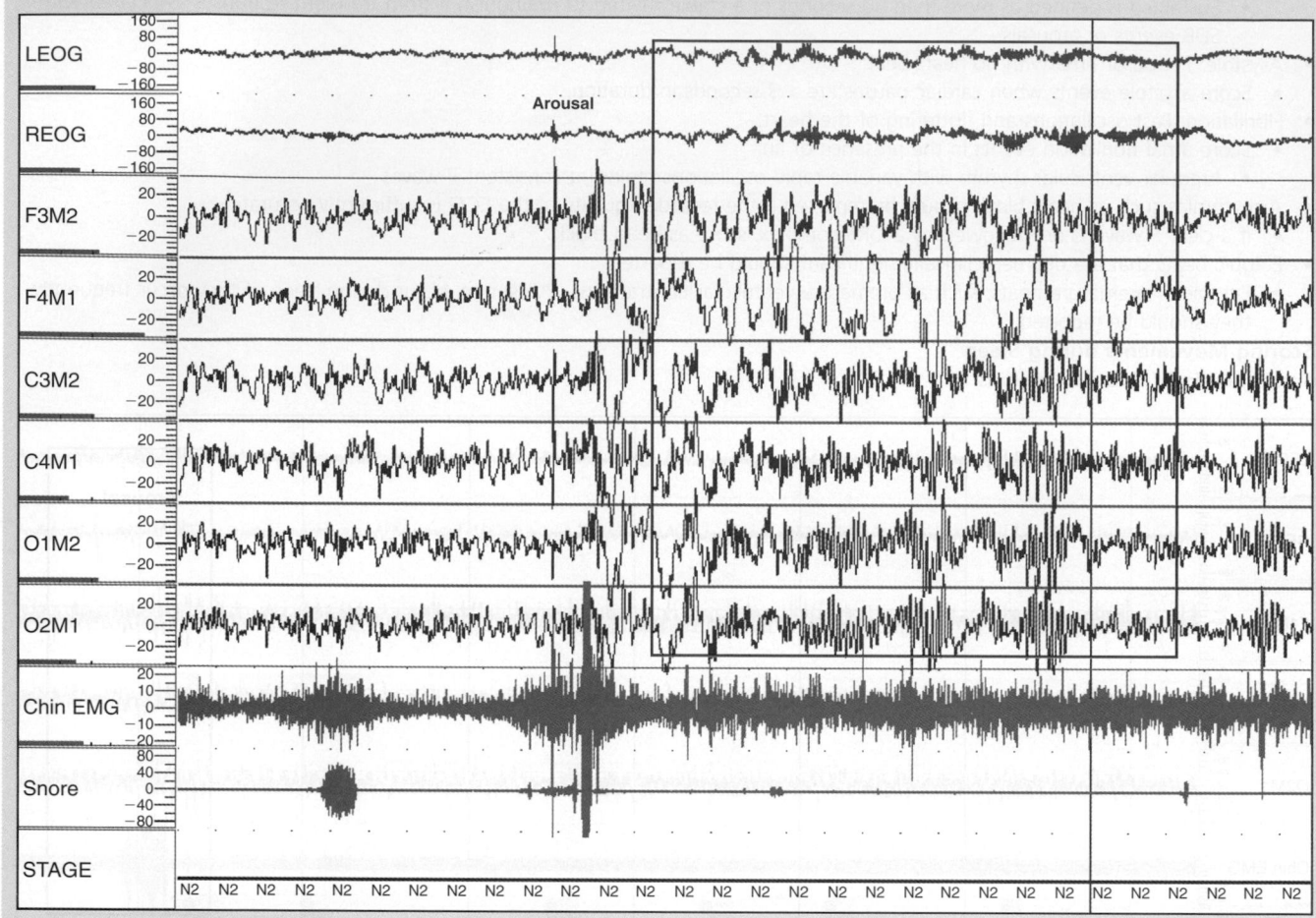

Bruxism. Note that events have been captured by the reference electrodes M1 and M2, EOG, and front electrodes, and occur with an arousal following a respiratory event related arousal (RERA), 1-minute screen. (With permission from Wendi M. Nugent, GateWay Community College, Phoenix, AZ.)

- Tonic (clenching) or phasic contractions (chewing) of the jaw during sleep
  - Additional masseter muscle monitoring may be helpful
- Hypnagogic foot tremor (HFT):
  - Bursts of foot jiggling upon falling asleep
- Excessive fragmentary myoclonus (EFM):
  - Twitching in fingers, toes, or corners of the mouth during sleep
  - May need to add electrodes to affected areas to monitor
- REM sleep behavior disorder:
  - Sustained or excessive muscle activity recorded during REM sleep in the chin or limb EMG electrodes
  - Patients may become mobile during testing, so care should be taken to protect the patient in the sleep lab
- Rhythmic movement disorder:
  - Four or more individual movements combine to make a cluster
  - May need to add electrodes to affected areas to monitor

BOX 28-8	**Calculation for Sleep Latency**

The time from lights out to the start of the first epoch of sleep, "lights out," is defined as the time at which the patient is allowed to fall asleep and marks the start of data that will be staged and analyzed. The first epoch of sleep occurs when more than 50% of the epoch demonstrates N1 or any other stage of sleep. The calculation for sleep latency (convention of staging sleep in sequential 30-second epochs) is:

Epoch for N1 or any other stage of sleep – Epoch for lights out
  = Sleep onset in epochs ÷ 2 = Sleep onset in minutes

Example:
Lights out epoch 25
N1 epoch 45
Sleep latency 45 – 25 = 20 epochs
20 epochs ÷ 2 = 10 minutes
(OR)
Lights out epoch 25
N2 epoch 60
Sleep latency = 60 – 25 = 35 epochs
35 epochs ÷ 2 = 17.5 minutes

BOX 28-9	**Calculation for REM Latency**

The time from sleep onset to the start of stage R is the REM latency. The calculation for REM latency (Convention of staging sleep in sequential 30-second epochs) is:

Epoch for stage R – Epoch for sleep onset
  = REM onset in epochs ÷ 2 = REM onset in minutes

Example:
Sleep onset epoch 45
R onset epoch 225
REM latency = 225 – 45 = 180 epochs
180 epochs ÷ 2 = 90 minutes

BOX 28-10	**Required Data to Calculate the Apnea Hypopnea Index (AHI)**

- Total sleep time (typically expressed in minutes). Divide by 60 to determine time in hours.
- Total number of apneas and hypopneas

Example:
Total Sleep Time 321 minutes or 5.35 hours
Total number of apneas and hypopneas—154
154 ÷ 5.35 = 28.8 events per hour of sleep
AHA = 28.8
Total sleep time = TST

BOX 28-11	**Required Data to Calculate Respiratory Disturbance Index (RDI)**

- Total sleep time (typically expressed in minutes). Divide by 60 to determine time in hours.
- Total number of apneas, hypopneas, and respiratory event related arousals (RERAs)

Example:
Total sleep time—321 minutes or 5.35 hours
Total number of apneas, hypopneas, and RERAs—325
325 ÷ 5.35 = 60.7 events per hour of sleep
RDI = 60.7

Bibliography

To learn more about the field of polysomnography, the American Academy of Sleep Medicine (AASM) and the American Association of Sleep Technologists (AAST) have provided learning tools to further your knowledge and expertise.
AASM Manual for the Scoring of Sleep and Associated Events 2007 and October 2012 update to scoring respiratory events: http://www.aasmnet.org. Accessed.
American Association of Sleep Technologists: http://www.aastweb.org. Accessed
Avidan AY, Barkoukis TJ: *Review of sleep medicine*, ed 3, Philadelphia, 2012, Philadelphia.
Berry RM: *Fundamentals of sleep medicine*, St. Louis, MO, 2011, Mosby.
Chokroverty S: *Sleep disorders medicine, basic science, technical considerations, and clinical aspects*, ed 3, Philadelphia, 2009, Saunders.
Kryger M, Roth T, Dement W: *Principles and practice of sleep medicine*, ed 5, Philadelphia, PA, 2011, Saunders.
Lee-Chong TL, Mattice C, Brooks R: *Fundamentals of sleep technology*, ed 2, Philadelphia, PA, 2012, Lippincott, Williams and Wilkins.
Spiro SG, Silvestri GA Agust A: *Clinical respiratory medicine*, ed 4, Philadelphia, 2012, Saunders.
Standardized terminology, techniques and scoring system for sleep stages of human subjects. Proposed supplements and amendments to A manual of Rechtschaffen & Kales standard, *Psychiat Clin Neurosci* 55:305-310, 2001.

The following information was collected during the polysomnogram. Calculate the required parameters based on the data given. Each PSG epoch is 30 seconds.

	Time	Epoch
Amplifier Calibration		24
Biocalibration		30
Lights-out	22:55	55
N1		72
N2		95
N3		None
REM		268
Lights-on		525

1. What is the total recording time expressed in hours? (Show the steps.)

_____

_____

2. What is the sleep latency expressed in minutes? (Show the steps.)

_____

_____

3. What is the REM latency expressed in minutes? (Show the steps.)

_____

_____

4. A patient had 280 epochs of sleep recorded. The subject slept 10% of the time in the supine position. There were 7 obstructive apneas, 2 mixed apneas, 45 hypopneas, and 130 respiratory related arousal events during the sleep period. While supine, the patient experienced 7 obstructive apneas, 2 mixed apneas, 30 hypopneas, and 100 respiratory event related arousals (RERAs).

a. What is the patient's apnea–hypopnea index (AHI)? (Show the steps.)

_____

_____

b. What is the patient's respiratory disturbance index (RDI)?

_____

_____

c. What is the patient's supine AHI?

_____

_____

Self-Assessment Questions

1. EEG wave form identification is dependent on:
   A. Amplitude, frequency, duration, and morphology
   B. Size of the subject's head
   C. Movement of the eyes during REM sleep
   D. Stage of sleep

2. The NREM–REM cycle during normal sleep occurs approximately:
   A. Every 30 minutes
   B. Every 90 minutes
   C. Every 120 minutes
   D. Every 190 minutes

3. Multiple Sleep Latency Test (MSLT) is:
   A. A series of nap studies, in which the patient is asked to remain awake for as long as possible while relaxing in an environment of low light and no outside stimulation
   B. A series of nap studies, in which the patient is asked to try to sleep
   C. A series of nap studies, in which the patient is asked to dream as much as possible
   D. A series of nap studies, in which the patient is asked to sleep while multiple events take place in the room

4. Maintenance of Wakefulness Test (MWT) is:
   A. A series of sleep trials, in which the patient is asked to remain awake for as long as possible while relaxing in an environment of low light and no outside stimulation
   B. A series of sleep trials, in which the patient is asked to try to sleep
   C. A series of sleep trials, in which the patient is asked to dream as much as possible
   D. A series of sleep trials, in which the patient is asked to sleep while there are multiple events taking place in the room

5. EEG is the abbreviation for:
   A. Electroocculogram
   B. Electromyogram
   C. Electrocardiogram
   D. Electroencephalogram

6. EOG is the abbreviation for
   A. Electroocculogram
   B. Electromyogram
   C. Electrocardiogram
   D. Electroencephalogram

7. EMG is the abbreviation for:
   A. Electroocculogram
   B. Electromyogram
   C. Electrocardiogram
   D. Electroencephalogram

8. The method for applying scalp electrodes for polysomnography is:
   A. International 10-20 System
   B. Measuring from ear to ear and applying electrodes spaced evenly every inch
   C. Feeling for skull landmarks and spacing the electrodes evenly
   D. Estimating the circumference of the head and applying electrodes every 10 to 20 cm

9. Nomenclature in the 10-20 System is based on:
   A. Alphabetical order
   B. Numeric order
   C. 10% to 20% of the measurements made
   D. Alphabetical characters refer to the area of brain being recorded, and numerals refer to the brain hemisphere and proximity to midline

10. Which of the following ancillary devices are included in respiratory event monitoring?
    A. Thermister and respiratory inductance plethysmography (RIP) belts
    B. Thermister or thermocouple, pressure transducer, and RIP belts
    C. Thermocouple, pressure transducer, and RIP belts
    D. Pressure transducer and RIP belts

11. For limb movement monitoring, the AASM recommends:
    A. One leg lead on each shin bone
    B. One leg lead on the right and left anterior tibialis muscles
    C. Two leg leads each on the left and right anterior tibialis muscle
    D. One leg lead on the left anterior tibialis and one arm lead on the right flexor carpi ulnaris muscle

CASE STUDY 28-1

Sherry, a 54-year-old female, presented to the clinic for evaluation of excessive daytime sleepiness, snoring, and nonrefreshing sleep. Her primary care physician had been treating her hypertension for years and has informed the patient that her blood pressure has been increasing steadily for the past 2 years and had not responded to changes made in her angiotensin-converting enzyme (ACE)-inhibitors in an attempt to normalize her blood pressure. During her office visit, Sherry's height was measured at 62 inches, and her weight was recorded at 175 pounds. History and physical examination revealed a healthy female with no medical conditions other than chronic, uncontrolled hypertension. Sherry's physical examination revealed her to be moderately obese, and a nasal examination revealed a mildly deviated septum, although Sherry denied symptoms of chronic nasal obstruction. An examination of her throat revealed enlarged tonsils, a large uvula, and crowding of the soft tissues at the back of her throat. During her interview, Sherry revealed that her bed partner noted loud snoring, and Sherry acknowledged that her own snoring would at times awaken her from sleep. Sherry's Epworth Sleepiness Scale score was 13 out of 24. The primary care physician recommended polysomnography to determine if her reported snoring and possible sleep apnea might be the underlying cause of her hypertension and referred her to the sleep clinic. The PSG study would be conducted in split-night fashion to allow for PAP titration if the patient demonstrated obstructive sleep apnea of greater than 10 events per hour in the first 2 hours of the night.

A polysomnographic study was scheduled. Upon arrival at the sleep center, Sherry was introduced to the staff and shown to her testing room. The technologist reviewed the testing preparation and procedure. The technologist explained sleep-disordered breathing and the recommended treatment if she were to demonstrate obstructive sleep apnea. Sherry was allowed to try several PAP interfaces and PAP pressure at 4 cmH$_2$O. With encouragement and minor changes to the interface, Sherry became comfortable with PAP and was willing to try it if testing indicated that she met the criteria for a PAP trial. Following standard PSG monitoring application procedures, Sherry was ready to begin the overnight study. The PSG recording was initiated at 21:45, and requisite calibrations were performed and documented. Once Sherry was comfortable in bed, the technologist reassured Sherry that she would be observed and that the technologist would be available during the night if she needed any assistance. The technologist then asked Sherry to close her eyes and try to sleep. Sherry was in the supine position. "Lights out" was documented at 21:59 at epoch 100.

Sleep onset was documented at epoch 160. Sherry progressed through non-REM sleep stages until REM was first documented at epoch 320 and subsequently ended at epoch 350. During this recording time, the technologist noted that Sherry changed her body position from supine to her left side at epoch 210 without awakening. She remained on her left side until epoch 350, at which time she experienced a brief awakening and resumed the supine position. Documentation of loud snoring and a mixture of obstructive apnea, hypopneas, and respiratory event related arousals (RERAs) were noted. The respiratory events were associated with oxygen desaturations. Sleep-related breathing events scored in NREM sleep included 2 obstructive apneas, 17 hypopneas with oxygen desaturation of 5% from baseline, and 26 RERAs. Sleep-related breathing events scored in REM sleep included 12 obstructive apneas, 16 hypopneas with oxygen desaturation of 8% from baseline, and no RERAs. Sleep resumed at epoch 356 and quickly reverted back to REM sleep at epoch 366. Sleep-related breathing events became more pronounced, with obstructive apneas dominating the events. She remained in REM while supine until snoring disturbed her sleep at epoch 388, at which time she awakened and requested assistance to use the restroom.

After assisting with the restroom break and assuring Sherry that the study was proceeding as expected, the technologist determined that Sherry met the criteria for the initiation of PAP therapy. Sherry was fitted with the PAP interface chosen prior to bedtime and PAP pressure was initiated at 4 cmH$_2$O. The technologist resumed the study at epoch 398, and Sherry settled into a comfortable supine position and tried to sleep. After a few minor adjustments with the PAP interface, Sherry became very relaxed, and sleep resumed at epoch 414. The technologist noted that hypopneas, RERAs, and snoring continued to occur at 4 cmH$_2$O and increased the PAP pressure to 5 cmH$_2$O at epoch 434. Increasing the pressure resolved the hypopneas, but the PAP flow channel continued to demonstrate a flattened waveform during inspiration and mild snoring remained. The technologist increased the PAP pressure to 6 cmH$_2$O at epoch 444. The increase in pressure resolved the RERAs and snoring. Sherry appeared to sleep comfortably without respiratory events or sleep arousals, and the technologist continued to monitor her. REM was documented at epoch 494, and during the REM phase, reemergence of hypopneas was noted with desaturations to SpO$_2$ of 86% during events. The PAP pressure was increased to 7 cmH$_2$O at epoch 525, with resolution of the sleep-related breathing event desaturations. Sherry was sleeping soundly, although an increase in the interface leak was reported through the PAP device display. The increased leak did not result in arousal from sleep or breathing events, so the technologist decided not to intervene and risk waking Sherry. The study ended at 06:25 and was considered a successful PAP titration following the diagnosis of obstructive sleep apnea. Sherry was awakened and disconnected from all monitoring devices. Her post-sleep questionnaire indicated that she felt improvement in her sleep quality after the initiation of PAP therapy.

1. Calculate initial sleep latency (minutes).

_____

_____

2. Calculate initial REM latency (minutes).

_____

_____

3. Calculate pretreatment respiratory disturbance index (RDI) and apnea–hypopnea index (AHI).

_____

_____

4. Calculate sleep latency after PAP initiation (minutes).

_____

_____

5. What is the recommended PAP prescription?

_____

_____

6. What recommendations could the technologist make regarding leaks observed during the titration?

_____

_____

7. Was the titration successful? Did the primary care physician correctly assume that Sherry's uncontrolled hypertension might be the result of underlying sleep-disordered breathing?

_____

_____

The Procedural Assessments for all Polysomnographic checklists can be found online at http://evolve.elsevier.com/Hinski/respcarelabmanual/

Respiratory Care in Alternative Settings and Transport

▪ OBJECTIVES

Upon the completion of the chapter activities and content review topics, the student should be able to:

1. Describe the alternative care settings in which a respiratory care is performed.
2. Identify eligibility for home oxygen therapy.
3. Describe proper guidelines for discharge planning.
4. Describe how a respiratory therapist helps ensure an effective discharge plan.
5. Explain the use of oxygen therapy in the home care setting using different oxygen systems.
6. Explain how to select, assemble, and monitor equipment used for invasive ventilator care in the alternative setting.
7. Instruct the family or patient caregivers on basic patient assessment.
8. Teach home tracheostomy care and suctioning.

▪ KEY TERMS

- Alternative settings
- Compressed oxygen
- Discharge planning
- Liquid oxygen
- Long term acute care hospital (LTACH)
- Oxygen concentrator
- Skilled nursing facility (SNF)

▪ CONTENT REVIEW TOPICS

- Capped-rental items
- Demand-flow regulator
- Durable medical equipment

- Duration of flow calculations for compressed and liquid oxygen
- Noninvasive positive pressure ventilation in the alternative setting
- Reimbursement policies

▪ PROCEDURAL ASSESSMENTS

29-1 Discharge Planning
29-2 Using Home Oxygen Equipment
29-3 Invasive Ventilatory Support in the Alternative Settings
29-4 Teaching Home Tracheostomy Care and Suctioning

▪ EQUIPMENT

- Oxygen concentrator
- Portable ventilator
- Ventilator circuits
- Portable liquid oxygen cylinders
- Compressed oxygen cylinder
- Gloves
- Sterile suctioning kit
- Sterile gloves
- Tracheostomy

Patients receive care in a variety of settings following discharge from an acute care facility. As a respiratory therapist (RT), you may work outside the walls of an acute care hospital to provide the respiratory care to your patients in skilled nursing facilities (SNFs), long-term acute care hospitals (LTACHs), or even the patient's home. With oxygen therapy being the most common modality of respiratory care in the alternative setting, RTs are frequently responsible for home care visits and for helping patients with home oxygen issues and questions. This includes the use of oxygen with ventilators and the management of artificial airways. Oxygen is a drug and requires a prescription for its use in the alternative care setting. Eligibility for home oxygen therapy is based on a patient's documented hypoxemia Box 29-1.

> → **Reality Check** RTs work in the home setting, skilled nursing facilities, long-term acute care hospitals, rehabilitation facilities, and other subacute facilities. Care during air travel is also a possibility.

An example of the certificate of medical necessity from the Centers for Medicare and Medicaid Services is illustrated in Figure 29-1. This chapter will cover concepts and skills relating to discharge planning as well as oxygen and ventilatory support in the alternative setting. The sleep laboratory as an alternative setting is discussed in Chapter 28.

BOX 29-1	Medicare Qualification for Home Oxygen Therapy

Oxygen Therapy at Rest
- PaO_2 ≤55 mm Hg; or SaO_2 ≤89% at room air
- PaO_2 56 to 59 mm Hg; or SaO_2 ≤89% *and one of the following:*
  - Dependent edema suggesting congestive heart failure
  - Cor pulmonale or pulmonary hypertension confirmed on ECG, gated blood pool scanning, or pulmonary artery pressure measurement
  - Erythrocythemia confirmed by hematocrit >56%

Nocturnal Oxygen Therapy
- PaO_2 ≤56 mm Hg; or SaO_2 ≤89% at room air while awake *and one of the following:*
  - PaO_2 ≤55 mm Hg; or SaO_2 ≤88% during sleep
  - PaO_2 falls more than 10 mm Hg during sleep
  - SaO_2 falls more than 5% with signs and symptoms of hypoxemia during sleep

Exercise Oxygen Therapy
- PaO_2 ≤56 mm Hg; or SaO_2 ≤89% at room air while at rest *and one of the following:*
  - PaO_2 ≤55 mm Hg during exercise
  - SaO_2 ≤88% during exercise

PaO_2, Arterial oxygen tension (partial pressure); *SaO_2,* oxygen saturation in blood; *ECG,* electrocardiography.
(From Perry AG, Potter PA: *Clinical nursing skills and techniques,* ed 7, St. Louis, MO, 2010, Mosby.)

>> SKILL CHECK LISTS

29-1 Discharge Planning

The beginning of respiratory care in the alternative setting is discharge planning. For a successful transition from the acute care setting to an alternative one, an effective care plan should be in place to minimize the chance of readmission to the hospital and to maximize patient benefit. Guidelines have been published by the American Association for Respiratory Care (AARC) to direct RTs in providing a discharge care plan for their patients. Discharge planning should be a multidisciplinary team approach so that all of the patient's medical needs, from nutrition to respiratory care to follow-up care, can be addressed. The following is the step-by-step process for discharge planning.

> → **Reality Check** The physician is usually responsible for the initial order to discharge a patient, and the physician depends on the respiratory therapist to provide an accurate assessment of the patient's ability and needs as he or she transitions to an alternative setting.

Procedural Preparation
1. Review the patient's chart.
2. Verify transfer order to alternative setting.
3. Assess the patient and the family members for need for health teaching.
4. Collaborate with the physician and staff in other disciplines about the patient's need for referral for home health care services provided by an extended care facility.

Implementation
1. Perform patient evaluation, including the following:
   a. Assess the patient's medical condition.
   b. Evaluate the psychosocial condition of the patient and the family.
   c. Determine the respiratory and ventilatory support required.
   d. Evaluate the patient's physical and functional ability to perform activities of daily living.
   e. Set goals of care.
2. Perform a site evaluation for continuing care, including the following:
   a. Determine the number of personnel required.
   b. Evaluate the physical environment's safety and suitability.
   c. Establish the equipment and supplies needed.
   d. Evaluate financial resources.
3. Develop a multidisciplinary plan of care based on the patient's needs and goals, including the following:
   a. Plan for integration into the community.
   b. Plan for administration of medications.
   c. Determine patient self-care, when appropriate.
   d. Establish a method for ongoing assessment of outcomes.
   e. Determine the roles and responsibilities of the team members for daily care management.
   f. Establish a method to assess the growth and development of pediatric patients.
   g. Set up a documented mechanism for securing and training additional caregivers.
   h. Set up a mechanism for communication among all of the health care team members.
   i. Put an alternative emergency and contingency plan in place.
   j. Set up follow up plans.
   k. Plan for the use, maintenance, and troubleshooting of equipment.
   l. Set up the time for implementation.

Evaluation of Procedure
1. Ensure that the discharge plan meets the patient's goals.
2. Evaluate any readmissions following discharge plan failure.
3. Ensure that a discharge plan coordinator monitors the patient following discharge.
4. Modify the plan according to the patient's goals.

Documentation and Reporting
1. Assess progress, and conduct a follow-up.
2. Communicate with other disciplines involved in patient care.
3. Document all your findings.

29-2 Using Home Oxygen Equipment

Three sources for oxygen (O_2) therapy you will come across in the alternative setting are (1) compressed gas cylinders, (2) liquid systems, and (3) concentrators. Some safe home oxygen therapy principles are given in Box 29-2. Gas cylinders always provide 100% oxygen at any liter flow prescribed with the actual fractional amount of inspired oxygen (FiO_2)

DEPARTMENT OF HEALTH AND HUMAN SERVICES
CENTERS FOR MEDICARE & MEDICAID SERVICES

Form Approved
OMB No. 0938-0534

CERTIFICATE OF MEDICAL NECESSITY
CMS-484 — OXYGEN

DME 484.03

SECTION A   Certification Type/Date: INITIAL ___/___/___   REVISED ___/___/___   RECERTIFICATION___/___/___

PATIENT NAME, ADDRESS, TELEPHONE and HIC NUMBER

(___) ___ ___ - ___ ___ ___ ___   HICN _____

SUPPLIER NAME, ADDRESS, TELEPHONE and NSC or applicable NPI NUMBER/LEGACY NUMBER

(___) ___ ___ - ___ ___ ___ ___   NSC or NPI # _____

PLACE OF SERVICE_____	HCPCS CODE	PT DOB ___/___/___ Sex ___ (M/F)

NAME and ADDRESS of FACILITY
if applicable (see reverse)

_____
_____
_____

PHYSICIAN NAME, ADDRESS, TELEPHONE and applicable NPI NUMBER or UPIN

(___) ___ ___ - ___ ___ ___ ___   UPIN or NPI # _____

SECTION B   Information in This Section May Not Be Completed by the Supplier of the Items/Supplies.

EST. LENGTH OF NEED (# OF MONTHS): _____ 1–99 *(99=LIFETIME)*   DIAGNOSIS CODES (ICD-9): _____ _____ _____ _____

ANSWERS	ANSWER QUESTIONS 1–9. (Circle Y for Yes, N for No, or D for Does Not Apply, unless otherwise noted.)
a)_____mm Hg b)_____% c)___/___/___	1. Enter the result of most recent test taken on or before the certification date listed in Section A. Enter (a) arterial blood gas PO2 and/or (b) oxygen saturation test; (c) date of test.
1 2 3	2. Was the test in Question 1 performed (1) with the patient in a chronic stable state as an outpatient, (2) within two days prior to discharge from an inpatient facility to home, or (3) under other circumstances?
1 2 3	3. Circle the one number for the condition of the test in Question 1: (1) At Rest; (2) During Exercise; (3) During Sleep
Y N D	4. If you are ordering portable oxygen, is the patient mobile within the home? If you are not ordering portable oxygen, circle D.
_____LPM	5. Enter the highest oxygen flow rate ordered for this patient in liters per minute. If less than 1 LPM, enter a "X".
a)_____mm Hg b)_____% c)___/___/___	6. If greater than 4 LPM is prescribed, enter results of most recent test taken on 4 LPM. This may be an (a) arterial blood gas PO2 and/or (b) oxygen saturation test with patient in a chronic stable state. Enter date of test (c).
	ANSWER QUESTIONS 7-9 **ONLY** IF PO2 = 56–59 OR OXYGEN SATURATION = 89 IN QUESTION 1
Y N	7. Does the patient have dependent edema due to congestive heart failure?
Y N	8. Does the patient have cor pulmonale or pulmonary hypertension documented by P pulmonale on an EKG or by an echocardiogram, gated blood pool scan or direct pulmonary artery pressure measurement?
Y N	9. Does the patient have a hematocrit greater than 56%?

NAME OF PERSON ANSWERING SECTION B QUESTIONS, IF OTHER THAN PHYSICIAN (Please Print):
NAME: _____   TITLE: _____   EMPLOYER: _____

SECTION C   Narrative Description of Equipment and Cost

(1) Narrative description of all items, accessories and options ordered; (2) Supplier's charge and (3) Medicare Fee Schedule Allowance for each item, accessory and option. (See instructions on back.)

SECTION D   Physician Attestation and Signature/Date

I certify that I am the treating physician identified in Section A of this form. I have received Sections A, B and C of the Certificate of Medical Necessity (including charges for items ordered). Any statement on my letterhead attached hereto, has been reviewed and signed by me. I certify that the medical necessity information in Section B is true, accurate and complete, to the best of my knowledge, and I understand that any falsification, omission, or concealment of material fact in that section may subject me to civil or criminal liability.

PHYSICIAN'S SIGNATURE _____   DATE ___/___/___
Signature and Date Stamps Are Not Acceptable.

Form CMS-484 (09/05)

A

Figure 29-1 Certificate of Medical Necessity of Oxygen (1: Instructions for completion; 2: Form). (From Centers for Medicaid and Medicare Services (CMS): www. cms.gov. Accessed.)

INSTRUCTIONS FOR COMPLETING THE CERTIFICATE
OF MEDICAL NECESSITY FOR OXYGEN (CMS-484)

SECTION A: — (May be completed by the supplier)

CERTIFICATION TYPE/DATE: — If this is an initial certification for this patient, indicate this by placing date (MM/DD/YY) needed initially in the space marked "INITIAL." If this is a revised certification (to be completed when the physician changes the order, based on the patient's changing clinical needs), indicate the initial date needed in the space marked "INITIAL," and indicate the recertification date in the space marked "REVISED." If this is a recertification, indicate the initial date needed in the space marked "INITIAL," and indicate the recertification date in the space marked "RECERTIFICATION." Whether submitting a REVISED or a RECERTIFIED CMN, be sure to always furnish the INITIAL date as well as the REVISED or RECERTIFICATION date.

PATIENT INFORMATION: — Indicate the patient's name, permanent legal address, telephone number and his/her health insurance claim number (HICN) as it appears on his/her Medicare card and on the claim form.

SUPPLIER INFORMATION: — Indicate the name of your company (supplier name), address and telephone number along with the Medicare Supplier Number assigned to you by the National Supplier Clearinghouse (NSC) or applicable National Provider Identifier (NPI). If using the NPI Number, indicate this by using the qualifier XX followed by the 10-digit number. If using a legacy number, e.g. NSC number, use the qualifier 1C followed by the 10-digit number. (For example. 1Cxxxxxxxxx)

PLACE OF SERVICE: — Indicate the place in which the item is being used, i.e., patient's home is 12, skilled nursing facility (SNF) is 31, End Stage Renal Disease (ESRD) facility is 65, etc. Refer to the DMERC supplier manual for a complete list.

FACILITY NAME: — If the place of service is a facility, indicate the name and complete address of the facility.

HCPCS CODES: — List all HCPCS procedure codes for items ordered. Procedure codes that do not require certification should not be listed on the CMN.

PATIENT DOB, HEIGHT, WEIGHT AND SEX: — Indicate patient's date of birth (MM/DD/YY) and sex (male or female); height in inches and weight in pounds, if requested.

PHYSICIAN NAME, ADDRESS: — Indicate the PHYSICIAN'S name and complete mailing address.

PHYSICIAN INFORMATION: — Accurately indicate the treating physician's Unique Physician Identification Number (UPIN) or applicable National Provider Identifier (NPI). If using the NPI Number, indicate this by using the qualifier XX followed by the 10-digit number. If using UPIN number, use the qualifier 1G followed by the 6-digit number. (For example. 1Gxxxxxx)

PHYSICIAN'S TELEPHONE NO. — Indicate the telephone number where the physician can be contacted (preferably where records would be accessible pertaining to this patient) if more information is needed.

SECTION B: — (May not be completed by the supplier. While this section may be completed by a non-physician clinician, or a Physician employee, it must be reviewed, and the CMN signed (in Section D) by the treating practitioner.)

EST. LENGTH OF NEED: — Indicate the estimated length of need (the length of time the physician expects the patient to require use of the ordered item) by filling in the appropriate number of months. If the patient will require the item for the duration of his/her life, then enter "99".

DIAGNOSIS CODES: — In the first space, list the ICD9 code that represents the primary reason for ordering this item. List any additional ICD9 codes that would further describe the medical need for the item (up to 4 codes).

QUESTION SECTION: — This section is used to gather clinical information to help Medicare determine the medical necessity for the item(s) being ordered. Answer each question which applies to the items ordered, circling "Y" for yes, "N" for no, or "D" for does not apply.

NAME OF PERSON ANSWERING SECTION B QUESTIONS: — If a clinical professional other than the treating physician (e.g., home health nurse, physical therapist, dietician) or a physician employee answers the questions of Section B, he/she must print his/her name, give his/her professional title and the name of his/her employer where indicated. If the physician is answering the questions, this space may be left blank.

SECTION C: — (To be completed by the supplier)

NARRATIVE DESCRIPTION OF EQUIPMENT & COST: — Supplier gives (1) a narrative description of the item(s) ordered, as well as all options, accessories, supplies and drugs; (2) the supplier's charge for each item(s), options, accessories, supplies and drugs; and (3) the Medicare fee schedule allowance for each item(s), options, accessories, supplies and drugs, if applicable.

SECTION D: — (To be completed by the physician)

PHYSICIAN ATTESTATION: — The physician's signature certifies (1) the CMN which he/she is reviewing includes Sections A, B, C and D; (2) the answers in Section B are correct; and (3) the self-identifying information in Section A is correct.

PHYSICIAN SIGNATURE AND DATE: — After completion and/or review by the physician of Sections A, B and C, the physician's must sign and date the CMN in Section D, verifying the Attestation appearing in this Section. The physician's signature also certifies the items ordered are medically necessary for this patient.

According to the Paperwork Reduction Act of 1995, no persons are required to respond to a collection of information unless it displays a valid OMB control number. The valid OMB control number for this information collection is 0938-0534. The time required to complete this information collection is estimated to average 12 minutes per response, including the time to review instructions, search existing resources, gather the data needed, and complete and review the information collection. If you have any comments concerning the accuracy of the time estimate or suggestions for improving this form, please write to: CMS, Attn: PRA Reports Clearance Officer, 7500 Security Blvd. Baltimore, Maryland 21244.

DO NOT SUBMIT CLAIMS TO THIS ADDRESS. Please see http://www.medicare.gov/ for information on claim filing.

Form CMS-484 (09/05) INSTRUCTIONS

B

Figure 29-1, cont'd

BOX 29-2	Safe Home Oxygen Therapy Principles

Fire Safety
- Although oxygen is not flammable, it will support combustion, so do the following:
  - Use and store oxygen in a well-ventilated area.
  - Do *not* use petroleum-based ointments (e.g., Vaseline) around the nose, as it may cause burns.
  - Keep all oxygen equipment at least 8 feet from open flames (e.g., matches, lighters, fireplaces, stoves, space heaters, candles).
  - Do *not* allow smoking in the house.
  - Avoid using electrical appliances that produce sparks (e.g., electric razors).
  - Install smoke detectors.
  - Have accessible fire extinguishers.
  - Help the patient and the family plan a fire evacuation route.

Oxygen Storage and Handling
- Store the oxygen tanks upright in carts or stands to prevent tipping or falling.
- Place the tanks flat on the floor when not in use.
- Do *not* store oxygen tanks in the trunk of a car.
- When transporting oxygen, ensure that the tanks are secured properly in the passenger area with the windows opened 2 to 3 inches to allow for adequate ventilation.

Concentrator Safety
- Plug the concentrators into properly grounded outlets.
- Do *not* use extension cords, power strips, or multi-outlet adaptors.
- Ensure that the power supply or circuit meets or exceeds the amperage requirements.

Liquid Oxygen Safety
- Avoid direct contact with liquid oxygen, as it may cause frostbite.
- Do *not* touch connectors that are icy or frozen.
- Keep ambulatory tanks upright. Do *not* place them on their sides.

From Perry AG, Potter PA: *Clinical nursing skills and techniques*, ed 7, St. Louis, MO, 2010, Mosby.

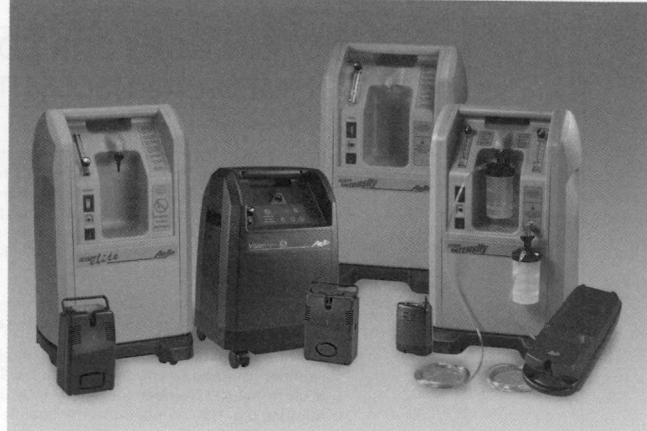

Figure 29-2 Oxygen concentrators for alternative settings (Courtesy AirSep. A Chart Industries Company, Buffalo, NY)

occur during transfilling or spillage of liquid oxygen if the unit is tipped. Liquid systems can deliver a high oxygen concentration but not 100%. The FIO_2 delivered depends on the flow rate.

Oxygen concentrators are electrically powered devices that separate oxygen out of room air. Pellets composed of inorganic sodium aluminum silicate absorb nitrogen, carbon dioxide, and water vapor from the air to produce concentrated oxygen. The nasal cannula is typically the delivery device of choice when using concentrators because masks require too much flow (Figure 29-2). Oxygen concentration decreases with increase in liter flow. The following is the step-by-step process for using home oxygen equipment.

> → **Reality Check** When choosing the oxygen delivery equipment that will be used in the alternative setting, remember to consider what it will be used for. Liquid oxygen and concentrators cannot be used with mechanical ventilators.

Procedural Preparation
1. Review the patient's chart.
2. Assess the patient's home environment for availability of adequate electrical power for the oxygen concentrator.
3. Assess the patient's or the caregiver's knowledge of oxygen therapy and ability to recognize signs and symptoms of hypoxia.
4. Determine the availability of readily available resource for assistance with home oxygen systems.
5. Determine the presence of a backup system in the event of a power failure.
6. Identify the patient using two patient identifiers.
7. Introduce yourself to the patient and the family.
8. Explain the procedure to the patient or the family.
9. Perform proper hand hygiene.

Implementation
1. Select the setting in the home where patient is more likely to use oxygen.
2. Place the oxygen delivery system in a safe place in the home.
3. Discuss safety measures and proper storage.

being delivered to the patient dependent on the delivery device used. Compressed gas cylinders are universally available and come in many sizes. Small cylinders are used during ambulation. However, they do have a limited gas volume when compared to larger cylinders, such as an H cylinder (H cylinder at 2 L/min will last a little more than 2 days). The cylinder may be heavy at times, and safety concerns and hazards such as fire or fracture of the cylinder stem do exist. Calculations of the duration of the supply of gas remaining in a compressed gas cylinder are provided in Chapter 14.

Liquid oxygen provides a large reservoir of gas in a very small space with 1 L of liquid oxygen equal to 840 L of gaseous oxygen. Typical home liquid system contains at maximum about 40 L of liquid oxygen (33,600 L of gaseous oxygen). Running at 2 L/min, a liquid oxygen source can last longer than 11 days. Some disadvantages are as follows: Some home care companies are reluctant to support its use because of high capital investment to purchase the equipment and the labor costs to refill them every 2 weeks. Thermal burns may

4. Demonstrate the steps for preparation and completion of oxygen therapy.
   a. Compressed oxygen system:
      i. Turn the cylinder valve counter-clockwise two to three turns with a wrench.
      ii. Check the cylinders by reading the amount on the pressure gauge.
      iii. Store the wrench with the oxygen tank or in another safe place.
   b. Oxygen concentrator system:
      i. Plug the concentrator into the appropriate outlet.
      ii. Turn on the power switch; the alarm will sound for a short period until it reaches the proper pressure.
   c. Liquid oxygen system:
      i. Check the liquid system by pressing the button and reading the dial on the stationary reservoir or the ambulatory tank.
      ii. Consult the equipment provider with regard to the instructions for refilling the ambulatory tank.
5. Connect the oxygen delivery device to the oxygen delivery system.
6. Adjust the liter flow, and place the device on the patient.
7. Perform hand hygiene.
8. Instruct the patient or the caregiver not to change the oxygen flow rate.
9. Instruct the patient to place a "No Smoking—Oxygen in Use" sign at each entrance to the home.
10. Provide and discuss the written materials regarding the system.
11. Instruct the patient or the caregiver on how to recognize the signs and symptoms of hypoxia and upper respiratory infection and when to notify the physician.

12. Discuss the emergency plan for dealing with respiratory distress, power failure, or a natural disaster.
13. Provide instructions with regard to activating 9-1-1.

Evaluation of Procedure

1. Monitor the oxygen delivery rate.
2. Evaluate the patient's or the caregiver's ability to administer oxygen therapy.
3. Evaluate any problem with oxygen delivery at home.
4. Have the patient or the caregiver verbalize safety guidelines and emergency plans.
5. Identify unexpected outcomes.

Documentation and Reporting

1. Record the teaching plan, and document the patient's learning.

29-3 Invasive Ventilatory Support in Alternative Settings

The development of small, portable ventilators has facilitated the move of ventilatory support from the intensive care unit (ICU) to the home and other alternative settings. Success in this modality requires several prerequisites, extensive planning, and caregiver education. These are listed in Table 29-1. The patient's needs, as well as the ease of operation and the dependability of the ventilator, are important when choosing the type of home ventilator. The RT or other caregiver should be completely familiar with the device. A manual resuscitation device with a mask should always be available at the patient's bedside. Caregivers must know how to use it and when to utilize emergency procedures and call 9-1-1. The following is

TABLE 29-1 Prerequisites, Planning, and Caregiver Education Requirements for Successful Home Ventilatory Support

Prerequisites	Planning	Caregiver Education
Willingness of family to accept responsibility	Family is consulted regarding feasibility.	Simple patient assessment
Adequacy of family and professional support	Physician writes appropriate orders.	Airway management and airway care
Overall viability of the home care plan	Physician and other team members discuss plan with family and caregivers.	CPT therapy
Stability of patient	Education and training are initiated and completed.	Medication administration
Adequacy of home setting	Patient and family are prepared for discharge.	Patient movement and ambulation
	Home layout is assessed with necessary changes made.	Equipment operation and maintenance
	Equipment and supplies are readied.	Equipment troubleshooting
	Discharge planner meets with team and makes final preparations.	Cleaning and disinfection
	Patient is discharged.	Emergency procedures
	Power company is notified regarding the presence of life-support equipment.	
	Ongoing and follow-up care is provided by visiting nurse, respiratory therapist (RT), and other health care professionals.	

the step-by-step process for invasive ventilatory support in alternative settings.

Procedural Preparation

1. Review the patient's chart.
2. Verify the physician's order or the facility's protocol for standard of care.
3. Obtain, clean, and inspect the appropriate equipment prior to entering the patient's room.
4. Follow PPE requirements, and observe standard precautions for any transmission-based isolation procedure.
5. Identify the patient using two patient identifiers.
6. Introduce yourself to the patient and to the family.
7. Explain the procedure to the patient and to the family, and acknowledge the patient's understanding.
8. Perform proper hand hygiene, and put on gloves, mask, and protective eyewear, as appropriate for the procedure.

Implementation

1. Demonstrate necessary infection control procedures to the patient, the family, or the caregiver.
2. Assess vital signs.
3. Instruct the family or the caregiver on the basic assessment to determine patient tolerance or distress.
4. Evaluate and ensure airway patency.
5. Instruct the caregiver while performing the following tasks:
   a. Set the initial vent settings according to protocol or the physician's orders.
   b. Set the alarms.
   c. Check all the accessory equipment.
   d. Charge the battery pack.
   e. Troubleshoot any problems.
   f. Clean or disinfect any equipment, as needed, based on the manufacturer's specifications.
6. Remove the supplies from the patient's room, and clean the area, as needed.
7. Remove PPE, and perform proper hand hygiene prior to leaving the patient's room.

Evaluation of Procedure

1. Establish a baseline, or compare with previous measurements.
2. Evaluate the emergency plan.
3. Develop an appropriate respiratory care plan based on assessment data.
4. Identify the need for any ventilatory setting changes:
   a. Contact the physician for change orders, or follow protocols.
5. Identify any unexpected outcomes.

Documentation and Reporting

1. Record your findings in the patient's chart.
2. Report any abnormal findings to the appropriate health care provider.

29-4 Teaching Home Tracheostomy Care and Suctioning

Teaching proper tracheostomy care ("trach care") and suction should begin in the acute care setting before a patient is

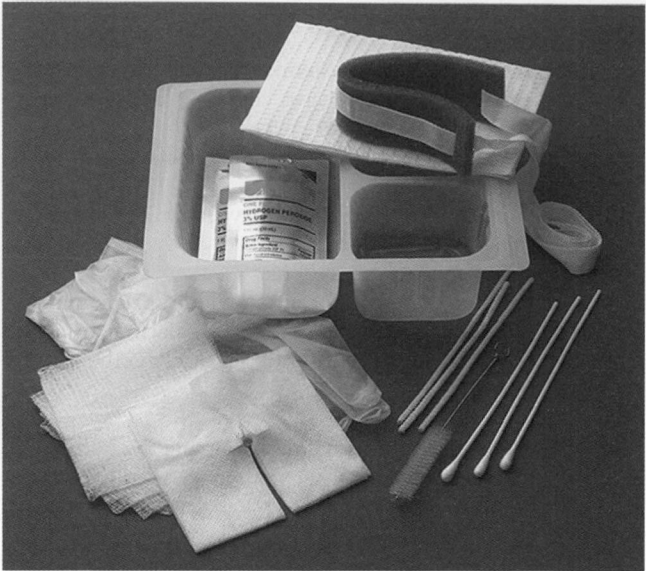

Figure 29-3 Equipment for tracheostomy care. (From Pierce L: *Management of the mechanically ventilated patient*, ed 2, St. Louis, MO, 2007, Saunders.)

BOX 29-3 **Indications for Suctioning and Tracheostomy Care**

Suctioning
- Gurgling tactile fremitus
- Wheezes or crackles on inspiration or expiration
- Restlessness
- Ineffective coughing
- Absent or diminished breath sounds
- Tachypnea
- Cyanosis
- Acutely decreased level of consciousness
- Hypertension or hypotension
- Tachycardia or bradycardia
- Acutely shallow respirations
- Acute dyspnea

Tracheostomy Care
- Presence of excessive peristomal secretions
- Excessive intratracheal secretions
- Soiled or damp tracheostomy dressings
- Diminished airway through tracheostomy tube

---

transferred to his or her home. The caregiver and the patient should be evaluated before the patient leaves the facility to ensure understanding of proper technique. The skill is learned quickly by some, but others may take longer to master it. Figure 29-3 illustrates a common tracheostomy care kit. Knowing when to suction and perform trach care is just as important as knowing how to perform it. Indications for trach care and suctioning are given in Box 29-3. The key point to remember is that the risk of infection should be minimized by using proper techniques. The following is the step-by-step process for teaching home tracheostomy care and suctioning.

Procedural Preparation

1. Review the patient's chart.
2. Verify the physician's order or the facility's protocol for standard of care.

3. Obtain, clean, and inspect the appropriate equipment prior to entering the patient's room.
4. Follow PPE requirements, and observe standard precautions for any transmission-based isolation procedure.
5. Identify the patient using two patient identifiers.
6. Introduce yourself to the patient and to the family.
7. Explain the procedure to the patient and to the family, and acknowledge the patient's understanding.
8. Assess the patient's or caregiver's ability to perform tracheostomy care and suctioning.
9. Perform proper hand hygiene, and put on gloves, mask, and protective eyewear, as appropriate for the procedure.

Implementation

1. Place the patient in a comfortable position.
2. Assess vital signs.
3. For suctioning:
   a. Put on sterile gloves.
   b. Instruct, demonstrate, and observe the steps of aseptic preparation and technique for suctioning tracheostomy tube.
   c. Preoxygenate the patient, if he or she is receiving supplemental oxygen.
   d. Instruct, demonstrate, and observe nasal and oral suctioning to be done as needed.
   e. Instruct the patient to take three deep breaths.
   f. Instruct, demonstrate, and observe disconnection and disposal of the suction catheter.
4. For tracheostomy care:
   a. Instruct, demonstrate, and observe the tracheostomy care technique.
   b. Instruct, demonstrate, and observe proper disposal of any used equipment in the appropriate container.
   c. Instruct, demonstrate, and observe proper disinfection of any reusable equipment.
5. Guide the caregiver during each step.
6. Remove the supplies from the patient's room, and clean the area, as needed.
7. Remove PPE, and perform proper hand hygiene prior to leaving the patient's room.

Evaluation of Procedure

1. Instruct the patient or the caregiver to state the signs and symptoms of complications from the procedure.
2. Observe the patient or the caregiver demonstrating proper techniques independently.
3. Instruct the patient or the caregiver about the steps to take in an emergency situation.

Documentation and Reporting

1. Record the instructions and skills demonstrated and the correctness of self-care or care delivered by the caregiver.
2. Report any abnormal findings to the appropriate health care provider.

Bibliography

Joint Commission on Accreditation of Healthcare Organizations: *2011 Comprehensive accreditation manual for long term care*, Oakbrook Terrace, IL, 2010, The Joint Commission.

Kacmarek RM, Stoller JK, Heuer AJ: *Egan's fundamentals of respiratory care*, ed 10, St. Louis, MO, 2013, Mosby.

Perry AG, Potter PA: *Clinical nursing skills & technique*, ed 7, St. Louis, MO, 2010, Mosby.

Spratt G, Petty T: Partnering for optimal respiratory home care: physicians working with respiratory therapist to optimally meet respiratory home care needs, *Respir Care* 46:475-488, 2001.

1. What six elements should be included in a prescription for oxygen therapy in the alternative care setting?

   a. _____

   b. _____

   c. _____

   d. _____

   e. _____

   f. _____

2. List the four indications for oxygen therapy in the home or alternative site health care facility.

   a. _____

   b. _____

   c. _____

   d. _____

3. List the seven precautions and possible complications of oxygen therapy in the home or alternative site health care facility?

   a. _____

   b. _____

   c. _____

   d. _____

   e. _____

   f. _____

   g. _____

4. Fill in the following chart comparing the advantages and disadvantages of major alternative oxygen supply systems:

System	Advantages	Disadvantages
Compressed oxygen		
Liquid oxygen system		
Oxygen concentrator		

5. List the two indications for long-term invasive mechanical ventilation in the home.

a. _____

b. _____

6. List the five contraindications to long-term invasive mechanical ventilation in the home.

a. _____

b. _____

c. _____

d. _____

e. _____

7. Obtain a home care ventilator. If one is not available, use an Internet or text resource to fill in the following chart:

VENTILATOR NAME:

Feature	Is it present in the ventilator? Circle yes or no.
Positive pressure tidal breaths	YES / NO
Mandatory rate	YES / NO
Flow or inspiratory-to-expiratory or inspiratory time	YES / NO
Positive end-expiratory pressure (PEEP)	YES / NO
Fractional inspired oxygen (FiO_2) to 1.0	YES / NO
Patient spontaneous breath	YES / NO
Breath-triggering mechanism	YES / NO
Flow-timing interaction	YES / NO
Feedback control	YES / NO

8. Using a mannequin and a tracheostomy tube, instruct a lab partner on how to perform tracheostomy care and suctioning. Have him or her sign below upon your successful demonstration, instruction, and observation of the task performed.

Signature: _____

Self-Assessment Questions

1. All of the following are examples of the most common alternative sites for providing health care *except:*
   A. Level 1 urban trauma centers
   B. Rehabilitation facilities
   C. Skilled nursing facilities
   D. Home care

2. Currently, most of respiratory care in the alternative setting is provided:
   A. In the home setting
   B. In skilled nursing facilities
   C. During air travel
   D. In rehabilitation facilities

3. Discharge planning is the responsibility of:
   A. Physicians
   B. Nurses
   C. Respiratory therapists
   D. All of the above

4. Components of the oxygen prescription include:
   1. Flow rate in L/min
   2. Duration of need
   3. Diagnosis
   4. Laboratory evidence provided by a home care company

   A. 1 and 3 only
   B. 1, 2, and 3 only
   C. 2, 3, and 4 only
   D. 1, 2, 3, and 4

5. The most common type of oxygen concentrator is:
   A. A molecular sieve
   B. Membrane technology
   C. Liquid
   D. Compressed gas tanks

6. Diseases involved in groups requiring ventilatory support in alternative sittings include:
   1. Amyotrophic lateral sclerosis
   2. Severe chronic obstructive pulmonary disease (COPD)
   3. Asthma
   4. Late-stage muscular dystrophy

   A. 1 and 3 only
   B. 2 and 3 only
   C. 1, 2, and 4 only
   D. 1, 2, 3, and 4

7. Which of the following would exclude a patient from being considered stable for ventilatory support in the alternative setting?
   A. PEEP requirement of 6 centimeters of water (cmH_2O)
   B. Tracheostomy tube
   C. FIO_2 requirements of 0.35
   D. Two hospital admissions in the past 3 weeks

8. Assessing the home environment for home care should include:
   A. Accessibility
   B. Equipment
   C. Environment
   D. All of the above

9. Durable medical equipment suppliers usually provide:
   1. Service 24 hours and 7 days a week
   2. Home instruction and follow-up by a pulmonologist
   3. Most forms of respiratory care
   4. Third-party insurance processing

   A. 1 and 2 only
   B. 2, 3, and 4 only
   C. 1, 2, and 3 only
   D. 1, 3, and 4 only

10. Compressed oxygen cylinders can provide 50 psi (pounds per square inch) working pressures for at home ventilators.
    A. True
    B. False

>> **CASE STUDY 29-1**

Mr. G is an 81-year-old male patient with COPD. His daughter is working with the physician and a RT to get him home oxygen therapy for his shortness of breath. His demographics and current laboratory values are listed below:

Mr. G
1234 Big Street Ave. Apt. 83
Hometown, AZ 12345
480-555-5555
Date of birth (DOB): 9/1/1932
   Last ABG on 1/1/2013 on room air: pH 7.35; $PaCO_2$ 45 mm Hg; HCO_3^- 36 mEq/L; PaO_2 61 mm Hg; SpO_2 83%

1. Does this patient qualify for home oxygen therapy?

   _____

   _____

2. If you believe that this patient qualifies for home oxygen therapy, fill in the Certificate of Medical Necessity (Figure 29-4). If you do not believe that he qualifies for home oxygen therapy, explain your reasons.

   _____

   _____

3. What are some accessibility, equipment, and environmental issues you would assess in the home environment for this patient before he receives home oxygen therapy?

   _____

   _____

DEPARTMENT OF HEALTH AND HUMAN SERVICES
CENTERS FOR MEDICARE & MEDICAID SERVICES

Form Approved
OMB No. 0938-0534

CERTIFICATE OF MEDICAL NECESSITY
CMS-484 — OXYGEN

DME 484.03

SECTION A	Certification Type/Date: INITIAL ___/___/___ REVISED ___/___/___ RECERTIFICATION___/___/___

PATIENT NAME, ADDRESS, TELEPHONE and HIC NUMBER	SUPPLIER NAME, ADDRESS, TELEPHONE and NSC or applicable NPI NUMBER/LEGACY NUMBER
(___) ___ - ___ HICN	(___) ___ - ___ NSC or NPI #_____

PLACE OF SERVICE_____	HCPCS CODE	PT DOB ___/___/___ Sex ___ (M/F)
NAME and ADDRESS of FACILITY *if applicable (see reverse)*		PHYSICIAN NAME, ADDRESS, TELEPHONE and applicable NPI NUMBER or UPIN
		(___) ___ - ___ UPIN or NPI #_____

SECTION B	Information in This Section May Not Be Completed by the Supplier of the Items/Supplies.

EST. LENGTH OF NEED (# OF MONTHS): _____ 1–99 (*99=LIFETIME*)   DIAGNOSIS CODES (ICD-9): _____ _____ _____ _____

ANSWERS	ANSWER QUESTIONS 1–9. (Circle Y for Yes, N for No, or D for Does Not Apply, unless otherwise noted.)
a)_____mm Hg b)_____% c)___/___/___	1. Enter the result of most recent test taken on or before the certification date listed in Section A. Enter (a) arterial blood gas PO2 and/or (b) oxygen saturation test; (c) date of test.
1 2 3	2. Was the test in Question 1 performed (1) with the patient in a chronic stable state as an outpatient, (2) within two days prior to discharge from an inpatient facility to home, or (3) under other circumstances?
1 2 3	3. Circle the one number for the condition of the test in Question 1: (1) At Rest; (2) During Exercise; (3) During Sleep
Y N D	4. If you are ordering portable oxygen, is the patient mobile within the home? If you are not ordering portable oxygen, circle D.
_____LPM	5. Enter the highest oxygen flow rate ordered for this patient in liters per minute. If less than 1 LPM, enter a "X".
a)_____mm Hg b)_____% c)___/___/___	6. If greater than 4 LPM is prescribed, enter results of most recent test taken on 4 LPM. This may be an (a) arterial blood gas PO2 and/or (b) oxygen saturation test with patient in a chronic stable state. Enter date of test (c).
	ANSWER QUESTIONS 7-9 **ONLY** IF PO2 = 56–59 OR OXYGEN SATURATION = 89 IN QUESTION 1
Y N	7. Does the patient have dependent edema due to congestive heart failure?
Y N	8. Does the patient have cor pulmonale or pulmonary hypertension documented by P pulmonale on an EKG or by an echocardiogram, gated blood pool scan or direct pulmonary artery pressure measurement?
Y N	9. Does the patient have a hematocrit greater than 56%?

NAME OF PERSON ANSWERING SECTION B QUESTIONS, IF OTHER THAN PHYSICIAN (Please Print):
NAME: _____ TITLE: _____ EMPLOYER: _____

SECTION C	Narrative Description of Equipment and Cost

(1) Narrative description of all items, accessories and options ordered; (2) Supplier's charge and (3) Medicare Fee Schedule Allowance for each item, accessory and option. (See instructions on back.)

SECTION D	Physician Attestation and Signature/Date

I certify that I am the treating physician identified in Section A of this form. I have received Sections A, B and C of the Certificate of Medical Necessity (including charges for items ordered). Any statement on my letterhead attached hereto, has been reviewed and signed by me. I certify that the medical necessity information in Section B is true, accurate and complete, to the best of my knowledge, and I understand that any falsification, omission, or concealment of material fact in that section may subject me to civil or criminal liability.

PHYSICIAN'S SIGNATURE _____ DATE ___/___/___
Signature and Date Stamps Are Not Acceptable.

Form CMS-484 (09/05)

Figure 29-4 Certificate of Medical Necessity for Oxygen. (From Centers for Medicaid and Medicare Services (CMS): www. cms.gov. Accessed.)

Interviewing and Preparing to Enter the Respiratory Care Profession

▪ OBJECTIVES

Upon the completion of the chapter activities and content review topics, the student should be able to:

1. Explain the credentialing process.
2. Identify specialty credentials.
3. Explain the licensure process.
4. Write a resume.
5. Construct a cover letter.
6. Identify the difference between a resumé and a curriculum vitae.
7. Prepare effectively for the interview process.
8. Use communication strategies during the interview process.

▪ KEY TERMS

- Certified respiratory therapist (CRT)
- Clinical simulation examination (CSE)
- Continuing Respiratory Care Education (CRCE)
- Credentials
- Curriculum vitae (CV)
- Licensure
- Registered respiratory therapist (RRT)
- Respiratory care practitioner (RCP)
- The National Board for Respiratory Care, Inc. (NBRC)

▪ CONTENT REVIEW TOPICS

- Licensure requirements for your state

I n the last few years, you have prepared, developed, and implemented a plan to become a successful respiratory therapist (RT). The positive attitude and the time management skills you applied toward school and clinical education can now be implemented to obtain a position as an RT. The Merriam-Webster dictionary defines a *profession* as "a calling requiring specialized knowledge and often long and intensive academic preparation." As you prepare to enter your new profession, you must remember that just because school is over, it does not mean that you can stop learning. Journals such as *Respiratory Care* are great resources. Also, becoming a member of the American Association for Respiratory Care (AARC) and your state respiratory care society is critical to your success and longevity as an RT.

Preparing to Enter the Field of Respiratory Care

Credentials and Licensure

Before you apply for a job as an RT, you must obtain your credentials. The National Board for Respiratory Care, Inc. (NBRC) is the certifying board that evaluates the professional competence of an RT. A list of all the NBRC examinations, as well as an examination awarded by the National Asthma Educator Certification Board (NAECB), is provided in Box 30-1.

First, you must obtain your credential as a certified respiratory therapist (CRT). This 3-hour entry-level examination consists of 160 multiple-choice questions. Twenty of these questions are pretest items and are not graded, and the other 140 questions are scored. The major content areas include clinical data, equipment, and therapeutic procedures. Presently, the cost to take this examination is $190, and the examination eligibility criteria are listed in Box 30-2.

> ✳ **Tip** Make sure you have a valid form of identification with you when you take your examination.

> → **Reality Check** Calculators cannot be used in credentialing examinations.

Once you are successful in passing the CRT examination, you need to take two separate examinations to become a Registered Respiratory Therapist (RRT): (1) a written examination and (2) a clinical simulation examination (CSE). The written portion is a 2-hour advanced-level examination consisting of 115 multiple-choice questions. Fifteen of these questions are pretest items and are not graded, and the other 100 questions are scored. The major content areas include the recall, application, and analysis of patient data, equipment, and therapeutic procedures. Presently, the cost to take this examination is $190. The CSE portion is a 4-hour examination consisting of 12 clinical simulations. Two of these simulations involve pretest problems, and the other 10 are scored. The CSE is intended to imitate the real world setting and be relevant to the clinical practice of respiratory care. The cost to take this examination is $200, and the examination eligibility criteria are listed in Box 30-3.

> ✳ **Tip** The format of the CRT and RRT examinations are expected to change. The CRT and RRT written examinations will be combined into one examination with different cut scores. The CSE will expand to 20 problems with shorter scenarios. You may refer to the NBRC website for up-to-date information.

BOX 30-1 NBRC Examinations

- Certified Respiratory Therapist (CRT)
  The Entry Level CRT Examination is designed to objectively measure essential knowledge, skills, and abilities required of entry-level respiratory therapists.
- Registered Respiratory Therapist (RRT)
  The Registry Examination System was developed to objectively measure essential knowledge, skills, and abilities required of advanced respiratory therapists and to set uniform standards for measuring such knowledge.
- Certified Pulmonary Function Technologist (CPFT)
  The Entry Level CPFT Examination is designed to objectively measure essential knowledge, skills, and abilities required of entry-level pulmonary function technologists at beginning practice.
- Registered Pulmonary Function Technologist (RPFT)
  The RPFT Examination is designed to objectively measure essential knowledge, skills, and abilities required of an advanced pulmonary function technologist.
- Neonatal/Pediatric Respiratory Care Specialist (CRT-NPS or RRT-NPS)
  The Neonatal/Pediatric Respiratory Care Specialty Examination is designed to objectively measure essential knowledge, skills, and abilities required of respiratory therapists in this specialty area.
- Adult Critical Care Specialty Examination (RRT-ACCS)
  The Adult Critical Care Specialty Examination is designed to objectively measure essential knowledge, skills, and abilities required of respiratory therapists in this specialty area.
- Sleep Disorders Testing and Therapeutic Intervention Respiratory Care Specialist (CRT-SDS or RRT-SDS)
  The Specialty Examination for Respiratory Therapists Performing Sleep Disorders Testing and Therapeutic Intervention is designed to objectively measure essential knowledge, skills, and abilities required of respiratory therapists in this specialty area.
- Credential awarded by the National Asthma Educator Certification Board (NAECB)
  - Asthma Educator Certification (AE-C) is the official designation of a certified asthma educator who has the necessary knowledge and skills to counsel patients in asthma management and has successfully passed the NAECB examination.

→ **Reality Check** If you do not successfully complete an examination, it is possible to retake the examination at an additional cost.

Once you have obtained the CRT or RRT credential, you will have to apply for licensure as a respiratory care practitioner (RCP) in the state where you wish to practice. At the present time, 49 states, the District of Columbia, and Puerto Rico require state licensure or other legal credentialing. Before you are able to practice, you must obtain the set requirements for your state.

→ **Reality Check** Alaska does not have licensure for RCPs.

BOX 30-2 Admission Requirements for CRT Examination Eligibility

1. Applicants shall be 18 years of age or older.
2. Applicants shall satisfy ONE of the following educational requirements:
   a. Applicants shall have a minimum of an associate degree from a respiratory therapist education program (1) supported or accredited by the Commission on Accreditation for Respiratory Care (CoARC), or (2) accredited by the Commission on Accreditation of Allied Health Education Programs (CAAHEP) and graduated on or before November 11, 2009.
   b. Applicants enrolled in an accredited respiratory therapy program in an institution offering a baccalaureate degree may be admitted to the CRT Examination with a "special certificate of completion" issued by a sponsoring educational institution. The CoARC will authorize such institutions to issue the "special certificate of completion" at the advanced-level following completion of the science, general academic, and respiratory therapy coursework commensurate with the requirements for accreditation.

The NBRC website offers information specific to your state licensing agency as well as a handbook for test candidates.

Resumé Writing

When applying for a position as an RT, you will be required to fill out an application and submit a resumé. A resumé should be a one- or two-page summary of your skills, experience, and education. When writing a resumé, use an easy-to-read font size (a 12-point font is usually adequate), and proofread it numerous times. If possible, get an instructor, peer, or someone from the career development office at your college or university to read it over and offer suggestions to improve the content, layout, or overall appearance. A resumé should be the tool that gets you an interview. Most hospitals and agencies have a human resource (HR) department that sifts through all the resumés for an RT job opening. Make your resumé stand out by using key words from the job description, and use short sentences or bulleted points to describe your educational background, clinical experience, volunteer activities, and your professional objectives.

✳ **Tip** The main difference between a resumé and a curriculum vitae (CV) is the length. A CV is longer (at least two pages) and more detailed and includes a summary of educational and academic backgrounds, including teaching and research experiences, any publications, awards and honors, and speaking engagements. A resumé will suffice for your initial job application.

✳ **Tip** Using professional objectives will help give potential employers an idea of where you want to go and how you intend to achieve those goals.

<table>
<tr><td>**BOX 30-3**</td><td>**Admission Requirements for RRT Examination Eligibility**</td></tr>
</table>

RRT4

1. Applicants shall be 18 years of age or older.
2. Applicants shall satisfy ONE of the following educational requirements:
   a. Be a certified respiratory therapist (CRT) having earned a minimum of an associate degree* from a respiratory therapist educational program (1) supported or accredited by the Commission on Accreditation for Respiratory Care (CoARC), or (2) accredited by the Commission on Accreditation of Allied Health Education Programs (CAAHEP) and graduated on or before November 11, 2009. Graduates of accredited 100-level respiratory therapist education programs are not eligible for admission to the RRT Examination under this admission provision.

   Or

   b. Be a CRT having been enrolled in an accredited respiratory therapy program in an institution offering a baccalaureate degree offering a "special certificate of completion" issued by a sponsoring educational institution. The CoARC will authorize such institutions to issue the "special certificate of completion" at the advanced level following completion of the science, general academic, and respiratory therapy coursework commensurate with the requirements for accreditation.

   Or

   c. Be a CRT certified by the NBRC and have 4 years of full-time clinical in respiratory therapy under licensed medical supervision following certification and prior to applying for the Registry Examination. In addition, the applicant shall have at least 62 semester hours of college credit from a college or university accredited by its regional association or its equivalent. The 62 semester hours of college credit must include the following courses: anatomy and physiology, chemistry, microbiology, physics, and mathematics.

   Or

   d. Be a CRT having earned a minimum of an associate degree from an accredited entry-level respiratory therapist educational program with 2 years of full-time, clinical experience in respiratory care under licensed medical supervision following certification and prior to applying for the examination.

   Or

   e. Be a CRT with a baccalaureate degree in an area other than respiratory care, including college credit level courses in anatomy and physiology, chemistry, mathematics, microbiology, and physics. In addition, they shall have 2 years of full-time clinical experience in respiratory care under licensed medical supervision following certification and before applying for the examination. In addition, the applicant shall have at least 62 semester hours of college credit from a college or university accredited by its regional association or its equivalent.

Prioritize your resumé with the most relevant information first. It should begin with your name in a bold font slightly larger than the rest of the resumé.

> **Reality Check** Make sure you have an appropriate email address that does not contain inappropriate words, phrases, numbers, or derogatory terms. An address that contains your name is best. If you have a gender neutral name, include the Miss, Mr., or Ms. prefix.

As a recent graduate, you will not have any prior work experience as an RT, so you must make certain to highlight the clinical experiences and skills you obtained during your education. Simply stating that you can do something will not catch the attention of a potential employer. You must explain how it will benefit the respiratory care department at that hospital or agency. This can be accomplished by tailoring your resumé for each specific hospital or agency you apply to.

> **Tip** Include academic achievements and student organizations you belong to on your resumé along with certifications such as ACLS, PALS, and AE-C.

Never include information about your hobbies, political affiliation, religion, or sexual orientation. All such information is irrelevant and will not help you get an interview. If you have difficulties writing a resumé, professional resumé writing assistance is available. Check with your college or university to find out if it can help. Figure 30-1 is an example of the resumé of a recent graduate from the respiratory care course.

Along with your resumé, you should send or attach a cover letter. A well-written cover letter is your first chance to make good impression and, hopefully, allows your resumé to "stick out" from those of other applicants. A cover letter should be specific to the respiratory care position and to the facility to which you are applying. Look at the job description and the facility's mission and vision statements. Use these along with the job posting requirements to highlight your skills and experiences. This will demonstrate why you are the best candidate for the position. A sample cover letter is given in Figure 30-2.

Interview

First and foremost, arrive a few minutes early for the interview. Call ahead of time and get the interviewer's name and the interview location. If more than one person is interviewing you, make sure you know which interviewer has the most authority, and address him or her first when introducing yourself. Bring copies of your resumé printed on white paper along with a list of references. Use your preferred personal title when introducing yourself to the interviewer(s). Respect professional and personal titles, and never address your interviewer by his or her first name. A smile and a handshake are appropriate gestures, and this courtesy will create a positive first impression. First impressions are important, so dress in business attire that is conservative and tasteful, and put your cell phone away and in the silent mode (Figure 30-3).

Jane Doe, RRT
1234 Main St. Phoenix, Arizona, 85034
Jane.Doe@email.com

EDUCATION

School Name, College of Health Care – Phoenix, AZ
May 2013

- B.S. in Respiratory Care

HEALTH CARE AND RELATED EXPERIENCE

Big Hospital – Phoenix, AZ *June 2008 - Present*
Patient transporter

- Transport patients to and from clinical, ancillary and support areas via wheelchair, stretcher or beds as requested to include transport of patients with oxygen tanks, intravenous pumps, drips and special equipment. With assistance, transfers patients to or from beds, wheelchairs or stretchers as needed. During discharge transports patients to hospital lobby and open doors.

EMS Agency – Seattle, WA *June 2002 - June 2005*
EMT

- Administers first-aid treatment to and transports sick or injured persons to medical facility, working as member of emergency medical team, monitors communication equipment to maintain contact with dispatcher, removes or assists in removal of victims from scene of accident or catastrophe, determines nature and extent of illness or injury, or magnitude of catastrophe, to establish first aid procedures to be followed or need for additional assistance, basing decisions on statements of persons involved, examination of victim or victims, and knowledge of emergency medical practice.

Professional Memberships, Licensure, and Certifications
- Registered Respiratory Therapist (RRT)
- Licensed Respiratory Care Practitioner, State of Arizona
- American Association for Respiratory Care (AARC)
- Advanced Cardiac Life Support (ACLS)
- Arizona State Society of Respiratory Care (AzSRC)

Offices Held

President of student respiratory care organization

Figure 30-1 Sample Resumé.

✱ **Tip** Review the mission and vision statements of the hospital or agency you are interviewing with prior to your interview. You should have knowledge of the relevant heath care topics and facts directly relating to that facility so that you will be able to discuss them during the interview.

→ **Reality Check** Always ask for permission before you use someone as a reference.

✱ **Tip** Physicians or anyone who has obtained a doctoral degree should always be addressed as *Doctor*. Women and men without doctoral degrees should be addressed as "Ms." or "Mr."

→ **Reality Check** Hugs are never appropriate during an interview.

You may be given a tour of the department, so make sure you wear comfortable shoes. Many employers frown on fake nails, body piercings, and visible tattoos. Remove any piercings and cover tattoos, if possible. A correlation exists between poor personal hygiene and transmissible diseases, so it is imperative that you display excellent grooming and personal hygiene by arriving at the interview looking clean and smelling fresh. Do not wear overpowering perfumes or colognes. Daily personal hygiene tips for the health care professional are listed in Box 30-4.

→ **Reality Check** Never chew gum during an interview.

Your Contact Information
Address
City, State, Zip Code
Phone Number
Cell Phone Number
Email

Employer Contact Information

Name
Title
Company
Address
City, State, Zip Code

Date

Dear Mr./Ms. XYZ or Dear selection committee,

I am very interested in the entry-level RRT position that is available at Big Hospital USA. I recently graduated from Respiratory University and am actively seeking employment with hospitals in the Phoenix area. My courses in respiratory care, pharmacology, and cardiopulmonary pathophysiology along with my student clinical experiences at your facility have given me a solid base upon which I plan to build my career in respiratory care.

During my respiratory school clinicals, I dealt with a variety of pulmonary patients, spent many hours in the critical care environment, and attended two rotations at your facility. The experience allowed me to learn important skills, develop the confidence needed to succeed in the respiratory care environment, and solidify my desire to work at your facility.

I have enclosed my resume for your review. Thank you for your time and consideration.

It would be a pleasure to interview with you and I look forward to hearing from you soon.

Sincerely,

Your Signature

Your Typed Name

Figure 30-2 Sample Cover Letter.

BOX 30-4   Daily Personal Hygiene Tips for the Health Care Professional

- Shower or bathe and shampoo daily.
- Use a deodorant. Avoid heavy perfumes and colognes.
- Choose a hair style that does not call attention. Avoid unnatural hair colors.
- Apply makeup moderately.
- Cut your fingernails short. Some hospitals do not allow acrylic or fake nails.
- Practice daily dental hygiene.
- Practice proper hand hygiene techniques all day.

During the interview process, maintain eye contact with your interviewer(s), and speak in a professional manner. Avoid using slang terms, and never use profanity. If you are nervous, you may stutter or speak too fast. Be aware of your tone and how it affects the person listening. You are attempting to enter the field of health care and must use medical terminology correctly. This will instill confidence in your interviewers and

mark you as a professional. If English is not your first language, you may need to speak more slowly. You should be aware of your facial expressions, body language, and nonverbal aspects that can come across during the interview. Aspects of body language that may convey a specific expression are listed in Box 30-5.

> **Reality Check** Ability to speak a language other than English is often desirable in health care.

During the interview, some facilities require you take a short examination on respiratory care topics, ranging from oxygen delivery to mechanical ventilation. Be prepared by reviewing some modalities that are common to the everyday practice of an RT. Last, but certainly not least, one of the most important aspects of the interview that is often neglected during interview preparation is having questions to ask the interviewer. They may ask you, "So, do you have any questions for me at this time?" Be prepared. Box 30-6 lists some broad questions that may help you during this portion of the

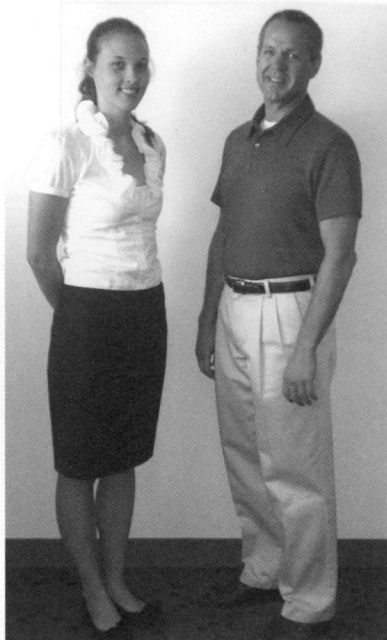

Figure 30-3 Looking professional is important for good first impressions. (From Elsevier: *Job readiness for health professionals: soft skills strategies for success*, St. Louis, MO, 2013, Mosby.)

BOX 30-5 Aspects of Body Language

- Eye contact
- Gestures
- Appearance
- Posture
- Tone of voice
- Pace of speech
- Volume of speech
- Facial expressions
- Smell
- Sound
- Respecting personal space
- Nonverbal vocalization such as sighing
- Twitching
- Being distracted

BOX 30-6 Sample questions for the interviewee

- How will I be trained once I start working here?
- How long is the orientation process?
- Do you offer advanced training for RTs?
- Do you encourage your employees to attend professional meetings?
- Are the RTs here currently involved in any research projects?
- As the director of the department, what organizations in the field of respiratory care are you involved in?

→ **Reality Check** Passing a physical examination and a drug test may be a condition of employment.

interview. Once the interview is over, thank the interviewer(s), and ask when and how you should expect to hear about the outcome of your interview and a possible job offer. It is always proper to write a thank-you note to the interviewer using a simply designed thank-you note format.

Starting Your Career

Once you have been offered a position as an RT, make sure that you follow through with all additional requirements such as physical examinations and drug tests that the new employer requires of you. Typically, new therapists will be hired to work the overnight shift. Do not expect to walk into a Monday-to-Friday, 9-to-5 position and work exclusively in the intensive care unit (ICU). You will have a period at work during which you follow a preceptor, get cleared to perform specific therapies (i.e., arterial line placement, mini-bronchoalveolar lavages [BALs]), which you may not have performed as a student.

As a respiratory care professional, you are obligated to meet all state licensure laws. To maintain your RCP license, you will be required to complete continuing education. The AARC defines Continuing Respiratory Care Education (CRCE) as "the variety of learning experiences meant to enhance the knowledge of respiratory therapists enabling them to provide safe, and effective respiratory care to patients." Many venues provide CRCEs. The AARC offers online CRCEs, national or state meetings, and educational institution–sponsored CRCEs, as well as product-related and sponsored events.

✱ **Tip** Contact your state board of respiratory care to ensure that you have attended the appropriate number of continuing respiratory care education (CRCE) courses to maintain your license.

Create positive expectations for yourself, and embrace your new role. You worked hard to achieve your credentials and become a professional. Welcome to the world of respiratory care!

Bibliography

American Association for Respiratory Care: *Continuing respiratory care education*: www.AARC.org. Accessed 2012.

Kacmarek RM, Stoller JK, Heuer AJ: *Egan's fundamentals of respiratory care*, ed 10, St. Louis, MO, 2013, Mosby.

Elsevier: *Job readiness for the health professionals*, St. Louis, MO, 2012, Mosby.

Student _____ Date _____

Instructor (Laboratory setting) _____ Date _____

Instructor (Clinical setting) _____ Date _____

Criteria for assessment success:

Student must obtain all **satisfactory (S)** scores to pass the procedural assessment. Any **unsatisfactory (U)** scores will result in failure of the procedural assessment.

Scoring:

Satisfactory (S): Procedural step performed correctly with no instructor prompting. Student-initiated correction is acceptable.

Unsatisfactory (U): Procedural step was performed incorrectly, omitted, or performed in a way that compromised patient care.

Not applicable (N/A): Procedural step was not indicated or necessary.

Evaluation:

	Peer Evaluation Laboratory Setting	Instructor Evaluation Laboratory Setting	Instructor Evaluation Clinical Setting
Procedural Preparation			
1. Reviews the patient chart.	S ☐ U ☐ N/A ☐	S ☐ U ☐ N/A ☐	S ☐ U ☐ N/A ☐
2. Verifies the physician's order or the facility's protocol for standard of care.	S ☐ U ☐ N/A ☐	S ☐ U ☐ N/A ☐	S ☐ U ☐ N/A ☐
3. Obtains, cleans, and inspects the appropriate equipment prior to entering the patient's room.	S ☐ U ☐ N/A ☐	S ☐ U ☐ N/A ☐	S ☐ U ☐ N/A ☐
4. Follows PPE requirements, and observes standard precautions for any transmission-based isolation procedure.	S ☐ U ☐ N/A ☐	S ☐ U ☐ N/A ☐	S ☐ U ☐ N/A ☐
5. Identifies the patient using two patient identifiers.	S ☐ U ☐ N/A ☐	S ☐ U ☐ N/A ☐	S ☐ U ☐ N/A ☐
6. Introduces self to the patient and to the family.	S ☐ U ☐ N/A ☐	S ☐ U ☐ N/A ☐	S ☐ U ☐ N/A ☐
7. Explains the procedure to the patient and to the family, and acknowledges the patient's understanding.	S ☐ U ☐ N/A ☐	S ☐ U ☐ N/A ☐	S ☐ U ☐ N/A ☐
8. Performs proper hand hygiene, and puts on gloves, mask, and protective eyewear, as appropriate for the procedure.	S ☐ U ☐ N/A ☐	S ☐ U ☐ N/A ☐	S ☐ U ☐ N/A ☐
Implementation			
1. Reports accurate, objective information in chronological order.	S ☐ U ☐ N/A ☐	S ☐ U ☐ N/A ☐	S ☐ U ☐ N/A ☐
2. Restores the patient's safety.	S ☐ U ☐ N/A ☐	S ☐ U ☐ N/A ☐	S ☐ U ☐ N/A ☐
3. Assesses the extent of injury.	S ☐ U ☐ N/A ☐	S ☐ U ☐ N/A ☐	S ☐ U ☐ N/A ☐
4. Notifies the proper medical personal needed to treat the patient if he or she is injured.	S ☐ U ☐ N/A ☐	S ☐ U ☐ N/A ☐	S ☐ U ☐ N/A ☐

Continued

	Peer Evaluation Laboratory Setting			Instructor Evaluation Laboratory Setting			Instructor Evaluation Clinical Setting		
5. If injured party is not a patient of the facility, refers him or her to the appropriate location for evaluation.	S ☐	U ☐	N/A ☐	S ☐	U ☐	N/A ☐	S ☐	U ☐	N/A ☐
6. If the injured party is a patient, assesses and implements any ordered therapies.	S ☐	U ☐	N/A ☐	S ☐	U ☐	N/A ☐	S ☐	U ☐	N/A ☐
Documentation and Reporting									
1. Completes an incident report promptly.	S ☐	U ☐	N/A ☐	S ☐	U ☐	N/A ☐	S ☐	U ☐	N/A ☐
2. Documents events of the incident in the patient's chart, if applicable.	S ☐	U ☐	N/A ☐	S ☐	U ☐	N/A ☐	S ☐	U ☐	N/A ☐
3. Delivers the report to the appropriate designated department.	S ☐	U ☐	N/A ☐	S ☐	U ☐	N/A ☐	S ☐	U ☐	N/A ☐

Comments:

_____

_____

_____

Signatures:

Student _____ Date Passed _____

Instructor (Laboratory Setting) _____ Date Passed _____

Student _____ Date Passed _____

Instructor (Clinical Setting) _____ Date Passed _____

Procedural Assessment 2-1

Case study presentation

Student _____ Date _____

Instructor (Laboratory setting) _____ Date _____

Location _____ Date _____

Criteria for assessment success:

Student must obtain a score of 75% or above to pass the procedural assessment. Scores under 75% result in failure of the procedural assessment.

Scoring:

Satisfactory (S): Section presented correctly or appropriately for student's level of knowledge. **2 pts.**

Unsatisfactory (U): Section incomplete or presented with incorrect information. **1 pt.**

Not included (N/I): Procedural step was not indicated or necessary. **0 pts.**

	Peer Evaluation	Instructor Evaluation
Procedural Preparation		
1. Chooses a patient with whom contact and respiratory assessment was performed.	S ☐ U ☐ N/I ☐	S ☐ U ☐ N/I ☐
2. Follows all facility protocols for patient interaction and interviews the patient, and collects all pertinent data for presentation.	S ☐ U ☐ N/I ☐	S ☐ U ☐ N/I ☐
3. Follows all PPE and observes standard precautions for any transmission-based isolation procedure and performs a physical assessment of the patient.	S ☐ U ☐ N/I ☐	S ☐ U ☐ N/I ☐
4. Prepares a PowerPoint presentation to aid in oral case study presentation.	S ☐ U ☐ N/I ☐	S ☐ U ☐ N/I ☐
5. Prepares any materials that will be needed by your audience.	S ☐ U ☐ N/I ☐	S ☐ U ☐ N/I ☐
Implementation		
1. Dresses professionally on the day of the presentation.	S ☐ U ☐ N/I ☐	S ☐ U ☐ N/I ☐
2. Identifies self to your audience.	S ☐ U ☐ N/I ☐	S ☐ U ☐ N/I ☐
3. States the patients age, gender, and pertinent demographic information.	S ☐ U ☐ N/I ☐	S ☐ U ☐ N/I ☐
4. States the chief complaint.	S ☐ U ☐ N/I ☐	S ☐ U ☐ N/I ☐
5. States the history of the patient's present illness.	S ☐ U ☐ N/I ☐	S ☐ U ☐ N/I ☐
6. States the admitting diagnosis.	S ☐ U ☐ N/I ☐	S ☐ U ☐ N/I ☐
7. States the past medical history and identifies the relevant pulmonary history.	S ☐ U ☐ N/I ☐	S ☐ U ☐ N/I ☐
8. States the patient's social and environmental histories.	S ☐ U ☐ N/I ☐	S ☐ U ☐ N/I ☐
9. Provides a well-ordered explanation of the physical assessment and a relevant review of systems information.	S ☐ U ☐ N/I ☐	S ☐ U ☐ N/I ☐
10. Provides and explains all laboratory data and radiologic test results.	S ☐ U ☐ N/I ☐	S ☐ U ☐ N/I ☐
11. Lists the patient's medications, with focus on the respiratory medications.	S ☐ U ☐ N/I ☐	S ☐ U ☐ N/I ☐
12. Describes the effect of the medications on the patient's respiratory condition.	S ☐ U ☐ N/I ☐	S ☐ U ☐ N/I ☐
13. Clearly describes all respiratory care modalities performed.	S ☐ U ☐ N/I ☐	S ☐ U ☐ N/I ☐

Continued

	Peer Evaluation	Instructor Evaluation
Evaluation of Procedure		
1. Compares the actual management of the patient with textbook management.	S ☐ U ☐ N/I ☐	S ☐ U ☐ N/I ☐
2. Develops appropriate respiratory care plan based on information and evaluates current care using CPGs.	S ☐ U ☐ N/I ☐	S ☐ U ☐ N/I ☐
3. Gives a patient update.	S ☐ U ☐ N/I ☐	S ☐ U ☐ N/I ☐
Documentation and Reporting		
1. Ensures that the PowerPoint or other media presentation material is easy to read, with no misspellings and no inappropriate use of acronyms.	S ☐ U ☐ N/I ☐	S ☐ U ☐ N/I ☐
2. No use of patient identifiers during presentation.	S ☐ U ☐ N/I ☐	S ☐ U ☐ N/I ☐
3. Did not criticize the care given by any of the health care providers involved in the care of the patient.	S ☐ U ☐ N/I ☐	S ☐ U ☐ N/I ☐
4. Presents the case study in a timely manor.	S ☐ U ☐ N/I ☐	S ☐ U ☐ N/I ☐
5. Submits the corresponding case study written paper according to rubric.	S ☐ U ☐ N/I ☐	S ☐ U ☐ N/I ☐
Procedural Assessment Rating	___pts/52 ___%	___pts/52 ___%

75%–100% = pass
Less than 75% = fail

Comments:

_____

_____

_____

Signatures:

Student _____ Date Passed _____

Instructor _____ Date Passed _____

Student _____ Date _____

Instructor (Laboratory setting)_____ Date _____

Instructor (Clinical setting) _____ Date _____

Criteria for assessment success:

Student must obtain all **satisfactory (S)** scores to pass the procedural evaluation. Any **unsatisfactory (U)** scores will result in failure of the procedural assessment.

Scoring:

Satisfactory (S): Procedural step performed correctly with no instructor prompting. Student-initiated correction is acceptable.

Unsatisfactory (U): Procedural step was performed incorrectly, omitted, or performed in a way that compromised patient care.

Not applicable (N/A): Procedural step was not indicated or necessary.

Evaluation:

	Peer Evaluation Laboratory Setting	Instructor Evaluation Laboratory Setting	Instructor Evaluation Clinical Setting
Procedural Preparation			
1. Reviews the patient's chart.	S ☐ U ☐ N/A ☐	S ☐ U ☐ N/A ☐	S ☐ U ☐ N/A ☐
2. Verifies the physician's order or the facility's protocol for standard of care.	S ☐ U ☐ N/A ☐	S ☐ U ☐ N/A ☐	S ☐ U ☐ N/A ☐
3. Obtains, cleans, and inspects the appropriate equipment prior to entering the patient's room.	S ☐ U ☐ N/A ☐	S ☐ U ☐ N/A ☐	S ☐ U ☐ N/A ☐
4. Follows PPE requirements, and observe standard precautions for any transmission-based isolation procedure.	S ☐ U ☐ N/A ☐	S ☐ U ☐ N/A ☐	S ☐ U ☐ N/A ☐
5. Identifies the patient using two patient identifiers.	S ☐ U ☐ N/A ☐	S ☐ U ☐ N/A ☐	S ☐ U ☐ N/A ☐
6. Introduces self to the patient and to the family.	S ☐ U ☐ N/A ☐	S ☐ U ☐ N/A ☐	S ☐ U ☐ N/A ☐
7. Explains the procedure to the patient and to the family, and acknowledges the patient's understanding.	S ☐ U ☐ N/A ☐	S ☐ U ☐ N/A ☐	S ☐ U ☐ N/A ☐
8. Performs proper hand hygiene, and puts on gloves, mask, and protective eyewear, as appropriate for the procedure.	S ☐ U ☐ N/A ☐	S ☐ U ☐ N/A ☐	S ☐ U ☐ N/A ☐
Implementation			
1. Completes a patient assessment, any interventions necessary, and notes the patient's response.	S ☐ U ☐ N/A ☐	S ☐ U ☐ N/A ☐	S ☐ U ☐ N/A ☐
2. Removes supplies from the patient's room, and cleans the area, as needed.	S ☐ U ☐ N/A ☐	S ☐ U ☐ N/A ☐	S ☐ U ☐ N/A ☐
3. Removes PPE, and observes standard precautions prior to leaving the patient's room.	S ☐ U ☐ N/A ☐	S ☐ U ☐ N/A ☐	S ☐ U ☐ N/A ☐
4. Uses appropriate forms, and maintain them in their proper location in the chart.	S ☐ U ☐ N/A ☐	S ☐ U ☐ N/A ☐	S ☐ U ☐ N/A ☐

Continued

	Peer Evaluation Laboratory Setting			Instructor Evaluation Laboratory Setting			Instructor Evaluation Clinical Setting		
5. Documents information in a timely manner. Iif using paper charting, ensures that these forms are legible.	S ☐	U ☐	N/A ☐	S ☐	U ☐	N/A ☐	S ☐	U ☐	N/A ☐
6. Includes significant patient status changes, findings, and progress toward any goals set.	S ☐	U ☐	N/A ☐	S ☐	U ☐	N/A ☐	S ☐	U ☐	N/A ☐
7. Signs the note according to policy.	S ☐	U ☐	N/A ☐	S ☐	U ☐	N/A ☐	S ☐	U ☐	N/A ☐

Documentation and Reporting

	Peer Evaluation Laboratory Setting			Instructor Evaluation Laboratory Setting			Instructor Evaluation Clinical Setting		
1. Reports any abnormal findings to the appropriate health care provider, and documents the provider's name and credentials.	S ☐	U ☐	N/A ☐	S ☐	U ☐	N/A ☐	S ☐	U ☐	N/A ☐

Comments:

_____

_____

_____

Signatures:

Student _____ Date Passed _____

Instructor (Laboratory Setting) _____ Date Passed _____

Student _____ Date Passed _____

Instructor (Clinical Setting) _____ Date Passed _____

Student _____ Date _____

Instructor (Laboratory setting) _____ Date _____

Instructor (Clinical setting) _____ Date _____

Location _____ Date _____

Criteria for assessment success:

Student must obtain all **satisfactory (S)** scores to pass the procedural evaluation. Any **unsatisfactory (U)** scores will result in failure of the procedural assessment.

Scoring:

Satisfactory (S): Procedural step performed correctly with no instructor prompting. Student-initiated correction is acceptable.

Unsatisfactory (U): Procedural step was performed incorrectly, omitted, or performed in a way that compromised patient care.

Not applicable (N/A): Procedural step was not indicated or necessary.

Evaluation:

	Peer Evaluation Laboratory Setting	Instructor Evaluation Laboratory Setting	Instructor Evaluation Clinical Setting
Procedural Preparation			
1. Reviews the patient's chart.	S ☐ U ☐ N/A ☐	S ☐ U ☐ N/A ☐	S ☐ U ☐ N/A ☐
2. Verifies the physician's order or the facility's protocol for standard of care.	S ☐ U ☐ N/A ☐	S ☐ U ☐ N/A ☐	S ☐ U ☐ N/A ☐
3. Obtains, cleans, and inspects the appropriate equipment prior to entering the patient's room.	S ☐ U ☐ N/A ☐	S ☐ U ☐ N/A ☐	S ☐ U ☐ N/A ☐
4. Follows PPE requirements, and observe standard precautions for any transmission-based isolation procedure.	S ☐ U ☐ N/A ☐	S ☐ U ☐ N/A ☐	S ☐ U ☐ N/A ☐
5. Identifies the patient using two patient identifiers.	S ☐ U ☐ N/A ☐	S ☐ U ☐ N/A ☐	S ☐ U ☐ N/A ☐
6. Introduces self to the patient and to the family.	S ☐ U ☐ N/A ☐	S ☐ U ☐ N/A ☐	S ☐ U ☐ N/A ☐
7. Explains the procedure to the patient and, as needed, to the family, and acknowledges the patient's understanding.	S ☐ U ☐ N/A ☐	S ☐ U ☐ N/A ☐	S ☐ U ☐ N/A ☐
8. Performs proper hand hygiene, and puts on gloves, mask, and protective eyewear, as appropriate for the procedure.	S ☐ U ☐ N/A ☐	S ☐ U ☐ N/A ☐	S ☐ U ☐ N/A ☐
9. Assesses the patient for risk of injury and determines the need for special transfer equipment.	S ☐ U ☐ N/A ☐	S ☐ U ☐ N/A ☐	S ☐ U ☐ N/A ☐
10. Assesses the patient for the presence of weakness, dizziness, or postural hypotension.	S ☐ U ☐ N/A ☐	S ☐ U ☐ N/A ☐	S ☐ U ☐ N/A ☐
11. Determines the number of people needed to safely transfer the patient.	S ☐ U ☐ N/A ☐	S ☐ U ☐ N/A ☐	S ☐ U ☐ N/A ☐

Continued

	Peer Evaluation Laboratory Setting			Instructor Evaluation Laboratory Setting			Instructor Evaluation Clinical Setting		

Implementation

1. Gathers pertinent information regarding the patient and his or her condition.	S ☐	U ☐	N/A ☐	S ☐	U ☐	N/A ☐	S ☐	U ☐	N/A ☐
2. Prioritizes the information.	S ☐	U ☐	N/A ☐	S ☐	U ☐	N/A ☐	S ☐	U ☐	N/A ☐
3. Prepares a detailed description of the patient's current status.	S ☐	U ☐	N/A ☐	S ☐	U ☐	N/A ☐	S ☐	U ☐	N/A ☐
4. Reports any significant needs or changes.	S ☐	U ☐	N/A ☐	S ☐	U ☐	N/A ☐	S ☐	U ☐	N/A ☐
5. Reports the patient's postoperative, postdiagnostic, or post–therapeutic procedure status.	S ☐	U ☐	N/A ☐	S ☐	U ☐	N/A ☐	S ☐	U ☐	N/A ☐
6. Makes a clear verbal report to oncoming staff.	S ☐	U ☐	N/A ☐	S ☐	U ☐	N/A ☐	S ☐	U ☐	N/A ☐
7. Respects the patient's privacy. Gives the report in the appropriate location.	S ☐	U ☐	N/A ☐	S ☐	U ☐	N/A ☐	S ☐	U ☐	N/A ☐

Comments:

_____

_____

_____

Signatures:

Student _____ Date Passed _____

Instructor (Laboratory Setting) _____ Date Passed _____

Student _____ Date Passed _____

Instructor (Clinical Setting) _____ Date Passed _____

Procedural Assessment 3-3

Student _____ Date _____

Instructor (Laboratory setting) _____ Date _____

Instructor (Clinical setting) _____ Date _____

Criteria for assessment success:

Student must obtain all **satisfactory (S)** scores to pass the procedural evaluation. Any **unsatisfactory (U)** scores will result in failure of the procedural assessment.

Scoring:

Satisfactory (S): Procedural step performed correctly with no instructor prompting. Student-initiated correction is acceptable.

Unsatisfactory (U): Procedural step was performed incorrectly, omitted, or performed in a way that compromised patient care.

Not applicable (N/A): Procedural step was not indicated or necessary.

Evaluation:

	Peer Evaluation Laboratory Setting	Instructor Evaluation Laboratory Setting	Instructor Evaluation Clinical Setting
Procedural Preparation			
1. Reviews the patient's chart.	S ☐ U ☐ N/A ☐	S ☐ U ☐ N/A ☐	S ☐ U ☐ N/A ☐
2. Verifies the physician's order or the facility's protocol for standard of care.	S ☐ U ☐ N/A ☐	S ☐ U ☐ N/A ☐	S ☐ U ☐ N/A ☐
3. Obtains, cleans, and inspecst the appropriate equipment prior to entering the patient's room.	S ☐ U ☐ N/A ☐	S ☐ U ☐ N/A ☐	S ☐ U ☐ N/A ☐
4. Follows PPE requirements, and observes standard precautions for any transmission-based isolation procedure.	S ☐ U ☐ N/A ☐	S ☐ U ☐ N/A ☐	S ☐ U ☐ N/A ☐
5. Identifies the patient using two patient identifiers.	S ☐ U ☐ N/A ☐	S ☐ U ☐ N/A ☐	S ☐ U ☐ N/A ☐
6. Introduces self to the patient and to the family.	S ☐ U ☐ N/A ☐	S ☐ U ☐ N/A ☐	S ☐ U ☐ N/A ☐
7. Explains the procedure to the patient and to the family, and acknowledges the patient's understanding.	S ☐ U ☐ N/A ☐	S ☐ U ☐ N/A ☐	S ☐ U ☐ N/A ☐
8. Performs proper hand hygiene, and puts on gloves, mask, and protective eyewear, as appropriate for the procedure.	S ☐ U ☐ N/A ☐	S ☐ U ☐ N/A ☐	S ☐ U ☐ N/A ☐
9. Assesses the patient for risk of injury, and determines the need for special transfer equipment.	S ☐ U ☐ N/A ☐	S ☐ U ☐ N/A ☐	S ☐ U ☐ N/A ☐
10. Assesses the patient for the presence of weakness, dizziness, or postural hypotension.	S ☐ U ☐ N/A ☐	S ☐ U ☐ N/A ☐	S ☐ U ☐ N/A ☐
11. Determines the number of people needed to safely transfer the patient.	S ☐ U ☐ N/A ☐	S ☐ U ☐ N/A ☐	S ☐ U ☐ N/A ☐

Continued

	Peer Evaluation Laboratory Setting	Instructor Evaluation Laboratory Setting	Instructor Evaluation Clinical Setting
Implementation			
1. Instructs the patient to breathe normally.	S ☐ U ☐ N/A ☐	S ☐ U ☐ N/A ☐	S ☐ U ☐ N/A ☐
2. Positions the bed in the low position.	S ☐ U ☐ N/A ☐	S ☐ U ☐ N/A ☐	S ☐ U ☐ N/A ☐
3. Ensures that all equipment (intravenous lines, oxygen tubing, etc.) is close to the patient so that it will not get dislodged.	S ☐ U ☐ N/A ☐	S ☐ U ☐ N/A ☐	S ☐ U ☐ N/A ☐
4. Assists the patient to a sitting position.	S ☐ U ☐ N/A ☐	S ☐ U ☐ N/A ☐	S ☐ U ☐ N/A ☐
5. Assists the patient to the sitting position, using an electrical bed.	S ☐ U ☐ N/A ☐	S ☐ U ☐ N/A ☐	S ☐ U ☐ N/A ☐
6. Assists the patient from the bed to the chair.	S ☐ U ☐ N/A ☐	S ☐ U ☐ N/A ☐	S ☐ U ☐ N/A ☐
7. Assists the patient in a horizontal transfer from the bed to the stretcher (or to a different bed).	S ☐ U ☐ N/A ☐	S ☐ U ☐ N/A ☐	S ☐ U ☐ N/A ☐
8. Removes the supplies from the patient's room, and cleans the area, as needed.	S ☐ U ☐ N/A ☐	S ☐ U ☐ N/A ☐	S ☐ U ☐ N/A ☐
9. Removes the PPE, and observes standard precautions prior to leaving the patient's room.	S ☐ U ☐ N/A ☐	S ☐ U ☐ N/A ☐	S ☐ U ☐ N/A ☐
Evaluation of Procedure			
1. Assesses the patient's vital signs.	S ☐ U ☐ N/A ☐	S ☐ U ☐ N/A ☐	S ☐ U ☐ N/A ☐
2. Asks the patient if he or she is feeling dizzy or experiencing any pain during the transfer.	S ☐ U ☐ N/A ☐	S ☐ U ☐ N/A ☐	S ☐ U ☐ N/A ☐
3. Identifies any unexpected outcomes.	S ☐ U ☐ N/A ☐	S ☐ U ☐ N/A ☐	S ☐ U ☐ N/A ☐
Documentation and Reporting			
1. Records the transfer procedure in the patient's chart.	S ☐ U ☐ N/A ☐	S ☐ U ☐ N/A ☐	S ☐ U ☐ N/A ☐
2. Reports any abnormal findings to the appropriate health care provider.	S ☐ U ☐ N/A ☐	S ☐ U ☐ N/A ☐	S ☐ U ☐ N/A ☐

Comments:

_____

_____

_____

Signatures:

Student _____ Date Passed _____

Instructor (Laboratory Setting) _____ Date Passed _____

Student _____ Date Passed _____

Instructor (Clinical Setting) _____ Date Passed _____

Procedural Assessment 4-1
Hand hygiene

Student _____ Date _____

Instructor (Laboratory setting) _____ Date _____

Instructor (Clinical setting) _____ Date _____

Criteria for assessment success:

Student must obtain all **satisfactory (S)** scores to pass the procedural evaluation. Any **unsatisfactory (U)** scores will result in failure of the procedural assessment.

Scoring:

Satisfactory (S): Procedural step performed correctly with no instructor prompting. Student-initiated correction is acceptable.

Unsatisfactory (U): Procedural step was performed incorrectly, omitted, or performed in a way that compromised patient care.

Not applicable (N/A): Procedural step was not indicated or necessary.

Evaluation:

	Peer Evaluation Laboratory Setting	Instructor Evaluation Laboratory Setting	Instructor Evaluation Clinical Setting
Procedural Preparation			
1. None	S ☐ U ☐ N/A ☐	S ☐ U ☐ N/A ☐	S ☐ U ☐ N/A ☐
Implementation			
1. Inspects forearms, hands, and fingers for cuts, abrasions, or breaks in skin.	S ☐ U ☐ N/A ☐	S ☐ U ☐ N/A ☐	S ☐ U ☐ N/A ☐
2. Inspects nails for length and condition.	S ☐ U ☐ N/A ☐	S ☐ U ☐ N/A ☐	S ☐ U ☐ N/A ☐
3. Removes jewelry and watch, or pushes watch and clothing above wrist area.	S ☐ U ☐ N/A ☐	S ☐ U ☐ N/A ☐	S ☐ U ☐ N/A ☐
4. Performs hand antisepsis using an instant alcohol waterless antiseptic product.	S ☐ U ☐ N/A ☐	S ☐ U ☐ N/A ☐	S ☐ U ☐ N/A ☐
5. Performs hand hygiene with antimicrobial soap and warm water.	S ☐ U ☐ N/A ☐	S ☐ U ☐ N/A ☐	S ☐ U ☐ N/A ☐
6. Avoids opening doors or touching objects with clean hands.	S ☐ U ☐ N/A ☐	S ☐ U ☐ N/A ☐	S ☐ U ☐ N/A ☐
Evaluation of Procedure			
1. Inspects the surface of hands and fingers.	S ☐ U ☐ N/A ☐	S ☐ U ☐ N/A ☐	S ☐ U ☐ N/A ☐
2. Identifies any unexpected outcomes.	S ☐ U ☐ N/A ☐	S ☐ U ☐ N/A ☐	S ☐ U ☐ N/A ☐

Comments:

_____

_____

_____

Signatures:

Student _____ Date Passed _____

Instructor (Laboratory Setting) _____ Date Passed _____

Student _____ Date Passed _____

Instructor (Clinical Setting) _____ Date Passed _____

Procedural Assessment 4-2

Sterile gloving

Student _____ Date _____

Instructor (Laboratory setting) _____ Date _____

Instructor (Clinical setting) _____ Date _____

Criteria for assessment success:

Student must obtain all **satisfactory (S)** scores to pass the procedural evaluation. Any **unsatisfactory (U)** scores will result in failure of the procedural assessment.

Scoring:

Satisfactory (S): Procedural step performed correctly with no instructor prompting. Student-initiated correction is acceptable.

Unsatisfactory (U): Procedural step was performed incorrectly, omitted, or performed in a way that compromised patient care.

Not applicable (N/A): Procedural step was not indicated or necessary.

Evaluation:

	Peer Evaluation Laboratory Setting	Instructor Evaluation Laboratory Setting	Instructor Evaluation Clinical Setting
Procedural Preparation			
1. Reviews the patient's chart.	S ☐ U ☐ N/A ☐	S ☐ U ☐ N/A ☐	S ☐ U ☐ N/A ☐
2. Examines the condition of the packaging and expiration date of gloves.	S ☐ U ☐ N/A ☐	S ☐ U ☐ N/A ☐	S ☐ U ☐ N/A ☐
3. Determines if the patient has any latex allergy.	S ☐ U ☐ N/A ☐	S ☐ U ☐ N/A ☐	S ☐ U ☐ N/A ☐
4. Selects the proper-sized gloves.	S ☐ U ☐ N/A ☐	S ☐ U ☐ N/A ☐	S ☐ U ☐ N/A ☐
Implementation			
1. Glove application.	S ☐ U ☐ N/A ☐	S ☐ U ☐ N/A ☐	S ☐ U ☐ N/A ☐
2. Glove removal and disposal.	S ☐ U ☐ N/A ☐	S ☐ U ☐ N/A ☐	S ☐ U ☐ N/A ☐
3. Performs proper hand hygiene.	S ☐ U ☐ N/A ☐	S ☐ U ☐ N/A ☐	S ☐ U ☐ N/A ☐
Evaluation of Procedure			
1. Identifies any unexpected outcomes.	S ☐ U ☐ N/A ☐	S ☐ U ☐ N/A ☐	S ☐ U ☐ N/A ☐
Documentation and Reporting			
1. Reports any exposure, according to the agency protocols.	S ☐ U ☐ N/A ☐	S ☐ U ☐ N/A ☐	S ☐ U ☐ N/A ☐

Comments:

_____

_____

_____

Signatures:

Student _____ Date Passed _____

Instructor (Laboratory Setting) _____ Date Passed _____

Student _____ Date Passed _____

Instructor (Clinical Setting) _____ Date Passed _____

Student _____ Date _____

Instructor (Laboratory setting) _____ Date _____

Instructor (Clinical setting) _____ Date _____

Criteria for assessment success:

Student must obtain all **satisfactory (S)** scores to pass the procedural evaluation. Any **unsatisfactory (U)** scores will result in failure of the procedural assessment.

Scoring:

Satisfactory (S): Procedural step performed correctly with no instructor prompting. Student-initiated correction is acceptable.

Unsatisfactory (U): Procedural step was performed incorrectly, omitted, or performed in a way that compromised patient care.

Not applicable (N/A): Procedural step was not indicated or necessary.

Evaluation:

	Peer Evaluation Laboratory Setting	Instructor Evaluation Laboratory Setting	Instructor Evaluation Clinical Setting
Procedural Preparation			
1. Reviews patient's chart.	S ☐ U ☐ N/A ☐	S ☐ U ☐ N/A ☐	S ☐ U ☐ N/A ☐
2. Determines need to apply cap, mask, or protective eyewear.	S ☐ U ☐ N/A ☐	S ☐ U ☐ N/A ☐	S ☐ U ☐ N/A ☐
3. Prepares and inspects equipment.	S ☐ U ☐ N/A ☐	S ☐ U ☐ N/A ☐	S ☐ U ☐ N/A ☐
4. Performs proper hand hygiene, and applies gloves.	S ☐ U ☐ N/A ☐	S ☐ U ☐ N/A ☐	S ☐ U ☐ N/A ☐
Implementation			
1. Applies cap: a. Secures long hair back or up.	S ☐ U ☐ N/A ☐	S ☐ U ☐ N/A ☐	S ☐ U ☐ N/A ☐
2. Applies mask.	S ☐ U ☐ N/A ☐	S ☐ U ☐ N/A ☐	S ☐ U ☐ N/A ☐
3. Applies protective eyewear: a. Applies eyewear or goggles comfortably, and ensures that vision is unobstructed.	S ☐ U ☐ N/A ☐	S ☐ U ☐ N/A ☐	S ☐ U ☐ N/A ☐
4. Disposes of the cap, mask, and protective eyewear.	S ☐ U ☐ N/A ☐	S ☐ U ☐ N/A ☐	S ☐ U ☐ N/A ☐
5. Performs proper hand hygiene.	S ☐ U ☐ N/A ☐	S ☐ U ☐ N/A ☐	S ☐ U ☐ N/A ☐
Evaluation of Procedure			
1. Identifies any unexpected outcomes.	S ☐ U ☐ N/A ☐	S ☐ U ☐ N/A ☐	S ☐ U ☐ N/A ☐
Documentation and Reporting			
1. Reports any exposure, according to agency protocols.	S ☐ U ☐ N/A ☐	S ☐ U ☐ N/A ☐	S ☐ U ☐ N/A ☐

Comments:

_____

_____

_____

Signatures:

Student _____ Date Passed _____

Instructor (Laboratory Setting) _____ Date Passed _____

Student _____ Date Passed _____

Instructor (Clinical Setting) _____ Date Passed _____

Procedural Assessment 4-4

Isolation precautions

Student _____ Date _____

Instructor (Laboratory setting) _____ Date _____

Instructor (Clinical setting) _____ Date _____

Criteria for assessment success:

Student must obtain all **satisfactory (S)** scores to pass the procedural evaluation. Any **unsatisfactory (U)** scores will result in failure of the procedural assessment.

Scoring:

Satisfactory (S): Procedural step performed correctly with no instructor prompting. Student-initiated correction is acceptable.

Unsatisfactory (U): Procedural step was performed incorrectly, omitted, or performed in a way that compromised patient care.

Not applicable (N/A): Procedural step was not indicated or necessary.

Evaluation:

	Peer Evaluation Laboratory Setting	Instructor Evaluation Laboratory Setting	Instructor Evaluation Clinical Setting
Procedural Preparation			
1. Reviews the patient's chart for the specific isolation category.	S ☐ U ☐ N/A ☐	S ☐ U ☐ N/A ☐	S ☐ U ☐ N/A ☐
2. Reviews pertinent laboratory test needs or results.	S ☐ U ☐ N/A ☐	S ☐ U ☐ N/A ☐	S ☐ U ☐ N/A ☐
3. Considers the type of care to be delivered to the patient.	S ☐ U ☐ N/A ☐	S ☐ U ☐ N/A ☐	S ☐ U ☐ N/A ☐
4. Obtains the proper-sized personal protective equipment (PPE).	S ☐ U ☐ N/A ☐	S ☐ U ☐ N/A ☐	S ☐ U ☐ N/A ☐
5. Places all needed materials near work area.	S ☐ U ☐ N/A ☐	S ☐ U ☐ N/A ☐	S ☐ U ☐ N/A ☐
Implementation			
1. Performs proper hand hygiene.	S ☐ U ☐ N/A ☐	S ☐ U ☐ N/A ☐	S ☐ U ☐ N/A ☐
2. Applies a gown.	S ☐ U ☐ N/A ☐	S ☐ U ☐ N/A ☐	S ☐ U ☐ N/A ☐
3. Applies cap, mask and protective eyewear (see PA 4-3).	S ☐ U ☐ N/A ☐	S ☐ U ☐ N/A ☐	S ☐ U ☐ N/A ☐
4. Applies gloves with the edges overlying the gown cuffs (see PA 4-2).	S ☐ U ☐ N/A ☐	S ☐ U ☐ N/A ☐	S ☐ U ☐ N/A ☐
5. Opens the door with his/her back to enter the patient's room.	S ☐ U ☐ N/A ☐	S ☐ U ☐ N/A ☐	S ☐ U ☐ N/A ☐
6. Explains the purpose of isolation and the necessary precautions to the patient and family.	S ☐ U ☐ N/A ☐	S ☐ U ☐ N/A ☐	S ☐ U ☐ N/A ☐
7. Removes all the isolation attire before leaving the room:			
a. Removes gloves, turning them inside out.	S ☐ U ☐ N/A ☐	S ☐ U ☐ N/A ☐	S ☐ U ☐ N/A ☐
b. Removes the mask and protective eyewear (see PA 4-4).	S ☐ U ☐ N/A ☐	S ☐ U ☐ N/A ☐	S ☐ U ☐ N/A ☐
c. Removes the gown.	S ☐ U ☐ N/A ☐	S ☐ U ☐ N/A ☐	S ☐ U ☐ N/A ☐

Continued

	Peer Evaluation Laboratory Setting			Instructor Evaluation Laboratory Setting			Instructor Evaluation Clinical Setting		
8. Disposes of all isolation attire appropriately.	S ☐	U ☐	N/A ☐	S ☐	U ☐	N/A ☐	S ☐	U ☐	N/A ☐
9. Performs proper hand hygiene before leaving the room and again outside room.	S ☐	U ☐	N/A ☐	S ☐	U ☐	N/A ☐	S ☐	U ☐	N/A ☐

Evaluation of Procedure

1. Identifies any unexpected outcomes.	S ☐	U ☐	N/A ☐	S ☐	U ☐	N/A ☐	S ☐	U ☐	N/A ☐

Documentation and Reporting

1. Reports any exposure, according to agency protocols.	S ☐	U ☐	N/A ☐	S ☐	U ☐	N/A ☐	S ☐	U ☐	N/A ☐

Comments:

_____

_____

_____

Signatures:

Student _____ Date Passed _____

Instructor (Laboratory Setting) _____ Date Passed _____

Student _____ Date Passed _____

Instructor (Clinical Setting) _____ Date Passed _____

Student _____ Date _____

Instructor (Laboratory setting) _____ Date _____

Instructor (Clinical setting) _____ Date _____

Criteria for assessment success:

Student must obtain all **satisfactory (S)** scores to pass the procedural evaluation. Any **unsatisfactory (U)** scores will result in failure of the procedural assessment.

Scoring:

Satisfactory (S): Procedural step performed correctly with no instructor prompting. Student-initiated correction is acceptable.

Unsatisfactory (U): Procedural step was performed incorrectly, omitted, or performed in a way that compromised patient care.

Not applicable (N/A): Procedural step was not indicated or necessary.

Evaluation:

	Peer Evaluation Laboratory Setting	Instructor Evaluation Laboratory Setting	Instructor Evaluation Clinical Setting
Procedural Preparation			
1. Reviews the patient's chart.	S ☐ U ☐ N/A ☐	S ☐ U ☐ N/A ☐	S ☐ U ☐ N/A ☐
2. Attends N-95 mask fitting to ensure the size required to protect you.	S ☐ U ☐ N/A ☐	S ☐ U ☐ N/A ☐	S ☐ U ☐ N/A ☐
3. Assesses the potential for TB infection.	S ☐ U ☐ N/A ☐	S ☐ U ☐ N/A ☐	S ☐ U ☐ N/A ☐
4. Verifies physician's order or the facility's protocol for standard of care.	S ☐ U ☐ N/A ☐	S ☐ U ☐ N/A ☐	S ☐ U ☐ N/A ☐
5. Obtains, cleans, and inspects the appropriate equipment prior to entering the patient's room.	S ☐ U ☐ N/A ☐	S ☐ U ☐ N/A ☐	S ☐ U ☐ N/A ☐
6. Follows PPE requirements, and observes standard precautions for any transmission-based isolation procedure.	S ☐ U ☐ N/A ☐	S ☐ U ☐ N/A ☐	S ☐ U ☐ N/A ☐
7. Identifies patient using two patient identifiers.	S ☐ U ☐ N/A ☐	S ☐ U ☐ N/A ☐	S ☐ U ☐ N/A ☐
8. Introduces self to the patient and to the family.	S ☐ U ☐ N/A ☐	S ☐ U ☐ N/A ☐	S ☐ U ☐ N/A ☐
9. Explains the procedure to the patient and to the family, and acknowledges the patient's understanding.	S ☐ U ☐ N/A ☐	S ☐ U ☐ N/A ☐	S ☐ U ☐ N/A ☐
10. Performs proper hand hygiene, and puts on gloves, mask, and protective eyewear, as appropriate for the procedure.	S ☐ U ☐ N/A ☐	S ☐ U ☐ N/A ☐	S ☐ U ☐ N/A ☐
Implementation			
1. Applies N-95 mask, and checks fit.	S ☐ U ☐ N/A ☐	S ☐ U ☐ N/A ☐	S ☐ U ☐ N/A ☐
2. Enters negative-pressure room, and closes the door.	S ☐ U ☐ N/A ☐	S ☐ U ☐ N/A ☐	S ☐ U ☐ N/A ☐
3. Explains the purpose of TB isolation to the patient and family.	S ☐ U ☐ N/A ☐	S ☐ U ☐ N/A ☐	S ☐ U ☐ N/A ☐

Continued

	Peer Evaluation Laboratory Setting	Instructor Evaluation Laboratory Setting	Instructor Evaluation Clinical Setting
4. Instructs the patient to always cover the mouth with a tissue when coughing and to wear a disposable surgical mask when leaving the room.	S □ U □ N/A □	S □ U □ N/A □	S □ U □ N/A □
5. Provides scheduled patient care.	S □ U □ N/A □	S □ U □ N/A □	S □ U □ N/A □
6. Closes the door when leaving the room.	S □ U □ N/A □	S □ U □ N/A □	S □ U □ N/A □
7. Removes the N-95 mask.	S □ U □ N/A □	S □ U □ N/A □	S □ U □ N/A □
8. Performs proper hand hygiene.	S □ U □ N/A □	S □ U □ N/A □	S □ U □ N/A □

Evaluation of Procedure

1. Assesses the patient's laboratory data for AFB smears or PPD placement.	S □ U □ N/A □	S □ U □ N/A □	S □ U □ N/A □
2. Asks the patient or family to identify how TB may have been contracted by the patient.	S □ U □ N/A □	S □ U □ N/A □	S □ U □ N/A □
3. Identifies any unexpected outcomes.	S □ U □ N/A □	S □ U □ N/A □	S □ U □ N/A □

Documentation and Reporting

1. Reports any abnormal findings to the appropriate health care provider.	S □ U □ N/A □	S □ U □ N/A □	S □ U □ N/A □

Comments:

_____

_____

_____

Signatures:

Student _____ Date Passed _____

Instructor (Laboratory Setting) _____ Date Passed _____

Student _____ Date Passed _____

Instructor (Clinical Setting) _____ Date Passed _____

Procedural Assessment 5-1 Taking a medical history

Student _____ Date _____

Instructor (Laboratory setting) _____ Date _____

Instructor (Clinical setting) _____ Date _____

Criteria for assessment success:

Student must obtain all **satisfactory (S)** scores to pass the procedural evaluation. Any **unsatisfactory (U)** scores will result in failure of the procedural assessment.

Scoring:

Satisfactory (S): Procedural step performed correctly with no instructor prompting. Student-initiated correction is acceptable.

Unsatisfactory (U): Procedural step was performed incorrectly, omitted, or performed in a way that compromised patient care.

Not applicable (N/A): Procedural step was not indicated or necessary.

Evaluation:

	Peer Evaluation Laboratory Setting	Instructor Evaluation Laboratory Setting	Instructor Evaluation Clinical Setting
Procedural Preparation			
1. Reviews the patient's chart.	S ☐ U ☐ N/A ☐	S ☐ U ☐ N/A ☐	S ☐ U ☐ N/A ☐
2. Verifies the physician's order or the facility's protocol for standard of care.	S ☐ U ☐ N/A ☐	S ☐ U ☐ N/A ☐	S ☐ U ☐ N/A ☐
3. Obtains, cleans, and inspects the appropriate equipment prior to entering the patient's room.	S ☐ U ☐ N/A ☐	S ☐ U ☐ N/A ☐	S ☐ U ☐ N/A ☐
4. Follows PPE requirements, and observes standard precautions for any transmission-based isolation procedure.	S ☐ U ☐ N/A ☐	S ☐ U ☐ N/A ☐	S ☐ U ☐ N/A ☐
5. Identifies the patient using two patient identifiers.	S ☐ U ☐ N/A ☐	S ☐ U ☐ N/A ☐	S ☐ U ☐ N/A ☐
6. Introduces self to the patient and to the family.	S ☐ U ☐ N/A ☐	S ☐ U ☐ N/A ☐	S ☐ U ☐ N/A ☐
7. Explains the procedure to the patient and to the family, and acknowledges the patient's understanding.	S ☐ U ☐ N/A ☐	S ☐ U ☐ N/A ☐	S ☐ U ☐ N/A ☐
8. Performs proper hand hygiene, and puts on gloves, mask, and protective eyewear, as appropriate for the procedure.	S ☐ U ☐ N/A ☐	S ☐ U ☐ N/A ☐	S ☐ U ☐ N/A ☐
Implementation			
1. In the social space, provides a brief introduction of self and role to the patient.	S ☐ U ☐ N/A ☐	S ☐ U ☐ N/A ☐	S ☐ U ☐ N/A ☐
2. Assesses the patient's level of consciousness (orientation to person, place, and time).	S ☐ U ☐ N/A ☐	S ☐ U ☐ N/A ☐	S ☐ U ☐ N/A ☐
3. Identifies patient respectfully using titles (e.g., Mr., Mrs., Ms.) and his or her last name.	S ☐ U ☐ N/A ☐	S ☐ U ☐ N/A ☐	S ☐ U ☐ N/A ☐

Continued

	Peer Evaluation Laboratory Setting	Instructor Evaluation Laboratory Setting	Instructor Evaluation Clinical Setting
4. Assesses for factors influencing communication (e.g., language barriers, hearing impairment, anxiety, etc.).	S ☐ U ☐ N/A ☐	S ☐ U ☐ N/A ☐	S ☐ U ☐ N/A ☐
5. Uses appropriate nonverbal behaviors and active listening skills while conducting the patient interview.	S ☐ U ☐ N/A ☐	S ☐ U ☐ N/A ☐	S ☐ U ☐ N/A ☐
6. Ensures patient privacy during the interview (e.g., closes the door, pulls the curtain, asks visitors to leave during assessments).	S ☐ U ☐ N/A ☐	S ☐ U ☐ N/A ☐	S ☐ U ☐ N/A ☐
7. Structures the interview in an orderly manner.	S ☐ U ☐ N/A ☐	S ☐ U ☐ N/A ☐	S ☐ U ☐ N/A ☐
8. Ensures patient comfort before leaving the room.	S ☐ U ☐ N/A ☐	S ☐ U ☐ N/A ☐	S ☐ U ☐ N/A ☐
9. Removes all supplies from patient's room, and cleans the area, as needed.	S ☐ U ☐ N/A ☐	S ☐ U ☐ N/A ☐	S ☐ U ☐ N/A ☐
10. Removes PPE, and performs proper hand hygiene prior to leaving the patient's room.	S ☐ U ☐ N/A ☐	S ☐ U ☐ N/A ☐	S ☐ U ☐ N/A ☐

Evaluation of Procedure

	Peer Evaluation Laboratory Setting	Instructor Evaluation Laboratory Setting	Instructor Evaluation Clinical Setting
1. Establishes a baseline, or compares with previous measurements.	S ☐ U ☐ N/A ☐	S ☐ U ☐ N/A ☐	S ☐ U ☐ N/A ☐
2. Develops appropriate respiratory care plan based on assessment data.	S ☐ U ☐ N/A ☐	S ☐ U ☐ N/A ☐	S ☐ U ☐ N/A ☐
3. Reviews the chart for the presence of an advance directive.	S ☐ U ☐ N/A ☐	S ☐ U ☐ N/A ☐	S ☐ U ☐ N/A ☐
4. Identifies any unexpected outcomes.	S ☐ U ☐ N/A ☐	S ☐ U ☐ N/A ☐	S ☐ U ☐ N/A ☐

Documentation and Reporting

	Peer Evaluation Laboratory Setting	Instructor Evaluation Laboratory Setting	Instructor Evaluation Clinical Setting
1. Records his or her findings in the patient's chart.	S ☐ U ☐ N/A ☐	S ☐ U ☐ N/A ☐	S ☐ U ☐ N/A ☐
2. Reports any abnormal findings to the appropriate health care provider.	S ☐ U ☐ N/A ☐	S ☐ U ☐ N/A ☐	S ☐ U ☐ N/A ☐

Comments:

_____

_____

_____

Signature:

Student _____ Date Passed _____

Instructor (Laboratory Setting) _____ Date Passed _____

Student _____ Date Passed _____

Instructor (Clinical Setting) _____ Date Passed _____

Procedural Assessment 5-2

Student _____ Date _____

Instructor (Laboratory setting) _____ Date _____

Instructor (Clinical setting) _____ Date _____

Criteria for assessment success:

Student must obtain all **satisfactory (S)** scores to pass the procedural evaluation. Any **unsatisfactory (U)** scores will result in failure of the procedural assessment.

Scoring:

Satisfactory (S): Procedural step performed correctly with no instructor prompting. Student-initiated correction is acceptable.

Unsatisfactory (U): Procedural step was performed incorrectly, omitted, or performed in a way that compromised patient care.

Not applicable (N/A): Procedural step was not indicated or necessary.

Evaluation:

	Peer Evaluation Laboratory Setting	Instructor Evaluation Laboratory Setting	Instructor Evaluation Clinical Setting
Procedural Preparation			
1. Reviews the patient's chart.	S ☐ U ☐ N/A ☐	S ☐ U ☐ N/A ☐	S ☐ U ☐ N/A ☐
2. Verifies the physician's order or the facility's protocol for standard of care.	S ☐ U ☐ N/A ☐	S ☐ U ☐ N/A ☐	S ☐ U ☐ N/A ☐
3. Obtains, cleans, and inspects the appropriate equipment prior to entering the patient's room.	S ☐ U ☐ N/A ☐	S ☐ U ☐ N/A ☐	S ☐ U ☐ N/A ☐
4. Follows PPE requirements, and observes standard precautions for any transmission-based isolation procedure.	S ☐ U ☐ N/A ☐	S ☐ U ☐ N/A ☐	S ☐ U ☐ N/A ☐
5. Identifies the patient using two patient identifiers.	S ☐ U ☐ N/A ☐	S ☐ U ☐ N/A ☐	S ☐ U ☐ N/A ☐
6. Introduces self to the patient and to the family.	S ☐ U ☐ N/A ☐	S ☐ U ☐ N/A ☐	S ☐ U ☐ N/A ☐
7. Explains the procedure to the patient and to the family, and acknowledges the patient's understanding.	S ☐ U ☐ N/A ☐	S ☐ U ☐ N/A ☐	S ☐ U ☐ N/A ☐
8. Performs proper hand hygiene, and puts on gloves, mask, and protective eyewear, as appropriate for the procedure.	S ☐ U ☐ N/A ☐	S ☐ U ☐ N/A ☐	S ☐ U ☐ N/A ☐
9. Mutes or turns off the patient's TV or radio. Ensures patient privacy.	S ☐ U ☐ N/A ☐	S ☐ U ☐ N/A ☐	S ☐ U ☐ N/A ☐
PULSE RATE: **Implementation**			
1. Positions the patient comfortably, and instructs him or her to breathe normally.	S ☐ U ☐ N/A ☐	S ☐ U ☐ N/A ☐	S ☐ U ☐ N/A ☐
2. Locates the preferred site, and palpates pulse rate for the appropriate amount of time: a. Determines the pulse rate, rhythm, and quality (Box 5-2).	S ☐ U ☐ N/A ☐	S ☐ U ☐ N/A ☐	S ☐ U ☐ N/A ☐

Continued

	Peer Evaluation Laboratory Setting	Instructor Evaluation Laboratory Setting	Instructor Evaluation Clinical Setting
RESPIRATORY RATE: **Implementation**			
1. Assesses the patient's respiratory rate, rhythm, and depth.	S ☐ U ☐ N/A ☐	S ☐ U ☐ N/A ☐	S ☐ U ☐ N/A ☐
EXAMINATION OF THORAX AND LUNGS: **Inspection**			
1. Inspects the chest visually, noting the thoracic configuration.	S ☐ U ☐ N/A ☐	S ☐ U ☐ N/A ☐	S ☐ U ☐ N/A ☐
2. Assesses breathing pattern and effort.	S ☐ U ☐ N/A ☐	S ☐ U ☐ N/A ☐	S ☐ U ☐ N/A ☐
Palpation			
1. Assesses for tactile fremitus, and evaluates the posterior, lateral, and anterior portions of the thorax.	S ☐ U ☐ N/A ☐	S ☐ U ☐ N/A ☐	S ☐ U ☐ N/A ☐
2. Assesses for chest wall symmetry during inhalation.	S ☐ U ☐ N/A ☐	S ☐ U ☐ N/A ☐	S ☐ U ☐ N/A ☐
3. Assesses for air leaks.	S ☐ U ☐ N/A ☐	S ☐ U ☐ N/A ☐	S ☐ U ☐ N/A ☐
Percussion			
1. Assesses the chest by percussion for excess fluid or tissue.	S ☐ U ☐ N/A ☐	S ☐ U ☐ N/A ☐	S ☐ U ☐ N/A ☐
Auscultation			
1. Starting from the posterior bases, auscultates each lung position bilaterally.	S ☐ U ☐ N/A ☐	S ☐ U ☐ N/A ☐	S ☐ U ☐ N/A ☐
2. Auscultates each position bilaterally on the lateral chest.	S ☐ U ☐ N/A ☐	S ☐ U ☐ N/A ☐	S ☐ U ☐ N/A ☐
3. Auscultates each position on the anterior chest.	S ☐ U ☐ N/A ☐	S ☐ U ☐ N/A ☐	S ☐ U ☐ N/A ☐
Implementation Continued			
4. Return the TV or radio to the previous sound level.	S ☐ U ☐ N/A ☐	S ☐ U ☐ N/A ☐	S ☐ U ☐ N/A ☐
5. Ensure patient comfort and safety.	S ☐ U ☐ N/A ☐	S ☐ U ☐ N/A ☐	S ☐ U ☐ N/A ☐
6. Remove the supplies from the patient's room, and clean the area, as needed.	S ☐ U ☐ N/A ☐	S ☐ U ☐ N/A ☐	S ☐ U ☐ N/A ☐
7. Remove the PPE, and perform proper hand hygiene prior to leaving the patient's room.	S ☐ U ☐ N/A ☐	S ☐ U ☐ N/A ☐	S ☐ U ☐ N/A ☐
Evaluation of Procedure			
1. Establishes a baseline of vital signs assessed, or compares with previous measurements.	S ☐ U ☐ N/A ☐	S ☐ U ☐ N/A ☐	S ☐ U ☐ N/A ☐
2. Notes any oxygen therapy needs or if changes in current therapy are indicated.	S ☐ U ☐ N/A ☐	S ☐ U ☐ N/A ☐	S ☐ U ☐ N/A ☐
3. Identifies any unexpected outcomes to the appropriate health care provider.	S ☐ U ☐ N/A ☐	S ☐ U ☐ N/A ☐	S ☐ U ☐ N/A ☐
Documentation and Reporting			
1. Describes and records the rhythm and quality of pulse rate, respiratory rate, and any auscultation findings in the patient's chart.	S ☐ U ☐ N/A ☐	S ☐ U ☐ N/A ☐	S ☐ U ☐ N/A ☐
2. Records oxygen therapy needs or if changes in current therapy are indicated.	S ☐ U ☐ N/A ☐	S ☐ U ☐ N/A ☐	S ☐ U ☐ N/A ☐
3. Reports any abnormal finding to appropriate health care provider.	S ☐ U ☐ N/A ☐	S ☐ U ☐ N/A ☐	S ☐ U ☐ N/A ☐

Comments:

_____

_____

_____

Signatures:

Student _____ Date Passed _____

Instructor (Laboratory Setting) _____ Date Passed _____

Student _____ Date Passed _____

Instructor (Clinical Setting) _____ Date Passed _____

Comments:

Signatures:

Student _____ Date Passed _____

Instructor (Laboratory Setting) _____ Date Passed _____

Student _____ Date Passed _____

Instructor (Clinical Setting) _____ Date Passed _____

Procedural Assessment 5-3   Performing pulse oximetry

Student _____ Date _____

Instructor (Laboratory setting) _____ Date _____

Instructor (Clinical setting) _____ Date _____

Criteria for assessment success:

Student must obtain all **satisfactory (S)** scores to pass the procedural evaluation. Any **unsatisfactory (U)** scores will result in failure of the procedural assessment.

Scoring:

Satisfactory (S): Procedural step performed correctly with no instructor prompting. Student-initiated correction is acceptable.

Unsatisfactory (U): Procedural step was performed incorrectly, omitted, or performed in a way that compromised patient care.

Not applicable (N/A): Procedural step was not indicated or necessary.

Evaluation:

	Peer Evaluation Laboratory Setting	Instructor Evaluation Laboratory Setting	Instructor Evaluation Clinical Setting
Procedural Preparation			
1. Reviews the patient's chart.	S ☐ U ☐ N/A ☐	S ☐ U ☐ N/A ☐	S ☐ U ☐ N/A ☐
2. Verifies the physician's order or the facility's protocol for standard of care.	S ☐ U ☐ N/A ☐	S ☐ U ☐ N/A ☐	S ☐ U ☐ N/A ☐
3. Obtains, cleans, and inspects the appropriate equipment prior to entering the patient's room.	S ☐ U ☐ N/A ☐	S ☐ U ☐ N/A ☐	S ☐ U ☐ N/A ☐
4. Follows PPE requirements, and observes standard precautions for any transmission-based isolation procedure.	S ☐ U ☐ N/A ☐	S ☐ U ☐ N/A ☐	S ☐ U ☐ N/A ☐
5. Identifies the patient using two patient identifiers.	S ☐ U ☐ N/A ☐	S ☐ U ☐ N/A ☐	S ☐ U ☐ N/A ☐
6. Introduces self to the patient and to the family.	S ☐ U ☐ N/A ☐	S ☐ U ☐ N/A ☐	S ☐ U ☐ N/A ☐
7. Explains the procedure to the patient and to the family, and acknowledges the patient's understanding.	S ☐ U ☐ N/A ☐	S ☐ U ☐ N/A ☐	S ☐ U ☐ N/A ☐
8. Performs proper hand hygiene, and puts on gloves, mask, and protective eyewear, as appropriate for the procedure.	S ☐ U ☐ N/A ☐	S ☐ U ☐ N/A ☐	S ☐ U ☐ N/A ☐
Implementation			
1. Positions the patient comfortably, and instructs him or her to breathe normally.	S ☐ U ☐ N/A ☐	S ☐ U ☐ N/A ☐	S ☐ U ☐ N/A ☐
2. Determines the most appropriate site to attach the probe.	S ☐ U ☐ N/A ☐	S ☐ U ☐ N/A ☐	S ☐ U ☐ N/A ☐
3. Turns on the pulse oximeter.	S ☐ U ☐ N/A ☐	S ☐ U ☐ N/A ☐	S ☐ U ☐ N/A ☐
4. Cleans the selected site with an alcohol pad.	S ☐ U ☐ N/A ☐	S ☐ U ☐ N/A ☐	S ☐ U ☐ N/A ☐
5. Attaches the probe to the selected site, and secures it.	S ☐ U ☐ N/A ☐	S ☐ U ☐ N/A ☐	S ☐ U ☐ N/A ☐

Continued

	Peer Evaluation Laboratory Setting			Instructor Evaluation Laboratory Setting			Instructor Evaluation Clinical Setting		
6. Observes the pulse waveform or intensity display, and correlates with the radial pulse rate.	S ☐	U ☐	N/A ☐	S ☐	U ☐	N/A ☐	S ☐	U ☐	N/A ☐
7. Sets the alarms, and monitors skin integrity if oximetry is continuous.	S ☐	U ☐	N/A ☐	S ☐	U ☐	N/A ☐	S ☐	U ☐	N/A ☐

Evaluation of Procedure

1. Establishes a pulse oximetry baseline, or compares with previous measurements.	S ☐	U ☐	N/A ☐	S ☐	U ☐	N/A ☐	S ☐	U ☐	N/A ☐
2. Notes any use of oxygen therapy.	S ☐	U ☐	N/A ☐	S ☐	U ☐	N/A ☐	S ☐	U ☐	N/A ☐
3. Identifies any unexpected outcomes.	S ☐	U ☐	N/A ☐	S ☐	U ☐	N/A ☐	S ☐	U ☐	N/A ☐
4. Correlates findings with arterial blood gas measurement.	S ☐	U ☐	N/A ☐	S ☐	U ☐	N/A ☐	S ☐	U ☐	N/A ☐

Documentation and Recording

1. Records pulse oximetry, pulse rate, and patient's current oxygen use and amount, if applicable.	S ☐	U ☐	N/A ☐	S ☐	U ☐	N/A ☐	S ☐	U ☐	N/A ☐
2. Records whether pulse oximetry is continuous or intermittent.	S ☐	U ☐	N/A ☐	S ☐	U ☐	N/A ☐	S ☐	U ☐	N/A ☐
3. Records the need for oxygen therapy or if changes in current therapy are indicated.	S ☐	U ☐	N/A ☐	S ☐	U ☐	N/A ☐	S ☐	U ☐	N/A ☐
4. Reports any abnormal findings to the appropriate health care provider.	S ☐	U ☐	N/A ☐	S ☐	U ☐	N/A ☐	S ☐	U ☐	N/A ☐

Comments:

_____

_____

_____

Signatures:

Student _____ Date Passed _____

Instructor (Laboratory Setting) _____ Date Passed _____

Student _____ Date Passed _____

Instructor (Clinical Setting) _____ Date Passed _____

Procedural Assessment 5-4

Student _____ Date _____

Instructor (Laboratory setting) _____ Date _____

Instructor (Clinical setting) _____ Date _____

Criteria for assessment success:

Student must obtain all **satisfactory (S)** scores to pass the procedural evaluation. Any **unsatisfactory (U)** scores will result in failure of the procedural assessment.

Scoring:

Satisfactory (S): Procedural step performed correctly with no instructor prompting. Student-initiated correction is acceptable.

Unsatisfactory (U): Procedural step was performed incorrectly, omitted, or performed in a way that compromised patient care.

Not applicable (N/A): Procedural step was not indicated or necessary.

Evaluation:

	Peer Evaluation Laboratory Setting	Instructor Evaluation Laboratory Setting	Instructor Evaluation Clinical Setting
Procedural Preparation			
1. Reviews the patient's chart.	S ☐ U ☐ N/A ☐	S ☐ U ☐ N/A ☐	S ☐ U ☐ N/A ☐
2. Verifies the physician's order or the facility's protocol for standard of care.	S ☐ U ☐ N/A ☐	S ☐ U ☐ N/A ☐	S ☐ U ☐ N/A ☐
3. Obtains, cleans, and inspects the appropriate equipment prior to entering the patient's room.	S ☐ U ☐ N/A ☐	S ☐ U ☐ N/A ☐	S ☐ U ☐ N/A ☐
4. Follows PPE requirements, and observes standard precautions for any transmission-based isolation procedure.	S ☐ U ☐ N/A ☐	S ☐ U ☐ N/A ☐	S ☐ U ☐ N/A ☐
5. Identifies the patient using two patient identifiers.	S ☐ U ☐ N/A ☐	S ☐ U ☐ N/A ☐	S ☐ U ☐ N/A ☐
6. Introduces self to the patient and to the family.	S ☐ U ☐ N/A ☐	S ☐ U ☐ N/A ☐	S ☐ U ☐ N/A ☐
7. Explains the procedure to the patient and to the family, and acknowledges the patient's understanding.	S ☐ U ☐ N/A ☐	S ☐ U ☐ N/A ☐	S ☐ U ☐ N/A ☐
8. Performs proper hand hygiene, and puts on gloves, mask, and protective eyewear, as appropriate for the procedure.	S ☐ U ☐ N/A ☐	S ☐ U ☐ N/A ☐	S ☐ U ☐ N/A ☐
9. Mutes or turns off the patient TV or radio, and ensures patient privacy.	S ☐ U ☐ N/A ☐	S ☐ U ☐ N/A ☐	S ☐ U ☐ N/A ☐
BLOOD PRESSURE **Implementation**			
1. Wraps a deflated cuff snugly around the patient's upper arm.	S ☐ U ☐ N/A ☐	S ☐ U ☐ N/A ☐	S ☐ U ☐ N/A ☐
2. While palpating the brachial artery for a pulse, inflates the cuff to approximately 30 mm Hg above the point at which the brachial pulse can no longer be felt (Figure 5-7).	S ☐ U ☐ N/A ☐	S ☐ U ☐ N/A ☐	S ☐ U ☐ N/A ☐

Continued

	Peer Evaluation Laboratory Setting	Instructor Evaluation Laboratory Setting	Instructor Evaluation Clinical Setting
3. Places the diaphragm portion of the stethoscope over the brachial artery, and slowly deflates the cuff at a rate of 2 mm Hg per second while observing the manometer.	S ☐ U ☐ N/A ☐	S ☐ U ☐ N/A ☐	S ☐ U ☐ N/A ☐
4. Notes the systolic pressure.	S ☐ U ☐ N/A ☐	S ☐ U ☐ N/A ☐	S ☐ U ☐ N/A ☐
5. Notes the diastolic pressure.	S ☐ U ☐ N/A ☐	S ☐ U ☐ N/A ☐	S ☐ U ☐ N/A ☐
6. Removes the cuff in a timely manner.	S ☐ U ☐ N/A ☐	S ☐ U ☐ N/A ☐	S ☐ U ☐ N/A ☐
7. Returns the TV or radio to the previous sound level.	S ☐ U ☐ N/A ☐	S ☐ U ☐ N/A ☐	S ☐ U ☐ N/A ☐
8. Ensures patient comfort and safety.	S ☐ U ☐ N/A ☐	S ☐ U ☐ N/A ☐	S ☐ U ☐ N/A ☐
9. Removes the supplies from the patient's room, and cleans the area, as needed.	S ☐ U ☐ N/A ☐	S ☐ U ☐ N/A ☐	S ☐ U ☐ N/A ☐
10. Removes the PPE, and performs proper hand hygiene prior to leaving the patient's room.	S ☐ U ☐ N/A ☐	S ☐ U ☐ N/A ☐	S ☐ U ☐ N/A ☐

TEMPERATURE
Implementation

1. Positions the patient comfortably and instructs him or her to breathe normally.	S ☐ U ☐ N/A ☐	S ☐ U ☐ N/A ☐	S ☐ U ☐ N/A ☐
2. Determines the most appropriate site to obtain temperature.	S ☐ U ☐ N/A ☐	S ☐ U ☐ N/A ☐	S ☐ U ☐ N/A ☐
3. Places the disposable sheath on the thermometer probe. Turns device on, and presses START.	S ☐ U ☐ N/A ☐	S ☐ U ☐ N/A ☐	S ☐ U ☐ N/A ☐
4. Takes the temperature.	S ☐ U ☐ N/A ☐	S ☐ U ☐ N/A ☐	S ☐ U ☐ N/A ☐

Evaluation of Procedure

1. Establishes a baseline of vital signs assessed, or compare with previous measurements.	S ☐ U ☐ N/A ☐	S ☐ U ☐ N/A ☐	S ☐ U ☐ N/A ☐
2. Notes any use of oxygen therapy.	S ☐ U ☐ N/A ☐	S ☐ U ☐ N/A ☐	S ☐ U ☐ N/A ☐
3. Identifies any unexpected outcomes.	S ☐ U ☐ N/A ☐	S ☐ U ☐ N/A ☐	S ☐ U ☐ N/A ☐

Documentation and Reporting

1. Records blood pressure and temperature readings in the patient's chart.	S ☐ U ☐ N/A ☐	S ☐ U ☐ N/A ☐	S ☐ U ☐ N/A ☐
2. Records the need for oxygen therapy or if changes in current therapy are indicated.	S ☐ U ☐ N/A ☐	S ☐ U ☐ N/A ☐	S ☐ U ☐ N/A ☐
3. Reports any abnormal findings to the appropriate health care provider.	S ☐ U ☐ N/A ☐	S ☐ U ☐ N/A ☐	S ☐ U ☐ N/A ☐

Comments:

_____

_____

Signatures:

Student _____ Date Passed _____

Instructor (Laboratory Setting) _____ Date Passed _____

Student _____ Date Passed _____

Instructor (Clinical Setting) _____ Date Passed _____

Procedural Assessment 6-1   Obtaining a 12-lead ECG

Student _____ Date _____

Instructor (Laboratory Setting) _____ Date _____

Instructor (Clinical Setting) _____ Date _____

Criteria for assessment success:

The student must obtain all **satisfactory (S)** scores to pass the procedural evaluation. Any **unsatisfactory (U)** scores will result in failure of the procedural assessment.

Scoring:

Satisfactory (S): Procedural step performed correctly with no instructor prompting. Student-initiated correction is acceptable.

Unsatisfactory (U): Procedural step was performed incorrectly, omitted, or performed in a way that compromised patient care.

Not applicable (N/A): Procedural step was not indicated or necessary.

Evaluation:

	Peer Evaluation Laboratory Setting	Instructor Evaluation Laboratory Setting	Instructor Evaluation Clinical Setting
Procedural Preparation			
1. Reviews the patient's chart.	S ☐ U ☐ N/A ☐	S ☐ U ☐ N/A ☐	S ☐ U ☐ N/A ☐
2. Verifies the physician's order or the facility's protocol for standard of care.	S ☐ U ☐ N/A ☐	S ☐ U ☐ N/A ☐	S ☐ U ☐ N/A ☐
3. Obtains, cleans, and inspects the appropriate equipment prior to entering the patient's room.	S ☐ U ☐ N/A ☐	S ☐ U ☐ N/A ☐	S ☐ U ☐ N/A ☐
4. Follows PPE requirements, and observes standard precautions for any transmission-based isolation procedure.	S ☐ U ☐ N/A ☐	S ☐ U ☐ N/A ☐	S ☐ U ☐ N/A ☐
5. Identifies the patient using two patient identifiers.	S ☐ U ☐ N/A ☐	S ☐ U ☐ N/A ☐	S ☐ U ☐ N/A ☐
6. Introduces self to the patient and to the family.	S ☐ U ☐ N/A ☐	S ☐ U ☐ N/A ☐	S ☐ U ☐ N/A ☐
7. Explains the procedure to the patient and to the family, and acknowledges the patient's understanding.	S ☐ U ☐ N/A ☐	S ☐ U ☐ N/A ☐	S ☐ U ☐ N/A ☐
8. Performs proper hand hygiene, and puts on gloves, mask, and protective eyewear, as appropriate for the procedure.	S ☐ U ☐ N/A ☐	S ☐ U ☐ N/A ☐	S ☐ U ☐ N/A ☐
Implementation			
1. Positions the patient in the semi-Fowler position, and instructs him or her to breathe normally.	S ☐ U ☐ N/A ☐	S ☐ U ☐ N/A ☐	S ☐ U ☐ N/A ☐
2. Provides privacy.	S ☐ U ☐ N/A ☐	S ☐ U ☐ N/A ☐	S ☐ U ☐ N/A ☐
3. Prepares the patient's skin, as needed.	S ☐ U ☐ N/A ☐	S ☐ U ☐ N/A ☐	S ☐ U ☐ N/A ☐
4. Applies self-sticking electrodes, and attaches leads to the chest and extremities.	S ☐ U ☐ N/A ☐	S ☐ U ☐ N/A ☐	S ☐ U ☐ N/A ☐

Continued

	Peer Evaluation Laboratory Setting			Instructor Evaluation Laboratory Setting			Instructor Evaluation Clinical Setting		
5. Turns on the ECG machine, and enters the patient's demographic information.	S □	U □	N/A □	S □	U □	N/A □	S □	U □	N/A □
6. Obtains a tracing.	S □	U □	N/A □	S □	U □	N/A □	S □	U □	N/A □
7. Inspects the printout for clarity, and repeats, if necessary.	S □	U □	N/A □	S □	U □	N/A □	S □	U □	N/A □
8. Disconnects the leads, cleanses skin, and repositions the patient.	S □	U □	N/A □	S □	U □	N/A □	S □	U □	N/A □
9. Discards any disposable equipment.	S □	U □	N/A □	S □	U □	N/A □	S □	U □	N/A □
10. Removes the supplies from the patient's room, and cleans the area, as needed.	S □	U □	N/A □	S □	U □	N/A □	S □	U □	N/A □
11. Removes the PPE, and performs proper hand hygiene prior to leaving the patient's room.	S □	U □	N/A □	S □	U □	N/A □	S □	U □	N/A □

Evaluation of Procedure

1. Establishes a baseline, or compares with previous measurements.	S □	U □	N/A □	S □	U □	N/A □	S □	U □	N/A □

Documentation and Reporting

1. Attaches the ECG tracing in the patient's chart.	S □	U □	N/A □	S □	U □	N/A □	S □	U □	N/A □
2. Reports or delivers the ECG tracing to the appropriate health care provider.	S □	U □	N/A □	S □	U □	N/A □	S □	U □	N/A □
3. Reports any abnormal findings immediately to the appropriate health care provider.	S □	U □	N/A □	S □	U □	N/A □	S □	U □	N/A □

Comments:

_____

_____

_____

Signatures:

Student _____ Date Passed _____

Instructor (Laboratory Setting) _____ Date Passed _____

Student _____ Date Passed _____

Instructor (Clinical Setting) _____ Date Passed _____

Procedural Assessment 6-2   ECG interpretation

Student _____ Date _____

Instructor (Laboratory Setting) _____ Date _____

Instructor (Clinical Setting) _____ Date _____

Criteria for assessment success:

The student must obtain all **satisfactory (S)** scores to pass the procedural evaluation. Any **unsatisfactory (U)** scores will result in failure of the procedural assessment.

Scoring:

Satisfactory (S): Procedural step performed correctly with no instructor prompting. Student-initiated correction is acceptable.

Unsatisfactory (U): Procedural step was performed incorrectly, omitted, or performed in a way that compromised patient care.

Not applicable (N/A): Procedural step was not indicated or necessary.

Evaluation:

Procedural Preparation	Peer Evaluation Laboratory Setting	Instructor Evaluation Laboratory Setting	Instructor Evaluation Clinical Setting
1. Reviews the patient's chart.	S ☐ U ☐ N/A ☐	S ☐ U ☐ N/A ☐	S ☐ U ☐ N/A ☐
2. Verifies the physician's order or the facility's protocol for standard of care.	S ☐ U ☐ N/A ☐	S ☐ U ☐ N/A ☐	S ☐ U ☐ N/A ☐
3. Obtains, cleans, and inspects the appropriate equipment prior to entering the patient's room.	S ☐ U ☐ N/A ☐	S ☐ U ☐ N/A ☐	S ☐ U ☐ N/A ☐
4. Follows PPE requirements, and observes standard precautions for any transmission-based isolation procedure.	S ☐ U ☐ N/A ☐	S ☐ U ☐ N/A ☐	S ☐ U ☐ N/A ☐
5. Identifies the patient using two patient identifiers.	S ☐ U ☐ N/A ☐	S ☐ U ☐ N/A ☐	S ☐ U ☐ N/A ☐
6. Introduces self to the patient and to the family.	S ☐ U ☐ N/A ☐	S ☐ U ☐ N/A ☐	S ☐ U ☐ N/A ☐
7. Explains the procedure to the patient and to the family, and acknowledges the patient's understanding.	S ☐ U ☐ N/A ☐	S ☐ U ☐ N/A ☐	S ☐ U ☐ N/A ☐
8. Performs proper hand hygiene and puts on gloves, mask and protective eyewear, as appropriate for procedure.	S ☐ U ☐ N/A ☐	S ☐ U ☐ N/A ☐	S ☐ U ☐ N/A ☐
9. Obtains a 12-lead ECG strip for interpretation.	S ☐ U ☐ N/A ☐	S ☐ U ☐ N/A ☐	S ☐ U ☐ N/A ☐
10. Assesses the ECG strip for artifact, if present, and determines the likely cause.	S ☐ U ☐ N/A ☐	S ☐ U ☐ N/A ☐	S ☐ U ☐ N/A ☐

Continued

	Peer Evaluation Laboratory Setting	Instructor Evaluation Laboratory Setting	Instructor Evaluation Clinical Setting

Implementation

1. Uses a 12-lead ECG strip and:

	Peer	Lab (Instr)	Clinical (Instr)
a. Evaluates the presence of a P wave.	S ☐ U ☐ N/A ☐	S ☐ U ☐ N/A ☐	S ☐ U ☐ N/A ☐
b. Evaluates the shape of the P wave, if present.	S ☐ U ☐ N/A ☐	S ☐ U ☐ N/A ☐	S ☐ U ☐ N/A ☐
c. Identifies the atrial rate.	S ☐ U ☐ N/A ☐	S ☐ U ☐ N/A ☐	S ☐ U ☐ N/A ☐
d. Identifies the ventricular rate.	S ☐ U ☐ N/A ☐	S ☐ U ☐ N/A ☐	S ☐ U ☐ N/A ☐
e. Measures the P–R interval.	S ☐ U ☐ N/A ☐	S ☐ U ☐ N/A ☐	S ☐ U ☐ N/A ☐
f. Evaluates the shape of the QRS complex.	S ☐ U ☐ N/A ☐	S ☐ U ☐ N/A ☐	S ☐ U ☐ N/A ☐
g. Measures the duration of the QRS complex.	S ☐ U ☐ N/A ☐	S ☐ U ☐ N/A ☐	S ☐ U ☐ N/A ☐
h. Evaluates the shape of the T wave.	S ☐ U ☐ N/A ☐	S ☐ U ☐ N/A ☐	S ☐ U ☐ N/A ☐
i. Evaluates the ST segment.	S ☐ U ☐ N/A ☐	S ☐ U ☐ N/A ☐	S ☐ U ☐ N/A ☐
j. Measures the R–R interval.	S ☐ U ☐ N/A ☐	S ☐ U ☐ N/A ☐	S ☐ U ☐ N/A ☐
k. Identifies the mean QRS axis.	S ☐ U ☐ N/A ☐	S ☐ U ☐ N/A ☐	S ☐ U ☐ N/A ☐
l. Identifies the presence of any ectopic beats.	S ☐ U ☐ N/A ☐	S ☐ U ☐ N/A ☐	S ☐ U ☐ N/A ☐

Evaluation of Procedure

	Peer	Lab (Instr)	Clinical (Instr)
1. Interprets the ECG strip correctly.	S ☐ U ☐ N/A ☐	S ☐ U ☐ N/A ☐	S ☐ U ☐ N/A ☐

Documentation and Reporting

	Peer	Lab (Instr)	Clinical (Instr)
1. Attaches the ECG tracing to the patient's chart.	S ☐ U ☐ N/A ☐	S ☐ U ☐ N/A ☐	S ☐ U ☐ N/A ☐
2. Reports or delivers the ECG tracing to the appropriate health care provider.	S ☐ U ☐ N/A ☐	S ☐ U ☐ N/A ☐	S ☐ U ☐ N/A ☐
3. Reports any abnormal findings immediately to the appropriate health care provider.	S ☐ U ☐ N/A ☐	S ☐ U ☐ N/A ☐	S ☐ U ☐ N/A ☐

Comments:

_____

_____

_____

Signatures:

Student _____ Date Passed _____

Instructor (Laboratory Setting) _____ Date Passed _____

Student _____ Date Passed _____

Instructor (Clinical Setting) _____ Date Passed _____

Student _____ Date _____

Instructor (Laboratory Setting) _____ Date _____

Instructor (Clinical Setting) _____ Date _____

Criteria for assessment success:

The student must obtain all **satisfactory (S)** scores to pass the procedural evaluation. Any **unsatisfactory (U)** scores will result in failure of the procedural assessment.

Scoring:

Satisfactory (S): Procedural step performed correctly with no instructor prompting. Student-initiated correction is acceptable.

Unsatisfactory (U): Procedural step was performed incorrectly, omitted, or performed in a way that compromised patient care.

Not applicable (N/A): Procedural step was not indicated or necessary.

Evaluation:

	Peer Evaluation Laboratory Setting	Instructor Evaluation Laboratory Setting	Instructor Evaluation Clinical Setting
Procedural Preparation			
1. Reviews the patient's chart.	S ☐ U ☐ N/A ☐	S ☐ U ☐ N/A ☐	S ☐ U ☐ N/A ☐
2. Verifies the physician's order or the facility's protocol for standard of care.	S ☐ U ☐ N/A ☐	S ☐ U ☐ N/A ☐	S ☐ U ☐ N/A ☐
3. Obtains, cleans, and inspects the appropriate equipment prior to entering the patient's room.	S ☐ U ☐ N/A ☐	S ☐ U ☐ N/A ☐	S ☐ U ☐ N/A ☐
4. Follows PPE requirements, and observes standard precautions for any transmission-based isolation procedure.	S ☐ U ☐ N/A ☐	S ☐ U ☐ N/A ☐	S ☐ U ☐ N/A ☐
5. Identifies the patient using two patient identifiers.	S ☐ U ☐ N/A ☐	S ☐ U ☐ N/A ☐	S ☐ U ☐ N/A ☐
6. Introduces self to the patient and to the family.	S ☐ U ☐ N/A ☐	S ☐ U ☐ N/A ☐	S ☐ U ☐ N/A ☐
7. Explains the procedure to the patient and to the family, and acknowledges the patient's understanding.	S ☐ U ☐ N/A ☐	S ☐ U ☐ N/A ☐	S ☐ U ☐ N/A ☐
8. Performs proper hand hygiene, and puts on gloves, mask, and protective eyewear, as appropriate for the procedure.	S ☐ U ☐ N/A ☐	S ☐ U ☐ N/A ☐	S ☐ U ☐ N/A ☐
Implementation			
1. Places the patient in the supine position, with the head of the bed no higher than 45 degrees.	S ☐ U ☐ N/A ☐	S ☐ U ☐ N/A ☐	S ☐ U ☐ N/A ☐
2. Opens the prepackaged pressure transducer kit.	S ☐ U ☐ N/A ☐	S ☐ U ☐ N/A ☐	S ☐ U ☐ N/A ☐
3. Tightens all the connections.	S ☐ U ☐ N/A ☐	S ☐ U ☐ N/A ☐	S ☐ U ☐ N/A ☐
4. Attaches the transducer clamp to the intravenous (IV) pole, and places the transducer inline with the patient's phlebostatic axis.	S ☐ U ☐ N/A ☐	S ☐ U ☐ N/A ☐	S ☐ U ☐ N/A ☐
5. Opens the bag of heparinized saline, and inserts it into the pressure bag.	S ☐ U ☐ N/A ☐	S ☐ U ☐ N/A ☐	S ☐ U ☐ N/A ☐
6. Spikes the bag, and hangs the bag from the IV pole.	S ☐ U ☐ N/A ☐	S ☐ U ☐ N/A ☐	S ☐ U ☐ N/A ☐

Continued

	Peer Evaluation Laboratory Setting			Instructor Evaluation Laboratory Setting			Instructor Evaluation Clinical Setting		
7. Turns the stopcock off to the patient, and attaches the pressure tubing to the transducer stopcock.	S ☐	U ☐	N/A ☐	S ☐	U ☐	N/A ☐	S ☐	U ☐	N/A ☐
8. Opens the roller clamp, and primes the drip chamber.	S ☐	U ☐	N/A ☐	S ☐	U ☐	N/A ☐	S ☐	U ☐	N/A ☐
9. Flushes the tubing and attaches it to the pressure transducer.	S ☐	U ☐	N/A ☐	S ☐	U ☐	N/A ☐	S ☐	U ☐	N/A ☐
10. Turns the stopcock off to the patient, and flushes through the transducer.	S ☐	U ☐	N/A ☐	S ☐	U ☐	N/A ☐	S ☐	U ☐	N/A ☐
11. Turns the stopcock so that it is open to the transducer.	S ☐	U ☐	N/A ☐	S ☐	U ☐	N/A ☐	S ☐	U ☐	N/A ☐
12. Inflates the pressure bag to 300 mm Hg	S ☐	U ☐	N/A ☐	S ☐	U ☐	N/A ☐	S ☐	U ☐	N/A ☐
13. Attaches the pressure tubing to the appropriate catheter port.	S ☐	U ☐	N/A ☐	S ☐	U ☐	N/A ☐	S ☐	U ☐	N/A ☐
14. Turns on the bedside monitor.	S ☐	U ☐	N/A ☐	S ☐	U ☐	N/A ☐	S ☐	U ☐	N/A ☐
15. Plugs the pressure cable into the appropriate monitor port.	S ☐	U ☐	N/A ☐	S ☐	U ☐	N/A ☐	S ☐	U ☐	N/A ☐
16. Turns on the chosen parameter (pulmonary artery [PA], right atrial [RA], arterial).	S ☐	U ☐	N/A ☐	S ☐	U ☐	N/A ☐	S ☐	U ☐	N/A ☐
17. Sets the appropriate scale.	S ☐	U ☐	N/A ☐	S ☐	U ☐	N/A ☐	S ☐	U ☐	N/A ☐
18. Levels the transducer and sets to zero.	S ☐	U ☐	N/A ☐	S ☐	U ☐	N/A ☐	S ☐	U ☐	N/A ☐
19. Removes the supplies from the patient's room, and cleans the area, as needed.	S ☐	U ☐	N/A ☐	S ☐	U ☐	N/A ☐	S ☐	U ☐	N/A ☐
20. Removes the PPE, and performs proper hand hygiene prior to leaving the patient's room.	S ☐	U ☐	N/A ☐	S ☐	U ☐	N/A ☐	S ☐	U ☐	N/A ☐

Evaluation of Procedure

1. Establishes a baseline, or compares with previous measurements.	S ☐	U ☐	N/A ☐	S ☐	U ☐	N/A ☐	S ☐	U ☐	N/A ☐
2. Develops the appropriate respiratory care plan based on assessment data.	S ☐	U ☐	N/A ☐	S ☐	U ☐	N/A ☐	S ☐	U ☐	N/A ☐
3. Identifies any unexpected outcomes.	S ☐	U ☐	N/A ☐	S ☐	U ☐	N/A ☐	S ☐	U ☐	N/A ☐
4. Correlates findings with noninvasive data, if applicable.	S ☐	U ☐	N/A ☐	S ☐	U ☐	N/A ☐	S ☐	U ☐	N/A ☐

Documentation and Reporting

1. Records findings in the patient's chart.	S ☐	U ☐	N/A ☐	S ☐	U ☐	N/A ☐	S ☐	U ☐	N/A ☐
2. Reports any abnormal findings to the appropriate health care provider.	S ☐	U ☐	N/A ☐	S ☐	U ☐	N/A ☐	S ☐	U ☐	N/A ☐

Comments:

_____

_____

_____

Signatures:

Student _____ Date Passed _____

Instructor (Laboratory Setting) _____ Date Passed _____

Student _____ Date Passed _____

Instructor (Clinical Setting) _____ Date Passed _____

Student _____ Date _____

Instructor (Laboratory Setting) _____ Date _____

Instructor (Clinical Setting) _____ Date _____

Criteria for assessment success:

The student must obtain all **satisfactory (S)** scores to pass the procedural evaluation. Any **unsatisfactory (U)** scores will result in failure of the procedural assessment.

Scoring:

Satisfactory (S): Procedural step performed correctly with no instructor prompting. Student-initiated correction is acceptable.

Unsatisfactory (U): Procedural step was performed incorrectly, omitted, or performed in a way that compromised patient care.

Not applicable (N/A): Procedural step was not indicated or necessary.

Evaluation:

	Peer Evaluation Laboratory Setting	Instructor Evaluation Laboratory Setting	Instructor Evaluation Clinical Setting
Procedural Preparation			
1. Reviews the patient's chart.	S ☐ U ☐ N/A ☐	S ☐ U ☐ N/A ☐	S ☐ U ☐ N/A ☐
2. Verifies the physician's order or the facility's protocol for standard of care.	S ☐ U ☐ N/A ☐	S ☐ U ☐ N/A ☐	S ☐ U ☐ N/A ☐
3. Obtains, cleans, and inspects the appropriate equipment prior to entering the patient's room.	S ☐ U ☐ N/A ☐	S ☐ U ☐ N/A ☐	S ☐ U ☐ N/A ☐
4. Follows PPE requirements, and observes standard precautions for any transmission-based isolation procedure.	S ☐ U ☐ N/A ☐	S ☐ U ☐ N/A ☐	S ☐ U ☐ N/A ☐
5. Identifies the patient using two patient identifiers.	S ☐ U ☐ N/A ☐	S ☐ U ☐ N/A ☐	S ☐ U ☐ N/A ☐
6. Introduces self to the patient and to the family.	S ☐ U ☐ N/A ☐	S ☐ U ☐ N/A ☐	S ☐ U ☐ N/A ☐
7. Explains the procedure to the patient and to the family, and acknowledges the patient's understanding.	S ☐ U ☐ N/A ☐	S ☐ U ☐ N/A ☐	S ☐ U ☐ N/A ☐
8. Performs proper hand hygiene, and puts on gloves, mask, and protective eyewear, as appropriate for the procedure.	S ☐ U ☐ N/A ☐	S ☐ U ☐ N/A ☐	S ☐ U ☐ N/A ☐
Implementation			
1. Positions the patient in a comfortable position.	S ☐ U ☐ N/A ☐	S ☐ U ☐ N/A ☐	S ☐ U ☐ N/A ☐
2. Assesses vital signs.	S ☐ U ☐ N/A ☐	S ☐ U ☐ N/A ☐	S ☐ U ☐ N/A ☐
3. Visually inspects the catheter.	S ☐ U ☐ N/A ☐	S ☐ U ☐ N/A ☐	S ☐ U ☐ N/A ☐
4. Assesses the arterial catheter insertion site and involved extremity for postinsertion complications.	S ☐ U ☐ N/A ☐	S ☐ U ☐ N/A ☐	S ☐ U ☐ N/A ☐
5. Sets the transducer to zero.	S ☐ U ☐ N/A ☐	S ☐ U ☐ N/A ☐	S ☐ U ☐ N/A ☐
6. Obtains the tracing.	S ☐ U ☐ N/A ☐	S ☐ U ☐ N/A ☐	S ☐ U ☐ N/A ☐

Continued

	Peer Evaluation Laboratory Setting			Instructor Evaluation Laboratory Setting			Instructor Evaluation Clinical Setting		
7. Assesses the waveform.	S ☐	U ☐	N/A ☐	S ☐	U ☐	N/A ☐	S ☐	U ☐	N/A ☐
8. Removes the supplies from the patient's room, and cleans the area, as needed.	S ☐	U ☐	N/A ☐	S ☐	U ☐	N/A ☐	S ☐	U ☐	N/A ☐
9. Removes the PPE, and performs proper hand hygiene prior to leaving the patient's room.	S ☐	U ☐	N/A ☐	S ☐	U ☐	N/A ☐	S ☐	U ☐	N/A ☐
Evaluation of Procedure									
1. Establishes a baseline, or compares with previous measurements.	S ☐	U ☐	N/A ☐	S ☐	U ☐	N/A ☐	S ☐	U ☐	N/A ☐
2. Attaches the tracing to the patient's chart, if applicable.	S ☐	U ☐	N/A ☐	S ☐	U ☐	N/A ☐	S ☐	U ☐	N/A ☐
3. Identifies any unexpected outcomes	S ☐	U ☐	N/A ☐	S ☐	U ☐	N/A ☐	S ☐	U ☐	N/A ☐
Documentation and Reporting									
1. Records findings in the patient's chart.	S ☐	U ☐	N/A ☐	S ☐	U ☐	N/A ☐	S ☐	U ☐	N/A ☐
2. Reports any abnormal findings to the appropriate health care provider.	S ☐	U ☐	N/A ☐	S ☐	U ☐	N/A ☐	S ☐	U ☐	N/A ☐

Comments:

_____

_____

_____

Signatures:

Student _____ Date Passed _____

Instructor (Laboratory Setting) _____ Date Passed _____

Student _____ Date Passed _____

Instructor (Clinical Setting) _____ Date Passed _____

Student _____ Date _____

Instructor (Laboratory Setting) _____ Date _____

Instructor (Clinical Setting) _____ Date _____

Criteria for assessment success:

The student must obtain all **satisfactory (S)** scores to pass the procedural evaluation. Any **unsatisfactory (U)** scores will result in failure of the procedural assessment.

Scoring:

Satisfactory (S): Procedural step performed correctly with no instructor prompting. Student-initiated correction is acceptable.

Unsatisfactory (U): Procedural step was performed incorrectly, omitted, or performed in a way that compromised patient care.

Not applicable (N/A): Procedural step was not indicated or necessary.

Evaluation:

	Peer Evaluation Laboratory Setting	Instructor Evaluation Laboratory Setting	Instructor Evaluation Clinical Setting
Procedural Preparation			
1. Reviews the patient's chart.	S ☐ U ☐ N/A ☐	S ☐ U ☐ N/A ☐	S ☐ U ☐ N/A ☐
2. Verifies the physician's order or the facility's protocol for standard of care.	S ☐ U ☐ N/A ☐	S ☐ U ☐ N/A ☐	S ☐ U ☐ N/A ☐
3. Obtains, cleans, and inspects the appropriate equipment prior to entering the patient's room.	S ☐ U ☐ N/A ☐	S ☐ U ☐ N/A ☐	S ☐ U ☐ N/A ☐
4. Follows PPE requirements, and observes standard precautions for any transmission-based isolation procedure.	S ☐ U ☐ N/A ☐	S ☐ U ☐ N/A ☐	S ☐ U ☐ N/A ☐
5. Identifies the patient using two patient identifiers.	S ☐ U ☐ N/A ☐	S ☐ U ☐ N/A ☐	S ☐ U ☐ N/A ☐
6. Introduces self to the patient and to the family.	S ☐ U ☐ N/A ☐	S ☐ U ☐ N/A ☐	S ☐ U ☐ N/A ☐
7. Explains the procedure to the patient and to the family, and acknowledges the patient's understanding.	S ☐ U ☐ N/A ☐	S ☐ U ☐ N/A ☐	S ☐ U ☐ N/A ☐
8. Performs proper hand hygiene, and puts on gloves, mask, and protective eyewear, as appropriate for the procedure.	S ☐ U ☐ N/A ☐	S ☐ U ☐ N/A ☐	S ☐ U ☐ N/A ☐
Implementation			
1. Places the patient in the supine position, with the head of the bed elevated no higher than 45 degrees.	S ☐ U ☐ N/A ☐	S ☐ U ☐ N/A ☐	S ☐ U ☐ N/A ☐
2. Assesses vital signs.	S ☐ U ☐ N/A ☐	S ☐ U ☐ N/A ☐	S ☐ U ☐ N/A ☐
3. Levels the air–fluid interface of the monitoring system at the level of the atria.	S ☐ U ☐ N/A ☐	S ☐ U ☐ N/A ☐	S ☐ U ☐ N/A ☐
4. Sets the transducer to zero.	S ☐ U ☐ N/A ☐	S ☐ U ☐ N/A ☐	S ☐ U ☐ N/A ☐

Continued

	Peer Evaluation Laboratory Setting			Instructor Evaluation Laboratory Setting			Instructor Evaluation Clinical Setting		
5. Runs the dual-channel ECG and CVP strip.	S ☐	U ☐	N/A ☐	S ☐	U ☐	N/A ☐	S ☐	U ☐	N/A ☐
6. Measures the pressures at the end of expiration.	S ☐	U ☐	N/A ☐	S ☐	U ☐	N/A ☐	S ☐	U ☐	N/A ☐
7. Reassesses vital signs.	S ☐	U ☐	N/A ☐	S ☐	U ☐	N/A ☐	S ☐	U ☐	N/A ☐
8. Removes the supplies from the patient's room, and cleans the area, as needed.	S ☐	U ☐	N/A ☐	S ☐	U ☐	N/A ☐	S ☐	U ☐	N/A ☐
9. Removes PPE, and performs proper hand hygiene prior to leaving the patient's room.	S ☐	U ☐	N/A ☐	S ☐	U ☐	N/A ☐	S ☐	U ☐	N/A ☐

Evaluation of Procedure

1. Establishes a baseline, or compares with previous measurements.	S ☐	U ☐	N/A ☐	S ☐	U ☐	N/A ☐	S ☐	U ☐	N/A ☐
2. Develops an appropriate respiratory care plan based on assessment data.	S ☐	U ☐	N/A ☐	S ☐	U ☐	N/A ☐	S ☐	U ☐	N/A ☐
3. Identifies any unexpected outcomes.	S ☐	U ☐	N/A ☐	S ☐	U ☐	N/A ☐	S ☐	U ☐	N/A ☐

Documentation and Reporting

1. Records findings in the patient's chart.	S ☐	U ☐	N/A ☐	S ☐	U ☐	N/A ☐	S ☐	U ☐	N/A ☐
2. Reports any abnormal findings to the appropriate health care provider.	S ☐	U ☐	N/A ☐	S ☐	U ☐	N/A ☐	S ☐	U ☐	N/A ☐

Comments:

_____

_____

_____

Signatures:

Student _____ Date Passed _____

Instructor (Laboratory Setting) _____ Date Passed _____

Student _____ Date Passed _____

Instructor (Clinical Setting) _____ Date Passed _____

Student _____ Date _____

Instructor (Laboratory Setting) _____ Date _____

Instructor (Clinical Setting) _____ Date _____

Evaluation:

	Peer Evaluation Laboratory Setting			Instructor Evaluation Laboratory Setting			Instructor Evaluation Clinical Setting		
Procedural Preparation									
1. Reviews the patient's chart.	S ☐	U ☐	N/A ☐	S ☐	U ☐	N/A ☐	S ☐	U ☐	N/A ☐
2. Verifies the physician's order or the facility's protocol for standard of care.	S ☐	U ☐	N/A ☐	S ☐	U ☐	N/A ☐	S ☐	U ☐	N/A ☐
3. Obtains, cleans, and inspects the appropriate equipment prior to entering the patient's room.	S ☐	U ☐	N/A ☐	S ☐	U ☐	N/A ☐	S ☐	U ☐	N/A ☐
4. Follows PPE requirements, and observes standard precautions for any transmission-based isolation procedure.	S ☐	U ☐	N/A ☐	S ☐	U ☐	N/A ☐	S ☐	U ☐	N/A ☐
5. Identifies the patient using two patient identifiers.	S ☐	U ☐	N/A ☐	S ☐	U ☐	N/A ☐	S ☐	U ☐	N/A ☐
6. Introduces self to the patient and to the family.	S ☐	U ☐	N/A ☐	S ☐	U ☐	N/A ☐	S ☐	U ☐	N/A ☐
7. Explains the procedure to the patient and to the family, and acknowledges the patient's understanding.	S ☐	U ☐	N/A ☐	S ☐	U ☐	N/A ☐	S ☐	U ☐	N/A ☐
8. Performs proper hand hygiene, and puts on gloves, mask, and protective eyewear, as appropriate for the procedure.	S ☐	U ☐	N/A ☐	S ☐	U ☐	N/A ☐	S ☐	U ☐	N/A ☐
Implementation									
1. Places the patient in a comfortable position.	S ☐	U ☐	N/A ☐	S ☐	U ☐	N/A ☐	S ☐	U ☐	N/A ☐
2. Assesses vital signs.	S ☐	U ☐	N/A ☐	S ☐	U ☐	N/A ☐	S ☐	U ☐	N/A ☐
3. Inspects the catheter for leaks or air bubbles.	S ☐	U ☐	N/A ☐	S ☐	U ☐	N/A ☐	S ☐	U ☐	N/A ☐
4. Cleanses the needleless cap at the top of the stopcock with alcohol or other antiseptic solution.	S ☐	U ☐	N/A ☐	S ☐	U ☐	N/A ☐	S ☐	U ☐	N/A ☐
5. Attaches the needleless blood sampling device to the capped stopcock of the monitoring system.	S ☐	U ☐	N/A ☐	S ☐	U ☐	N/A ☐	S ☐	U ☐	N/A ☐
6. Suspends the right atrial pressure or CVP monitoring alarm.	S ☐	U ☐	N/A ☐	S ☐	U ☐	N/A ☐	S ☐	U ☐	N/A ☐
7. Turns the stopcock off to the monitoring system, and flushes the system.	S ☐	U ☐	N/A ☐	S ☐	U ☐	N/A ☐	S ☐	U ☐	N/A ☐
8. Inserts a blood specimen tube into the blood sampling device.	S ☐	U ☐	N/A ☐	S ☐	U ☐	N/A ☐	S ☐	U ☐	N/A ☐
9. Removes the discarded blood specimen tube, and disposes of it appropriately.	S ☐	U ☐	N/A ☐	S ☐	U ☐	N/A ☐	S ☐	U ☐	N/A ☐
10. Inserts the blood specimen tube into the blood sampling device to obtain a specimen.	S ☐	U ☐	N/A ☐	S ☐	U ☐	N/A ☐	S ☐	U ☐	N/A ☐

Continued

	Peer Evaluation Laboratory Setting			Instructor Evaluation Laboratory Setting			Instructor Evaluation Clinical Setting		
11. Detaches the blood sampling device from the capped stopcock, and discards it appropriately.	S ☐	U ☐	N/A ☐	S ☐	U ☐	N/A ☐	S ☐	U ☐	N/A ☐
12. Cleanses the needleless cap at the top of the stopcock with alcohol or other antiseptic solution.	S ☐	U ☐	N/A ☐	S ☐	U ☐	N/A ☐	S ☐	U ☐	N/A ☐
13. Attaches a 10-mL syringe filled with sterile normal saline solution to the needleless capped stopcock.	S ☐	U ☐	N/A ☐	S ☐	U ☐	N/A ☐	S ☐	U ☐	N/A ☐
14. Gently flushes the normal saline solution into the needleless cap.	S ☐	U ☐	N/A ☐	S ☐	U ☐	N/A ☐	S ☐	U ☐	N/A ☐
15. Turns the stopcock off to the blood sampling device.	S ☐	U ☐	N/A ☐	S ☐	U ☐	N/A ☐	S ☐	U ☐	N/A ☐
16. Fast-flushes the remaining blood in the central venous catheter back into the patient.	S ☐	U ☐	N/A ☐	S ☐	U ☐	N/A ☐	S ☐	U ☐	N/A ☐
17. Observes the monitor for return of the right atrial pressure or CVP waveform.	S ☐	U ☐	N/A ☐	S ☐	U ☐	N/A ☐	S ☐	U ☐	N/A ☐
18. Turns the alarms on.	S ☐	U ☐	N/A ☐	S ☐	U ☐	N/A ☐	S ☐	U ☐	N/A ☐
19. Labels the specimen.	S ☐	U ☐	N/A ☐	S ☐	U ☐	N/A ☐	S ☐	U ☐	N/A ☐
20. Disposes of used supplies in the appropriate container.	S ☐	U ☐	N/A ☐	S ☐	U ☐	N/A ☐	S ☐	U ☐	N/A ☐
21. Sends the specimen for analysis.	S ☐	U ☐	N/A ☐	S ☐	U ☐	N/A ☐	S ☐	U ☐	N/A ☐
22. Removes the supplies from the patient's room, and cleans the area, as needed.	S ☐	U ☐	N/A ☐	S ☐	U ☐	N/A ☐	S ☐	U ☐	N/A ☐
23. Removes PPE, and performs proper hand hygiene prior to leaving the patient's room.	S ☐	U ☐	N/A ☐	S ☐	U ☐	N/A ☐	S ☐	U ☐	N/A ☐

Evaluation of Procedure

1. Establishes a baseline, or compares with previous measurements.	S ☐	U ☐	N/A ☐	S ☐	U ☐	N/A ☐	S ☐	U ☐	N/A ☐
2. Develops an appropriate respiratory care plan based on assessment data.	S ☐	U ☐	N/A ☐	S ☐	U ☐	N/A ☐	S ☐	U ☐	N/A ☐
3. Identifies any unexpected outcomes.	S ☐	U ☐	N/A ☐	S ☐	U ☐	N/A ☐	S ☐	U ☐	N/A ☐

Documentation and Reporting

1. Records findings in the patient's chart.	S ☐	U ☐	N/A ☐	S ☐	U ☐	N/A ☐	S ☐	U ☐	N/A ☐
2. Reports any abnormal findings to the appropriate health care provider.	S ☐	U ☐	N/A ☐	S ☐	U ☐	N/A ☐	S ☐	U ☐	N/A ☐

Comments:

_____

_____

_____

Signatures:

Student _____ Date Passed _____

Instructor (Laboratory Setting) _____ Date Passed _____

Student _____ Date Passed _____

Instructor (Clinical Setting) _____ Date Passed _____

Procedural Assessment 7-5 — Thermodilution

Student _____ Date _____

Instructor (Laboratory Setting) _____ Date _____

Instructor (Clinical Setting) _____ Date _____

Criteria for assessment success:

The student must obtain all **satisfactory (S)** scores to pass the procedural evaluation. Any **unsatisfactory (U)** scores will result in failure of the procedural assessment.

Scoring:

Satisfactory (S): Procedural step performed correctly with no instructor prompting. Student-initiated correction is acceptable.

Unsatisfactory (U): Procedural step was performed incorrectly, omitted, or performed in a way that compromised patient care.

Not applicable (N/A): Procedural step was not indicated or necessary.

Evaluation:

	Peer Evaluation Laboratory Setting	Instructor Evaluation Laboratory Setting	Instructor Evaluation Clinical Setting
Procedural Preparation			
1. Reviews the patient's chart.	S ☐ U ☐ N/A ☐	S ☐ U ☐ N/A ☐	S ☐ U ☐ N/A ☐
2. Verifies the physician's order or the facility's protocol for standard of care.	S ☐ U ☐ N/A ☐	S ☐ U ☐ N/A ☐	S ☐ U ☐ N/A ☐
3. Obtains, cleans, and inspects the appropriate equipment prior to entering the patient's room	S ☐ U ☐ N/A ☐	S ☐ U ☐ N/A ☐	S ☐ U ☐ N/A ☐
4. Follows PPE requirements, and observes standard precautions for any transmission-based isolation procedure.	S ☐ U ☐ N/A ☐	S ☐ U ☐ N/A ☐	S ☐ U ☐ N/A ☐
5. Identifies the patient using two patient identifiers.	S ☐ U ☐ N/A ☐	S ☐ U ☐ N/A ☐	S ☐ U ☐ N/A ☐
6. Introduces self to the patient and to the family.	S ☐ U ☐ N/A ☐	S ☐ U ☐ N/A ☐	S ☐ U ☐ N/A ☐
7. Explains the procedure to the patient and to the family, and acknowledges the patient's understanding.	S ☐ U ☐ N/A ☐	S ☐ U ☐ N/A ☐	S ☐ U ☐ N/A ☐
8. Performs proper hand hygiene, and puts on gloves, mask, and protective eyewear, as appropriate for the procedure.	S ☐ U ☐ N/A ☐	S ☐ U ☐ N/A ☐	S ☐ U ☐ N/A ☐
Implementation			
1. Places the patient in the supine position, with the head of the bed no higher than 20 degrees.	S ☐ U ☐ N/A ☐	S ☐ U ☐ N/A ☐	S ☐ U ☐ N/A ☐
2. Selects cold or room-temperature injectate.	S ☐ U ☐ N/A ☐	S ☐ U ☐ N/A ☐	S ☐ U ☐ N/A ☐
3. Selects the injectate bolus amount, typically 10 mL.	S ☐ U ☐ N/A ☐	S ☐ U ☐ N/A ☐	S ☐ U ☐ N/A ☐
4. Connects the CO cable to the PA catheter.	S ☐ U ☐ N/A ☐	S ☐ U ☐ N/A ☐	S ☐ U ☐ N/A ☐
5. Selects the computation constant.	S ☐ U ☐ N/A ☐	S ☐ U ☐ N/A ☐	S ☐ U ☐ N/A ☐
6. Connects and turns on the CO computer.	S ☐ U ☐ N/A ☐	S ☐ U ☐ N/A ☐	S ☐ U ☐ N/A ☐

Continued

	Peer Evaluation Laboratory Setting			Instructor Evaluation Laboratory Setting			Instructor Evaluation Clinical Setting		
7. Records the temperature of the injectate.	S ☐	U ☐	N/A ☐	S ☐	U ☐	N/A ☐	S ☐	U ☐	N/A ☐
8. Verifies the position of the PA catheter by assessing the RA and PA waveforms.	S ☐	U ☐	N/A ☐	S ☐	U ☐	N/A ☐	S ☐	U ☐	N/A ☐
9. Observes the patient's cardiac rate and rhythm.	S ☐	U ☐	N/A ☐	S ☐	U ☐	N/A ☐	S ☐	U ☐	N/A ☐
10. Aseptically connects the IV tubing to the injectate solution.	S ☐	U ☐	N/A ☐	S ☐	U ☐	N/A ☐	S ☐	U ☐	N/A ☐
11. Hangs the IV injectate solution on an IV pole, and primes the tubing.	S ☐	U ☐	N/A ☐	S ☐	U ☐	N/A ☐	S ☐	U ☐	N/A ☐
12. Removes the sterile cap from the proximal lumen of the PA catheter.	S ☐	U ☐	N/A ☐	S ☐	U ☐	N/A ☐	S ☐	U ☐	N/A ☐
13. Connects the injectate tubing to the proximal lumen of the PA catheter via a three-way stopcock.	S ☐	U ☐	N/A ☐	S ☐	U ☐	N/A ☐	S ☐	U ☐	N/A ☐
14. Connects the injectate syringe to the three-way stopcock.	S ☐	U ☐	N/A ☐	S ☐	U ☐	N/A ☐	S ☐	U ☐	N/A ☐
15. Connects the in-line temperature probe.	S ☐	U ☐	N/A ☐	S ☐	U ☐	N/A ☐	S ☐	U ☐	N/A ☐
16. If using cold injectate, sets up the cold injectate system.	S ☐	U ☐	N/A ☐	S ☐	U ☐	N/A ☐	S ☐	U ☐	N/A ☐
17. Turns the stopcock so that it is open to the injectate solution (closed to the patient), and withdraws 10 mL of the injectate solution into the syringe.	S ☐	U ☐	N/A ☐	S ☐	U ☐	N/A ☐	S ☐	U ☐	N/A ☐
18. Turns the stopcock so that it is closed to the injectate solution and open to the patient.	S ☐	U ☐	N/A ☐	S ☐	U ☐	N/A ☐	S ☐	U ☐	N/A ☐
19. Activates the CO computer.	S ☐	U ☐	N/A ☐	S ☐	U ☐	N/A ☐	S ☐	U ☐	N/A ☐
20. Observes for steady baseline temperature on the monitor screen.	S ☐	U ☐	N/A ☐	S ☐	U ☐	N/A ☐	S ☐	U ☐	N/A ☐
21. Observes the patient's respiratory pattern.	S ☐	U ☐	N/A ☐	S ☐	U ☐	N/A ☐	S ☐	U ☐	N/A ☐
22. Begins administering the injectate at end expiration to decrease variance in CO measurements caused by the respiratory cycle.	S ☐	U ☐	N/A ☐	S ☐	U ☐	N/A ☐	S ☐	U ☐	N/A ☐
23. Administers the injectate rapidly and smoothly in 4 seconds or less.	S ☐	U ☐	N/A ☐	S ☐	U ☐	N/A ☐	S ☐	U ☐	N/A ☐
24. Assesses the CO curve and value on the monitor screen.	S ☐	U ☐	N/A ☐	S ☐	U ☐	N/A ☐	S ☐	U ☐	N/A ☐
25. Repeats steps 17 through 24 up to three times for cold injectate and up to five times for room-temperature injectate.	S ☐	U ☐	N/A ☐	S ☐	U ☐	N/A ☐	S ☐	U ☐	N/A ☐
26. Determines the mean CO measurement.	S ☐	U ☐	N/A ☐	S ☐	U ☐	N/A ☐	S ☐	U ☐	N/A ☐
27. Returns the proximal stopcock at the RA lumen to the original position.	S ☐	U ☐	N/A ☐	S ☐	U ☐	N/A ☐	S ☐	U ☐	N/A ☐
28. Continues infusions delivered through the introducer or other central lines.	S ☐	U ☐	N/A ☐	S ☐	U ☐	N/A ☐	S ☐	U ☐	N/A ☐
29. Observes the PA and RA waveforms on the monitor.	S ☐	U ☐	N/A ☐	S ☐	U ☐	N/A ☐	S ☐	U ☐	N/A ☐
30. Appropriately discards used supplies.	S ☐	U ☐	N/A ☐	S ☐	U ☐	N/A ☐	S ☐	U ☐	N/A ☐
31. Removes PPE, and performs proper hand hygiene prior to leaving the patient's room.	S ☐	U ☐	N/A ☐	S ☐	U ☐	N/A ☐	S ☐	U ☐	N/A ☐

	Peer Evaluation Laboratory Setting	Instructor Evaluation Laboratory Setting	Instructor Evaluation Clinical Setting
Evaluation of Procedure			
1. Establishes baseline, or compares with previous measurements.	S ☐ U ☐ N/A ☐	S ☐ U ☐ N/A ☐	S ☐ U ☐ N/A ☐
2. Develops an appropriate respiratory care plan based on assessment data.	S ☐ U ☐ N/A ☐	S ☐ U ☐ N/A ☐	S ☐ U ☐ N/A ☐
3. Identifies any unexpected outcomes.	S ☐ U ☐ N/A ☐	S ☐ U ☐ N/A ☐	S ☐ U ☐ N/A ☐
Documentation and Reporting			
1. Records findings in the patient's chart.	S ☐ U ☐ N/A ☐	S ☐ U ☐ N/A ☐	S ☐ U ☐ N/A ☐
2. Reports any abnormal findings to the appropriate health care provider.	S ☐ U ☐ N/A ☐	S ☐ U ☐ N/A ☐	S ☐ U ☐ N/A ☐

Comments:

_____

_____

_____

Signatures:

Student _____ Date Passed _____

Instructor (Laboratory Setting) _____ Date Passed _____

Student _____ Date Passed _____

Instructor (Clinical Setting) _____ Date Passed _____

Student _____ Date _____

Instructor (Laboratory Setting) _____ Date _____

Instructor (Clinical Setting) _____ Date _____

Criteria for assessment success:

The student must obtain all **satisfactory (S)** scores to pass the procedural evaluation. Any **unsatisfactory (U)** scores will result in failure of the procedural assessment.

Scoring:

Satisfactory (S): Procedural step performed correctly with no instructor prompting. Student-initiated correction is acceptable.

Unsatisfactory (U): Procedural step was performed incorrectly, omitted, or performed in a way that compromised patient care.

Not applicable (N/A): Procedural step was not indicated or necessary.

Evaluation:

	Peer Evaluation Laboratory Setting	Instructor Evaluation Laboratory Setting	Instructor Evaluation Clinical Setting
Procedural Preparation			
1. Reviews the patient's chart.	S ☐ U ☐ N/A ☐	S ☐ U ☐ N/A ☐	S ☐ U ☐ N/A ☐
2. Verifies the physician's order or the facility's protocol for standard of care.	S ☐ U ☐ N/A ☐	S ☐ U ☐ N/A ☐	S ☐ U ☐ N/A ☐
3. Obtains, cleans, and inspects the appropriate equipment prior to entering the patient's room.	S ☐ U ☐ N/A ☐	S ☐ U ☐ N/A ☐	S ☐ U ☐ N/A ☐
4. Follows PPE requirements, and observes standard precautions for any transmission-based isolation procedure.	S ☐ U ☐ N/A ☐	S ☐ U ☐ N/A ☐	S ☐ U ☐ N/A ☐
5. Identifies the patient using two patient identifiers.	S ☐ U ☐ N/A ☐	S ☐ U ☐ N/A ☐	S ☐ U ☐ N/A ☐
6. Introduces self to the patient and to the family.	S ☐ U ☐ N/A ☐	S ☐ U ☐ N/A ☐	S ☐ U ☐ N/A ☐
7. Explains the procedure to the patient and to the family, and acknowledges the patient's understanding.	S ☐ U ☐ N/A ☐	S ☐ U ☐ N/A ☐	S ☐ U ☐ N/A ☐
8. Performs proper hand hygiene, and puts on gloves, mask, and protective eyewear, as appropriate for the procedure.	S ☐ U ☐ N/A ☐	S ☐ U ☐ N/A ☐	S ☐ U ☐ N/A ☐
Implementation			
1. Identifies the problem waveform: **Overdamped**			
a. Checks the patient for hypotension.	S ☐ U ☐ N/A ☐	S ☐ U ☐ N/A ☐	S ☐ U ☐ N/A ☐
b. Performs a dynamic response test.	S ☐ U ☐ N/A ☐	S ☐ U ☐ N/A ☐	S ☐ U ☐ N/A ☐
c. Ensures that the flush bag has fluid and a maintained pressure of 300 mm Hg.	S ☐ U ☐ N/A ☐	S ☐ U ☐ N/A ☐	S ☐ U ☐ N/A ☐
d. Checks the positioning of the arterial line.	S ☐ U ☐ N/A ☐	S ☐ U ☐ N/A ☐	S ☐ U ☐ N/A ☐
e. Checks the system for air bubbles.	S ☐ U ☐ N/A ☐	S ☐ U ☐ N/A ☐	S ☐ U ☐ N/A ☐
f. Checks the tubing system for disconnections or leaks.	S ☐ U ☐ N/A ☐	S ☐ U ☐ N/A ☐	S ☐ U ☐ N/A ☐
g. Checks for appropriate rigid tubing	S ☐ U ☐ N/A ☐	S ☐ U ☐ N/A ☐	S ☐ U ☐ N/A ☐

Continued

	Peer Evaluation Laboratory Setting			Instructor Evaluation Laboratory Setting			Instructor Evaluation Clinical Setting		
h. Aspirates before flushing, if applicable.	S ☐	U ☐	N/A ☐	S ☐	U ☐	N/A ☐	S ☐	U ☐	N/A ☐
i. Flushes the line clear.	S ☐	U ☐	N/A ☐	S ☐	U ☐	N/A ☐	S ☐	U ☐	N/A ☐
Underdamped									
a. Performs a dynamic response test.	S ☐	U ☐	N/A ☐	S ☐	U ☐	N/A ☐	S ☐	U ☐	N/A ☐
b. Checks the system for air bubbles.	S ☐	U ☐	N/A ☐	S ☐	U ☐	N/A ☐	S ☐	U ☐	N/A ☐
c. Checks the length of the pressurized tubing system.	S ☐	U ☐	N/A ☐	S ☐	U ☐	N/A ☐	S ☐	U ☐	N/A ☐
2. Reassesses vital signs.	S ☐	U ☐	N/A ☐	S ☐	U ☐	N/A ☐	S ☐	U ☐	N/A ☐
3. Removes the supplies from the patient's room, and cleans the area, as needed.	S ☐	U ☐	N/A ☐	S ☐	U ☐	N/A ☐	S ☐	U ☐	N/A ☐
4. Removes the PPE, and performs proper hand hygiene prior to leaving the patient's room.	S ☐	U ☐	N/A ☐	S ☐	U ☐	N/A ☐	S ☐	U ☐	N/A ☐

Evaluation of Procedure

1. Establishes a baseline, or compares with previous measurements.	S ☐	U ☐	N/A ☐	S ☐	U ☐	N/A ☐	S ☐	U ☐	N/A ☐
2. Reevaluates blood pressure, if needed:	S ☐	U ☐	N/A ☐	S ☐	U ☐	N/A ☐	S ☐	U ☐	N/A ☐
3. Identifies any unexpected outcomes.	S ☐	U ☐	N/A ☐	S ☐	U ☐	N/A ☐	S ☐	U ☐	N/A ☐

Documentation and Reporting

1. Records findings in the patient's chart.	S ☐	U ☐	N/A ☐	S ☐	U ☐	N/A ☐	S ☐	U ☐	N/A ☐
2. Reports any abnormal findings to the appropriate health care provider.	S ☐	U ☐	N/A ☐	S ☐	U ☐	N/A ☐	S ☐	U ☐	N/A ☐

Comments:

_____

_____

_____

Signatures:

Student _____ Date Passed _____

Instructor (Laboratory Setting) _____ Date Passed _____

Student _____ Date Passed _____

Instructor (Clinical Setting) _____ Date Passed _____

Student _____ Date _____

Instructor (Laboratory Setting) _____ Date _____

Instructor (Clinical Setting) _____ Date _____

Criteria for assessment success:
The student must obtain all **satisfactory (S)** scores to pass the procedural evaluation. Any **unsatisfactory (U)** scores will result in failure of the procedural assessment.

Scoring:
Satisfactory (S): Procedural step performed correctly with no instructor prompting. Student-initiated correction is acceptable.
Unsatisfactory (U): Procedural step was performed incorrectly, omitted, or performed in a way that compromised patient care.
Not applicable (N/A): Procedural step was not indicated or necessary.

Evaluation:

	Peer Evaluation Laboratory Setting	Instructor Evaluation Laboratory Setting	Instructor Evaluation Clinical Setting
Procedural Preparation			
1. Reviews the patient's chart.	S ☐ U ☐ N/A ☐	S ☐ U ☐ N/A ☐	S ☐ U ☐ N/A ☐
2. Verifies the physician's order or the facility's protocol for standard of care.	S ☐ U ☐ N/A ☐	S ☐ U ☐ N/A ☐	S ☐ U ☐ N/A ☐
3. Obtains, cleans, and inspects the appropriate equipment prior to entering the patient's room.	S ☐ U ☐ N/A ☐	S ☐ U ☐ N/A ☐	S ☐ U ☐ N/A ☐
4. Follows PPE requirements, and observes standard precautions for any transmission-based isolation procedure.	S ☐ U ☐ N/A ☐	S ☐ U ☐ N/A ☐	S ☐ U ☐ N/A ☐
5. Identifies the patient using two patient identifiers.	S ☐ U ☐ N/A ☐	S ☐ U ☐ N/A ☐	S ☐ U ☐ N/A ☐
6. Introduces self to the patient and to the family.	S ☐ U ☐ N/A ☐	S ☐ U ☐ N/A ☐	S ☐ U ☐ N/A ☐
7. Explains the procedure to the patient and to the family, and acknowledges the patient's understanding.	S ☐ U ☐ N/A ☐	S ☐ U ☐ N/A ☐	S ☐ U ☐ N/A ☐
8. Performs proper hand hygiene, and puts on gloves, mask, and protective eyewear, as appropriate for the procedure.	S ☐ U ☐ N/A ☐	S ☐ U ☐ N/A ☐	S ☐ U ☐ N/A ☐
Implementation			
1. Places the patient in a comfortable position, and instructs him or her to breathe normally.	S ☐ U ☐ N/A ☐	S ☐ U ☐ N/A ☐	S ☐ U ☐ N/A ☐
2. Assesses vital signs.	S ☐ U ☐ N/A ☐	S ☐ U ☐ N/A ☐	S ☐ U ☐ N/A ☐
3. Instructs the patient to form a tight fist or raise the arm above heart level for several seconds.	S ☐ U ☐ N/A ☐	S ☐ U ☐ N/A ☐	S ☐ U ☐ N/A ☐

Continued

	Peer Evaluation Laboratory Setting	Instructor Evaluation Laboratory Setting	Instructor Evaluation Clinical Setting
4. Applies direct pressure to the radial and ulnar arteries, thus obstructing arterial blood flow to the hand, while the patient opens and closes the fist rapidly several times.	S ☐ U ☐ N/A ☐	S ☐ U ☐ N/A ☐	S ☐ U ☐ N/A ☐
5. Instructs the patient to open the hand or keep the arm above heart level with the radial artery compressed.	S ☐ U ☐ N/A ☐	S ☐ U ☐ N/A ☐	S ☐ U ☐ N/A ☐
6. Examines the palmar surface for an erythematous blush or pallor within 6 seconds.	S ☐ U ☐ N/A ☐	S ☐ U ☐ N/A ☐	S ☐ U ☐ N/A ☐
7. Removes the supplies from the patient's room, and cleans the area, as needed.	S ☐ U ☐ N/A ☐	S ☐ U ☐ N/A ☐	S ☐ U ☐ N/A ☐
8. Removes PPE, and performs proper hand hygiene prior to leaving the patient's room.	S ☐ U ☐ N/A ☐	S ☐ U ☐ N/A ☐	S ☐ U ☐ N/A ☐

Evaluation of Procedure

1. Establishes a baseline, or compares previous measurements.	S ☐ U ☐ N/A ☐	S ☐ U ☐ N/A ☐	S ☐ U ☐ N/A ☐
2. Identifies any unexpected outcomes.	S ☐ U ☐ N/A ☐	S ☐ U ☐ N/A ☐	S ☐ U ☐ N/A ☐
3. Evaluates alternative site for arterial puncture if the Allen's test is negative.	S ☐ U ☐ N/A ☐	S ☐ U ☐ N/A ☐	S ☐ U ☐ N/A ☐

Documentation and Reporting

1. Records findings in the patient's chart.	S ☐ U ☐ N/A ☐	S ☐ U ☐ N/A ☐	S ☐ U ☐ N/A ☐
2. Reports any abnormal findings to the appropriate health care provider.	S ☐ U ☐ N/A ☐	S ☐ U ☐ N/A ☐	S ☐ U ☐ N/A ☐

Comments:

_____

_____

_____

Signatures:

Student _____ Date Passed _____

Instructor (Laboratory Setting) _____ Date Passed _____

Student _____ Date Passed _____

Instructor (Clinical Setting) _____ Date Passed _____

Student _____ Date _____

Instructor (Laboratory Setting) _____ Date _____

Instructor (Clinical Setting) _____ Date _____

Evaluation:

	Peer Evaluation Laboratory Setting			Instructor Evaluation Laboratory Setting			Instructor Evaluation Clinical Setting		
Procedural Preparation									
1. Reviews the patient's chart.	S ☐	U ☐	N/A ☐	S ☐	U ☐	N/A ☐	S ☐	U ☐	N/A ☐
2. Verifies the physician's order or the facility's protocol for standard of care.	S ☐	U ☐	N/A ☐	S ☐	U ☐	N/A ☐	S ☐	U ☐	N/A ☐
3. Obtains, cleans, and inspects the appropriate equipment prior to entering the patient's room.	S ☐	U ☐	N/A ☐	S ☐	U ☐	N/A ☐	S ☐	U ☐	N/A ☐
4. Follows PPE requirements, and observes standard precautions for any transmission-based isolation procedure.	S ☐	U ☐	N/A ☐	S ☐	U ☐	N/A ☐	S ☐	U ☐	N/A ☐
5. Identifies the patient using two patient identifiers.	S ☐	U ☐	N/A ☐	S ☐	U ☐	N/A ☐	S ☐	U ☐	N/A ☐
6. Introduces self to the patient and to the family.	S ☐	U ☐	N/A ☐	S ☐	U ☐	N/A ☐	S ☐	U ☐	N/A ☐
7. Explains the procedure to the patient and to the family, and acknowledges the patient's understanding.	S ☐	U ☐	N/A ☐	S ☐	U ☐	N/A ☐	S ☐	U ☐	N/A ☐
8. Performs proper hand hygiene, and puts on gloves, mask, and protective eyewear, as appropriate for the procedure.	S ☐	U ☐	N/A ☐	S ☐	U ☐	N/A ☐	S ☐	U ☐	N/A ☐
Implementation									
1. Positions the patient by extending the patient's wrist approximately 30 degrees, and instructs him or her to breathe normally.	S ☐	U ☐	N/A ☐	S ☐	U ☐	N/A ☐	S ☐	U ☐	N/A ☐
2. Assesses vital signs, and estimates the oxygen concentration or FIO_2 that the patient is receiving.	S ☐	U ☐	N/A ☐	S ☐	U ☐	N/A ☐	S ☐	U ☐	N/A ☐
3. Performs an Allen's test, if radial artery puncture is used (see PA 8-1).	S ☐	U ☐	N/A ☐	S ☐	U ☐	N/A ☐	S ☐	U ☐	N/A ☐
4. Cleans the site thoroughly with 70% isopropyl alcohol or an equivalent antiseptic.	S ☐	U ☐	N/A ☐	S ☐	U ☐	N/A ☐	S ☐	U ☐	N/A ☐
5. Uses a preheparinized blood gas kit syringe, or heparinizes a syringe and expels the excess.	S ☐	U ☐	N/A ☐	S ☐	U ☐	N/A ☐	S ☐	U ☐	N/A ☐
6. Palpates and secures the artery with one hand.	S ☐	U ☐	N/A ☐	S ☐	U ☐	N/A ☐	S ☐	U ☐	N/A ☐
7. Inserts the needle.	S ☐	U ☐	N/A ☐	S ☐	U ☐	N/A ☐	S ☐	U ☐	N/A ☐
8. Allows 1 mL of blood to fill the syringe.	S ☐	U ☐	N/A ☐	S ☐	U ☐	N/A ☐	S ☐	U ☐	N/A ☐
9. Removes the needle and syringe from the artery.	S ☐	U ☐	N/A ☐	S ☐	U ☐	N/A ☐	S ☐	U ☐	N/A ☐
10. Applies firm pressure to the puncture site with sterile gauze until the bleeding stops.	S ☐	U ☐	N/A ☐	S ☐	U ☐	N/A ☐	S ☐	U ☐	N/A ☐

Continued

	Peer Evaluation Laboratory Setting			Instructor Evaluation Laboratory Setting			Instructor Evaluation Clinical Setting		
11. Applies dressing or bandage to the puncture site.	S ☐	U ☐	N/A ☐	S ☐	U ☐	N/A ☐	S ☐	U ☐	N/A ☐
12. Expels any air bubbles from the sample, and caps or plugs the syringe.	S ☐	U ☐	N/A ☐	S ☐	U ☐	N/A ☐	S ☐	U ☐	N/A ☐
13. Mixes the sample by rolling and inverting the syringe.	S ☐	U ☐	N/A ☐	S ☐	U ☐	N/A ☐	S ☐	U ☐	N/A ☐
14. Places the sample in a transport container, or on ice if specimen will not be analyzed within 10 to 30 minutes.	S ☐	U ☐	N/A ☐	S ☐	U ☐	N/A ☐	S ☐	U ☐	N/A ☐
15. Attaches the correct patient identification label and laboratory requisition to the side of the specimen container and a patient identification label on the syringe.	S ☐	U ☐	N/A ☐	S ☐	U ☐	N/A ☐	S ☐	U ☐	N/A ☐
16. Removes the supplies from the patient's room, and cleans the area, as needed.	S ☐	U ☐	N/A ☐	S ☐	U ☐	N/A ☐	S ☐	U ☐	N/A ☐
17. Removes PPE, and performs proper hand hygiene prior to leaving the patient's room.	S ☐	U ☐	N/A ☐	S ☐	U ☐	N/A ☐	S ☐	U ☐	N/A ☐

Evaluation of Procedure

	Peer Evaluation Laboratory Setting			Instructor Evaluation Laboratory Setting			Instructor Evaluation Clinical Setting		
1. Establishes a baseline, or compares previous measurements.	S ☐	U ☐	N/A ☐	S ☐	U ☐	N/A ☐	S ☐	U ☐	N/A ☐
2. Develops an appropriate respiratory care plan based on assessment data.	S ☐	U ☐	N/A ☐	S ☐	U ☐	N/A ☐	S ☐	U ☐	N/A ☐
3. Notes any use of oxygen therapy.	S ☐	U ☐	N/A ☐	S ☐	U ☐	N/A ☐	S ☐	U ☐	N/A ☐
4. Checks the puncture site after 20 minutes for hematoma and adequacy of distal circulation.	S ☐	U ☐	N/A ☐	S ☐	U ☐	N/A ☐	S ☐	U ☐	N/A ☐
5. Identifies any unexpected outcomes.	S ☐	U ☐	N/A ☐	S ☐	U ☐	N/A ☐	S ☐	U ☐	N/A ☐
6. Correlates findings with SpO_2, if available.	S ☐	U ☐	N/A ☐	S ☐	U ☐	N/A ☐	S ☐	U ☐	N/A ☐

Documentation and Reporting

	Peer Evaluation Laboratory Setting			Instructor Evaluation Laboratory Setting			Instructor Evaluation Clinical Setting		
1. Documents the procedure, and records findings in the patient's chart.	S ☐	U ☐	N/A ☐	S ☐	U ☐	N/A ☐	S ☐	U ☐	N/A ☐
2. Reports any abnormal findings to the appropriate health care provider.	S ☐	U ☐	N/A ☐	S ☐	U ☐	N/A ☐	S ☐	U ☐	N/A ☐

Comments:

_____

_____

_____

Signatures:

Student _____ Date Passed _____

Instructor (Laboratory Setting) _____ Date Passed _____

Student _____ Date Passed _____

Instructor (Clinical Setting) _____ Date Passed _____

Procedural Assessment 8-3

Placing a radial arterial line

Student _____ Date _____

Instructor (Laboratory Setting) _____ Date _____

Instructor (Clinical Setting) _____ Date _____

Evaluation:

	Peer Evaluation Laboratory Setting			Instructor Evaluation Laboratory Setting			Instructor Evaluation Clinical Setting		
Procedural Preparation									
1. Reviews the patient's chart.	S ☐	U ☐	N/A ☐	S ☐	U ☐	N/A ☐	S ☐	U ☐	N/A ☐
2. Verifies the physician's order or the facility's protocol for standard of care.	S ☐	U ☐	N/A ☐	S ☐	U ☐	N/A ☐	S ☐	U ☐	N/A ☐
3. Obtains, cleans, and inspects the appropriate equipment prior to entering the patient's room.	S ☐	U ☐	N/A ☐	S ☐	U ☐	N/A ☐	S ☐	U ☐	N/A ☐
4. Follows PPE requirements, and observes standard precautions for any transmission-based isolation procedure.	S ☐	U ☐	N/A ☐	S ☐	U ☐	N/A ☐	S ☐	U ☐	N/A ☐
5. Identifies the patient using two patient identifiers.	S ☐	U ☐	N/A ☐	S ☐	U ☐	N/A ☐	S ☐	U ☐	N/A ☐
6. Introduces self to the patient and to the family.	S ☐	U ☐	N/A ☐	S ☐	U ☐	N/A ☐	S ☐	U ☐	N/A ☐
7. Explains the procedure to the patient and to the family, and acknowledges the patient's understanding.	S ☐	U ☐	N/A ☐	S ☐	U ☐	N/A ☐	S ☐	U ☐	N/A ☐
8. Performs proper hand hygiene, ands put on gloves, mask, and protective eyewear, as appropriate for the procedure.	S ☐	U ☐	N/A ☐	S ☐	U ☐	N/A ☐	S ☐	U ☐	N/A ☐
Implementation									
1. Places the patient in a comfortable position that gives adequate access to the placement site, and instructs him or her to breathe normally.	S ☐	U ☐	N/A ☐	S ☐	U ☐	N/A ☐	S ☐	U ☐	N/A ☐
2. Assesses vital signs.	S ☐	U ☐	N/A ☐	S ☐	U ☐	N/A ☐	S ☐	U ☐	N/A ☐
3. Performs an Allen's test (see PA 8-1).	S ☐	U ☐	N/A ☐	S ☐	U ☐	N/A ☐	S ☐	U ☐	N/A ☐
4. Positions the patient's wrist and hand.	S ☐	U ☐	N/A ☐	S ☐	U ☐	N/A ☐	S ☐	U ☐	N/A ☐
5. Applies sterile gloves and protective eyewear.	S ☐	U ☐	N/A ☐	S ☐	U ☐	N/A ☐	S ☐	U ☐	N/A ☐
6. Prepares the entry site with betadine, chlorhexidine, or other skin cleanser.	S ☐	U ☐	N/A ☐	S ☐	U ☐	N/A ☐	S ☐	U ☐	N/A ☐
7. Applies sterile drape at the entry site.	S ☐	U ☐	N/A ☐	S ☐	U ☐	N/A ☐	S ☐	U ☐	N/A ☐
8. Identifies the radial artery.	S ☐	U ☐	N/A ☐	S ☐	U ☐	N/A ☐	S ☐	U ☐	N/A ☐
9. Stabilizes the artery by pulling skin taut.	S ☐	U ☐	N/A ☐	S ☐	U ☐	N/A ☐	S ☐	U ☐	N/A ☐
10. Using sterile technique, inserts the arterial needle into the skin.	S ☐	U ☐	N/A ☐	S ☐	U ☐	N/A ☐	S ☐	U ☐	N/A ☐
11. Advances the needle into the artery until spontaneous pulsatile bright red blood enters the column.	S ☐	U ☐	N/A ☐	S ☐	U ☐	N/A ☐	S ☐	U ☐	N/A ☐

Continued

	Peer Evaluation Laboratory Setting			Instructor Evaluation Laboratory Setting			Instructor Evaluation Clinical Setting		
12. Advances the guidewire.	S ☐	U ☐	N/A ☐	S ☐	U ☐	N/A ☐	S ☐	U ☐	N/A ☐
13. Advances the plastic catheter over the guidewire.	S ☐	U ☐	N/A ☐	S ☐	U ☐	N/A ☐	S ☐	U ☐	N/A ☐
14. Connects to the pressure tubing and transducer.	S ☐	U ☐	N/A ☐	S ☐	U ☐	N/A ☐	S ☐	U ☐	N/A ☐
15. Levels and sets the transducer to zero, and verifies the arterial waveform.	S ☐	U ☐	N/A ☐	S ☐	U ☐	N/A ☐	S ☐	U ☐	N/A ☐
16. Cleans the area of any blood; allows the site to dry.	S ☐	U ☐	N/A ☐	S ☐	U ☐	N/A ☐	S ☐	U ☐	N/A ☐
17. Applies Benzoin to the cleansed area, and allows the site to dry and become tacky.	S ☐	U ☐	N/A ☐	S ☐	U ☐	N/A ☐	S ☐	U ☐	N/A ☐
18. Secures the arterial line with tape or steri-strips, and covers with a Tegaderm dressing.	S ☐	U ☐	N/A ☐	S ☐	U ☐	N/A ☐	S ☐	U ☐	N/A ☐
19. Secures the tubing to prevent it from being pulled.	S ☐	U ☐	N/A ☐	S ☐	U ☐	N/A ☐	S ☐	U ☐	N/A ☐
20. Removes the supplies from the patient's room, and cleans the area, as needed.	S ☐	U ☐	N/A ☐	S ☐	U ☐	N/A ☐	S ☐	U ☐	N/A ☐
21. Removes PPE, and performs proper hand hygiene prior to leaving the patient's room.	S ☐	U ☐	N/A ☐	S ☐	U ☐	N/A ☐	S ☐	U ☐	N/A ☐

Evaluation of Procedure

	Peer Evaluation Laboratory Setting			Instructor Evaluation Laboratory Setting			Instructor Evaluation Clinical Setting		
1. Establishes a baseline, or compares with previous measurements.	S ☐	U ☐	N/A ☐	S ☐	U ☐	N/A ☐	S ☐	U ☐	N/A ☐
2. Develops an appropriate respiratory care plan based on assessment data.	S ☐	U ☐	N/A ☐	S ☐	U ☐	N/A ☐	S ☐	U ☐	N/A ☐
3. Identifies any unexpected outcomes.	S ☐	U ☐	N/A ☐	S ☐	U ☐	N/A ☐	S ☐	U ☐	N/A ☐

Documentation and Reporting

	Peer Evaluation Laboratory Setting			Instructor Evaluation Laboratory Setting			Instructor Evaluation Clinical Setting		
1. Records findings in the patient's chart.	S ☐	U ☐	N/A ☐	S ☐	U ☐	N/A ☐	S ☐	U ☐	N/A ☐
2. Reports any abnormal findings to the appropriate health care provider.	S ☐	U ☐	N/A ☐	S ☐	U ☐	N/A ☐	S ☐	U ☐	N/A ☐

Comments:

_____

_____

_____

_____

Signatures:

Student _____ Date Passed _____

Instructor (Laboratory Setting) _____ Date Passed _____

Student _____ Date Passed _____

Instructor (Clinical Setting) _____ Date Passed _____

Procedural Assessment 8-4

Blood sampling from an indwelling arterial catheter

Student _____ Date _____

Instructor (Laboratory Setting) _____ Date _____

Instructor (Clinical Setting) _____ Date _____

Evaluation:

	Peer Evaluation Laboratory Setting	Instructor Evaluation Laboratory Setting	Instructor Evaluation Clinical Setting
Procedural Preparation			
1. Reviews the patient's chart.	S ☐ U ☐ N/A ☐	S ☐ U ☐ N/A ☐	S ☐ U ☐ N/A ☐
2. Verifies the physician's order or the facility's protocol for standard of care.	S ☐ U ☐ N/A ☐	S ☐ U ☐ N/A ☐	S ☐ U ☐ N/A ☐
3. Obtains, cleans, and inspects the appropriate equipment prior to entering the patient's room.	S ☐ U ☐ N/A ☐	S ☐ U ☐ N/A ☐	S ☐ U ☐ N/A ☐
4. Follows PPE requirements, and observes standard precautions for any transmission-based isolation procedure.	S ☐ U ☐ N/A ☐	S ☐ U ☐ N/A ☐	S ☐ U ☐ N/A ☐
5. Identifies the patient using two patient identifiers.	S ☐ U ☐ N/A ☐	S ☐ U ☐ N/A ☐	S ☐ U ☐ N/A ☐
6. Introduces self to the patient and to the family.	S ☐ U ☐ N/A ☐	S ☐ U ☐ N/A ☐	S ☐ U ☐ N/A ☐
7. Explains the procedure to the patient and to the family, and acknowledges the patient's understanding.	S ☐ U ☐ N/A ☐	S ☐ U ☐ N/A ☐	S ☐ U ☐ N/A ☐
8. Performs proper hand hygiene, and puts on gloves, mask, and protective eyewear, as appropriate for the procedure.	S ☐ U ☐ N/A ☐	S ☐ U ☐ N/A ☐	S ☐ U ☐ N/A ☐
Implementation			
1. Places the patient in a comfortable position, and instructs him or her to breathe normally.	S ☐ U ☐ N/A ☐	S ☐ U ☐ N/A ☐	S ☐ U ☐ N/A ☐
2. Assesses vital signs, and estimates the oxygen concentration or FIO_2 that the patient is receiving.	S ☐ U ☐ N/A ☐	S ☐ U ☐ N/A ☐	S ☐ U ☐ N/A ☐
3. Attaches the waste syringe to the stopcock port.	S ☐ U ☐ N/A ☐	S ☐ U ☐ N/A ☐	S ☐ U ☐ N/A ☐
4. Positions the stopcock so that blood flows into the syringe and the IV flush solution.	S ☐ U ☐ N/A ☐	S ☐ U ☐ N/A ☐	S ☐ U ☐ N/A ☐
5. Aspirates 2 mL of fluid or blood.	S ☐ U ☐ N/A ☐	S ☐ U ☐ N/A ☐	S ☐ U ☐ N/A ☐
6. Repositions the stopcock to close off all the ports.	S ☐ U ☐ N/A ☐	S ☐ U ☐ N/A ☐	S ☐ U ☐ N/A ☐
7. Disconnects and disposes of waste syringe.	S ☐ U ☐ N/A ☐	S ☐ U ☐ N/A ☐	S ☐ U ☐ N/A ☐
8. Attaches a new heparinized syringe to the sampling port.	S ☐ U ☐ N/A ☐	S ☐ U ☐ N/A ☐	S ☐ U ☐ N/A ☐
9. Positions the stopcock so that blood flows into the sample syringe, and closes the IV flush port.	S ☐ U ☐ N/A ☐	S ☐ U ☐ N/A ☐	S ☐ U ☐ N/A ☐
10. Fills syringe with 2 mL of blood.	S ☐ U ☐ N/A ☐	S ☐ U ☐ N/A ☐	S ☐ U ☐ N/A ☐
11. Repositions the stopcock to close the sampling port, and opens the IV flush port.	S ☐ U ☐ N/A ☐	S ☐ U ☐ N/A ☐	S ☐ U ☐ N/A ☐

Continued

	Peer Evaluation Laboratory Setting			Instructor Evaluation Laboratory Setting			Instructor Evaluation Clinical Setting		
12. Disconnects the sample syringe.	S ☐	U ☐	N/A ☐	S ☐	U ☐	N/A ☐	S ☐	U ☐	N/A ☐
13. Expels any air bubbles from sample, and caps.	S ☐	U ☐	N/A ☐	S ☐	U ☐	N/A ☐	S ☐	U ☐	N/A ☐
14. Rolls the syringe to mix.	S ☐	U ☐	N/A ☐	S ☐	U ☐	N/A ☐	S ☐	U ☐	N/A ☐
15. Confirms that the stopcock port is open to the IV flush bag and the catheter.	S ☐	U ☐	N/A ☐	S ☐	U ☐	N/A ☐	S ☐	U ☐	N/A ☐
16. Confirms undampened pulse pressure waveform on the monitor.	S ☐	U ☐	N/A ☐	S ☐	U ☐	N/A ☐	S ☐	U ☐	N/A ☐
17. Places the sample syringe in an appropriate container, or on ice if necessary.	S ☐	U ☐	N/A ☐	S ☐	U ☐	N/A ☐	S ☐	U ☐	N/A ☐
18. Removes the supplies from the patient's room, and cleans the area, as needed.	S ☐	U ☐	N/A ☐	S ☐	U ☐	N/A ☐	S ☐	U ☐	N/A ☐
19. Removes PPE, and performs proper hand hygiene prior to leaving the patient's room.	S ☐	U ☐	N/A ☐	S ☐	U ☐	N/A ☐	S ☐	U ☐	N/A ☐

Evaluation of Procedure

	Peer Evaluation Laboratory Setting			Instructor Evaluation Laboratory Setting			Instructor Evaluation Clinical Setting		
1. Establishes a baseline, or compares with previous measurements.	S ☐	U ☐	N/A ☐	S ☐	U ☐	N/A ☐	S ☐	U ☐	N/A ☐
2. Develops an appropriate respiratory care plan based on assessment data.	S ☐	U ☐	N/A ☐	S ☐	U ☐	N/A ☐	S ☐	U ☐	N/A ☐
3. Makes changes to FIO$_2$, if indicated.	S ☐	U ☐	N/A ☐	S ☐	U ☐	N/A ☐	S ☐	U ☐	N/A ☐
4. Identifies any unexpected outcomes.	S ☐	U ☐	N/A ☐	S ☐	U ☐	N/A ☐	S ☐	U ☐	N/A ☐
5. Correlates findings with noninvasive measurements, if applicable.	S ☐	U ☐	N/A ☐	S ☐	U ☐	N/A ☐	S ☐	U ☐	N/A ☐

Documentation and Reporting

	Peer Evaluation Laboratory Setting			Instructor Evaluation Laboratory Setting			Instructor Evaluation Clinical Setting		
1. Records findings in the patient's chart.	S ☐	U ☐	N/A ☐	S ☐	U ☐	N/A ☐	S ☐	U ☐	N/A ☐
2. Reports any abnormal findings to the appropriate health care provider.	S ☐	U ☐	N/A ☐	S ☐	U ☐	N/A ☐	S ☐	U ☐	N/A ☐

Comments:

_____

_____

_____

Signatures:

Student _____ Date Passed _____

Instructor (Laboratory Setting) _____ Date Passed _____

Student _____ Date Passed _____

Instructor (Clinical Setting) _____ Date Passed _____

Procedural Assessment 8-5 Capillary blood sampling

Student _____ Date _____

Instructor (Laboratory Setting) _____ Date _____

Instructor (Clinical Setting) _____ Date _____

Criteria for assessment success:

The student must obtain all **satisfactory (S)** scores to pass the procedural evaluation. Any **unsatisfactory (U)** scores will result in failure of the procedural assessment.

Scoring:

Satisfactory (S): Procedural step performed correctly with no instructor prompting. Student-initiated correction is acceptable.

Unsatisfactory (U): Procedural step was performed incorrectly, omitted, or performed in a way that compromised patient care.

Not applicable (N/A): Procedural step was not indicated or necessary.

Evaluation:

	Peer Evaluation Laboratory Setting	Instructor Evaluation Laboratory Setting	Instructor Evaluation Clinical Setting
Procedural Preparation			
1. Reviews the patient's chart.	S ☐ U ☐ N/A ☐	S ☐ U ☐ N/A ☐	S ☐ U ☐ N/A ☐
2. Verifies the physician's order or the facility's protocol for standard of care.	S ☐ U ☐ N/A ☐	S ☐ U ☐ N/A ☐	S ☐ U ☐ N/A ☐
3. Obtains, cleans, and inspects the appropriate equipment prior to entering the patient's room.	S ☐ U ☐ N/A ☐	S ☐ U ☐ N/A ☐	S ☐ U ☐ N/A ☐
4. Follows PPE requirements, and observes standard precautions for any transmission-based isolation procedure.	S ☐ U ☐ N/A ☐	S ☐ U ☐ N/A ☐	S ☐ U ☐ N/A ☐
5. Identifies the patient using two patient identifiers.	S ☐ U ☐ N/A ☐	S ☐ U ☐ N/A ☐	S ☐ U ☐ N/A ☐
6. Introduces self to the patient and to the family.	S ☐ U ☐ N/A ☐	S ☐ U ☐ N/A ☐	S ☐ U ☐ N/A ☐
7. Explains the procedure to the patient and to the family, and acknowledges the patient's understanding.	S ☐ U ☐ N/A ☐	S ☐ U ☐ N/A ☐	S ☐ U ☐ N/A ☐
8. Performs proper hand hygiene, and puts on gloves, mask, and protective eyewear, as appropriate for the procedure.	S ☐ U ☐ N/A ☐	S ☐ U ☐ N/A ☐	S ☐ U ☐ N/A ☐
Implementation			
1. Places the patient in a comfortable position, and selects the site.	S ☐ U ☐ N/A ☐	S ☐ U ☐ N/A ☐	S ☐ U ☐ N/A ☐
2. Assesses vital signs, and estimates the oxygen concentration or FIO$_2$ that the patient is receiving.	S ☐ U ☐ N/A ☐	S ☐ U ☐ N/A ☐	S ☐ U ☐ N/A ☐
3. Warms the site to 42°C for 10 minutes by using a compress, heat lamp, or commercial hot pack.	S ☐ U ☐ N/A ☐	S ☐ U ☐ N/A ☐	S ☐ U ☐ N/A ☐
4. Cleans skin with an antiseptic solution.	S ☐ U ☐ N/A ☐	S ☐ U ☐ N/A ☐	S ☐ U ☐ N/A ☐

Continued

	Peer Evaluation Laboratory Setting			Instructor Evaluation Laboratory Setting			Instructor Evaluation Clinical Setting		
5. Punctures the skin with the lancet.	S ☐	U ☐	N/A ☐	S ☐	U ☐	N/A ☐	S ☐	U ☐	N/A ☐
6. Wipes away the first drop of blood, and observes free flow.	S ☐	U ☐	N/A ☐	S ☐	U ☐	N/A ☐	S ☐	U ☐	N/A ☐
7. Fills the sample tube from the middle of the blood drop until the tube is completely full.	S ☐	U ☐	N/A ☐	S ☐	U ☐	N/A ☐	S ☐	U ☐	N/A ☐
8. Places the metal flea in the capillary tube, and seals the tube ends.	S ☐	U ☐	N/A ☐	S ☐	U ☐	N/A ☐	S ☐	U ☐	N/A ☐
9. Tapes sterile cotton or a bandage over the puncture wound.	S ☐	U ☐	N/A ☐	S ☐	U ☐	N/A ☐	S ☐	U ☐	N/A ☐
10. Mixes the sample by moving the magnet back and forth along the capillary tube.	S ☐	U ☐	N/A ☐	S ☐	U ☐	N/A ☐	S ☐	U ☐	N/A ☐
11. Chills the sample immediately, or analyzes it within 10 to 15 minutes if left at room temperature.	S ☐	U ☐	N/A ☐	S ☐	U ☐	N/A ☐	S ☐	U ☐	N/A ☐
12. Removes the supplies from the patient's room, and cleans the area, as needed.	S ☐	U ☐	N/A ☐	S ☐	U ☐	N/A ☐	S ☐	U ☐	N/A ☐
13. Removes the PPE, and performs proper hand hygiene prior to leaving the patient's room.	S ☐	U ☐	N/A ☐	S ☐	U ☐	N/A ☐	S ☐	U ☐	N/A ☐

Evaluation of Procedure

1. Establishes a baseline, or compares with previous measurements.	S ☐	U ☐	N/A ☐	S ☐	U ☐	N/A ☐	S ☐	U ☐	N/A ☐
2. Develops an appropriate respiratory care plan based on assessment data.	S ☐	U ☐	N/A ☐	S ☐	U ☐	N/A ☐	S ☐	U ☐	N/A ☐
3. Notes any use of oxygen therapy.	S ☐	U ☐	N/A ☐	S ☐	U ☐	N/A ☐	S ☐	U ☐	N/A ☐
4. Identifies any unexpected outcomes.	S ☐	U ☐	N/A ☐	S ☐	U ☐	N/A ☐	S ☐	U ☐	N/A ☐

Documentation and Reporting

1. Records findings in the patient's chart.	S ☐	U ☐	N/A ☐	S ☐	U ☐	N/A ☐	S ☐	U ☐	N/A ☐
2. Reports any abnormal findings to the appropriate health care provider.	S ☐	U ☐	N/A ☐	S ☐	U ☐	N/A ☐	S ☐	U ☐	N/A ☐

Comments:

_____

_____

_____

Signatures:

Student _____ Date Passed _____

Instructor (Laboratory Setting) _____ Date Passed _____

Student _____ Date Passed _____

Instructor (Clinical Setting) _____ Date Passed _____

Procedural Assessment 8-6

Monitoring transcutaneous blood gas

Student _____ Date _____

Instructor (Laboratory Setting) _____ Date _____

Instructor (Clinical Setting) _____ Date _____

Criteria for assessment success:

The student must obtain all **satisfactory (S)** scores to pass the procedural evaluation. Any **unsatisfactory (U)** scores will result in failure of the procedural assessment.

Scoring:

Satisfactory (S): Procedural step performed correctly with no instructor prompting. Student-initiated correction is acceptable.

Unsatisfactory (U): Procedural step was performed incorrectly, omitted, or performed in a way that compromised patient care.

Not applicable (N/A): Procedural step was not indicated or necessary.

Evaluation:

	Peer Evaluation Laboratory Setting	Instructor Evaluation Laboratory Setting	Instructor Evaluation Clinical Setting
Procedural Preparation			
1. Reviews the patient's chart.	S ☐ U ☐ N/A ☐	S ☐ U ☐ N/A ☐	S ☐ U ☐ N/A ☐
2. Verifies the physician's order or the facility's protocol for standard of care.	S ☐ U ☐ N/A ☐	S ☐ U ☐ N/A ☐	S ☐ U ☐ N/A ☐
3. Obtains, cleans, and inspects the appropriate equipment prior to entering the patient's room.	S ☐ U ☐ N/A ☐	S ☐ U ☐ N/A ☐	S ☐ U ☐ N/A ☐
4. Follows PPE requirements, and observes standard precautions for any transmission-based isolation procedure.	S ☐ U ☐ N/A ☐	S ☐ U ☐ N/A ☐	S ☐ U ☐ N/A ☐
5. Identifies the patient using two patient identifiers.	S ☐ U ☐ N/A ☐	S ☐ U ☐ N/A ☐	S ☐ U ☐ N/A ☐
6. Introduces self to the patient and to the family.	S ☐ U ☐ N/A ☐	S ☐ U ☐ N/A ☐	S ☐ U ☐ N/A ☐
7. Explains the procedure to the patient and to the family, and acknowledges the patient's understanding.	S ☐ U ☐ N/A ☐	S ☐ U ☐ N/A ☐	S ☐ U ☐ N/A ☐
8. Performs proper hand hygiene, and puts on gloves, mask, and protective eyewear, as appropriate for the procedure.	S ☐ U ☐ N/A ☐	S ☐ U ☐ N/A ☐	S ☐ U ☐ N/A ☐
Implementation			
1. Places the patient in a comfortable position.	S ☐ U ☐ N/A ☐	S ☐ U ☐ N/A ☐	S ☐ U ☐ N/A ☐
2. Places the monitor at the bedside, and turns it on, as specified by the manufacturer.	S ☐ U ☐ N/A ☐	S ☐ U ☐ N/A ☐	S ☐ U ☐ N/A ☐
3. Assesses vital signs, and estimates the oxygen concentration or FIO_2 that the patient is receiving.	S ☐ U ☐ N/A ☐	S ☐ U ☐ N/A ☐	S ☐ U ☐ N/A ☐
4. Selects the monitoring site.	S ☐ U ☐ N/A ☐	S ☐ U ☐ N/A ☐	S ☐ U ☐ N/A ☐
5. Prepares the sensor.	S ☐ U ☐ N/A ☐	S ☐ U ☐ N/A ☐	S ☐ U ☐ N/A ☐

Continued

	Peer Evaluation Laboratory Setting	Instructor Evaluation Laboratory Setting	Instructor Evaluation Clinical Setting
6. Selects the appropriate probe temperature.	S ☐ U ☐ N/A ☐	S ☐ U ☐ N/A ☐	S ☐ U ☐ N/A ☐
7. Prepares the monitoring site.	S ☐ U ☐ N/A ☐	S ☐ U ☐ N/A ☐	S ☐ U ☐ N/A ☐
8. Attaches the probe to the patient.	S ☐ U ☐ N/A ☐	S ☐ U ☐ N/A ☐	S ☐ U ☐ N/A ☐
9. Allows for stabilization time.	S ☐ U ☐ N/A ☐	S ☐ U ☐ N/A ☐	S ☐ U ☐ N/A ☐
10. Sets the alarms.	S ☐ U ☐ N/A ☐	S ☐ U ☐ N/A ☐	S ☐ U ☐ N/A ☐
11. Removes the supplies from the patient's room, and cleans the area, as needed.	S ☐ U ☐ N/A ☐	S ☐ U ☐ N/A ☐	S ☐ U ☐ N/A ☐
12. Removes PPE, and performs proper hand hygiene prior to leaving the patient's room.	S ☐ U ☐ N/A ☐	S ☐ U ☐ N/A ☐	S ☐ U ☐ N/A ☐

Evaluation of Procedure

1. Establishes a baseline, or compares with previous measurements.	S ☐ U ☐ N/A ☐	S ☐ U ☐ N/A ☐	S ☐ U ☐ N/A ☐
2. Develops an appropriate respiratory care plan based on assessment data.	S ☐ U ☐ N/A ☐	S ☐ U ☐ N/A ☐	S ☐ U ☐ N/A ☐
3. Correlates with ABG measurements, if applicable.	S ☐ U ☐ N/A ☐	S ☐ U ☐ N/A ☐	S ☐ U ☐ N/A ☐
4. Identifies any unexpected outcomes.	S ☐ U ☐ N/A ☐	S ☐ U ☐ N/A ☐	S ☐ U ☐ N/A ☐
5. Establishes the probe site change time, and documents it.	S ☐ U ☐ N/A ☐	S ☐ U ☐ N/A ☐	S ☐ U ☐ N/A ☐
6. Monitors the probe site for complications.	S ☐ U ☐ N/A ☐	S ☐ U ☐ N/A ☐	S ☐ U ☐ N/A ☐

Documentation and Reporting

1. Records findings in the patient's chart.	S ☐ U ☐ N/A ☐	S ☐ U ☐ N/A ☐	S ☐ U ☐ N/A ☐
2. Reports any abnormal findings to the appropriate health care provider.	S ☐ U ☐ N/A ☐	S ☐ U ☐ N/A ☐	S ☐ U ☐ N/A ☐

Comments:

_____

_____

_____

Signatures:

Student _____ Date Passed _____

Instructor (Laboratory Setting) _____ Date Passed _____

Student _____ Date Passed _____

Instructor (Clinical Setting) _____ Date Passed _____

Student _____ Date _____

Instructor (Laboratory Setting) _____ Date _____

Instructor (Clinical Setting) _____ Date _____

Criteria for assessment success:

The student must obtain all **satisfactory (S)** scores to pass the procedural evaluation. Any **unsatisfactory (U)** scores will result in failure of the procedural assessment.

Scoring:

Satisfactory (S): Procedural step performed correctly with no instructor prompting. Student-initiated correction is acceptable.

Unsatisfactory (U): Procedural step was performed incorrectly, omitted, or performed in a way that compromised patient care.

Not applicable (N/A): Procedural step was not indicated or necessary.

Evaluation:

	Peer Evaluation Laboratory Setting	Instructor Evaluation Laboratory Setting	Instructor Evaluation Clinical Setting
Procedural Preparation			
1. Reviews the patient's chart.	S ☐ U ☐ N/A ☐	S ☐ U ☐ N/A ☐	S ☐ U ☐ N/A ☐
2. Verifies the physician's order or the facility's protocol for standard of care.	S ☐ U ☐ N/A ☐	S ☐ U ☐ N/A ☐	S ☐ U ☐ N/A ☐
3. Obtains, cleans, and inspects the appropriate equipment prior to entering the patient's room.	S ☐ U ☐ N/A ☐	S ☐ U ☐ N/A ☐	S ☐ U ☐ N/A ☐
4. Follows PPE requirements, and observes standard precautions for any transmission based isolation procedure.	S ☐ U ☐ N/A ☐	S ☐ U ☐ N/A ☐	S ☐ U ☐ N/A ☐
5. Identifies the patient using two patient identifiers.	S ☐ U ☐ N/A ☐	S ☐ U ☐ N/A ☐	S ☐ U ☐ N/A ☐
6. Introduces self to the patient and to the family.	S ☐ U ☐ N/A ☐	S ☐ U ☐ N/A ☐	S ☐ U ☐ N/A ☐
7. Explains the procedure to the patient and to the family, and acknowledges the patient's understanding.	S ☐ U ☐ N/A ☐	S ☐ U ☐ N/A ☐	S ☐ U ☐ N/A ☐
8. Performs proper hand hygiene, and puts on gloves, mask, and protective eyewear, as appropriate for the procedure.	S ☐ U ☐ N/A ☐	S ☐ U ☐ N/A ☐	S ☐ U ☐ N/A ☐
Implementation			
1. Assesses vital signs, and estimates the oxygen concentration or FIO_2 that the patient is receiving.	S ☐ U ☐ N/A ☐	S ☐ U ☐ N/A ☐	S ☐ U ☐ N/A ☐
2. Connects the monitor to the electrical outlet.	S ☐ U ☐ N/A ☐	S ☐ U ☐ N/A ☐	S ☐ U ☐ N/A ☐
3. Calibrates the monitor to the known CO_2 level.	S ☐ U ☐ N/A ☐	S ☐ U ☐ N/A ☐	S ☐ U ☐ N/A ☐
4. Connects the monitor to the patient's airway. a. Directly to the airway for a mainstream monitor. b. Uses an adapter for a sidestream monitor.	S ☐ U ☐ N/A ☐ S ☐ U ☐ N/A ☐	S ☐ U ☐ N/A ☐ S ☐ U ☐ N/A ☐	S ☐ U ☐ N/A ☐ S ☐ U ☐ N/A ☐
5. Reassesses vital signs.	S ☐ U ☐ N/A ☐	S ☐ U ☐ N/A ☐	S ☐ U ☐ N/A ☐

Continued

	Peer Evaluation Laboratory Setting			Instructor Evaluation Laboratory Setting			Instructor Evaluation Clinical Setting		
6. Removes the supplies from the patient's room, and cleans the area, as needed.	S □	U □	N/A □	S □	U □	N/A □	S □	U □	N/A □
7. Removes PPE, and performs proper hand hygiene prior to leaving the patient's room.	S □	U □	N/A □	S □	U □	N/A □	S □	U □	N/A □

Evaluation of Procedure

1. Establishes a baseline, or compares with previous measurements.	S □	U □	N/A □	S □	U □	N/A □	S □	U □	N/A □
2. Correlates findings with an arterial $PaCO_2$ measurement.	S □	U □	N/A □	S □	U □	N/A □	S □	U □	N/A □
3. Develops an appropriate respiratory care plan based on assessment data.	S □	U □	N/A □	S □	U □	N/A □	S □	U □	N/A □
4. Identifies any unexpected outcomes.	S □	U □	N/A □	S □	U □	N/A □	S □	U □	N/A □

Documentation and Reporting

1. Records findings in the patient's chart.	S □	U □	N/A □	S □	U □	N/A □	S □	U □	N/A □
2. Reports any abnormal findings to the appropriate health care provider.	S □	U □	N/A □	S □	U □	N/A □	S □	U □	N/A □

Comments:

_____

_____

_____

Signatures:

Student _____ Date Passed _____

Instructor (Laboratory Setting) _____ Date Passed _____

Student _____ Date Passed _____

Instructor (Clinical Setting) _____ Date Passed _____

Student _____ Date _____

Instructor (Laboratory Setting) _____ Date _____

Instructor (Clinical Setting) _____ Date _____

Evaluation:

	Peer Evaluation Laboratory Setting	Instructor Evaluation Laboratory Setting	Instructor Evaluation Clinical Setting
Procedural Preparation			
1. Reviews the patient's chart.	S ☐ U ☐ N/A ☐	S ☐ U ☐ N/A ☐	S ☐ U ☐ N/A ☐
2. Verifies the physician's order or the facility's protocol for standard of care.	S ☐ U ☐ N/A ☐	S ☐ U ☐ N/A ☐	S ☐ U ☐ N/A ☐
3. Obtains, cleans, and inspects the appropriate equipment prior to entering the patient's room.	S ☐ U ☐ N/A ☐	S ☐ U ☐ N/A ☐	S ☐ U ☐ N/A ☐
4. Follows PPE requirements, and observes standard precautions for any transmission-based isolation procedure.	S ☐ U ☐ N/A ☐	S ☐ U ☐ N/A ☐	S ☐ U ☐ N/A ☐
5. Identifies the patient using two patient identifiers.	S ☐ U ☐ N/A ☐	S ☐ U ☐ N/A ☐	S ☐ U ☐ N/A ☐
6. Introduces self to the patient and to the family.	S ☐ U ☐ N/A ☐	S ☐ U ☐ N/A ☐	S ☐ U ☐ N/A ☐
7. Explains the procedure to the patient and to the family, and acknowledges the patient's understanding.	S ☐ U ☐ N/A ☐	S ☐ U ☐ N/A ☐	S ☐ U ☐ N/A ☐
8. Performs proper hand hygiene, and puts on gloves, mask, and protective eyewear, as appropriates for the procedure.	S ☐ U ☐ N/A ☐	S ☐ U ☐ N/A ☐	S ☐ U ☐ N/A ☐
Implementation			
1. Places the patient in the sitting or high-Fowler position.	S ☐ U ☐ N/A ☐	S ☐ U ☐ N/A ☐	S ☐ U ☐ N/A ☐
2. Assesses vital signs.	S ☐ U ☐ N/A ☐	S ☐ U ☐ N/A ☐	S ☐ U ☐ N/A ☐
3. Provides instruction and demonstrates the tests to the patient before administering them.	S ☐ U ☐ N/A ☐	S ☐ U ☐ N/A ☐	S ☐ U ☐ N/A ☐
4. Positions the nose clips, if applicable.	S ☐ U ☐ N/A ☐	S ☐ U ☐ N/A ☐	S ☐ U ☐ N/A ☐
5. Positions the mouthpiece in the patient's mouth, resting it on the top of the tongue.	S ☐ U ☐ N/A ☐	S ☐ U ☐ N/A ☐	S ☐ U ☐ N/A ☐
6. Instructs the patient to gently bite down with his or her teeth and to seal the lips firmly around the mouthpiece.	S ☐ U ☐ N/A ☐	S ☐ U ☐ N/A ☐	S ☐ U ☐ N/A ☐
7. Places the spirometer hose or flow sensor in the patient's hand, and instructs him or her to breaths quietly for several breaths.	S ☐ U ☐ N/A ☐	S ☐ U ☐ N/A ☐	S ☐ U ☐ N/A ☐
8. Instructs patient to perform VC.	S ☐ U ☐ N/A ☐	S ☐ U ☐ N/A ☐	S ☐ U ☐ N/A ☐
9. Instructs patient to perform IC.	S ☐ U ☐ N/A ☐	S ☐ U ☐ N/A ☐	S ☐ U ☐ N/A ☐

Continued

	Peer Evaluation Laboratory Setting			Instructor Evaluation Laboratory Setting			Instructor Evaluation Clinical Setting		
10. Instructs patient to perform ERV.	S ☐	U ☐	N/A ☐	S ☐	U ☐	N/A ☐	S ☐	U ☐	N/A ☐
11. Ensures that the patient performs the procedure until acceptability and repeatability criteria are achieved.	S ☐	U ☐	N/A ☐	S ☐	U ☐	N/A ☐	S ☐	U ☐	N/A ☐
12. Removes the supplies from the patient's room, and cleans the area, as needed.	S ☐	U ☐	N/A ☐	S ☐	U ☐	N/A ☐	S ☐	U ☐	N/A ☐
13. Removes the PPE, and performs proper hand hygiene prior to leaving the patient's room.	S ☐	U ☐	N/A ☐	S ☐	U ☐	N/A ☐	S ☐	U ☐	N/A ☐

Evaluation of Procedure

	Peer Evaluation Laboratory Setting			Instructor Evaluation Laboratory Setting			Instructor Evaluation Clinical Setting		
1. Establishes a baseline, or compares with previous measurements.	S ☐	U ☐	N/A ☐	S ☐	U ☐	N/A ☐	S ☐	U ☐	N/A ☐
2. Assesses the patient during the test to identify any distress or physical complications.	S ☐	U ☐	N/A ☐	S ☐	U ☐	N/A ☐	S ☐	U ☐	N/A ☐
3. Interprets the results.	S ☐	U ☐	N/A ☐	S ☐	U ☐	N/A ☐	S ☐	U ☐	N/A ☐
4. Develops an appropriate respiratory care plan based on assessment data.	S ☐	U ☐	N/A ☐	S ☐	U ☐	N/A ☐	S ☐	U ☐	N/A ☐
5. Identifies any unexpected outcomes.	S ☐	U ☐	N/A ☐	S ☐	U ☐	N/A ☐	S ☐	U ☐	N/A ☐

Documentation and Reporting

	Peer Evaluation Laboratory Setting			Instructor Evaluation Laboratory Setting			Instructor Evaluation Clinical Setting		
1. Records findings in the patient's chart as percent of the predicted, BTPS.	S ☐	U ☐	N/A ☐	S ☐	U ☐	N/A ☐	S ☐	U ☐	N/A ☐
2. Reports any abnormal findings to the appropriate health care provider.	S ☐	U ☐	N/A ☐	S ☐	U ☐	N/A ☐	S ☐	U ☐	N/A ☐

Comments:

_____

_____

_____

Signatures:

Student _____ Date Passed _____

Instructor (Laboratory Setting) _____ Date Passed _____

Student _____ Date Passed _____

Instructor (Clinical Setting) _____ Date Passed _____

Student _____ Date _____

Instructor (Laboratory Setting) _____ Date _____

Instructor (Clinical Setting) _____ Date _____

Evaluation:

	Peer Evaluation Laboratory Setting	Instructor Evaluation Laboratory Setting	Instructor Evaluation Clinical Setting
Procedural Preparation			
1. Reviews the patient's chart.	S ☐ U ☐ N/A ☐	S ☐ U ☐ N/A ☐	S ☐ U ☐ N/A ☐
2. Verifies the physician's order or the facility's protocol for standard of care.	S ☐ U ☐ N/A ☐	S ☐ U ☐ N/A ☐	S ☐ U ☐ N/A ☐
3. Obtains, cleans, and inspects the appropriate equipment prior to entering the patient's room.	S ☐ U ☐ N/A ☐	S ☐ U ☐ N/A ☐	S ☐ U ☐ N/A ☐
4. Follows PPE requirements, and observes standard precautions for any transmission-based isolation procedure.	S ☐ U ☐ N/A ☐	S ☐ U ☐ N/A ☐	S ☐ U ☐ N/A ☐
5. Identifies the patient using two patient identifiers.	S ☐ U ☐ N/A ☐	S ☐ U ☐ N/A ☐	S ☐ U ☐ N/A ☐
6. Introduces self to the patient and to the family.	S ☐ U ☐ N/A ☐	S ☐ U ☐ N/A ☐	S ☐ U ☐ N/A ☐
7. Explains the procedure to the patient and to the family, and acknowledges the patient's understanding.	S ☐ U ☐ N/A ☐	S ☐ U ☐ N/A ☐	S ☐ U ☐ N/A ☐
8. Performs proper hand hygiene, and puts on gloves, mask, and protective eyewear, as appropriate for the procedure.	S ☐ U ☐ N/A ☐	S ☐ U ☐ N/A ☐	S ☐ U ☐ N/A ☐
Implementation			
1. Places the patient in the sitting or high-Fowler position or sitting upright with feet flat on the floor.	S ☐ U ☐ N/A ☐	S ☐ U ☐ N/A ☐	S ☐ U ☐ N/A ☐
2. Assesses vital signs.	S ☐ U ☐ N/A ☐	S ☐ U ☐ N/A ☐	S ☐ U ☐ N/A ☐
3. Instructs and demonstrates the tests to the patient before administering them.	S ☐ U ☐ N/A ☐	S ☐ U ☐ N/A ☐	S ☐ U ☐ N/A ☐
4. Positions nose clips, if applicable.	S ☐ U ☐ N/A ☐	S ☐ U ☐ N/A ☐	S ☐ U ☐ N/A ☐
5. Positions the mouthpiece to rest on the top of the patient's tongue.	S ☐ U ☐ N/A ☐	S ☐ U ☐ N/A ☐	S ☐ U ☐ N/A ☐
6. Instructs the patient to gently bite down with the teeth and to seal the lips firmly around the mouthpiece.	S ☐ U ☐ N/A ☐	S ☐ U ☐ N/A ☐	S ☐ U ☐ N/A ☐
7. Places the spirometer hose or flow sensor in the patient's hand, and instructs him or her to breathe quietly for several breaths.	S ☐ U ☐ N/A ☐	S ☐ U ☐ N/A ☐	S ☐ U ☐ N/A ☐
8. Instructs the patient to take a maximal inspiration and then to blast air out forcefully.	S ☐ U ☐ N/A ☐	S ☐ U ☐ N/A ☐	S ☐ U ☐ N/A ☐
9. Encourages the patient to continue to blow.	S ☐ U ☐ N/A ☐	S ☐ U ☐ N/A ☐	S ☐ U ☐ N/A ☐

Continued

	Peer Evaluation Laboratory Setting	Instructor Evaluation Laboratory Setting	Instructor Evaluation Clinical Setting
10. Ensures that the patient performs procedure until acceptability and repeatability criteria are achieved.	S ☐ U ☐ N/A ☐	S ☐ U ☐ N/A ☐	S ☐ U ☐ N/A ☐
11. Removes the supplies from the patient's room, and cleans the area, as needed.	S ☐ U ☐ N/A ☐	S ☐ U ☐ N/A ☐	S ☐ U ☐ N/A ☐
12. Removes the PPE, and performs proper hand hygiene prior to leaving the patient's room.	S ☐ U ☐ N/A ☐	S ☐ U ☐ N/A ☐	S ☐ U ☐ N/A ☐

Evaluation of Procedure

1. Establishes a baseline, or compares with previous measurements.	S ☐ U ☐ N/A ☐	S ☐ U ☐ N/A ☐	S ☐ U ☐ N/A ☐
2. Assesses the patient during the test to identify any distress or physical complications.	S ☐ U ☐ N/A ☐	S ☐ U ☐ N/A ☐	S ☐ U ☐ N/A ☐
3. Interprets the results.	S ☐ U ☐ N/A ☐	S ☐ U ☐ N/A ☐	S ☐ U ☐ N/A ☐
4. Develops an appropriate respiratory care plan based on assessment data.	S ☐ U ☐ N/A ☐	S ☐ U ☐ N/A ☐	S ☐ U ☐ N/A ☐
5. Identifies any unexpected outcomes.	S ☐ U ☐ N/A ☐	S ☐ U ☐ N/A ☐	S ☐ U ☐ N/A ☐

Documentation and Reporting

1. Records findings in the patient's chart as percent of the predicted, BTPS.	S ☐ U ☐ N/A ☐	S ☐ U ☐ N/A ☐	S ☐ U ☐ N/A ☐
2. Reports any abnormal findings to the appropriate health care provider.	S ☐ U ☐ N/A ☐	S ☐ U ☐ N/A ☐	S ☐ U ☐ N/A ☐

Comments:

_____

_____

_____

Signatures:

Student _____ Date Passed _____

Instructor (Laboratory Setting) _____ Date Passed _____

Student _____ Date Passed _____

Instructor (Clinical Setting) _____ Date Passed _____

Student _____ Date _____

Instructor (Laboratory Setting) _____ Date _____

Instructor (Clinical Setting) _____ Date _____

Evaluation:

	Peer Evaluation Laboratory Setting	Instructor Evaluation Laboratory Setting	Instructor Evaluation Clinical Setting
Procedural Preparation			
1. Reviews the patient's chart.	S ☐ U ☐ N/A ☐	S ☐ U ☐ N/A ☐	S ☐ U ☐ N/A ☐
2. Verifies the physician's order or the facility's protocol for standard of care.	S ☐ U ☐ N/A ☐	S ☐ U ☐ N/A ☐	S ☐ U ☐ N/A ☐
3. Obtains, cleans, and inspects the appropriate equipment prior to entering the patient's room.	S ☐ U ☐ N/A ☐	S ☐ U ☐ N/A ☐	S ☐ U ☐ N/A ☐
4. Follows PPE requirements, and observes standard precautions for any transmission-based isolation procedure.	S ☐ U ☐ N/A ☐	S ☐ U ☐ N/A ☐	S ☐ U ☐ N/A ☐
5. Identifies the patient using two patient identifiers.	S ☐ U ☐ N/A ☐	S ☐ U ☐ N/A ☐	S ☐ U ☐ N/A ☐
6. Introduces self to the patient and to the family.	S ☐ U ☐ N/A ☐	S ☐ U ☐ N/A ☐	S ☐ U ☐ N/A ☐
7. Explains the procedure to the patient and to the family, and acknowledges the patient's understanding.	S ☐ U ☐ N/A ☐	S ☐ U ☐ N/A ☐	S ☐ U ☐ N/A ☐
8. Performs proper hand hygiene, and puts on gloves, mask, and protective eyewear, as appropriate for the procedure.	S ☐ U ☐ N/A ☐	S ☐ U ☐ N/A ☐	S ☐ U ☐ N/A ☐
Implementation			
1. Places the patient in a sitting or high-Fowler's position.	S ☐ U ☐ N/A ☐	S ☐ U ☐ N/A ☐	S ☐ U ☐ N/A ☐
2. Assesses vital signs.	S ☐ U ☐ N/A ☐	S ☐ U ☐ N/A ☐	S ☐ U ☐ N/A ☐
3. Provides instruction and demonstrates the tests to the patient before administering them.	S ☐ U ☐ N/A ☐	S ☐ U ☐ N/A ☐	S ☐ U ☐ N/A ☐
4. Positions nose clips.	S ☐ U ☐ N/A ☐	S ☐ U ☐ N/A ☐	S ☐ U ☐ N/A ☐
5. Positions the mouthpiece in the patient's mouth to rest on the top of the patient's tongue.	S ☐ U ☐ N/A ☐	S ☐ U ☐ N/A ☐	S ☐ U ☐ N/A ☐
6. Instructs patient to gently bite down with the teeth and seal the lips firmly around the mouthpiece.	S ☐ U ☐ N/A ☐	S ☐ U ☐ N/A ☐	S ☐ U ☐ N/A ☐
7. Places the spirometer hose or flow sensor in the patient's hand, and instructs him or her to breathe quietly for several breaths.	S ☐ U ☐ N/A ☐	S ☐ U ☐ N/A ☐	S ☐ U ☐ N/A ☐
8. For MEFV and MIFV: a. Instructs the patient to inspire fully and then exhale as rapidly as possible.	S ☐ U ☐ N/A ☐	S ☐ U ☐ N/A ☐	S ☐ U ☐ N/A ☐
b. Instructs the patient to inspire as rapidly as possible from the maximal expiratory level back to maximal inspiration.	S ☐ U ☐ N/A ☐	S ☐ U ☐ N/A ☐	S ☐ U ☐ N/A ☐

Continued

	Peer Evaluation Laboratory Setting			Instructor Evaluation Laboratory Setting			Instructor Evaluation Clinical Setting		
9. Ensures that the patient performs the procedure until acceptability and repeatability criteria are achieved.	S ☐	U ☐	N/A ☐	S ☐	U ☐	N/A ☐	S ☐	U ☐	N/A ☐
10. Removes the supplies from the patient's room, and cleans the area, as needed.	S ☐	U ☐	N/A ☐	S ☐	U ☐	N/A ☐	S ☐	U ☐	N/A ☐
11. Removes PPE, and performs proper hand hygiene prior to leaving the patient's room.	S ☐	U ☐	N/A ☐	S ☐	U ☐	N/A ☐	S ☐	U ☐	N/A ☐

Evaluation of Procedure

1. Establishes a baseline, or compares with previous measurements.	S ☐	U ☐	N/A ☐	S ☐	U ☐	N/A ☐	S ☐	U ☐	N/A ☐
2. Assesses the patient during the test to identify any distress or physical complications.	S ☐	U ☐	N/A ☐	S ☐	U ☐	N/A ☐	S ☐	U ☐	N/A ☐
3. Interprets the results.	S ☐	U ☐	N/A ☐	S ☐	U ☐	N/A ☐	S ☐	U ☐	N/A ☐
4. Develops an appropriate respiratory care plan based on assessment data.	S ☐	U ☐	N/A ☐	S ☐	U ☐	N/A ☐	S ☐	U ☐	N/A ☐
5. Identifies any unexpected outcomes.	S ☐	U ☐	N/A ☐	S ☐	U ☐	N/A ☐	S ☐	U ☐	N/A ☐

Documentation and Reporting

1. Records findings in the patient's chart as percent of predicted, BTPS.	S ☐	U ☐	N/A ☐	S ☐	U ☐	N/A ☐	S ☐	U ☐	N/A ☐
2. Reports any abnormal findings to the appropriate health care provider.	S ☐	U ☐	N/A ☐	S ☐	U ☐	N/A ☐	S ☐	U ☐	N/A ☐

Comments:

_____

_____

_____

Signatures:

Student _____ Date Passed _____

Instructor (Laboratory Setting) _____ Date Passed _____

Student _____ Date Passed _____

Instructor (Clinical Setting) _____ Date Passed _____

Student _____ Date _____

Instructor (Laboratory Setting) _____ Date _____

Instructor (Clinical Setting) _____ Date _____

Criteria for assessment success:

The student must obtain all **satisfactory (S)** scores to pass the procedural evaluation. Any **unsatisfactory (U)** scores will result in failure of the procedural assessment.

Scoring:

Satisfactory (S): Procedural step performed correctly with no instructor prompting. Student-initiated correction is acceptable.

Unsatisfactory (U): Procedural step was performed incorrectly, omitted, or performed in a way that compromised patient care.

Not applicable (N/A): Procedural step was not indicated or necessary.

Evaluation:

	Peer Evaluation Laboratory Setting	Instructor Evaluation Laboratory Setting	Instructor Evaluation Clinical Setting
Procedural Preparation			
1. Reviews the patient's chart.	S ☐ U ☐ N/A ☐	S ☐ U ☐ N/A ☐	S ☐ U ☐ N/A ☐
Implementation			
1. Confirms the patient's name and the date the chest radiograph was taken.	S ☐ U ☐ N/A ☐	S ☐ U ☐ N/A ☐	S ☐ U ☐ N/A ☐
2. Identifies the type of film.	S ☐ U ☐ N/A ☐	S ☐ U ☐ N/A ☐	S ☐ U ☐ N/A ☐
3. Looks for markers, and notes the position of the patient.	S ☐ U ☐ N/A ☐	S ☐ U ☐ N/A ☐	S ☐ U ☐ N/A ☐
4. Evaluates the quality of the radiograph.	S ☐ U ☐ N/A ☐	S ☐ U ☐ N/A ☐	S ☐ U ☐ N/A ☐
5. Evaluates the airway.	S ☐ U ☐ N/A ☐	S ☐ U ☐ N/A ☐	S ☐ U ☐ N/A ☐
6. Evaluates the cardiac silhouette.	S ☐ U ☐ N/A ☐	S ☐ U ☐ N/A ☐	S ☐ U ☐ N/A ☐
7. Evaluates the bones.	S ☐ U ☐ N/A ☐	S ☐ U ☐ N/A ☐	S ☐ U ☐ N/A ☐
8. Evaluates the hemidiaphragms and lung edges.	S ☐ U ☐ N/A ☐	S ☐ U ☐ N/A ☐	S ☐ U ☐ N/A ☐
9. Evaluates the lung fields.	S ☐ U ☐ N/A ☐	S ☐ U ☐ N/A ☐	S ☐ U ☐ N/A ☐
10. Evaluates the hilum.	S ☐ U ☐ N/A ☐	S ☐ U ☐ N/A ☐	S ☐ U ☐ N/A ☐
11. Evaluates soft tissue.	S ☐ U ☐ N/A ☐	S ☐ U ☐ N/A ☐	S ☐ U ☐ N/A ☐
12. Evaluates for the presence of instrumentation.	S ☐ U ☐ N/A ☐	S ☐ U ☐ N/A ☐	S ☐ U ☐ N/A ☐
Evaluation of Procedure			
1. Establishes a baseline, or compares with previous measurements.	S ☐ U ☐ N/A ☐	S ☐ U ☐ N/A ☐	S ☐ U ☐ N/A ☐
2. Trends the data if multiple radiographs are available.	S ☐ U ☐ N/A ☐	S ☐ U ☐ N/A ☐	S ☐ U ☐ N/A ☐

Continued

	Peer Evaluation Laboratory Setting	Instructor Evaluation Laboratory Setting	Instructor Evaluation Clinical Setting
3. Develops an appropriate respiratory care plan based on assessment data.	S ☐ U ☐ N/A ☐	S ☐ U ☐ N/A ☐	S ☐ U ☐ N/A ☐
4. Interprets from general data to specific data.	S ☐ U ☐ N/A ☐	S ☐ U ☐ N/A ☐	S ☐ U ☐ N/A ☐

Documentation and Reporting

1. Reports any abnormal findings to the appropriate health care provider.	S ☐ U ☐ N/A ☐	S ☐ U ☐ N/A ☐	S ☐ U ☐ N/A ☐

Comments:

_____

_____

_____

Signatures:

Student _____ Date Passed _____

Instructor (Laboratory Setting) _____ Date Passed _____

Student _____ Date Passed _____

Instructor (Clinical Setting) _____ Date Passed _____

Student _____ Date _____

Instructor (Laboratory Setting) _____ Date _____

Instructor (Clinical Setting) _____ Date _____

Criteria for assessment success:

The student must obtain all **satisfactory (S)** scores to pass the procedural evaluation. Any **unsatisfactory (U)** scores will result in failure of the procedural assessment.

Scoring:

Satisfactory (S): Procedural step performed correctly with no instructor prompting. Student-initiated correction is acceptable.

Unsatisfactory (U): Procedural step was performed incorrectly, omitted, or performed in a way that compromised patient care.

Not applicable (N/A): Procedural step was not indicated or necessary.

Evaluation:

	Peer Evaluation Laboratory Setting	Instructor Evaluation Laboratory Setting	Instructor Evaluation Clinical Setting
Procedural Preparation			
1. Reviews the patient's chart.	S ☐ U ☐ N/A ☐	S ☐ U ☐ N/A ☐	S ☐ U ☐ N/A ☐
2. Verifies the physician's order or the facility's protocol for standard of care.	S ☐ U ☐ N/A ☐	S ☐ U ☐ N/A ☐	S ☐ U ☐ N/A ☐
3. Obtains, cleans, and inspects the appropriate equipment prior to entering the patient's room.	S ☐ U ☐ N/A ☐	S ☐ U ☐ N/A ☐	S ☐ U ☐ N/A ☐
4. Follows PPE requirements, and observes standard precautions for any transmission-based isolation procedure.	S ☐ U ☐ N/A ☐	S ☐ U ☐ N/A ☐	S ☐ U ☐ N/A ☐
5. Identifies the patient using two patient identifiers.	S ☐ U ☐ N/A ☐	S ☐ U ☐ N/A ☐	S ☐ U ☐ N/A ☐
6. Introduces self to the patient and to the family.	S ☐ U ☐ N/A ☐	S ☐ U ☐ N/A ☐	S ☐ U ☐ N/A ☐
7. Explains the procedure to the patient and to the family, and acknowledges the patient's understanding.	S ☐ U ☐ N/A ☐	S ☐ U ☐ N/A ☐	S ☐ U ☐ N/A ☐
8. Performs proper hand hygiene, and puts on gloves, mask, and protective eyewear, as appropriate for the procedure.	S ☐ U ☐ N/A ☐	S ☐ U ☐ N/A ☐	S ☐ U ☐ N/A ☐
Implementation			
1. Places the patient in a comfortable position, and instructs him or her to breathe normally.	S ☐ U ☐ N/A ☐	S ☐ U ☐ N/A ☐	S ☐ U ☐ N/A ☐
2. Assesses vital signs and symptoms of upper airway obstruction requiring oropharyngeal suctioning.	S ☐ U ☐ N/A ☐	S ☐ U ☐ N/A ☐	S ☐ U ☐ N/A ☐
3. Connects the tubing and turns on suction device.	S ☐ U ☐ N/A ☐	S ☐ U ☐ N/A ☐	S ☐ U ☐ N/A ☐
4. Removes the oxygen mask, if present.	S ☐ U ☐ N/A ☐	S ☐ U ☐ N/A ☐	S ☐ U ☐ N/A ☐
5. Inserts the rigid tonsillar device, the Yankauer, or the catheter into patient's mouth.	S ☐ U ☐ N/A ☐	S ☐ U ☐ N/A ☐	S ☐ U ☐ N/A ☐

Continued

	Peer Evaluation Laboratory Setting			Instructor Evaluation Laboratory Setting			Instructor Evaluation Clinical Setting		
6. Covers, if needed, the thumb-control valve, and suctions the patient's mouth.	S ☐	U ☐	N/A ☐	S ☐	U ☐	N/A ☐	S ☐	U ☐	N/A ☐
7. Rinses the catheter, and turns off the suction device.	S ☐	U ☐	N/A ☐	S ☐	U ☐	N/A ☐	S ☐	U ☐	N/A ☐
8. Wipes the patient's face, if needed.	S ☐	U ☐	N/A ☐	S ☐	U ☐	N/A ☐	S ☐	U ☐	N/A ☐
9. If removed, replaces patient's oxygen mask.	S ☐	U ☐	N/A ☐	S ☐	U ☐	N/A ☐	S ☐	U ☐	N/A ☐
10. Removes the supplies from the patient's room, and cleans the area, as needed.	S ☐	U ☐	N/A ☐	S ☐	U ☐	N/A ☐	S ☐	U ☐	N/A ☐
11. Removes PPE, and performs proper hand hygiene prior to leaving the patient's room.	S ☐	U ☐	N/A ☐	S ☐	U ☐	N/A ☐	S ☐	U ☐	N/A ☐

Evaluation of Procedure

1. Establishes a baseline, or compares the patient's respiratory assessment before and after suctioning.	S ☐	U ☐	N/A ☐	S ☐	U ☐	N/A ☐	S ☐	U ☐	N/A ☐
2. Repeats suctioning, if needed.	S ☐	U ☐	N/A ☐	S ☐	U ☐	N/A ☐	S ☐	U ☐	N/A ☐
3. Repositions the patient.									
4. Identifies any unexpected outcomes.	S ☐	U ☐	N/A ☐	S ☐	U ☐	N/A ☐	S ☐	U ☐	N/A ☐

Documentation and Reporting

1. Records findings in the patient's chart.	S ☐	U ☐	N/A ☐	S ☐	U ☐	N/A ☐	S ☐	U ☐	N/A ☐
2. Reports any abnormal findings to the appropriate health care provider.	S ☐	U ☐	N/A ☐	S ☐	U ☐	N/A ☐	S ☐	U ☐	N/A ☐

Comments:

_____

_____

_____

Signatures:

Student _____ Date Passed _____

Instructor (Laboratory Setting) _____ Date Passed _____

Student _____ Date Passed _____

Instructor (Clinical Setting) _____ Date Passed _____

Procedural Assessment 11-2

Endotracheal tube suctioning

Student _____ Date _____

Instructor (Laboratory Setting) _____ Date _____

Instructor (Clinical Setting) _____ Date _____

Criteria for assessment success:

The student must obtain all **satisfactory (S)** scores to pass the procedural evaluation. Any **unsatisfactory (U)** scores will result in failure of the procedural assessment.

Scoring:

Satisfactory (S): Procedural step performed correctly with no instructor prompting. Student-initiated correction is acceptable.

Unsatisfactory (U): Procedural step was performed incorrectly, omitted, or performed in a way that compromised patient care.

Not applicable (N/A): Procedural step was not indicated or necessary.

Evaluation:

	Peer Evaluation Laboratory Setting	Instructor Evaluation Laboratory Setting	Instructor Evaluation Clinical Setting
Procedural Preparation			
1. Reviews the patient's chart.	S ☐ U ☐ N/A ☐	S ☐ U ☐ N/A ☐	S ☐ U ☐ N/A ☐
2. Verifies the physician's order or the facility's protocol for standard of care.	S ☐ U ☐ N/A ☐	S ☐ U ☐ N/A ☐	S ☐ U ☐ N/A ☐
3. Obtains, cleans, and inspects the appropriate equipment prior to entering the patient's room.	S ☐ U ☐ N/A ☐	S ☐ U ☐ N/A ☐	S ☐ U ☐ N/A ☐
4. Follows PPE requirements, and observes standard precautions for any transmission-based isolation procedure.	S ☐ U ☐ N/A ☐	S ☐ U ☐ N/A ☐	S ☐ U ☐ N/A ☐
5. Identifies the patient using two patient identifiers.	S ☐ U ☐ N/A ☐	S ☐ U ☐ N/A ☐	S ☐ U ☐ N/A ☐
6. Introduces self to the patient and to the family.	S ☐ U ☐ N/A ☐	S ☐ U ☐ N/A ☐	S ☐ U ☐ N/A ☐
7. Explains the procedure to the patient and to the family, and acknowledges the patient's understanding.	S ☐ U ☐ N/A ☐	S ☐ U ☐ N/A ☐	S ☐ U ☐ N/A ☐
8. Performs proper hand hygiene, and puts on gloves, mask, and protective eyewear, as appropriate for the procedure.	S ☐ U ☐ N/A ☐	S ☐ U ☐ N/A ☐	S ☐ U ☐ N/A ☐
Implementation			
1. Positions the patient.	S ☐ U ☐ N/A ☐	S ☐ U ☐ N/A ☐	S ☐ U ☐ N/A ☐
2. Assesses vital signs and need for suctioning.	S ☐ U ☐ N/A ☐	S ☐ U ☐ N/A ☐	S ☐ U ☐ N/A ☐
3. Hyperoxygenates the patient, according to institutional protocol and the patient's condition.	S ☐ U ☐ N/A ☐	S ☐ U ☐ N/A ☐	S ☐ U ☐ N/A ☐
4. Performs closed in-line suctioning.	S ☐ U ☐ N/A ☐	S ☐ U ☐ N/A ☐	S ☐ U ☐ N/A ☐
5. Hyperoxygenates the patient by using the same method as step 3.	S ☐ U ☐ N/A ☐	S ☐ U ☐ N/A ☐	S ☐ U ☐ N/A ☐
6. Performs oropharyngeal suctioning, if indicated (see PA 11-1).	S ☐ U ☐ N/A ☐	S ☐ U ☐ N/A ☐	S ☐ U ☐ N/A ☐

Continued

	Peer Evaluation Laboratory Setting			Instructor Evaluation Laboratory Setting			Instructor Evaluation Clinical Setting		
7. Removes the supplies from the patient's room, and cleans the area, as needed.	S ☐	U ☐	N/A ☐	S ☐	U ☐	N/A ☐	S ☐	U ☐	N/A ☐
8. Removes PPE, and performs proper hand hygiene prior to leaving the patient's room.	S ☐	U ☐	N/A ☐	S ☐	U ☐	N/A ☐	S ☐	U ☐	N/A ☐

Evaluation of Procedure

1. Establishes a baseline, or compares the patient's respiratory assessment before and after suctioning.	S ☐	U ☐	N/A ☐	S ☐	U ☐	N/A ☐	S ☐	U ☐	N/A ☐
2. Repeats suctioning, if needed.	S ☐	U ☐	N/A ☐	S ☐	U ☐	N/A ☐	S ☐	U ☐	N/A ☐
3. Repositions the patient, if needed.	S ☐	U ☐	N/A ☐	S ☐	U ☐	N/A ☐	S ☐	U ☐	N/A ☐
4. Identifies any unexpected outcomes.	S ☐	U ☐	N/A ☐	S ☐	U ☐	N/A ☐	S ☐	U ☐	N/A ☐

Documentation and Reporting

1. Records findings in the patient's chart.	S ☐	U ☐	N/A ☐	S ☐	U ☐	N/A ☐	S ☐	U ☐	N/A ☐
2. Reports any abnormal findings to the appropriate health care provider.	S ☐	U ☐	N/A ☐	S ☐	U ☐	N/A ☐	S ☐	U ☐	N/A ☐

Comments:

_____

_____

_____

Signatures:

Student _____ Date Passed _____

Instructor (Laboratory Setting) _____ Date Passed _____

Student _____ Date Passed _____

Instructor (Clinical Setting) _____ Date Passed _____

Procedural Assessment 11-3   Nasotracheal suctioning

Student _____ Date _____

Instructor (Laboratory Setting) _____ Date _____

Instructor (Clinical Setting) _____ Date _____

Criteria for assessment success:

The student must obtain all **satisfactory (S)** scores to pass the procedural evaluation. Any **unsatisfactory (U)** scores will result in failure of the procedural assessment.

Scoring:

Satisfactory (S): Procedural step performed correctly with no instructor prompting. Student-initiated correction is acceptable.

Unsatisfactory (U): Procedural step was performed incorrectly, omitted, or performed in a way that compromised patient care.

Not applicable (N/A): Procedural step was not indicated or necessary.

Evaluation:

	Peer Evaluation Laboratory Setting	Instructor Evaluation Laboratory Setting	Instructor Evaluation Clinical Setting
Procedural Preparation			
1. Reviews the patient's chart.	S ☐ U ☐ N/A ☐	S ☐ U ☐ N/A ☐	S ☐ U ☐ N/A ☐
2. Verifies the physician's order or the facility's protocol for standard of care.	S ☐ U ☐ N/A ☐	S ☐ U ☐ N/A ☐	S ☐ U ☐ N/A ☐
3. Obtains, cleans, and inspects the appropriate equipment prior to entering the patient's room.	S ☐ U ☐ N/A ☐	S ☐ U ☐ N/A ☐	S ☐ U ☐ N/A ☐
4. Follows PPE requirements, and observes standard precautions for any transmission-based isolation procedure.	S ☐ U ☐ N/A ☐	S ☐ U ☐ N/A ☐	S ☐ U ☐ N/A ☐
5. Identifies the patient using two patient identifiers.	S ☐ U ☐ N/A ☐	S ☐ U ☐ N/A ☐	S ☐ U ☐ N/A ☐
6. Introduces self to the patient and to the family.	S ☐ U ☐ N/A ☐	S ☐ U ☐ N/A ☐	S ☐ U ☐ N/A ☐
7. Explains the procedure to the patient and to the family, and acknowledges the patient's understanding.	S ☐ U ☐ N/A ☐	S ☐ U ☐ N/A ☐	S ☐ U ☐ N/A ☐
8. Performs proper hand hygiene, and puts on gloves, mask, and protective eyewear, as appropriate for the procedure.	S ☐ U ☐ N/A ☐	S ☐ U ☐ N/A ☐	S ☐ U ☐ N/A ☐
Implementation			
1. Places the patient in a comfortable position, and instructs him or her to breathe normally.	S ☐ U ☐ N/A ☐	S ☐ U ☐ N/A ☐	S ☐ U ☐ N/A ☐
2. Assesses vital signs and need for suctioning.	S ☐ U ☐ N/A ☐	S ☐ U ☐ N/A ☐	S ☐ U ☐ N/A ☐
3. Assembles and checks the equipment.	S ☐ U ☐ N/A ☐	S ☐ U ☐ N/A ☐	S ☐ U ☐ N/A ☐
4. Preoxygenates patient, as indicated.	S ☐ U ☐ N/A ☐	S ☐ U ☐ N/A ☐	S ☐ U ☐ N/A ☐
5. Removes the oxygen delivery device, if present.	S ☐ U ☐ N/A ☐	S ☐ U ☐ N/A ☐	S ☐ U ☐ N/A ☐
6. Coats the distal end of suction catheter with a water-soluble lubricant.	S ☐ U ☐ N/A ☐	S ☐ U ☐ N/A ☐	S ☐ U ☐ N/A ☐
7. Applies sterile glove to the dominant hand.	S ☐ U ☐ N/A ☐	S ☐ U ☐ N/A ☐	S ☐ U ☐ N/A ☐

Continued

	Peer Evaluation Laboratory Setting			Instructor Evaluation Laboratory Setting			Instructor Evaluation Clinical Setting		
8. Inserts the catheter gently through the nostril, directs it toward the septum and floor of the nasal cavity, twists the catheter to ease insertion, if needed.	S ☐	U ☐	N/A ☐	S ☐	U ☐	N/A ☐	S ☐	U ☐	N/A ☐
9. Has the patient assume a "sniffing" position.	S ☐	U ☐	N/A ☐	S ☐	U ☐	N/A ☐	S ☐	U ☐	N/A ☐
10. Advances the catheter until resistance is felt or the patient coughs.	S ☐	U ☐	N/A ☐	S ☐	U ☐	N/A ☐	S ☐	U ☐	N/A ☐
11. Applies suction while withdrawing catheter for no more than 15 seconds.	S ☐	U ☐	N/A ☐	S ☐	U ☐	N/A ☐	S ☐	U ☐	N/A ☐
12. Maintains sterile technique.	S ☐	U ☐	N/A ☐	S ☐	U ☐	N/A ☐	S ☐	U ☐	N/A ☐
13. Oxygenates according to procedure, as needed.	S ☐	U ☐	N/A ☐	S ☐	U ☐	N/A ☐	S ☐	U ☐	N/A ☐
14. Suctions the oropharynx, if needed (see PA 11-1).	S ☐	U ☐	N/A ☐	S ☐	U ☐	N/A ☐	S ☐	U ☐	N/A ☐
15. Removes the supplies from the patient's room, and cleans the area, as needed.	S ☐	U ☐	N/A ☐	S ☐	U ☐	N/A ☐	S ☐	U ☐	N/A ☐
16. Removes the PPE, and performs proper hand hygiene prior to leaving the patient's room.	S ☐	U ☐	N/A ☐	S ☐	U ☐	N/A ☐	S ☐	U ☐	N/A ☐

Evaluation of Procedure

	Peer Evaluation Laboratory Setting			Instructor Evaluation Laboratory Setting			Instructor Evaluation Clinical Setting		
1. Establishes a baseline, or compares the patient's respiratory assessment before and after suctioning.	S ☐	U ☐	N/A ☐	S ☐	U ☐	N/A ☐	S ☐	U ☐	N/A ☐
2. Repeats suctioning, if needed.	S ☐	U ☐	N/A ☐	S ☐	U ☐	N/A ☐	S ☐	U ☐	N/A ☐
3. Repositions patient.	S ☐	U ☐	N/A ☐	S ☐	U ☐	N/A ☐	S ☐	U ☐	N/A ☐
4. Identifies any unexpected outcomes.	S ☐	U ☐	N/A ☐	S ☐	U ☐	N/A ☐	S ☐	U ☐	N/A ☐

Documentation and Reporting

	Peer Evaluation Laboratory Setting			Instructor Evaluation Laboratory Setting			Instructor Evaluation Clinical Setting		
1. Records findings in the patient's chart.	S ☐	U ☐	N/A ☐	S ☐	U ☐	N/A ☐	S ☐	U ☐	N/A ☐
2. Reports any abnormal findings to the appropriate health care provider.	S ☐	U ☐	N/A ☐	S ☐	U ☐	N/A ☐	S ☐	U ☐	N/A ☐

Comments:

_____

_____

_____

Signatures:

Student _____ Date Passed _____

Instructor (Laboratory Setting) _____ Date Passed _____

Student _____ Date Passed _____

Instructor (Clinical Setting) _____ Date Passed _____

Procedural Assessment 11-4

Collecting sputum samples by suctioning

Student _____ Date _____

Instructor (Laboratory Setting) _____ Date _____

Instructor (Clinical Setting) _____ Date _____

Criteria for assessment success:

The student must obtain all **satisfactory (S)** scores to pass the procedural evaluation. Any **unsatisfactory (U)** scores will result in failure of the procedural assessment.

Scoring:

Satisfactory (S): Procedural step performed correctly with no instructor prompting. Student-initiated correction is acceptable.

Unsatisfactory (U): Procedural step was performed incorrectly, omitted, or performed in a way that compromised patient care.

Not applicable (N/A): Procedural step was not indicated or necessary.

Evaluation:

	Peer Evaluation Laboratory Setting	Instructor Evaluation Laboratory Setting	Instructor Evaluation Clinical Setting
Procedural Preparation			
1. Reviews the patient's chart.	S ☐ U ☐ N/A ☐	S ☐ U ☐ N/A ☐	S ☐ U ☐ N/A ☐
2. Verifies the physician's order or the facility's protocol for standard of care.	S ☐ U ☐ N/A ☐	S ☐ U ☐ N/A ☐	S ☐ U ☐ N/A ☐
3. Obtains, cleans, and inspects the appropriate equipment prior to entering the patient's room.	S ☐ U ☐ N/A ☐	S ☐ U ☐ N/A ☐	S ☐ U ☐ N/A ☐
4. Follows PPE requirements, and observes standard precautions for any transmission-based isolation procedure.	S ☐ U ☐ N/A ☐	S ☐ U ☐ N/A ☐	S ☐ U ☐ N/A ☐
5. Identifies the patient using two patient identifiers.	S ☐ U ☐ N/A ☐	S ☐ U ☐ N/A ☐	S ☐ U ☐ N/A ☐
6. Introduces self to the patient and to the family.	S ☐ U ☐ N/A ☐	S ☐ U ☐ N/A ☐	S ☐ U ☐ N/A ☐
7. Explains the procedure to the patient and to the family, and acknowledges the patient's understanding.	S ☐ U ☐ N/A ☐	S ☐ U ☐ N/A ☐	S ☐ U ☐ N/A ☐
8. Performs proper hand hygiene, and puts on gloves, mask, and protective eyewear, as appropriate for the procedure.	S ☐ U ☐ N/A ☐	S ☐ U ☐ N/A ☐	S ☐ U ☐ N/A ☐
Implementation			
1. Places the patient in a comfortable position, and instructs him or her to breathe normally.	S ☐ U ☐ N/A ☐	S ☐ U ☐ N/A ☐	S ☐ U ☐ N/A ☐
2. Assesses vital signs.	S ☐ U ☐ N/A ☐	S ☐ U ☐ N/A ☐	S ☐ U ☐ N/A ☐
3. Places a new catheter just before a suction sample is taken, if a closed suction system is being used.	S ☐ U ☐ N/A ☐	S ☐ U ☐ N/A ☐	S ☐ U ☐ N/A ☐
4. Applies sterile glove to the dominant hand.	S ☐ U ☐ N/A ☐	S ☐ U ☐ N/A ☐	S ☐ U ☐ N/A ☐
5. Inserts the specimen trap without applying suction.	S ☐ U ☐ N/A ☐	S ☐ U ☐ N/A ☐	S ☐ U ☐ N/A ☐
6. Suctions for no more than 15 seconds.	S ☐ U ☐ N/A ☐	S ☐ U ☐ N/A ☐	S ☐ U ☐ N/A ☐

Continued

	Peer Evaluation Laboratory Setting			Instructor Evaluation Laboratory Setting			Instructor Evaluation Clinical Setting		
7. Collects 2 to 10 mL of sputum, and labels, per facility's policy.	S ☐	U ☐	N/A ☐	S ☐	U ☐	N/A ☐	S ☐	U ☐	N/A ☐
8. Detaches the catheter from the sputum trap, and covers, while maintaining sterile technique.	S ☐	U ☐	N/A ☐	S ☐	U ☐	N/A ☐	S ☐	U ☐	N/A ☐
9. Removes the supplies from the patient's room, and cleans the area, as needed.	S ☐	U ☐	N/A ☐	S ☐	U ☐	N/A ☐	S ☐	U ☐	N/A ☐
10. Removes PPE, and performs proper hand hygiene prior to leaving the patient's room.	S ☐	U ☐	N/A ☐	S ☐	U ☐	N/A ☐	S ☐	U ☐	N/A ☐

Evaluation of Procedure

1. Establishes a baseline, or compares the patient's respiratory assessment before and after suctioning.	S ☐	U ☐	N/A ☐	S ☐	U ☐	N/A ☐	S ☐	U ☐	N/A ☐
2. Repeats suctioning, if needed.	S ☐	U ☐	N/A ☐	S ☐	U ☐	N/A ☐	S ☐	U ☐	N/A ☐
3. Repositions the patient.	S ☐	U ☐	N/A ☐	S ☐	U ☐	N/A ☐	S ☐	U ☐	N/A ☐
4. Identifies any unexpected outcomes.	S ☐	U ☐	N/A ☐	S ☐	U ☐	N/A ☐	S ☐	U ☐	N/A ☐

Documentation and Reporting

1. Records findings in the patient's chart.	S ☐	U ☐	N/A ☐	S ☐	U ☐	N/A ☐	S ☐	U ☐	N/A ☐
2. Reports any abnormal findings to the appropriate health care provider.	S ☐	U ☐	N/A ☐	S ☐	U ☐	N/A ☐	S ☐	U ☐	N/A ☐

Comments:

_____

_____

_____

Signatures:

Student _____ Date Passed _____

Instructor (Laboratory Setting) _____ Date Passed _____

Student _____ Date Passed _____

Instructor (Clinical Setting) _____ Date Passed _____

Procedural Assessment 11-5

Inserting an oropharyngeal airway

Student _____ Date _____

Instructor (Laboratory Setting) _____ Date _____

Instructor (Clinical Setting) _____ Date _____

Criteria for assessment success:

The student must obtain all **satisfactory (S)** scores to pass the procedural evaluation. Any **unsatisfactory (U)** scores will result in failure of the procedural assessment.

Scoring:

Satisfactory (S): Procedural step performed correctly with no instructor prompting. Student-initiated correction is acceptable.

Unsatisfactory (U): Procedural step was performed incorrectly, omitted, or performed in a way that compromised patient care.

Not applicable (N/A): Procedural step was not indicated or necessary.

Evaluation:

	Peer Evaluation Laboratory Setting	Instructor Evaluation Laboratory Setting	Instructor Evaluation Clinical Setting
Procedural Preparation			
1. Reviews the patient's chart.	S ☐ U ☐ N/A ☐	S ☐ U ☐ N/A ☐	S ☐ U ☐ N/A ☐
2. Verifies the physician's order or the facility's protocol for standard of care.	S ☐ U ☐ N/A ☐	S ☐ U ☐ N/A ☐	S ☐ U ☐ N/A ☐
3. Obtains, cleans, and inspects the appropriate equipment prior to entering the patient's room.	S ☐ U ☐ N/A ☐	S ☐ U ☐ N/A ☐	S ☐ U ☐ N/A ☐
4. Follows PPE requirements, and observes standard precautions for any transmission-based isolation procedure.	S ☐ U ☐ N/A ☐	S ☐ U ☐ N/A ☐	S ☐ U ☐ N/A ☐
5. Identifies the patient using two patient identifiers.	S ☐ U ☐ N/A ☐	S ☐ U ☐ N/A ☐	S ☐ U ☐ N/A ☐
6. Introduces self to the patient and to the family.	S ☐ U ☐ N/A ☐	S ☐ U ☐ N/A ☐	S ☐ U ☐ N/A ☐
7. Explains the procedure to the patient and to the family, and acknowledges the patient's understanding.	S ☐ U ☐ N/A ☐	S ☐ U ☐ N/A ☐	S ☐ U ☐ N/A ☐
8. Performs proper hand hygiene, and puts on gloves, mask, and protective eyewear, as appropriate for the procedure.	S ☐ U ☐ N/A ☐	S ☐ U ☐ N/A ☐	S ☐ U ☐ N/A ☐
Implementation			
1. Positions the patient.	S ☐ U ☐ N/A ☐	S ☐ U ☐ N/A ☐	S ☐ U ☐ N/A ☐
2. Assesses vital signs and for presence of a gag reflex.	S ☐ U ☐ N/A ☐	S ☐ U ☐ N/A ☐	S ☐ U ☐ N/A ☐
3. Opens the patient's mouth.	S ☐ U ☐ N/A ☐	S ☐ U ☐ N/A ☐	S ☐ U ☐ N/A ☐
4. Inserts the oral airway with curved end up and to one side of the oropharynx, and turns the airway over after reaching the back of the throat.	S ☐ U ☐ N/A ☐	S ☐ U ☐ N/A ☐	S ☐ U ☐ N/A ☐
5. Suctions the airway, if needed (see PA 11-1).	S ☐ U ☐ N/A ☐	S ☐ U ☐ N/A ☐	S ☐ U ☐ N/A ☐
6. Removes the supplies from the patient's room, and cleans the area, as needed.	S ☐ U ☐ N/A ☐	S ☐ U ☐ N/A ☐	S ☐ U ☐ N/A ☐

Continued

	Peer Evaluation Laboratory Setting			Instructor Evaluation Laboratory Setting			Instructor Evaluation Clinical Setting		
7. Removes PPE, and performs proper hand hygiene prior to leaving the patient's room.	S ☐	U ☐	N/A ☐	S ☐	U ☐	N/A ☐	S ☐	U ☐	N/A ☐

Evaluation of Procedure

1. Establishes a baseline, or compares the patient's respiratory assessment before and after oral airway insertion.	S ☐	U ☐	N/A ☐	S ☐	U ☐	N/A ☐	S ☐	U ☐	N/A ☐
2. Determines the use of airway (i.e., bite block or intermittent until endotracheal intubation is used to secure airway) (see PA 11-6).	S ☐	U ☐	N/A ☐	S ☐	U ☐	N/A ☐	S ☐	U ☐	N/A ☐
3. Repositions the patient, if needed.	S ☐	U ☐	N/A ☐	S ☐	U ☐	N/A ☐	S ☐	U ☐	N/A ☐
4. Identifies any unexpected outcomes.	S ☐	U ☐	N/A ☐	S ☐	U ☐	N/A ☐	S ☐	U ☐	N/A ☐

Documentation and Reporting

1. Records findings in the patient's chart.	S ☐	U ☐	N/A ☐	S ☐	U ☐	N/A ☐	S ☐	U ☐	N/A ☐
2. Reports any abnormal findings to the appropriate health care provider.	S ☐	U ☐	N/A ☐	S ☐	U ☐	N/A ☐	S ☐	U ☐	N/A ☐

Comments:

_____

_____

_____

Signatures:

Student _____ Date Passed _____

Instructor (Laboratory Setting) _____ Date Passed _____

Student _____ Date Passed _____

Instructor (Clinical Setting) _____ Date Passed _____

Procedural Assessment 11-6

Student _____ Date _____

Instructor (Laboratory Setting) _____ Date _____

Instructor (Clinical Setting) _____ Date _____

Criteria for assessment success:

The student must obtain all **satisfactory (S)** scores to pass the procedural evaluation. Any **unsatisfactory (U)** scores will result in failure of the procedural assessment.

Scoring:

Satisfactory (S): Procedural step performed correctly with no instructor prompting. Student-initiated correction is acceptable.

Unsatisfactory (U): Procedural step was performed incorrectly, omitted, or performed in a way that compromised patient care.

Not applicable (N/A): Procedural step was not indicated or necessary.

Evaluation:

	Peer Evaluation Laboratory Setting	Instructor Evaluation Laboratory Setting	Instructor Evaluation Clinical Setting
Procedural Preparation			
1. Reviews the patient's chart.	S ☐ U ☐ N/A ☐	S ☐ U ☐ N/A ☐	S ☐ U ☐ N/A ☐
2. Verifies the physician's order or the facility's protocol for standard of care.	S ☐ U ☐ N/A ☐	S ☐ U ☐ N/A ☐	S ☐ U ☐ N/A ☐
3. Obtains, cleans, and inspects the appropriate equipment prior to entering the patient's room.	S ☐ U ☐ N/A ☐	S ☐ U ☐ N/A ☐	S ☐ U ☐ N/A ☐
4. Follows PPE requirements, and observes standard precautions for any transmission-based isolation procedure.	S ☐ U ☐ N/A ☐	S ☐ U ☐ N/A ☐	S ☐ U ☐ N/A ☐
5. Identifies the patient using two patient identifiers.	S ☐ U ☐ N/A ☐	S ☐ U ☐ N/A ☐	S ☐ U ☐ N/A ☐
6. Introduces self to the patient and to the family.	S ☐ U ☐ N/A ☐	S ☐ U ☐ N/A ☐	S ☐ U ☐ N/A ☐
7. Explains the procedure to the patient and to the family, and acknowledges the patient's understanding.	S ☐ U ☐ N/A ☐	S ☐ U ☐ N/A ☐	S ☐ U ☐ N/A ☐
8. Performs proper hand hygiene, and puts on gloves, mask, and protective eyewear, as appropriate for the procedure.	S ☐ U ☐ N/A ☐	S ☐ U ☐ N/A ☐	S ☐ U ☐ N/A ☐
Implementation			
1. Positions the patient.	S ☐ U ☐ N/A ☐	S ☐ U ☐ N/A ☐	S ☐ U ☐ N/A ☐
2. Manually ventilates and oxygenates the patient with bag-mask device and 100% oxygen, and suctions, if needed (see PA 11-1).	S ☐ U ☐ N/A ☐	S ☐ U ☐ N/A ☐	S ☐ U ☐ N/A ☐
3. Inserts the laryngoscope correctly.	S ☐ U ☐ N/A ☐	S ☐ U ☐ N/A ☐	S ☐ U ☐ N/A ☐
4. Inserts the endotracheal tube within 15 seconds, and inflates the cuff per the facility's policy.	S ☐ U ☐ N/A ☐	S ☐ U ☐ N/A ☐	S ☐ U ☐ N/A ☐

Continued

	Peer Evaluation Laboratory Setting			Instructor Evaluation Laboratory Setting			Instructor Evaluation Clinical Setting		
5. Ventilates with a bag-mask device, and assesses for proper tube placement:									
a. Visualizes the tube passing through the cords.	S ☐	U ☐	N/A ☐	S ☐	U ☐	N/A ☐	S ☐	U ☐	N/A ☐
b. Uses CO_2 detector.	S ☐	U ☐	N/A ☐	S ☐	U ☐	N/A ☐	S ☐	U ☐	N/A ☐
c. Visualizes condensation in the tube.	S ☐	U ☐	N/A ☐	S ☐	U ☐	N/A ☐	S ☐	U ☐	N/A ☐
6. Visualizes equal chest-rise.	S ☐	U ☐	N/A ☐	S ☐	U ☐	N/A ☐	S ☐	U ☐	N/A ☐
7. Auscultates the epigastric region.	S ☐	U ☐	N/A ☐	S ☐	U ☐	N/A ☐	S ☐	U ☐	N/A ☐
8. Auscultates the left and then the right lung fields.	S ☐	U ☐	N/A ☐	S ☐	U ☐	N/A ☐	S ☐	U ☐	N/A ☐
9. Secures the tube.	S ☐	U ☐	N/A ☐	S ☐	U ☐	N/A ☐	S ☐	U ☐	N/A ☐
10. Orders a chest radiograph to confirm placement.	S ☐	U ☐	N/A ☐	S ☐	U ☐	N/A ☐	S ☐	U ☐	N/A ☐
11. Orders the proper ventilator settings (see PA 22-1).	S ☐	U ☐	N/A ☐	S ☐	U ☐	N/A ☐	S ☐	U ☐	N/A ☐
12. Removes the supplies from the patient's room, and cleans the area, as needed.	S ☐	U ☐	N/A ☐	S ☐	U ☐	N/A ☐	S ☐	U ☐	N/A ☐
13. Removes PPE, and performs proper hand hygiene prior to leaving the patient's room.	S ☐	U ☐	N/A ☐	S ☐	U ☐	N/A ☐	S ☐	U ☐	N/A ☐

Evaluation of Procedure

1. Ensures appropriate ventilation and oxygenation.	S ☐	U ☐	N/A ☐	S ☐	U ☐	N/A ☐	S ☐	U ☐	N/A ☐
2. Identifies any unexpected outcomes.	S ☐	U ☐	N/A ☐	S ☐	U ☐	N/A ☐	S ☐	U ☐	N/A ☐

Documentation and Reporting

1. Records findings in the patient's chart.	S ☐	U ☐	N/A ☐	S ☐	U ☐	N/A ☐	S ☐	U ☐	N/A ☐
2. Reports any abnormal findings to the appropriate health care provider.	S ☐	U ☐	N/A ☐	S ☐	U ☐	N/A ☐	S ☐	U ☐	N/A ☐

Comments:

_____

_____

_____

Signatures:

Student _____ Date Passed _____

Instructor (Laboratory Setting) _____ Date Passed _____

Student _____ Date Passed _____

Instructor (Clinical Setting) _____ Date Passed _____

     Nasotracheal intubation

Student _____ Date _____

Instructor (Laboratory Setting) _____ Date _____

Instructor (Clinical Setting) _____ Date _____

Criteria for assessment success:

The Student must obtain all **satisfactory (S)** scores to pass the procedural evaluation. Any **unsatisfactory (U)** scores will result in failure of the procedural assessment.

Scoring:

Satisfactory (S): Procedural step performed correctly with no instructor prompting. Student-initiated correction is acceptable.

Unsatisfactory (U): Procedural step was performed incorrectly, omitted, or performed in a way that compromised patient care.

Not applicable (N/A): Procedural step was not indicated or necessary.

Evaluation:

	Peer Evaluation Laboratory Setting	Instructor Evaluation Laboratory Setting	Instructor Evaluation Clinical Setting
Procedural Preparation			
1. Reviews the patient's chart.	S ☐ U ☐ N/A ☐	S ☐ U ☐ N/A ☐	S ☐ U ☐ N/A ☐
2. Verifies the physician's order or the facility's protocol for standard of care.	S ☐ U ☐ N/A ☐	S ☐ U ☐ N/A ☐	S ☐ U ☐ N/A ☐
3. Obtains, cleans, and inspects the appropriate equipment prior to entering the patient's room.	S ☐ U ☐ N/A ☐	S ☐ U ☐ N/A ☐	S ☐ U ☐ N/A ☐
4. Follows PPE requirements, and observes standard precautions for any transmission-based isolation procedure.	S ☐ U ☐ N/A ☐	S ☐ U ☐ N/A ☐	S ☐ U ☐ N/A ☐
5. Identifies the patient using two patient identifiers.	S ☐ U ☐ N/A ☐	S ☐ U ☐ N/A ☐	S ☐ U ☐ N/A ☐
6. Introduces self to the patient and to the family.	S ☐ U ☐ N/A ☐	S ☐ U ☐ N/A ☐	S ☐ U ☐ N/A ☐
7. Explains the procedure to the patient and to the family, and acknowledges the patient's understanding.	S ☐ U ☐ N/A ☐	S ☐ U ☐ N/A ☐	S ☐ U ☐ N/A ☐
8. Performs proper hand hygiene, and puts on gloves, mask, and protective eyewear, as appropriate for the procedure.	S ☐ U ☐ N/A ☐	S ☐ U ☐ N/A ☐	S ☐ U ☐ N/A ☐
Implementation			
1. Positions the patient.	S ☐ U ☐ N/A ☐	S ☐ U ☐ N/A ☐	S ☐ U ☐ N/A ☐
2. Manually ventilates and oxygenates the patient with a bag-mask device and 100% oxygen.	S ☐ U ☐ N/A ☐	S ☐ U ☐ N/A ☐	S ☐ U ☐ N/A ☐
3. Applies appropriate medication to the nasal mucosa.	S ☐ U ☐ N/A ☐	S ☐ U ☐ N/A ☐	S ☐ U ☐ N/A ☐
4. Lubricates the tube with water-soluble gel.	S ☐ U ☐ N/A ☐	S ☐ U ☐ N/A ☐	S ☐ U ☐ N/A ☐
5. Inserts the tube properly by using direct visualization or blind passage technique, and inflates the cuff per the facility's policy.	S ☐ U ☐ N/A ☐	S ☐ U ☐ N/A ☐	S ☐ U ☐ N/A ☐

Continued

	Peer Evaluation Laboratory Setting	Instructor Evaluation Laboratory Setting	Instructor Evaluation Clinical Setting
6. Ventilates with a bag-mask device, and assesses for proper tube placement:			
a. Visualizes tube passing through the cords.	S ☐ U ☐ N/A ☐	S ☐ U ☐ N/A ☐	S ☐ U ☐ N/A ☐
b. Uses an end-tidal CO_2 detector.	S ☐ U ☐ N/A ☐	S ☐ U ☐ N/A ☐	S ☐ U ☐ N/A ☐
7. Visualizes equal chest-rise.	S ☐ U ☐ N/A ☐	S ☐ U ☐ N/A ☐	S ☐ U ☐ N/A ☐
8. Auscultates the epigastric region.	S ☐ U ☐ N/A ☐	S ☐ U ☐ N/A ☐	S ☐ U ☐ N/A ☐
9. Auscultates the left and then the right lung fields.	S ☐ U ☐ N/A ☐	S ☐ U ☐ N/A ☐	S ☐ U ☐ N/A ☐
10. Secures the tube.	S ☐ U ☐ N/A ☐	S ☐ U ☐ N/A ☐	S ☐ U ☐ N/A ☐
11. Orders a chest radiograph to confirm placement.	S ☐ U ☐ N/A ☐	S ☐ U ☐ N/A ☐	S ☐ U ☐ N/A ☐
12. Orders proper ventilator settings (see PA 22-1).	S ☐ U ☐ N/A ☐	S ☐ U ☐ N/A ☐	S ☐ U ☐ N/A ☐
13. Removes the supplies from the patient's room, and cleans the area, as needed.	S ☐ U ☐ N/A ☐	S ☐ U ☐ N/A ☐	S ☐ U ☐ N/A ☐
14. Removes PPE, and performs proper hand hygiene prior to leaving the patient's room.	S ☐ U ☐ N/A ☐	S ☐ U ☐ N/A ☐	S ☐ U ☐ N/A ☐

Evaluation of Procedure

1. Ensures appropriate ventilation and oxygenation.	S ☐ U ☐ N/A ☐	S ☐ U ☐ N/A ☐	S ☐ U ☐ N/A ☐
2. Identifies any unexpected outcomes.	S ☐ U ☐ N/A ☐	S ☐ U ☐ N/A ☐	S ☐ U ☐ N/A ☐

Documentation and Reporting

1. Records findings in the patient's chart.	S ☐ U ☐ N/A ☐	S ☐ U ☐ N/A ☐	S ☐ U ☐ N/A ☐
2. Reports any abnormal findings to the appropriate health care provider.	S ☐ U ☐ N/A ☐	S ☐ U ☐ N/A ☐	S ☐ U ☐ N/A ☐

Comments:

_____

_____

_____

Signatures:

Student _____ Date Passed _____

Instructor (Laboratory Setting) _____ Date Passed _____

Student _____ Date Passed _____

Instructor (Clinical Setting) _____ Date Passed _____

Student _____ Date _____

Instructor (Laboratory Setting) _____ Date _____

Instructor (Clinical Setting) _____ Date _____

Evaluation:

	Peer Evaluation Laboratory Setting			Instructor Evaluation Laboratory Setting			Instructor Evaluation Clinical Setting		
Procedural Preparation									
1. Reviews the patient's chart.	S ☐	U ☐	N/A ☐	S ☐	U ☐	N/A ☐	S ☐	U ☐	N/A ☐
2. Verifies the physician's order or the facility's protocol for standard of care.	S ☐	U ☐	N/A ☐	S ☐	U ☐	N/A ☐	S ☐	U ☐	N/A ☐
3. Obtains, cleans, and inspects the appropriate equipment prior to entering the patient's room.	S ☐	U ☐	N/A ☐	S ☐	U ☐	N/A ☐	S ☐	U ☐	N/A ☐
4. Follows PPE requirements, and observes standard precautions for any transmission-based isolation procedure.	S ☐	U ☐	N/A ☐	S ☐	U ☐	N/A ☐	S ☐	U ☐	N/A ☐
5. Identifies the patient using two patient identifiers.	S ☐	U ☐	N/A ☐	S ☐	U ☐	N/A ☐	S ☐	U ☐	N/A ☐
6. Introduces self to the patient and to the family.	S ☐	U ☐	N/A ☐	S ☐	U ☐	N/A ☐	S ☐	U ☐	N/A ☐
7. Explains the procedure to the patient and to the family, and acknowledges the patient's understanding.	S ☐	U ☐	N/A ☐	S ☐	U ☐	N/A ☐	S ☐	U ☐	N/A ☐
8. Performs proper hand hygiene, and puts on gloves, mask, and protective eyewear, as appropriate for the procedure.	S ☐	U ☐	N/A ☐	S ☐	U ☐	N/A ☐	S ☐	U ☐	N/A ☐
Implementation									
1. Positions the patient.	S ☐	U ☐	N/A ☐	S ☐	U ☐	N/A ☐	S ☐	U ☐	N/A ☐
2. Assesses vital signs.	S ☐	U ☐	N/A ☐	S ☐	U ☐	N/A ☐	S ☐	U ☐	N/A ☐
3. Manually ventilates and oxygenates the patient with bag-mask device and 100% oxygen.	S ☐	U ☐	N/A ☐	S ☐	U ☐	N/A ☐	S ☐	U ☐	N/A ☐
4. Suctions the airway, if needed (see PA 11-1).	S ☐	U ☐	N/A ☐	S ☐	U ☐	N/A ☐	S ☐	U ☐	N/A ☐
5. Performs LMA placement:									
a. Lubricates the posterior surface of the mask with water-soluble gel.	S ☐	U ☐	N/A ☐	S ☐	U ☐	N/A ☐	S ☐	U ☐	N/A ☐
b. Ensures that the cuff is fully deflated.	S ☐	U ☐	N/A ☐	S ☐	U ☐	N/A ☐	S ☐	U ☐	N/A ☐
c. Uses the index finger to guide insertion of the laryngeal mask along the palate and down into the oropharynx.	S ☐	U ☐	N/A ☐	S ☐	U ☐	N/A ☐	S ☐	U ☐	N/A ☐
d. Inflates the cuff to a maximum of 60 cmH$_2$O.	S ☐	U ☐	N/A ☐	S ☐	U ☐	N/A ☐	S ☐	U ☐	N/A ☐
6. Performs double-lumen airway placement:									
a. Inserts blindly through the oropharynx into the trachea or esophagus.	S ☐	U ☐	N/A ☐	S ☐	U ☐	N/A ☐	S ☐	U ☐	N/A ☐
b. Inflates the distal cuff with 12 to 15 mL	S ☐	U ☐	N/A ☐	S ☐	U ☐	N/A ☐	S ☐	U ☐	N/A ☐
c. Auscultates the chest and abdomen for breath sounds or gurgling in the epigastrium.	S ☐	U ☐	N/A ☐	S ☐	U ☐	N/A ☐	S ☐	U ☐	N/A ☐
d. In the case of a tracheal entry, inflates both cuffs (the proximal cuff with 85 to 100 mL of air and the distal with 15 mL of air) to prevent air from escaping through the esophagus.	S ☐	U ☐	N/A ☐	S ☐	U ☐	N/A ☐	S ☐	U ☐	N/A ☐

Continued

	Peer Evaluation Laboratory Setting	Instructor Evaluation Laboratory Setting	Instructor Evaluation Clinical Setting
7. Manually ventilates the patient.	S ☐ U ☐ N/A ☐	S ☐ U ☐ N/A ☐	S ☐ U ☐ N/A ☐
8. Visualizes equal chest-rise.			
9. Auscultates the epigastric region.	S ☐ U ☐ N/A ☐	S ☐ U ☐ N/A ☐	S ☐ U ☐ N/A ☐
10. Auscultates left and then right lung fields.	S ☐ U ☐ N/A ☐	S ☐ U ☐ N/A ☐	S ☐ U ☐ N/A ☐
11. Secures the tube.	S ☐ U ☐ N/A ☐	S ☐ U ☐ N/A ☐	S ☐ U ☐ N/A ☐
12. Removes the supplies from the patient's room, and cleans the area, as needed.	S ☐ U ☐ N/A ☐	S ☐ U ☐ N/A ☐	S ☐ U ☐ N/A ☐
13. Removes the PPE, and performs proper hand hygiene prior to leaving the patient's room.	S ☐ U ☐ N/A ☐	S ☐ U ☐ N/A ☐	S ☐ U ☐ N/A ☐

Evaluation of Procedure

1. Ensures appropriate ventilation and oxygenation.	S ☐ U ☐ N/A ☐	S ☐ U ☐ N/A ☐	S ☐ U ☐ N/A ☐
2. Identifies the unexpected outcomes.	S ☐ U ☐ N/A ☐	S ☐ U ☐ N/A ☐	S ☐ U ☐ N/A ☐
3. Uses a temporary airway until endotracheal intubation can be performed.	S ☐ U ☐ N/A ☐	S ☐ U ☐ N/A ☐	S ☐ U ☐ N/A ☐

Documentation and Reporting

1. Records findings in the patient's chart.	S ☐ U ☐ N/A ☐	S ☐ U ☐ N/A ☐	S ☐ U ☐ N/A ☐
2. Reports any abnormal findings to the appropriate health care provider.	S ☐ U ☐ N/A ☐	S ☐ U ☐ N/A ☐	S ☐ U ☐ N/A ☐

Comments:

_____

_____

_____

Signatures:

Student _____ Date Passed _____

Instructor (Laboratory Setting) _____ Date Passed _____

Student _____ Date Passed _____

Instructor (Clinical Setting) _____ Date Passed _____

Procedural Assessment 11-9 Endotracheal tube care

Student _____ Date _____

Instructor (Laboratory Setting) _____ Date _____

Instructor (Clinical Setting) _____ Date _____

Criteria for assessment success:

The student must obtain all **satisfactory (S)** scores to pass the procedural evaluation. Any **unsatisfactory (U)** scores will result in failure of the procedural assessment.

Scoring:

Satisfactory (S): Procedural step performed correctly with no instructor prompting. Student-initiated correction is acceptable.

Unsatisfactory (U): Procedural step was performed incorrectly, omitted, or performed in a way that compromised patient care.

Not applicable (N/A): Procedural step was not indicated or necessary.

Evaluation:

	Peer Evaluation Laboratory Setting	Instructor Evaluation Laboratory Setting	Instructor Evaluation Clinical Setting
Procedural Preparation			
1. Reviews the patient's chart.	S ☐ U ☐ N/A ☐	S ☐ U ☐ N/A ☐	S ☐ U ☐ N/A ☐
2. Verifies the physician's order or the facility's protocol for standard of care.	S ☐ U ☐ N/A ☐	S ☐ U ☐ N/A ☐	S ☐ U ☐ N/A ☐
3. Obtains, cleans, and inspects the appropriate equipment prior to entering the patient's room.	S ☐ U ☐ N/A ☐	S ☐ U ☐ N/A ☐	S ☐ U ☐ N/A ☐
4. Follows PPE requirements, and observes standard precautions for any transmission-based isolation procedure.	S ☐ U ☐ N/A ☐	S ☐ U ☐ N/A ☐	S ☐ U ☐ N/A ☐
5. Identifies the patient using two patient identifiers.	S ☐ U ☐ N/A ☐	S ☐ U ☐ N/A ☐	S ☐ U ☐ N/A ☐
6. Introduces self to the patient and to the family.	S ☐ U ☐ N/A ☐	S ☐ U ☐ N/A ☐	S ☐ U ☐ N/A ☐
7. Explains the procedure to the patient and to the family, and acknowledges the patient's understanding.	S ☐ U ☐ N/A ☐	S ☐ U ☐ N/A ☐	S ☐ U ☐ N/A ☐
8. Performs proper hand hygiene, and puts on gloves, mask, and protective eyewear, as appropriate for the procedure.	S ☐ U ☐ N/A ☐	S ☐ U ☐ N/A ☐	S ☐ U ☐ N/A ☐
Implementation			
1. Places the patient in a comfortable position; observes for signs and symptoms of need to perform ETT care and oral hygiene.	S ☐ U ☐ N/A ☐	S ☐ U ☐ N/A ☐	S ☐ U ☐ N/A ☐
2. Assesses vital signs and baseline ventilation.	S ☐ U ☐ N/A ☐	S ☐ U ☐ N/A ☐	S ☐ U ☐ N/A ☐
3. Assesses ETT depth.	S ☐ U ☐ N/A ☐	S ☐ U ☐ N/A ☐	S ☐ U ☐ N/A ☐
4. Places a towel across the patient's chest.	S ☐ U ☐ N/A ☐	S ☐ U ☐ N/A ☐	S ☐ U ☐ N/A ☐
5. Performs oropharyngeal suctioning (see PA 11-1).	S ☐ U ☐ N/A ☐	S ☐ U ☐ N/A ☐	S ☐ U ☐ N/A ☐

Continued

	Peer Evaluation Laboratory Setting			Instructor Evaluation Laboratory Setting			Instructor Evaluation Clinical Setting		
6. Removes the old tape or device from the tube and the patient's face with the dominant hand while stabilizing the ETT with the other hand.	S ☐	U ☐	N/A ☐	S ☐	U ☐	N/A ☐	S ☐	U ☐	N/A ☐
7. Cleans the adhesive from the patient's face.	S ☐	U ☐	N/A ☐	S ☐	U ☐	N/A ☐	S ☐	U ☐	N/A ☐
8. Removes the oral airway or bite block, and places it on the towel.	S ☐	U ☐	N/A ☐	S ☐	U ☐	N/A ☐	S ☐	U ☐	N/A ☐
9. Cleans the patient's mouth and teeth on both sides of the ETT using a brush or foam swab.	S ☐	U ☐	N/A ☐	S ☐	U ☐	N/A ☐	S ☐	U ☐	N/A ☐
10. Suctions the residue.	S ☐	U ☐	N/A ☐	S ☐	U ☐	N/A ☐	S ☐	U ☐	N/A ☐
11. Cleans the patient's face.	S ☐	U ☐	N/A ☐	S ☐	U ☐	N/A ☐	S ☐	U ☐	N/A ☐
12. Applies skin protectant.	S ☐	U ☐	N/A ☐	S ☐	U ☐	N/A ☐	S ☐	U ☐	N/A ☐
13. Secures the ETT with tape or commercial tube-holding device.	S ☐	U ☐	N/A ☐	S ☐	U ☐	N/A ☐	S ☐	U ☐	N/A ☐
14. Cleans and reinserts the oral airway or bite block.	S ☐	U ☐	N/A ☐	S ☐	U ☐	N/A ☐	S ☐	U ☐	N/A ☐
15. Reassesses the patient.	S ☐	U ☐	N/A ☐	S ☐	U ☐	N/A ☐	S ☐	U ☐	N/A ☐
16. Removes the supplies from the patient's room, and cleans the area, as needed.	S ☐	U ☐	N/A ☐	S ☐	U ☐	N/A ☐	S ☐	U ☐	N/A ☐
17. Removes PPE, and performs proper hand hygiene prior to leaving the patient's room.	S ☐	U ☐	N/A ☐	S ☐	U ☐	N/A ☐	S ☐	U ☐	N/A ☐

Evaluation of Procedure

1. Compares the assessments before and after the procedure.	S ☐	U ☐	N/A ☐	S ☐	U ☐	N/A ☐	S ☐	U ☐	N/A ☐
2. Notes the depth and position of the ETT.	S ☐	U ☐	N/A ☐	S ☐	U ☐	N/A ☐	S ☐	U ☐	N/A ☐
3. Ensures that the ETT is secure.	S ☐	U ☐	N/A ☐	S ☐	U ☐	N/A ☐	S ☐	U ☐	N/A ☐
4. Notes any skin damage or breakdown.	S ☐	U ☐	N/A ☐	S ☐	U ☐	N/A ☐	S ☐	U ☐	N/A ☐
5. Identifies any unexpected outcomes.	S ☐	U ☐	N/A ☐	S ☐	U ☐	N/A ☐	S ☐	U ☐	N/A ☐

Documentation and Reporting

1. Records findings in the patient's chart.	S ☐	U ☐	N/A ☐	S ☐	U ☐	N/A ☐	S ☐	U ☐	N/A ☐
2. Reports any abnormal findings to the appropriate health care provider.	S ☐	U ☐	N/A ☐	S ☐	U ☐	N/A ☐	S ☐	U ☐	N/A ☐

Comments:

_____

_____

_____

Signatures:

Student _____ Date Passed _____

Instructor (Laboratory Setting) _____ Date Passed _____

Student _____ Date Passed _____

Instructor (Clinical Setting) _____ Date Passed _____

Student _____ Date _____

Instructor (Laboratory Setting) _____ Date _____

Instructor (Clinical Setting) _____ Date _____

Criteria for assessment success:

The student must obtain all **satisfactory (S)** scores to pass the procedural evaluation. Any **unsatisfactory (U)** scores will result in failure of the procedural assessment.

Scoring:

Satisfactory (S): Procedural step performed correctly with no instructor prompting. Student-initiated correction is acceptable.

Unsatisfactory (U): Procedural step was performed incorrectly, omitted, or performed in a way that compromised patient care.

Not applicable (N/A): Procedural step was not indicated or necessary.

Evaluation:

	Peer Evaluation Laboratory Setting	Instructor Evaluation Laboratory Setting	Instructor Evaluation Clinical Setting
Procedural Preparation			
1. Reviews the patient's chart.	S ☐ U ☐ N/A ☐	S ☐ U ☐ N/A ☐	S ☐ U ☐ N/A ☐
2. Verifies the physician's order or the facility's protocol for standard of care.	S ☐ U ☐ N/A ☐	S ☐ U ☐ N/A ☐	S ☐ U ☐ N/A ☐
3. Obtains, cleans, and inspects the appropriate equipment prior to entering the patient's room.	S ☐ U ☐ N/A ☐	S ☐ U ☐ N/A ☐	S ☐ U ☐ N/A ☐
4. Follows PPE requirements, and observes standard precautions for any transmission-based isolation procedure.	S ☐ U ☐ N/A ☐	S ☐ U ☐ N/A ☐	S ☐ U ☐ N/A ☐
5. Identifies the patient using two patient identifiers.	S ☐ U ☐ N/A ☐	S ☐ U ☐ N/A ☐	S ☐ U ☐ N/A ☐
6. Introduces self to the patient and to the family.	S ☐ U ☐ N/A ☐	S ☐ U ☐ N/A ☐	S ☐ U ☐ N/A ☐
7. Explains the procedure to the patient and to the family, and acknowledges the patient's understanding.	S ☐ U ☐ N/A ☐	S ☐ U ☐ N/A ☐	S ☐ U ☐ N/A ☐
8. Performs proper hand hygiene, and puts on gloves, mask, and protective eyewear, as appropriate for the procedure.	S ☐ U ☐ N/A ☐	S ☐ U ☐ N/A ☐	S ☐ U ☐ N/A ☐
Implementation			
1. Positions the patient, and locates the pilot balloon; ensures that a 10-mL syringe is available.	S ☐ U ☐ N/A ☐	S ☐ U ☐ N/A ☐	S ☐ U ☐ N/A ☐
2. Assesses vital signs.	S ☐ U ☐ N/A ☐	S ☐ U ☐ N/A ☐	S ☐ U ☐ N/A ☐
3. Measures the cuff pressure.	S ☐ U ☐ N/A ☐	S ☐ U ☐ N/A ☐	S ☐ U ☐ N/A ☐
4. Adjusts the cuff pressure to 20 to 30 cm H_2O.	S ☐ U ☐ N/A ☐	S ☐ U ☐ N/A ☐	S ☐ U ☐ N/A ☐
5. Removes the three-way stopcock or cufflator from the inflation valve when measurements are completed.	S ☐ U ☐ N/A ☐	S ☐ U ☐ N/A ☐	S ☐ U ☐ N/A ☐

Continued

	Peer Evaluation Laboratory Setting			Instructor Evaluation Laboratory Setting			Instructor Evaluation Clinical Setting		
6. Removes the supplies from the patient's room, and cleans the area, as needed.	S ☐	U ☐	N/A ☐	S ☐	U ☐	N/A ☐	S ☐	U ☐	N/A ☐
7. Removes PPE, and performs proper hand hygiene prior to leaving the patient's room.	S ☐	U ☐	N/A ☐	S ☐	U ☐	N/A ☐	S ☐	U ☐	N/A ☐

Evaluation of Procedure

1. Establishes a baseline, or compares with previous measurements.	S ☐	U ☐	N/A ☐	S ☐	U ☐	N/A ☐	S ☐	U ☐	N/A ☐
2. Identifies any unexpected outcomes.	S ☐	U ☐	N/A ☐	S ☐	U ☐	N/A ☐	S ☐	U ☐	N/A ☐

Documentation and Reporting

1. Records findings in the patient's chart.	S ☐	U ☐	N/A ☐	S ☐	U ☐	N/A ☐	S ☐	U ☐	N/A ☐
2. Reports any abnormal findings to the appropriate health care provider.	S ☐	U ☐	N/A ☐	S ☐	U ☐	N/A ☐	S ☐	U ☐	N/A ☐

Comments:

_____

_____

_____

Signatures:

Student _____ Date Passed _____

Instructor (Laboratory Setting) _____ Date Passed _____

Student _____ Date Passed _____

Instructor (Clinical Setting) _____ Date Passed _____

Student _____ Date _____

Instructor (Laboratory Setting) _____ Date _____

Instructor (Clinical Setting) _____ Date _____

Criteria for assessment success:

The student must obtain all **satisfactory (S)** scores to pass the procedural evaluation. Any **unsatisfactory (U)** scores will result in failure of the procedural assessment.

Scoring:

Satisfactory (S): Procedural step performed correctly with no instructor prompting. Student-initiated correction is acceptable.

Unsatisfactory (U): Procedural step was performed incorrectly, omitted, or performed in a way that compromised patient care.

Not applicable (N/A): Procedural step was not indicated or necessary.

Evaluation:

	Peer Evaluation Laboratory Setting	Instructor Evaluation Laboratory Setting	Instructor Evaluation Clinical Setting
Procedural Preparation			
1. Reviews the patient's chart.	S ☐ U ☐ N/A ☐	S ☐ U ☐ N/A ☐	S ☐ U ☐ N/A ☐
2. Verifies the physician's order or the facility's protocol for standard of care.	S ☐ U ☐ N/A ☐	S ☐ U ☐ N/A ☐	S ☐ U ☐ N/A ☐
3. Obtains, cleans, and inspects the appropriate equipment prior to entering the patient's room.	S ☐ U ☐ N/A ☐	S ☐ U ☐ N/A ☐	S ☐ U ☐ N/A ☐
4. Follows PPE requirements, and observes standard precautions for any transmission-based isolation procedure.	S ☐ U ☐ N/A ☐	S ☐ U ☐ N/A ☐	S ☐ U ☐ N/A ☐
5. Identifies the patient using two patient identifiers.	S ☐ U ☐ N/A ☐	S ☐ U ☐ N/A ☐	S ☐ U ☐ N/A ☐
6. Introduces self to the patient and to the family.	S ☐ U ☐ N/A ☐	S ☐ U ☐ N/A ☐	S ☐ U ☐ N/A ☐
7. Explains the procedure to the patient and to the family, and acknowledges the patient's understanding.	S ☐ U ☐ N/A ☐	S ☐ U ☐ N/A ☐	S ☐ U ☐ N/A ☐
8. Performs proper hand hygiene, and puts on gloves, mask, and protective eyewear, as appropriate for the procedure.	S ☐ U ☐ N/A ☐	S ☐ U ☐ N/A ☐	S ☐ U ☐ N/A ☐
Implementation			
1. Places the patient in a comfortable position, and instructs him or her to breathe normally.	S ☐ U ☐ N/A ☐	S ☐ U ☐ N/A ☐	S ☐ U ☐ N/A ☐
2. Assesses vital signs.	S ☐ U ☐ N/A ☐	S ☐ U ☐ N/A ☐	S ☐ U ☐ N/A ☐
3. Suctions the patient, as needed (see PA 11-1).	S ☐ U ☐ N/A ☐	S ☐ U ☐ N/A ☐	S ☐ U ☐ N/A ☐
4. Removes the inner cannula, and reinserts a new cannula.	S ☐ U ☐ N/A ☐	S ☐ U ☐ N/A ☐	S ☐ U ☐ N/A ☐
5. Removes the dressing and tracheostomy ties.	S ☐ U ☐ N/A ☐	S ☐ U ☐ N/A ☐	S ☐ U ☐ N/A ☐
6. Cleans the stoma with an appropriate cleanser or sterile water.	S ☐ U ☐ N/A ☐	S ☐ U ☐ N/A ☐	S ☐ U ☐ N/A ☐
7. Applies new dressing and tracheostomy ties.	S ☐ U ☐ N/A ☐	S ☐ U ☐ N/A ☐	S ☐ U ☐ N/A ☐

Continued

	Peer Evaluation Laboratory Setting			Instructor Evaluation Laboratory Setting			Instructor Evaluation Clinical Setting		
8. Removes the supplies from the patient's room, and cleans the area, as needed.	S ☐	U ☐	N/A ☐	S ☐	U ☐	N/A ☐	S ☐	U ☐	N/A ☐
9. Removes PPE, and performs proper hand hygiene prior to leaving the patient's room.	S ☐	U ☐	N/A ☐	S ☐	U ☐	N/A ☐	S ☐	U ☐	N/A ☐

Evaluation of Procedure

1. Ensures stability of the tracheostomy tube throughout the procedure.	S ☐	U ☐	N/A ☐	S ☐	U ☐	N/A ☐	S ☐	U ☐	N/A ☐
2. Notes any increase in need for oxygen therapy throughout the procedure.	S ☐	U ☐	N/A ☐	S ☐	U ☐	N/A ☐	S ☐	U ☐	N/A ☐
3. Returns the patient to previous therapy.	S ☐	U ☐	N/A ☐	S ☐	U ☐	N/A ☐	S ☐	U ☐	N/A ☐
4. Identifies any unexpected outcomes.	S ☐	U ☐	N/A ☐	S ☐	U ☐	N/A ☐	S ☐	U ☐	N/A ☐

Documentation and Reporting

1. Records findings in the patient's chart.	S ☐	U ☐	N/A ☐	S ☐	U ☐	N/A ☐	S ☐	U ☐	N/A ☐
2. Reports any abnormal findings to the appropriate health care provider.	S ☐	U ☐	N/A ☐	S ☐	U ☐	N/A ☐	S ☐	U ☐	N/A ☐

Comments:

_____

_____

_____

Signatures:

Student _____ Date Passed _____

Instructor (Laboratory Setting) _____ Date Passed _____

Student _____ Date Passed _____

Instructor (Clinical Setting) _____ Date Passed _____

Procedural Assessment 11-12

Student _____ Date _____

Instructor (Laboratory Setting) _____ Date _____

Instructor (Clinical Setting) _____ Date _____

Criteria for assessment success:

Student must obtain all **satisfactory (S)** scores in order to pass the procedural evaluation. Any **unsatisfactory (U)** scores will result in failure of the procedural assessment.

Scoring:

Satisfactory (S): Procedural step performed correctly with no instructor prompting. Student-initiated correction is acceptable.

Unsatisfactory (U): Procedural step was performed incorrectly, omitted, or performed in a way that compromised patient care.

Not applicable (N/A): Procedural step was not indicated or necessary.

Evaluation:

	Peer Evaluation Laboratory Setting	Instructor Evaluation Laboratory Setting	Instructor Evaluation Clinical Setting
Procedural Preparation			
1. Reviews the patient's chart.	S ☐ U ☐ N/A ☐	S ☐ U ☐ N/A ☐	S ☐ U ☐ N/A ☐
2. Verifies the physician's order or the facility's protocol for standard of care.	S ☐ U ☐ N/A ☐	S ☐ U ☐ N/A ☐	S ☐ U ☐ N/A ☐
3. Obtains, cleans, and inspects the appropriate equipment prior to entering the patient's room.	S ☐ U ☐ N/A ☐	S ☐ U ☐ N/A ☐	S ☐ U ☐ N/A ☐
4. Follows PPE requirements, and observes standard precautions for any transmission-based isolation procedure.	S ☐ U ☐ N/A ☐	S ☐ U ☐ N/A ☐	S ☐ U ☐ N/A ☐
5. Identifies the patient using two patient identifiers.	S ☐ U ☐ N/A ☐	S ☐ U ☐ N/A ☐	S ☐ U ☐ N/A ☐
6. Introduces self to the patient and to the family	S ☐ U ☐ N/A ☐	S ☐ U ☐ N/A ☐	S ☐ U ☐ N/A ☐
7. Explains the procedure to the patient and to the family, and acknowledges the patient's understanding.	S ☐ U ☐ N/A ☐	S ☐ U ☐ N/A ☐	S ☐ U ☐ N/A ☐
8. Performs proper hand hygiene, and puts on gloves, mask, and protective eyewear, as appropriate for the procedure.	S ☐ U ☐ N/A ☐	S ☐ U ☐ N/A ☐	S ☐ U ☐ N/A ☐
Implementation			
1. Positions the patient comfortably in a comfortable semi-Fowler position and instructs them to breathe normally.	S ☐ U ☐ N/A ☐	S ☐ U ☐ N/A ☐	S ☐ U ☐ N/A ☐
2. Assesses vital signs.	S ☐ U ☐ N/A ☐	S ☐ U ☐ N/A ☐	S ☐ U ☐ N/A ☐
3. Performs suctioning (see PA 11-2).	S ☐ U ☐ N/A ☐	S ☐ U ☐ N/A ☐	S ☐ U ☐ N/A ☐
4. Prepares and inspects new tracheostomy tube; places in a prepared sterile field.	S ☐ U ☐ N/A ☐	S ☐ U ☐ N/A ☐	S ☐ U ☐ N/A ☐
5. Removes inner cannula of the new tracheostomy tube and inserts obturator into outer cannula.	S ☐ U ☐ N/A ☐	S ☐ U ☐ N/A ☐	S ☐ U ☐ N/A ☐
6. Attaches clean ties to one side of the phalange and checks integrity of cuff by inflating it; then deflates it.	S ☐ U ☐ N/A ☐	S ☐ U ☐ N/A ☐	S ☐ U ☐ N/A ☐

Continued

	Peer Evaluation Laboratory Setting			Instructor Evaluation Laboratory Setting			Instructor Evaluation Clinical Setting		
7. Applies sterile water-soluble lubricant to tip of new tracheostomy tube.	S ☐	U ☐	N/A ☐	S ☐	U ☐	N/A ☐	S ☐	U ☐	N/A ☐
8. On the patient's current tracheostomy; loosens ties and deflates cuff, if inflated.	S ☐	U ☐	N/A ☐	S ☐	U ☐	N/A ☐	S ☐	U ☐	N/A ☐
9. Removes any oxygen or humidity device.	S ☐	U ☐	N/A ☐	S ☐	U ☐	N/A ☐	S ☐	U ☐	N/A ☐
10. Removes old tracheostomy tube.	S ☐	U ☐	N/A ☐	S ☐	U ☐	N/A ☐	S ☐	U ☐	N/A ☐
11. Puts on sterile gloves.	S ☐	U ☐	N/A ☐	S ☐	U ☐	N/A ☐	S ☐	U ☐	N/A ☐
12. Pushes new tracheostomy tube into tracheostomy site, using gentle force.	S ☐	U ☐	N/A ☐	S ☐	U ☐	N/A ☐	S ☐	U ☐	N/A ☐
13. Removes obturator; allows air to flow; then inserts inner cannula.	S ☐	U ☐	N/A ☐	S ☐	U ☐	N/A ☐	S ☐	U ☐	N/A ☐
14. Attaches new tracheostomy ties; inflates cuff and places dressing around stoma, if necessary.	S ☐	U ☐	N/A ☐	S ☐	U ☐	N/A ☐	S ☐	U ☐	N/A ☐
15. Reapplies oxygen or humidity device.	S ☐	U ☐	N/A ☐	S ☐	U ☐	N/A ☐	S ☐	U ☐	N/A ☐
16. Removes the supplies from the patient's room, and cleans the area, as needed.	S ☐	U ☐	N/A ☐	S ☐	U ☐	N/A ☐	S ☐	U ☐	N/A ☐
17. Removes the PPE, and performs proper hand hygiene prior to leaving the patient's room.	S ☐	U ☐	N/A ☐	S ☐	U ☐	N/A ☐	S ☐	U ☐	N/A ☐

Evaluation of Procedure

1. Establishes a baseline, or compares the patient's respiratory assessment before and after tracheostomy tube change.	S ☐	U ☐	N/A ☐	S ☐	U ☐	N/A ☐	S ☐	U ☐	N/A ☐
2. Ensures spare tracheostomy of same size, the size below, and the manual resuscitation bag are available at the patient's bedside.	S ☐	U ☐	N/A ☐	S ☐	U ☐	N/A ☐	S ☐	U ☐	N/A ☐
3. Identifies any unexpected outcomes.	S ☐	U ☐	N/A ☐	S ☐	U ☐	N/A ☐	S ☐	U ☐	N/A ☐

Documentation and Reporting

1. Records findings in the patient's chart.	S ☐	U ☐	N/A ☐	S ☐	U ☐	N/A ☐	S ☐	U ☐	N/A ☐
2. Reports any abnormal findings to the appropriate health care provider.	S ☐	U ☐	N/A ☐	S ☐	U ☐	N/A ☐	S ☐	U ☐	N/A ☐

Comments:

_____

_____

_____

Signatures:

Student _____ Date Passed _____

Instructor (Laboratory Setting) _____ Date Passed _____

Student _____ Date Passed _____

Instructor (Clinical Setting) _____ Date Passed _____

Student _____ Date _____

Instructor (Laboratory Setting) _____ Date _____

Instructor (Clinical Setting) _____ Date _____

Criteria for assessment success:

The student must obtain all **satisfactory (S)** scores to pass the procedural evaluation. Any **unsatisfactory (U)** scores will result in failure of the procedural assessment.

Scoring:

Satisfactory (S): Procedural step performed correctly with no instructor prompting. Student-initiated correction is acceptable.

Unsatisfactory (U): Procedural step was performed incorrectly, omitted, or performed in a way that compromised patient care.

Not applicable (N/A): Procedural step was not indicated or necessary.

Evaluation:

	Peer Evaluation Laboratory Setting	Instructor Evaluation Laboratory Setting	Instructor Evaluation Clinical Setting
Procedural Preparation			
1. Reviews the patient's chart.	S ☐ U ☐ N/A ☐	S ☐ U ☐ N/A ☐	S ☐ U ☐ N/A ☐
2. Verifies the physician's order or the facility's protocol for standard of care.	S ☐ U ☐ N/A ☐	S ☐ U ☐ N/A ☐	S ☐ U ☐ N/A ☐
3. Obtains, cleans, and inspects the appropriate equipment prior to entering the patient's room.	S ☐ U ☐ N/A ☐	S ☐ U ☐ N/A ☐	S ☐ U ☐ N/A ☐
4. Follows PPE requirements, and observes standard precautions for any transmission-based isolation procedure.	S ☐ U ☐ N/A ☐	S ☐ U ☐ N/A ☐	S ☐ U ☐ N/A ☐
5. Identifies the patient using two patient identifiers.	S ☐ U ☐ N/A ☐	S ☐ U ☐ N/A ☐	S ☐ U ☐ N/A ☐
6. Introduces self to the patient and to the family.	S ☐ U ☐ N/A ☐	S ☐ U ☐ N/A ☐	S ☐ U ☐ N/A ☐
7. Explains the procedure to the patient and to the family, and acknowledges the patient's understanding.	S ☐ U ☐ N/A ☐	S ☐ U ☐ N/A ☐	S ☐ U ☐ N/A ☐
8. Performs proper hand hygiene, and puts on gloves, mask, and protective eyewear, as appropriate for the procedure.	S ☐ U ☐ N/A ☐	S ☐ U ☐ N/A ☐	S ☐ U ☐ N/A ☐
Implementation			
1. Places the patient in a comfortable position, and instructs him or her to breathe normally.	S ☐ U ☐ N/A ☐	S ☐ U ☐ N/A ☐	S ☐ U ☐ N/A ☐
2. Assesses vital signs.	S ☐ U ☐ N/A ☐	S ☐ U ☐ N/A ☐	S ☐ U ☐ N/A ☐
3. Suctions the patient's airway (see PA 11-1, 11-2, and 11-3).	S ☐ U ☐ N/A ☐	S ☐ U ☐ N/A ☐	S ☐ U ☐ N/A ☐
4. Hyperoxygenates the patient for 1 to 2 minutes before the extubation procedure.	S ☐ U ☐ N/A ☐	S ☐ U ☐ N/A ☐	S ☐ U ☐ N/A ☐
5. Deflates the cuff, and listens for leaks; if no leak is present, reinflates the cuff, and contacts the physician.	S ☐ U ☐ N/A ☐	S ☐ U ☐ N/A ☐	S ☐ U ☐ N/A ☐
6. Removes the tape or commercial tube holder.	S ☐ U ☐ N/A ☐	S ☐ U ☐ N/A ☐	S ☐ U ☐ N/A ☐

Continued

	Peer Evaluation Laboratory Setting			Instructor Evaluation Laboratory Setting			Instructor Evaluation Clinical Setting		
7. Removes the tube.	S ☐	U ☐	N/A ☐	S ☐	U ☐	N/A ☐	S ☐	U ☐	N/A ☐
8. Applies appropriate oxygen and humidity therapy; has racemic epinephrine ready.	S ☐	U ☐	N/A ☐	S ☐	U ☐	N/A ☐	S ☐	U ☐	N/A ☐
9. Auscultates the patient, and confirms that no stridor is present.	S ☐	U ☐	N/A ☐	S ☐	U ☐	N/A ☐	S ☐	U ☐	N/A ☐
10. Removes the supplies from the patient's room, and cleans the area, as needed.	S ☐	U ☐	N/A ☐	S ☐	U ☐	N/A ☐	S ☐	U ☐	N/A ☐
11. Removes PPE, and performs proper hand hygiene prior to leaving the patient's room.	S ☐	U ☐	N/A ☐	S ☐	U ☐	N/A ☐	S ☐	U ☐	N/A ☐

Evaluation of Procedure

1. Ensures that no immediate complications result from extubation.	S ☐	U ☐	N/A ☐	S ☐	U ☐	N/A ☐	S ☐	U ☐	N/A ☐
2. Notes any use of oxygen or humidity therapy.	S ☐	U ☐	N/A ☐	S ☐	U ☐	N/A ☐	S ☐	U ☐	N/A ☐
3. Identifies any unexpected outcomes.	S ☐	U ☐	N/A ☐	S ☐	U ☐	N/A ☐	S ☐	U ☐	N/A ☐

Documentation and Reporting

1. Records findings in the patient's chart.	S ☐	U ☐	N/A ☐	S ☐	U ☐	N/A ☐	S ☐	U ☐	N/A ☐
2. Reports any abnormal findings to the appropriate health care provider.	S ☐	U ☐	N/A ☐	S ☐	U ☐	N/A ☐	S ☐	U ☐	N/A ☐

Comments:

_____

_____

_____

Signatures:

Student _____ Date Passed _____

Instructor (Laboratory Setting) _____ Date Passed _____

Student _____ Date Passed _____

Instructor (Clinical Setting) _____ Date Passed _____

Procedural Assessment 11-14

Student _____ Date _____

Instructor (Laboratory Setting) _____ Date _____

Instructor (Clinical Setting) _____ Date _____

Evaluation:

	Peer Evaluation Laboratory Setting			Instructor Evaluation Laboratory Setting			Instructor Evaluation Clinical Setting		
Procedural Preparation									
1. Reviews the patient's chart.	S ☐	U ☐	N/A ☐	S ☐	U ☐	N/A ☐	S ☐	U ☐	N/A ☐
2. Verifies the physician's order or the facility's protocol for standard of care.	S ☐	U ☐	N/A ☐	S ☐	U ☐	N/A ☐	S ☐	U ☐	N/A ☐
3. Obtains, cleans, and inspects the appropriate equipment prior to entering the patient's room.	S ☐	U ☐	N/A ☐	S ☐	U ☐	N/A ☐	S ☐	U ☐	N/A ☐
4. Follows PPE requirements, and observes standard precautions for any transmission-based isolation procedure.	S ☐	U ☐	N/A ☐	S ☐	U ☐	N/A ☐	S ☐	U ☐	N/A ☐
5. Identifies the patient using two patient identifiers.	S ☐	U ☐	N/A ☐	S ☐	U ☐	N/A ☐	S ☐	U ☐	N/A ☐
6. Introduces self to the patient and to the family.	S ☐	U ☐	N/A ☐	S ☐	U ☐	N/A ☐	S ☐	U ☐	N/A ☐
7. Explains the procedure to the patient and to the family, and acknowledges the patient's understanding.	S ☐	U ☐	N/A ☐	S ☐	U ☐	N/A ☐	S ☐	U ☐	N/A ☐
8. Performs proper hand hygiene, and puts on gloves, mask, and protective eyewear, as appropriate for the procedure.	S ☐	U ☐	N/A ☐	S ☐	U ☐	N/A ☐	S ☐	U ☐	N/A ☐
9. Assesses the respiratory status.	S ☐	U ☐	N/A ☐	S ☐	U ☐	N/A ☐	S ☐	U ☐	N/A ☐
10. Determines the time the patient last ingested food.	S ☐	U ☐	N/A ☐	S ☐	U ☐	N/A ☐	S ☐	U ☐	N/A ☐
Implementation									
1. Assesses IV access; establishes a new IV line, if required (see PA 24-3).	S ☐	U ☐	N/A ☐	S ☐	U ☐	N/A ☐	S ☐	U ☐	N/A ☐
2. Prepares any patient monitoring equipment (see PA 5-3 and 6-1).	S ☐	U ☐	N/A ☐	S ☐	U ☐	N/A ☐	S ☐	U ☐	N/A ☐
3. Assists the patient in maintaining the required position.	S ☐	U ☐	N/A ☐	S ☐	U ☐	N/A ☐	S ☐	U ☐	N/A ☐
4. Turns off the alarms, if the patient is currently receiving mechanical ventilation.	S ☐	U ☐	N/A ☐	S ☐	U ☐	N/A ☐	S ☐	U ☐	N/A ☐
5. Places the suction catheter near the patient's mouth.	S ☐	U ☐	N/A ☐	S ☐	U ☐	N/A ☐	S ☐	U ☐	N/A ☐
6. Instructs the patient not to swallow as the local anesthetic is sprayed.	S ☐	U ☐	N/A ☐	S ☐	U ☐	N/A ☐	S ☐	U ☐	N/A ☐
7. Attaches the bronchoscope to the machine to provide light.	S ☐	U ☐	N/A ☐	S ☐	U ☐	N/A ☐	S ☐	U ☐	N/A ☐
8. Explains each step to the patient as it occurs.	S ☐	U ☐	N/A ☐	S ☐	U ☐	N/A ☐	S ☐	U ☐	N/A ☐
9. Reassesses the respiratory status continually throughout the procedure.	S ☐	U ☐	N/A ☐	S ☐	U ☐	N/A ☐	S ☐	U ☐	N/A ☐
10. Notes the characteristics of suctioned material.	S ☐	U ☐	N/A ☐	S ☐	U ☐	N/A ☐	S ☐	U ☐	N/A ☐
11. Labels all specimens collected.	S ☐	U ☐	N/A ☐	S ☐	U ☐	N/A ☐	S ☐	U ☐	N/A ☐

Continued

	Peer Evaluation Laboratory Setting			Instructor Evaluation Laboratory Setting			Instructor Evaluation Clinical Setting		
12. Wipes the patient's mouth and nose to remove the lubricant after the bronchoscope has been removed.	S ☐	U ☐	N/A ☐	S ☐	U ☐	N/A ☐	S ☐	U ☐	N/A ☐
13. Returns the alarm settings to acceptable range, if the patient is receiving mechanical ventilation.	S ☐	U ☐	N/A ☐	S ☐	U ☐	N/A ☐	S ☐	U ☐	N/A ☐
14. Removes the supplies from the patient's room, and cleans the area, as needed.	S ☐	U ☐	N/A ☐	S ☐	U ☐	N/A ☐	S ☐	U ☐	N/A ☐
15. Cleans and disinfects the bronchoscope per the manufacturer specifications.	S ☐	U ☐	N/A ☐	S ☐	U ☐	N/A ☐	S ☐	U ☐	N/A ☐
16. Removes PPE, and performs proper hand hygiene prior to leaving the patient's room.	S ☐	U ☐	N/A ☐	S ☐	U ☐	N/A ☐	S ☐	U ☐	N/A ☐

Evaluation of Procedure

1. Observes sputum production.	S ☐	U ☐	N/A ☐	S ☐	U ☐	N/A ☐	S ☐	U ☐	N/A ☐
2. Develops an appropriate respiratory care plan based on assessment data.	S ☐	U ☐	N/A ☐	S ☐	U ☐	N/A ☐	S ☐	U ☐	N/A ☐
3. Notes any use of oxygen therapy or ventilator changes, if applicable.	S ☐	U ☐	N/A ☐	S ☐	U ☐	N/A ☐	S ☐	U ☐	N/A ☐
4. Notes the monitoring devices used during the procedure.	S ☐	U ☐	N/A ☐	S ☐	U ☐	N/A ☐	S ☐	U ☐	N/A ☐
5. Identifies any unexpected outcomes.	S ☐	U ☐	N/A ☐	S ☐	U ☐	N/A ☐	S ☐	U ☐	N/A ☐
6. Correlates findings with other lab findings.	S ☐	U ☐	N/A ☐	S ☐	U ☐	N/A ☐	S ☐	U ☐	N/A ☐

Documentation and Reporting

1. Records findings in the patient's chart.	S ☐	U ☐	N/A ☐	S ☐	U ☐	N/A ☐	S ☐	U ☐	N/A ☐
2. Reports any abnormal findings to the appropriate health care provider.	S ☐	U ☐	N/A ☐	S ☐	U ☐	N/A ☐	S ☐	U ☐	N/A ☐

Comments:

_____

_____

_____

Signatures:

Student _____ Date Passed _____

Instructor (Laboratory Setting) _____ Date Passed _____

Student _____ Date Passed _____

Instructor (Clinical Setting) _____ Date Passed _____

Procedural Assessment 12-1 — Code management

Student _____ Date _____

Instructor (Laboratory Setting) _____ Date _____

Instructor (Clinical Setting) _____ Date _____

Criteria for assessment success:

The student must obtain all **satisfactory (S)** scores to pass the procedural evaluation. Any **unsatisfactory (U)** scores will result in failure of the procedural assessment.

Scoring:

Satisfactory (S): Procedural step performed correctly with no instructor prompting. Student-initiated correction is acceptable.

Unsatisfactory (U): Procedural step was performed incorrectly, omitted, or performed in a way that compromised patient care.

Not applicable (N/A): Procedural step was not indicated or necessary.

Evaluation:

	Peer Evaluation Laboratory Setting	Instructor Evaluation Laboratory Setting	Instructor Evaluation Clinical Setting
Procedural Preparation			
1. Follows PPE requirements and performs proper hand hygiene, and puts on gloves, mask, and protective eyewear, as appropriate for the procedure.	S ☐ U ☐ N/A ☐	S ☐ U ☐ N/A ☐	S ☐ U ☐ N/A ☐
2. Establishes unresponsiveness.	S ☐ U ☐ N/A ☐	S ☐ U ☐ N/A ☐	S ☐ U ☐ N/A ☐
3. Initiates code notification procedures based on his or her facility's protocol for standard of care.	S ☐ U ☐ N/A ☐	S ☐ U ☐ N/A ☐	S ☐ U ☐ N/A ☐
Implementation			
1. Restores circulation:			
a. Determines pulselessness.	S ☐ U ☐ N/A ☐	S ☐ U ☐ N/A ☐	S ☐ U ☐ N/A ☐
b. Performs chest compressions.	S ☐ U ☐ N/A ☐	S ☐ U ☐ N/A ☐	S ☐ U ☐ N/A ☐
2. Restores the airway:			
a. Inspects for any neck or facial trauma.	S ☐ U ☐ N/A ☐	S ☐ U ☐ N/A ☐	S ☐ U ☐ N/A ☐
b. Performs either the head-tilt or chin-lift method or the jaw thrust maneuver to open the airway.	S ☐ U ☐ N/A ☐	S ☐ U ☐ N/A ☐	S ☐ U ☐ N/A ☐
c. Performs oropharyngeal suctioning, if needed (see PA 11-1).	S ☐ U ☐ N/A ☐	S ☐ U ☐ N/A ☐	S ☐ U ☐ N/A ☐
d. Inserts the oropharyngeal airway (see PA 11-5).	S ☐ U ☐ N/A ☐	S ☐ U ☐ N/A ☐	S ☐ U ☐ N/A ☐
3. Restores breathing:			
a. Performs the appropriate method for artificial ventilation (see PA 11-8).	S ☐ U ☐ N/A ☐	S ☐ U ☐ N/A ☐	S ☐ U ☐ N/A ☐
4. For defibrillation:			
a. Applies and uses AED (see PA 12-3).	S ☐ U ☐ N/A ☐	S ☐ U ☐ N/A ☐	S ☐ U ☐ N/A ☐
5. Removes the supplies from the patient's room, and cleans the area, as needed.	S ☐ U ☐ N/A ☐	S ☐ U ☐ N/A ☐	S ☐ U ☐ N/A ☐
6. Removes PPE, and performs proper hand hygiene prior to leaving the patient's room.	S ☐ U ☐ N/A ☐	S ☐ U ☐ N/A ☐	S ☐ U ☐ N/A ☐

Continued

	Peer Evaluation Laboratory Setting			Instructor Evaluation Laboratory Setting			Instructor Evaluation Clinical Setting		
Evaluation of Procedure									
1. Reassesses the patient throughout code management.	S ☐	U ☐	N/A ☐	S ☐	U ☐	N/A ☐	S ☐	U ☐	N/A ☐
2. Observes for any spontaneous return of respirations or pulse.	S ☐	U ☐	N/A ☐	S ☐	U ☐	N/A ☐	S ☐	U ☐	N/A ☐
3. Develops an appropriate respiratory care plan based on assessment data.	S ☐	U ☐	N/A ☐	S ☐	U ☐	N/A ☐	S ☐	U ☐	N/A ☐
4. Identifies the causes of sudden cardiac or respiratory arrest.	S ☐	U ☐	N/A ☐	S ☐	U ☐	N/A ☐	S ☐	U ☐	N/A ☐
5. Identifies any unexpected outcomes.	S ☐	U ☐	N/A ☐	S ☐	U ☐	N/A ☐	S ☐	U ☐	N/A ☐
Documentation and Reporting									
1. Records the location of the respiratory or cardiac arrest.	S ☐	U ☐	N/A ☐	S ☐	U ☐	N/A ☐	S ☐	U ☐	N/A ☐
2. Records findings in the patient's chart.	S ☐	U ☐	N/A ☐	S ☐	U ☐	N/A ☐	S ☐	U ☐	N/A ☐
3. Records the arrest situation per your facility's protocol.	S ☐	U ☐	N/A ☐	S ☐	U ☐	N/A ☐	S ☐	U ☐	N/A ☐

Comments:

_____

_____

_____

Signatures:

Student _____ Date Passed _____

Instructor (Laboratory Setting) _____ Date Passed _____

Student _____ Date Passed _____

Instructor (Clinical Setting) _____ Date Passed _____

Procedural Assessment 12-2

Student _____   Date _____

Instructor (Laboratory Setting) _____   Date _____

Instructor (Clinical Setting) _____   Date _____

Criteria for assessment success:

The student must obtain all **satisfactory (S)** scores to pass the procedural evaluation. Any **unsatisfactory (U)** scores will result in failure of the procedural assessment.

Scoring:

Satisfactory (S): Procedural step performed correctly with no instructor prompting. Student-initiated correction is acceptable.

Unsatisfactory (U): Procedural step was performed incorrectly, omitted, or performed in a way that compromised patient care.

Not applicable (N/A): Procedural step was not indicated or necessary.

Evaluation:

	Peer Evaluation Laboratory Setting	Instructor Evaluation Laboratory Setting	Instructor Evaluation Clinical Setting
Procedural Preparation			
1. Reviews the patient's chart.	S ☐ U ☐ N/A ☐	S ☐ U ☐ N/A ☐	S ☐ U ☐ N/A ☐
2. Verifies the physician's order or the facility's protocol for standard of care.	S ☐ U ☐ N/A ☐	S ☐ U ☐ N/A ☐	S ☐ U ☐ N/A ☐
3. Obtains, cleans, and inspects the appropriate equipment prior to entering the patient's room.	S ☐ U ☐ N/A ☐	S ☐ U ☐ N/A ☐	S ☐ U ☐ N/A ☐
4. Follows PPE requirements, and observes standard precautions for any transmission-based isolation procedure.	S ☐ U ☐ N/A ☐	S ☐ U ☐ N/A ☐	S ☐ U ☐ N/A ☐
5. Identifies the patient using two patient identifiers.	S ☐ U ☐ N/A ☐	S ☐ U ☐ N/A ☐	S ☐ U ☐ N/A ☐
6. Introduces self to the patient and to the family.	S ☐ U ☐ N/A ☐	S ☐ U ☐ N/A ☐	S ☐ U ☐ N/A ☐
7. Explains the procedure to the patient and to the family, and acknowledges the patient's understanding.	S ☐ U ☐ N/A ☐	S ☐ U ☐ N/A ☐	S ☐ U ☐ N/A ☐
8. Performs proper hand hygiene, and puts on gloves, mask, and protective eyewear, as appropriate for the procedure.	S ☐ U ☐ N/A ☐	S ☐ U ☐ N/A ☐	S ☐ U ☐ N/A ☐
Implementation			
1. Positions the patient.	S ☐ U ☐ N/A ☐	S ☐ U ☐ N/A ☐	S ☐ U ☐ N/A ☐
2. Clears the airway of secretions, vomitus, and foreign objects (see PAs 11-1, 11-2, and 11-3).	S ☐ U ☐ N/A ☐	S ☐ U ☐ N/A ☐	S ☐ U ☐ N/A ☐
3. Inserts an oropharyngeal airway (see PA 11-5).	S ☐ U ☐ N/A ☐	S ☐ U ☐ N/A ☐	S ☐ U ☐ N/A ☐
4. Connects the device to an oxygen source, and sets the flowmeter to 15 liters per minute (L/min).	S ☐ U ☐ N/A ☐	S ☐ U ☐ N/A ☐	S ☐ U ☐ N/A ☐
5. Places the mask on the patient's face; makes a tight seal, or applies a manual resuscitator to the artificial airway device.	S ☐ U ☐ N/A ☐	S ☐ U ☐ N/A ☐	S ☐ U ☐ N/A ☐
6. Compresses the bag to ventilate at the appropriate volume and rate, based on the patient's age and size.	S ☐ U ☐ N/A ☐	S ☐ U ☐ N/A ☐	S ☐ U ☐ N/A ☐

Continued

	Peer Evaluation Laboratory Setting			Instructor Evaluation Laboratory Setting			Instructor Evaluation Clinical Setting		
7. Assesses the adequacy of ventilation.	S ☐	U ☐	N/A ☐	S ☐	U ☐	N/A ☐	S ☐	U ☐	N/A ☐
8. Removes the supplies from the patient's room, and cleans the area, as needed.	S ☐	U ☐	N/A ☐	S ☐	U ☐	N/A ☐	S ☐	U ☐	N/A ☐
9. Removes PPE, and performs proper hand hygiene prior to leaving the patient's room.	S ☐	U ☐	N/A ☐	S ☐	U ☐	N/A ☐	S ☐	U ☐	N/A ☐

Evaluation of Procedure

	Peer Evaluation Laboratory Setting			Instructor Evaluation Laboratory Setting			Instructor Evaluation Clinical Setting		
1. Reassesses the patient for adequate ventilation, and repositions to open the airway, as necessary.	S ☐	U ☐	N/A ☐	S ☐	U ☐	N/A ☐	S ☐	U ☐	N/A ☐
2. Develops an appropriate respiratory care plan based on assessment data.	S ☐	U ☐	N/A ☐	S ☐	U ☐	N/A ☐	S ☐	U ☐	N/A ☐
3. Identifies any unexpected outcomes.	S ☐	U ☐	N/A ☐	S ☐	U ☐	N/A ☐	S ☐	U ☐	N/A ☐

Documentation and Reporting

	Peer Evaluation Laboratory Setting			Instructor Evaluation Laboratory Setting			Instructor Evaluation Clinical Setting		
1. Records the location of the respiratory or cardiopulmonary arrest.	S ☐	U ☐	N/A ☐	S ☐	U ☐	N/A ☐	S ☐	U ☐	N/A ☐
2. Records findings in the patient's chart.	S ☐	U ☐	N/A ☐	S ☐	U ☐	N/A ☐	S ☐	U ☐	N/A ☐
3. Reports the arrest situation per facility's protocol.	S ☐	U ☐	N/A ☐	S ☐	U ☐	N/A ☐	S ☐	U ☐	N/A ☐

Comments:

_____

_____

_____

Signatures:

Student _____ Date Passed _____

Instructor (Laboratory Setting) _____ Date Passed _____

Student _____ Date Passed _____

Instructor (Clinical Setting) _____ Date Passed _____

Student _____ Date _____

Instructor (Laboratory Setting) _____ Date _____

Instructor (Clinical Setting) _____ Date _____

Criteria for assessment success:

The student must obtain all **satisfactory (S)** scores to pass the procedural evaluation. Any **unsatisfactory (U)** scores will result in failure of the procedural assessment.

Scoring:

Satisfactory (S): Procedural step performed correctly with no instructor prompting. Student-initiated correction is acceptable.

Unsatisfactory (U): Procedural step was performed incorrectly, omitted, or performed in a way that compromised patient care.

Not applicable (N/A): Procedural step was not indicated or necessary.

Evaluation:

	Peer Evaluation Laboratory Setting	Instructor Evaluation Laboratory Setting	Instructor Evaluation Clinical Setting
Procedural Preparation			
1. Ensures that an automated external defibillator (AED) is available and functions properly.	S ☐ U ☐ N/A ☐	S ☐ U ☐ N/A ☐	S ☐ U ☐ N/A ☐
2. Follows PPE requirements and performs proper hand hygiene, and puts on gloves, mask, and protective eye wear.	S ☐ U ☐ N/A ☐	S ☐ U ☐ N/A ☐	S ☐ U ☐ N/A ☐
3. Establishes unresponsiveness.	S ☐ U ☐ N/A ☐	S ☐ U ☐ N/A ☐	S ☐ U ☐ N/A ☐
4. Initiates code notification procedures based on the agency's protocol for standard of care.	S ☐ U ☐ N/A ☐	S ☐ U ☐ N/A ☐	S ☐ U ☐ N/A ☐
5. Starts CPR until the AED arrives.	S ☐ U ☐ N/A ☐	S ☐ U ☐ N/A ☐	S ☐ U ☐ N/A ☐
Implementation			
1. Places the AED near the patient's head.	S ☐ U ☐ N/A ☐	S ☐ U ☐ N/A ☐	S ☐ U ☐ N/A ☐
2. Turns on the power.	S ☐ U ☐ N/A ☐	S ☐ U ☐ N/A ☐	S ☐ U ☐ N/A ☐
3. Attaches pads per device instructions.	S ☐ U ☐ N/A ☐	S ☐ U ☐ N/A ☐	S ☐ U ☐ N/A ☐
4. Clears rescuers away from the patient.	S ☐ U ☐ N/A ☐	S ☐ U ☐ N/A ☐	S ☐ U ☐ N/A ☐
5. Allows the AED time to analyze the rhythm.	S ☐ U ☐ N/A ☐	S ☐ U ☐ N/A ☐	S ☐ U ☐ N/A ☐
6. Delivers shock as indicated by the AED.	S ☐ U ☐ N/A ☐	S ☐ U ☐ N/A ☐	S ☐ U ☐ N/A ☐
7. Continues chest compressions for 2 minutes.	S ☐ U ☐ N/A ☐	S ☐ U ☐ N/A ☐	S ☐ U ☐ N/A ☐
8. Allows the AED to resume analysis of the rhythm.	S ☐ U ☐ N/A ☐	S ☐ U ☐ N/A ☐	S ☐ U ☐ N/A ☐
9. Repeats steps 4 through 7 until ROSC or the physician pronounces death.	S ☐ U ☐ N/A ☐	S ☐ U ☐ N/A ☐	S ☐ U ☐ N/A ☐
10. Removes the supplies from the patient's room, and cleans the area, as needed.	S ☐ U ☐ N/A ☐	S ☐ U ☐ N/A ☐	S ☐ U ☐ N/A ☐

Continued

	Peer Evaluation Laboratory Setting			Instructor Evaluation Laboratory Setting			Instructor Evaluation Clinical Setting		
11. Removes PPE, and performs proper hand hygiene prior to leaving the patient's room.	S ☐	U ☐	N/A ☐	S ☐	U ☐	N/A ☐	S ☐	U ☐	N/A ☐

Evaluation of Procedure

1. Observes for any ROSC.	S ☐	U ☐	N/A ☐	S ☐	U ☐	N/A ☐	S ☐	U ☐	N/A ☐
2. Develops an appropriate respiratory care plan based on assessment data.	S ☐	U ☐	N/A ☐	S ☐	U ☐	N/A ☐	S ☐	U ☐	N/A ☐
3. Identifies the causes of sudden cardiac arrest.	S ☐	U ☐	N/A ☐	S ☐	U ☐	N/A ☐	S ☐	U ☐	N/A ☐
4. Identifies any unexpected outcomes.	S ☐	U ☐	N/A ☐	S ☐	U ☐	N/A ☐	S ☐	U ☐	N/A ☐

Documentation and Reporting

1. Records the location of the respiratory or cardiopulmonary arrest, time and number of AED shocks, medications given, procedures performed, cardiac rhythm, and use of CPR.	S ☐	U ☐	N/A ☐	S ☐	U ☐	N/A ☐	S ☐	U ☐	N/A ☐
2. Records findings in the patient's chart.	S ☐	U ☐	N/A ☐	S ☐	U ☐	N/A ☐	S ☐	U ☐	N/A ☐
3. Records the arrest situation per facility's protocol.	S ☐	U ☐	N/A ☐	S ☐	U ☐	N/A ☐	S ☐	U ☐	N/A ☐

Comments:

_____

_____

_____

Signatures:

Student _____ Date Passed _____

Instructor (Laboratory Setting) _____ Date Passed _____

Student _____ Date Passed _____

Instructor (Clinical Setting) _____ Date Passed _____

Student _____ Date _____

Instructor (Laboratory Setting) _____ Date _____

Instructor (Clinical Setting) _____ Date _____

Criteria for assessment success:

The student must obtain all **satisfactory (S)** scores to pass the procedural evaluation. Any **unsatisfactory (U)** scores will result in failure of the procedural assessment.

Scoring:

Satisfactory (S): Procedural step performed correctly with no instructor prompting. Student-initiated correction is acceptable.

Unsatisfactory (U): Procedural step was performed incorrectly, omitted, or performed in a way that compromised patient care.

Not applicable (N/A): Procedural step was not indicated or necessary.

Evaluation:

	Peer Evaluation Laboratory Setting	Instructor Evaluation Laboratory Setting	Instructor Evaluation Clinical Setting
Procedural Preparation			
1. Reviews the patient's chart.	S ☐ U ☐ N/A ☐	S ☐ U ☐ N/A ☐	S ☐ U ☐ N/A ☐
2. Verifies the physician's order or the facility's protocol for standard of care.	S ☐ U ☐ N/A ☐	S ☐ U ☐ N/A ☐	S ☐ U ☐ N/A ☐
3. Obtains, cleans, and inspects the appropriate equipment prior to entering the patient's room.	S ☐ U ☐ N/A ☐	S ☐ U ☐ N/A ☐	S ☐ U ☐ N/A ☐
4. Follows PPE requirements, and observes standard precautions for any transmission-based isolation procedure.	S ☐ U ☐ N/A ☐	S ☐ U ☐ N/A ☐	S ☐ U ☐ N/A ☐
5. Identifies the patient using two patient identifiers.	S ☐ U ☐ N/A ☐	S ☐ U ☐ N/A ☐	S ☐ U ☐ N/A ☐
6. Introduces self to the patient and to the family.	S ☐ U ☐ N/A ☐	S ☐ U ☐ N/A ☐	S ☐ U ☐ N/A ☐
7. Explains the procedure to the patient and to the family, and acknowledges the patient's understanding.	S ☐ U ☐ N/A ☐	S ☐ U ☐ N/A ☐	S ☐ U ☐ N/A ☐
8. Performs proper hand hygiene, and puts on gloves, mask, and protective eyewear, as appropriate for the procedure.	S ☐ U ☐ N/A ☐	S ☐ U ☐ N/A ☐	S ☐ U ☐ N/A ☐
Implementation			
1. Positions the patient's head, tilting it slightly backward.	S ☐ U ☐ N/A ☐	S ☐ U ☐ N/A ☐	S ☐ U ☐ N/A ☐
2. Lubricates the nasopharyngeal airway with water-soluble gel.	S ☐ U ☐ N/A ☐	S ☐ U ☐ N/A ☐	S ☐ U ☐ N/A ☐
3. Positions the airway perpendicular to the frontal plane of the patient's face.	S ☐ U ☐ N/A ☐	S ☐ U ☐ N/A ☐	S ☐ U ☐ N/A ☐
4. Advances the airway slowly through the inferior meatus, with the beveled edge facing the septum.	S ☐ U ☐ N/A ☐	S ☐ U ☐ N/A ☐	S ☐ U ☐ N/A ☐
5. Visualizes and confirms placement by using a tongue depressor.	S ☐ U ☐ N/A ☐	S ☐ U ☐ N/A ☐	S ☐ U ☐ N/A ☐
6. Suctions the airway, if needed (see PA 11-3).	S ☐ U ☐ N/A ☐	S ☐ U ☐ N/A ☐	S ☐ U ☐ N/A ☐

Continued

	Peer Evaluation Laboratory Setting	Instructor Evaluation Laboratory Setting	Instructor Evaluation Clinical Setting
7. Removes the supplies from the patient's room, and cleans the area, as needed.	S ☐ U ☐ N/A ☐	S ☐ U ☐ N/A ☐	S ☐ U ☐ N/A ☐
8. Removes PPE, and performs proper hand hygiene prior to leaving the patient's room.	S ☐ U ☐ N/A ☐	S ☐ U ☐ N/A ☐	S ☐ U ☐ N/A ☐

Evaluation of Procedure

1. Establishes a baseline, or compares the patient's respiratory assessment before and after oral airway insertion.	S ☐ U ☐ N/A ☐	S ☐ U ☐ N/A ☐	S ☐ U ☐ N/A ☐
2. Determines the use of airway, placed temporarily for nasotracheal suctioning, intermittently or until endotracheal intubation is used to secure the airway (see PA 11-6).	S ☐ U ☐ N/A ☐	S ☐ U ☐ N/A ☐	S ☐ U ☐ N/A ☐
3. Repositions the patient.	S ☐ U ☐ N/A ☐	S ☐ U ☐ N/A ☐	S ☐ U ☐ N/A ☐
4. Identifies any unexpected outcomes.	S ☐ U ☐ N/A ☐	S ☐ U ☐ N/A ☐	S ☐ U ☐ N/A ☐

Documentation and Reporting

1. Records findings in the patient's chart.	S ☐ U ☐ N/A ☐	S ☐ U ☐ N/A ☐	S ☐ U ☐ N/A ☐
2. Reports any abnormal findings to the appropriate health care provider.	S ☐ U ☐ N/A ☐	S ☐ U ☐ N/A ☐	S ☐ U ☐ N/A ☐

Comments:

_____

_____

_____

Signatures:

Student _____ Date Passed _____

Instructor (Laboratory Setting) _____ Date Passed _____

Student _____ Date Passed _____

Instructor (Clinical Setting) _____ Date Passed _____

Procedural Assessment 13-1

Student _____ Date _____

Instructor (Laboratory Setting) _____ Date _____

Instructor (Clinical Setting) _____ Date _____

Criteria for assessment success:

The student must obtain all **satisfactory (S)** scores to pass the procedural evaluation. Any **unsatisfactory (U)** scores will result in failure of the procedural assessment.

Scoring:

Satisfactory (S): Procedural step performed correctly with no instructor prompting. Student-initiated correction is acceptable.

Unsatisfactory (U): Procedural step was performed incorrectly, omitted, or performed in a way that compromised patient care.

Not applicable (N/A): Procedural step was not indicated or necessary.

Evaluation:

	Peer Evaluation Laboratory Setting	Instructor Evaluation Laboratory Setting	Instructor Evaluation Clinical Setting
Procedural Preparation			
1. Reviews the patient's chart.	S ☐ U ☐ N/A ☐	S ☐ U ☐ N/A ☐	S ☐ U ☐ N/A ☐
2. Verifies the physician's order or the facility's protocol for standard of care.	S ☐ U ☐ N/A ☐	S ☐ U ☐ N/A ☐	S ☐ U ☐ N/A ☐
3. Obtains, cleans, and inspects the appropriate equipment prior to entering the patient's room.	S ☐ U ☐ N/A ☐	S ☐ U ☐ N/A ☐	S ☐ U ☐ N/A ☐
4. Follows PPE requirements, and observes standard precautions for any transmission-based isolation procedure.	S ☐ U ☐ N/A ☐	S ☐ U ☐ N/A ☐	S ☐ U ☐ N/A ☐
5. Identifies the patient using two patient identifiers.	S ☐ U ☐ N/A ☐	S ☐ U ☐ N/A ☐	S ☐ U ☐ N/A ☐
6. Introduces self to the patient and to the family.	S ☐ U ☐ N/A ☐	S ☐ U ☐ N/A ☐	S ☐ U ☐ N/A ☐
7. Explains the procedure to the patient and to the family, and acknowledges the patient's understanding.	S ☐ U ☐ N/A ☐	S ☐ U ☐ N/A ☐	S ☐ U ☐ N/A ☐
8. Performs proper hand hygiene, and puts on gloves, mask, and protective eyewear, as appropriate for the procedure.	S ☐ U ☐ N/A ☐	S ☐ U ☐ N/A ☐	S ☐ U ☐ N/A ☐
Implementation			
1. Places the patient in a comfortable position.	S ☐ U ☐ N/A ☐	S ☐ U ☐ N/A ☐	S ☐ U ☐ N/A ☐
2. Assesses vital signs.	S ☐ U ☐ N/A ☐	S ☐ U ☐ N/A ☐	S ☐ U ☐ N/A ☐
3. Assesses the need for humidification.	S ☐ U ☐ N/A ☐	S ☐ U ☐ N/A ☐	S ☐ U ☐ N/A ☐
4. Fills the reservoir with sterile water.	S ☐ U ☐ N/A ☐	S ☐ U ☐ N/A ☐	S ☐ U ☐ N/A ☐
5. Attaches the humidifier to the flowmeter.	S ☐ U ☐ N/A ☐	S ☐ U ☐ N/A ☐	S ☐ U ☐ N/A ☐
6. Attaches the small-bore tube of the oxygen delivery device to the humidifier.	S ☐ U ☐ N/A ☐	S ☐ U ☐ N/A ☐	S ☐ U ☐ N/A ☐

Continued

	Peer Evaluation Laboratory Setting			Instructor Evaluation Laboratory Setting			Instructor Evaluation Clinical Setting		
7. Adjusts oxygen to the desired flow.	S ☐	U ☐	N/A ☐	S ☐	U ☐	N/A ☐	S ☐	U ☐	N/A ☐
8. Positions the oxygen delivery device on the patient.	S ☐	U ☐	N/A ☐	S ☐	U ☐	N/A ☐	S ☐	U ☐	N/A ☐
9. Ensures that the patient is comfortable with the device.	S ☐	U ☐	N/A ☐	S ☐	U ☐	N/A ☐	S ☐	U ☐	N/A ☐
10. Removes the supplies from the patient's room, and cleans the area, as needed.	S ☐	U ☐	N/A ☐	S ☐	U ☐	N/A ☐	S ☐	U ☐	N/A ☐
11. Removes PPE, and performs proper hand hygiene prior to leaving the patient's room.	S ☐	U ☐	N/A ☐	S ☐	U ☐	N/A ☐	S ☐	U ☐	N/A ☐

Evaluation of Procedure

	Peer Evaluation Laboratory Setting			Instructor Evaluation Laboratory Setting			Instructor Evaluation Clinical Setting		
1. Evaluates the patient's comfort with the humidification device.	S ☐	U ☐	N/A ☐	S ☐	U ☐	N/A ☐	S ☐	U ☐	N/A ☐
2. Monitors the fluid levels of the humidification device.	S ☐	U ☐	N/A ☐	S ☐	U ☐	N/A ☐	S ☐	U ☐	N/A ☐
3. Identifies any unexpected outcomes.	S ☐	U ☐	N/A ☐	S ☐	U ☐	N/A ☐	S ☐	U ☐	N/A ☐

Documentation and Reporting

	Peer Evaluation Laboratory Setting			Instructor Evaluation Laboratory Setting			Instructor Evaluation Clinical Setting		
1. Records humidification use in the patient's chart.	S ☐	U ☐	N/A ☐	S ☐	U ☐	N/A ☐	S ☐	U ☐	N/A ☐
2. Reports any changes or additions of humidification therapy to the appropriate health care provider.	S ☐	U ☐	N/A ☐	S ☐	U ☐	N/A ☐	S ☐	U ☐	N/A ☐
3. Reports any abnormal findings to the appropriate health care provider.	S ☐	U ☐	N/A ☐	S ☐	U ☐	N/A ☐	S ☐	U ☐	N/A ☐

Comments:

_____

_____

_____

Signatures:

Student _____ Date Passed _____

Instructor (Laboratory Setting) _____ Date Passed _____

Student _____ Date Passed _____

Instructor (Clinical Setting) _____ Date Passed _____

Procedural Assessment 13-2

Student _____ Date _____

Instructor (Laboratory Setting) _____ Date _____

Instructor (Clinical Setting) _____ Date _____

Criteria for assessment success:

The student must obtain all **satisfactory (S)** scores to pass the procedural evaluation. Any **unsatisfactory (U)** scores will result in failure of the procedural assessment.

Scoring:

Satisfactory (S): Procedural step performed correctly with no instructor prompting. Student-initiated correction is acceptable.

Unsatisfactory (U): Procedural step was performed incorrectly, omitted, or performed in a way that compromised patient care.

Not applicable (N/A): Procedural step was not indicated or necessary.

Evaluation:

	Peer Evaluation Laboratory Setting	Instructor Evaluation Laboratory Setting	Instructor Evaluation Clinical Setting
Procedural Preparation			
1. Reviews the patient's chart.	S ☐ U ☐ N/A ☐	S ☐ U ☐ N/A ☐	S ☐ U ☐ N/A ☐
2. Verifies the physician's order or the facility's protocol for standard of care.	S ☐ U ☐ N/A ☐	S ☐ U ☐ N/A ☐	S ☐ U ☐ N/A ☐
3. Obtains, cleans, and inspects the appropriate equipment prior to entering the patient's room.	S ☐ U ☐ N/A ☐	S ☐ U ☐ N/A ☐	S ☐ U ☐ N/A ☐
4. Follows PPE requirements, and observes standard precautions for any transmission-based isolation procedure.	S ☐ U ☐ N/A ☐	S ☐ U ☐ N/A ☐	S ☐ U ☐ N/A ☐
5. Identifies the patient using two patient identifiers.	S ☐ U ☐ N/A ☐	S ☐ U ☐ N/A ☐	S ☐ U ☐ N/A ☐
6. Introduces self to the patient and to the family.	S ☐ U ☐ N/A ☐	S ☐ U ☐ N/A ☐	S ☐ U ☐ N/A ☐
7. Explains the procedure to the patient and to the family, and acknowledges the patient's understanding.	S ☐ U ☐ N/A ☐	S ☐ U ☐ N/A ☐	S ☐ U ☐ N/A ☐
8. Performs proper hand hygiene, and puts on gloves, mask, and protective eyewear, as appropriate for the procedure.	S ☐ U ☐ N/A ☐	S ☐ U ☐ N/A ☐	S ☐ U ☐ N/A ☐
Implementation			
1. Place the patient in a comfortable position.	S ☐ U ☐ N/A ☐	S ☐ U ☐ N/A ☐	S ☐ U ☐ N/A ☐
2. Assesses vital signs.	S ☐ U ☐ N/A ☐	S ☐ U ☐ N/A ☐	S ☐ U ☐ N/A ☐
3. Assesses the need for humidification.	S ☐ U ☐ N/A ☐	S ☐ U ☐ N/A ☐	S ☐ U ☐ N/A ☐
4. Fills the reservoir with sterile water.	S ☐ U ☐ N/A ☐	S ☐ U ☐ N/A ☐	S ☐ U ☐ N/A ☐
5. Attaches the humidifier to the flowmeter.	S ☐ U ☐ N/A ☐	S ☐ U ☐ N/A ☐	S ☐ U ☐ N/A ☐
6. Attaches the large-bore tube of the oxygen delivery device to the humidifier.	S ☐ U ☐ N/A ☐	S ☐ U ☐ N/A ☐	S ☐ U ☐ N/A ☐
7. Adjusts oxygen to the desired flow and FIO$_2$.	S ☐ U ☐ N/A ☐	S ☐ U ☐ N/A ☐	S ☐ U ☐ N/A ☐

Continued

	Peer Evaluation Laboratory Setting			Instructor Evaluation Laboratory Setting			Instructor Evaluation Clinical Setting		
8. Positions the oxygen delivery device on the patient.	S ☐	U ☐	N/A ☐	S ☐	U ☐	N/A ☐	S ☐	U ☐	N/A ☐
9. Ensures patient comfort with the device.	S ☐	U ☐	N/A ☐	S ☐	U ☐	N/A ☐	S ☐	U ☐	N/A ☐
10. Removes the supplies from the patient's room, and cleans the area, as needed.	S ☐	U ☐	N/A ☐	S ☐	U ☐	N/A ☐	S ☐	U ☐	N/A ☐
11. Removes PPE, and performs proper hand hygiene prior to leaving the patient's room.	S ☐	U ☐	N/A ☐	S ☐	U ☐	N/A ☐	S ☐	U ☐	N/A ☐

Evaluation of Procedure

1. Evaluates the patient's comfort with the humidification device.	S ☐	U ☐	N/A ☐	S ☐	U ☐	N/A ☐	S ☐	U ☐	N/A ☐
2. Monitors the fluid levels of the humidification device.	S ☐	U ☐	N/A ☐	S ☐	U ☐	N/A ☐	S ☐	U ☐	N/A ☐
3. Analyzes FIO_2 delivery per facility's protocol.	S ☐	U ☐	N/A ☐	S ☐	U ☐	N/A ☐	S ☐	U ☐	N/A ☐
4. Evaluates the need for a water trap.	S ☐	U ☐	N/A ☐	S ☐	U ☐	N/A ☐	S ☐	U ☐	N/A ☐
5. Identifies any unexpected outcomes.	S ☐	U ☐	N/A ☐	S ☐	U ☐	N/A ☐	S ☐	U ☐	N/A ☐

Documentation and Reporting

1. Records humidification use in the patient's chart.	S ☐	U ☐	N/A ☐	S ☐	U ☐	N/A ☐	S ☐	U ☐	N/A ☐
2. Reports any changes or additions of humidification therapy to the appropriate health care provider.	S ☐	U ☐	N/A ☐	S ☐	U ☐	N/A ☐	S ☐	U ☐	N/A ☐
3. Reports any abnormal findings to the appropriate health care provider.	S ☐	U ☐	N/A ☐	S ☐	U ☐	N/A ☐	S ☐	U ☐	N/A ☐

Comments:

_____

_____

_____

Signatures:

Student _____ Date Passed _____

Instructor (Laboratory Setting) _____ Date Passed _____

Student _____ Date Passed _____

Instructor (Clinical Setting) _____ Date Passed _____

Procedural Assessment 13-3   Sputum induction

Student _____ Date _____

Instructor (Laboratory Setting) _____ Date _____

Instructor (Clinical Setting) _____ Date _____

Evaluation:

	Peer Evaluation Laboratory Setting			Instructor Evaluation Laboratory Setting			Instructor Evaluation Clinical Setting		
Procedural Preparation									
1. Reviews the patient's chart.	S ☐	U ☐	N/A ☐	S ☐	U ☐	N/A ☐	S ☐	U ☐	N/A ☐
2. Verifies the physician's order or the facility's protocol for standard of care.	S ☐	U ☐	N/A ☐	S ☐	U ☐	N/A ☐	S ☐	U ☐	N/A ☐
3. Obtains, cleans, and inspects the appropriate equipment prior to entering the patient's room.	S ☐	U ☐	N/A ☐	S ☐	U ☐	N/A ☐	S ☐	U ☐	N/A ☐
4. Follows PPE requirements, and observes standard precautions for any transmission-based isolation procedure.	S ☐	U ☐	N/A ☐	S ☐	U ☐	N/A ☐	S ☐	U ☐	N/A ☐
5. Identifies the patient using two patient identifiers.	S ☐	U ☐	N/A ☐	S ☐	U ☐	N/A ☐	S ☐	U ☐	N/A ☐
6. Introduces self to the patient and to the family.	S ☐	U ☐	N/A ☐	S ☐	U ☐	N/A ☐	S ☐	U ☐	N/A ☐
7. Explains the procedure to the patient and to the family, and acknowledges the patient's understanding.	S ☐	U ☐	N/A ☐	S ☐	U ☐	N/A ☐	S ☐	U ☐	N/A ☐
8. Performs proper hand hygiene, and puts on gloves, mask, and protective eyewear, as appropriate for the procedure.	S ☐	U ☐	N/A ☐	S ☐	U ☐	N/A ☐	S ☐	U ☐	N/A ☐
Implementation									
1. Places the patient in a comfortable position.	S ☐	U ☐	N/A ☐	S ☐	U ☐	N/A ☐	S ☐	U ☐	N/A ☐
2. Assesses vital signs.	S ☐	U ☐	N/A ☐	S ☐	U ☐	N/A ☐	S ☐	U ☐	N/A ☐
3. Provides the patient with the opportunity to rinse the mouth with water before the sample is taken.	S ☐	U ☐	N/A ☐	S ☐	U ☐	N/A ☐	S ☐	U ☐	N/A ☐
4. Ensures that the patient has an effective cough.	S ☐	U ☐	N/A ☐	S ☐	U ☐	N/A ☐	S ☐	U ☐	N/A ☐
5. Fills the appropriate delivery device with hypertonic saline.	S ☐	U ☐	N/A ☐	S ☐	U ☐	N/A ☐	S ☐	U ☐	N/A ☐
6. Positions the delivery device on the patient.	S ☐	U ☐	N/A ☐	S ☐	U ☐	N/A ☐	S ☐	U ☐	N/A ☐
7. Assesses the patient for bronchospasm or adverse reaction to therapy.	S ☐	U ☐	N/A ☐	S ☐	U ☐	N/A ☐	S ☐	U ☐	N/A ☐
8. Instructs the patient to periodically stop therapy to cough.	S ☐	U ☐	N/A ☐	S ☐	U ☐	N/A ☐	S ☐	U ☐	N/A ☐
9. Attaches the correct patient identification label and laboratory requisition to the side of the specimen container.	S ☐	U ☐	N/A ☐	S ☐	U ☐	N/A ☐	S ☐	U ☐	N/A ☐
10. Encloses the specimen container in a plastic biohazard bag.	S ☐	U ☐	N/A ☐	S ☐	U ☐	N/A ☐	S ☐	U ☐	N/A ☐
11. Offers the patient tissue to wipe the mouth followed by mouth care, if needed.	S ☐	U ☐	N/A ☐	S ☐	U ☐	N/A ☐	S ☐	U ☐	N/A ☐

Continued

	Peer Evaluation Laboratory Setting			Instructor Evaluation Laboratory Setting			Instructor Evaluation Clinical Setting		
12. Removes the supplies from the patient's room, and cleans the area, as needed.	S ☐	U ☐	N/A ☐	S ☐	U ☐	N/A ☐	S ☐	U ☐	N/A ☐
13. Removes PPE, and performs proper hand hygiene prior to leaving the patient's room.	S ☐	U ☐	N/A ☐	S ☐	U ☐	N/A ☐	S ☐	U ☐	N/A ☐
14. Sends the specimen immediately to the laboratory, according to the facility protocols.	S ☐	U ☐	N/A ☐	S ☐	U ☐	N/A ☐	S ☐	U ☐	N/A ☐
Evaluation of Procedure									
1. Assesses the patient frequently during therapy for bronchospasm.	S ☐	U ☐	N/A ☐	S ☐	U ☐	N/A ☐	S ☐	U ☐	N/A ☐
2. Develops an appropriate respiratory care plan based on sputum data.	S ☐	U ☐	N/A ☐	S ☐	U ☐	N/A ☐	S ☐	U ☐	N/A ☐
3. Identifies any unexpected outcomes.	S ☐	U ☐	N/A ☐	S ☐	U ☐	N/A ☐	S ☐	U ☐	N/A ☐
Documentation and Reporting									
1. Records the time the sample was obtained in the patient's chart.	S ☐	U ☐	N/A ☐	S ☐	U ☐	N/A ☐	S ☐	U ☐	N/A ☐
2. Reports any abnormal findings to the appropriate health care provider.	S ☐	U ☐	N/A ☐	S ☐	U ☐	N/A ☐	S ☐	U ☐	N/A ☐

Comments:

_____

_____

_____

Signatures:

Student _____ Date Passed _____

Instructor (Laboratory Setting) _____ Date Passed _____

Student _____ Date Passed _____

Instructor (Clinical Setting) _____ Date Passed _____

Student _____ Date _____

Instructor (Laboratory Setting) _____ Date _____

Instructor (Clinical Setting) _____ Date _____

Criteria for assessment success:

The student must obtain all **satisfactory (S)** scores to pass the procedural evaluation. Any **unsatisfactory (U)** scores will result in failure of the procedural assessment.

Scoring:

Satisfactory (S): Procedural step performed correctly with no instructor prompting. Student-initiated correction is acceptable.

Unsatisfactory (U): Procedural step was performed incorrectly, omitted, or performed in a way that compromised patient care.

Not applicable (N/A): Procedural step was not indicated or necessary.

Evaluation:

	Peer Evaluation Laboratory Setting	Instructor Evaluation Laboratory Setting	Instructor Evaluation Clinical Setting
Procedural Preparation			
1. Reviews the patient's chart.	S ☐ U ☐ N/A ☐	S ☐ U ☐ N/A ☐	S ☐ U ☐ N/A ☐
2. Verifies the physician's order or the facility's protocol for standard of care.	S ☐ U ☐ N/A ☐	S ☐ U ☐ N/A ☐	S ☐ U ☐ N/A ☐
3. Obtains, cleans, and inspects the appropriate equipment prior to entering the patient's room.	S ☐ U ☐ N/A ☐	S ☐ U ☐ N/A ☐	S ☐ U ☐ N/A ☐
4. Follows PPE requirements, and observes standard precautions for any transmission-based isolation procedure.	S ☐ U ☐ N/A ☐	S ☐ U ☐ N/A ☐	S ☐ U ☐ N/A ☐
5. Identifies the patient using two patient identifiers.	S ☐ U ☐ N/A ☐	S ☐ U ☐ N/A ☐	S ☐ U ☐ N/A ☐
6. Introduces self to the patient and to the family.	S ☐ U ☐ N/A ☐	S ☐ U ☐ N/A ☐	S ☐ U ☐ N/A ☐
7. Explains the procedure to the patient and to the family, and acknowledges the patient's understanding.	S ☐ U ☐ N/A ☐	S ☐ U ☐ N/A ☐	S ☐ U ☐ N/A ☐
8. Performs proper hand hygiene, and puts on gloves, mask, and protective eyewear, as appropriate for the procedure.	S ☐ U ☐ N/A ☐	S ☐ U ☐ N/A ☐	S ☐ U ☐ N/A ☐
Implementation			
1. Assesses vital signs.	S ☐ U ☐ N/A ☐	S ☐ U ☐ N/A ☐	S ☐ U ☐ N/A ☐
2. Determines the appropriate humidification device. **Heat Moisture Exchanger (HME)**			
a. Rules out any contraindications for use.	S ☐ U ☐ N/A ☐	S ☐ U ☐ N/A ☐	S ☐ U ☐ N/A ☐
b. Attaches a 15-mm ID (inner diameter) opening to the endotracheal or tracheostomy tube.	S ☐ U ☐ N/A ☐	S ☐ U ☐ N/A ☐	S ☐ U ☐ N/A ☐
c. Attaches a 22-mm ID opening to the ventilator circuit.	S ☐ U ☐ N/A ☐	S ☐ U ☐ N/A ☐	S ☐ U ☐ N/A ☐
d. Ensures that all the connections are secure.	S ☐ U ☐ N/A ☐	S ☐ U ☐ N/A ☐	S ☐ U ☐ N/A ☐

Continued

	Peer Evaluation Laboratory Setting			Instructor Evaluation Laboratory Setting			Instructor Evaluation Clinical Setting		
Heated Humidification (HH)									
a. Sets up per the manufacturer's instructions.	S ☐	U ☐	N/A ☐	S ☐	U ☐	N/A ☐	S ☐	U ☐	N/A ☐
b. Maintains the water level.	S ☐	U ☐	N/A ☐	S ☐	U ☐	N/A ☐	S ☐	U ☐	N/A ☐
c. Secures both temperature probes in place.	S ☐	U ☐	N/A ☐	S ☐	U ☐	N/A ☐	S ☐	U ☐	N/A ☐
d. Sets to deliver inspired gas at 33°C ± 2°C measured at the airway opening.	S ☐	U ☐	N/A ☐	S ☐	U ☐	N/A ☐	S ☐	U ☐	N/A ☐
e. Inserts a water trap at the lowest point in the circuit (both inspiratory and expiratory limbs).	S ☐	U ☐	N/A ☐	S ☐	U ☐	N/A ☐	S ☐	U ☐	N/A ☐
f. Ensures that the connections are secure.	S ☐	U ☐	N/A ☐	S ☐	U ☐	N/A ☐	S ☐	U ☐	N/A ☐
g. Sets high (no higher than 37°C) and low (no lower than 30°C) temperature alarms.	S ☐	U ☐	N/A ☐	S ☐	U ☐	N/A ☐	S ☐	U ☐	N/A ☐
Heated Wire Circuits									
a. Places the temperature probe outside the incubator or away from the radiant warmer.	S ☐	U ☐	N/A ☐	S ☐	U ☐	N/A ☐	S ☐	U ☐	N/A ☐
3. Performs patient–ventilator system assessment, as needed.	S ☐	U ☐	N/A ☐	S ☐	U ☐	N/A ☐	S ☐	U ☐	N/A ☐
4. Removes the supplies from the patient's room, and cleans the area, as needed.	S ☐	U ☐	N/A ☐	S ☐	U ☐	N/A ☐	S ☐	U ☐	N/A ☐
5. Removes PPE, and performs proper hand hygiene prior to leaving the patient's room.	S ☐	U ☐	N/A ☐	S ☐	U ☐	N/A ☐	S ☐	U ☐	N/A ☐
Evaluation of Procedure									
1. Evaluates the choice of the humidification device.	S ☐	U ☐	N/A ☐	S ☐	U ☐	N/A ☐	S ☐	U ☐	N/A ☐
2. Ensures proper conditioning of the inspired gas.	S ☐	U ☐	N/A ☐	S ☐	U ☐	N/A ☐	S ☐	U ☐	N/A ☐
3. Identifies any unexpected outcomes.	S ☐	U ☐	N/A ☐	S ☐	U ☐	N/A ☐	S ☐	U ☐	N/A ☐
Documentation and Reporting									
1. Records the humidification device used in the patient's chart.	S ☐	U ☐	N/A ☐	S ☐	U ☐	N/A ☐	S ☐	U ☐	N/A ☐
2. Records the quantity, consistency, and characteristics of secretions.	S ☐	U ☐	N/A ☐	S ☐	U ☐	N/A ☐	S ☐	U ☐	N/A ☐
3. Reports any abnormal findings to the appropriate health care provider.	S ☐	U ☐	N/A ☐	S ☐	U ☐	N/A ☐	S ☐	U ☐	N/A ☐

Comments:

_____

_____

_____

Signatures:

Student _____ Date Passed _____

Instructor (Laboratory Setting) _____ Date Passed _____

Student _____ Date Passed _____

Instructor (Clinical Setting) _____ Date Passed _____

Procedural Assessment 14-1 — Using an oxygen cylinder

Student _____ Date _____

Instructor (Laboratory Setting) _____ Date _____

Instructor (Clinical Setting) _____ Date _____

Criteria for assessment success:

The student must obtain all **satisfactory (S)** scores to pass the procedural evaluation. Any **unsatisfactory (U)** scores will result in failure of the procedural assessment.

Scoring:

Satisfactory (S): Procedural step performed correctly with no instructor prompting. Student-initiated correction is acceptable.

Unsatisfactory (U): Procedural step was performed incorrectly, omitted, or performed in a way that compromised patient care.

Not applicable (N/A): Procedural step was not indicated or necessary.

Evaluation:

	Peer Evaluation Laboratory Setting	Instructor Evaluation Laboratory Setting	Instructor Evaluation Clinical Setting
Procedural Preparation			
1. Obtains the appropriate medical gas cylinder depending on the need.	S ☐ U ☐ N/A ☐	S ☐ U ☐ N/A ☐	S ☐ U ☐ N/A ☐
2. Verifies content according to label and color.	S ☐ U ☐ N/A ☐	S ☐ U ☐ N/A ☐	S ☐ U ☐ N/A ☐
3. Obtains the correct regulator for the cylinder.	S ☐ U ☐ N/A ☐	S ☐ U ☐ N/A ☐	S ☐ U ☐ N/A ☐
Implementation			
1. Releases the safety strap or chain.	S ☐ U ☐ N/A ☐	S ☐ U ☐ N/A ☐	S ☐ U ☐ N/A ☐
2. Moves the cylinder onto the cart safely, and secures it.	S ☐ U ☐ N/A ☐	S ☐ U ☐ N/A ☐	S ☐ U ☐ N/A ☐
3. Moves the cart to the desired location for delivery of gas.	S ☐ U ☐ N/A ☐	S ☐ U ☐ N/A ☐	S ☐ U ☐ N/A ☐
4. Secures the cylinder in the new location, if it is removed from the cart.	S ☐ U ☐ N/A ☐	S ☐ U ☐ N/A ☐	S ☐ U ☐ N/A ☐
5. Removes the protective cap or wrap.	S ☐ U ☐ N/A ☐	S ☐ U ☐ N/A ☐	S ☐ U ☐ N/A ☐
6. Ensures the safety of bystanders by turning the valve away from persons present.	S ☐ U ☐ N/A ☐	S ☐ U ☐ N/A ☐	S ☐ U ☐ N/A ☐
7. Gives a verbal warning about the cylinder being cracked.	S ☐ U ☐ N/A ☐	S ☐ U ☐ N/A ☐	S ☐ U ☐ N/A ☐
8. Looks at the valve or the regulator inlet to confirm that it is contaminant free.	S ☐ U ☐ N/A ☐	S ☐ U ☐ N/A ☐	S ☐ U ☐ N/A ☐
9. Cracks the cylinder.	S ☐ U ☐ N/A ☐	S ☐ U ☐ N/A ☐	S ☐ U ☐ N/A ☐
10. Connects the regulator to the cylinder firmly, and opens the cylinder.	S ☐ U ☐ N/A ☐	S ☐ U ☐ N/A ☐	S ☐ U ☐ N/A ☐
11. Corrects any leaks.	S ☐ U ☐ N/A ☐	S ☐ U ☐ N/A ☐	S ☐ U ☐ N/A ☐
12. Following use, closes the cylinder valve, bleeds, and disconnects the regulator.	S ☐ U ☐ N/A ☐	S ☐ U ☐ N/A ☐	S ☐ U ☐ N/A ☐

Continued

	Peer Evaluation Laboratory Setting			Instructor Evaluation Laboratory Setting			Instructor Evaluation Clinical Setting		
13. Places the safety cap back on the cylinder, and returns it to the appropriate storage location.	S ☐	U ☐	N/A ☐	S ☐	U ☐	N/A ☐	S ☐	U ☐	N/A ☐

Evaluation of Procedure

1. Correctly calculates the duration of flow.	S ☐	U ☐	N/A ☐	S ☐	U ☐	N/A ☐	S ☐	U ☐	N/A ☐
2. Identifies any unexpected outcomes.	S ☐	U ☐	N/A ☐	S ☐	U ☐	N/A ☐	S ☐	U ☐	N/A ☐

Documentation and Reporting

1. Records the beginning pressures and the time cylinder use began in the patient's chart.	S ☐	U ☐	N/A ☐	S ☐	U ☐	N/A ☐	S ☐	U ☐	N/A ☐

Comments:

_____

_____

_____

Signatures:

Student _____ Date Passed _____

Instructor (Laboratory Setting) _____ Date Passed _____

Student _____ Date Passed _____

Instructor (Clinical Setting) _____ Date Passed _____

Procedural Assessment 14-2

Using a liquid oxygen system

Student _____ Date _____

Instructor (Laboratory Setting) _____ Date _____

Instructor (Clinical Setting) _____ Date _____

Criteria for assessment success:

The student must obtain all **satisfactory (S)** scores to pass the procedural evaluation. Any **unsatisfactory (U)** scores will result in failure of the procedural assessment.

Scoring:

Satisfactory (S): Procedural step performed correctly with no instructor prompting. Student-initiated correction is acceptable.

Unsatisfactory (U): Procedural step was performed incorrectly, omitted, or performed in a way that compromised patient care.

Not applicable (N/A): Procedural step was not indicated or necessary.

Evaluation:

	Peer Evaluation Laboratory Setting	Instructor Evaluation Laboratory Setting	Instructor Evaluation Clinical Setting
Procedural Preparation			
1. Weighs the portable system to determine if filling is needed.	S ☐ U ☐ N/A ☐	S ☐ U ☐ N/A ☐	S ☐ U ☐ N/A ☐
2. Confirms that all safety rules are followed.	S ☐ U ☐ N/A ☐	S ☐ U ☐ N/A ☐	S ☐ U ☐ N/A ☐
Implementation			
1. Connects the portable system to the stationary system.	S ☐ U ☐ N/A ☐	S ☐ U ☐ N/A ☐	S ☐ U ☐ N/A ☐
2. Opens the gas vent valve.	S ☐ U ☐ N/A ☐	S ☐ U ☐ N/A ☐	S ☐ U ☐ N/A ☐
3. Observes the venting through the gas vent port, and closes the gas vent valve.	S ☐ U ☐ N/A ☐	S ☐ U ☐ N/A ☐	S ☐ U ☐ N/A ☐
4. Disconnects the portable system from the stationary system.	S ☐ U ☐ N/A ☐	S ☐ U ☐ N/A ☐	S ☐ U ☐ N/A ☐
5. Confirms that the portable system is full.	S ☐ U ☐ N/A ☐	S ☐ U ☐ N/A ☐	S ☐ U ☐ N/A ☐
Evaluation of Procedure			
1. Calculates the duration of flow.	S ☐ U ☐ N/A ☐	S ☐ U ☐ N/A ☐	S ☐ U ☐ N/A ☐
2. Identifies any unexpected outcomes.	S ☐ U ☐ N/A ☐	S ☐ U ☐ N/A ☐	S ☐ U ☐ N/A ☐
Documentation and Reporting			
1. Records the liter flow and oxygen delivery device in the chart, if applicable.	S ☐ U ☐ N/A ☐	S ☐ U ☐ N/A ☐	S ☐ U ☐ N/A ☐

Comments:

_____

_____

_____

_____

Signatures:

Student _____   Date Passed _____

Instructor (Laboratory Setting) _____   Date Passed _____

Student _____   Date Passed _____

Instructor (Clinical Setting) _____   Date Passed _____

Student _____ Date _____

Instructor (Laboratory Setting) _____ Date _____

Instructor (Clinical Setting) _____ Date _____

Criteria for assessment success:

The student must obtain all **satisfactory (S)** scores to pass the procedural evaluation. Any **unsatisfactory (U)** scores will result in failure of the procedural assessment.

Scoring:

Satisfactory (S): Procedural step performed correctly with no instructor prompting. Student-initiated correction is acceptable.

Unsatisfactory (U): Procedural step was performed incorrectly, omitted, or performed in a way that compromised patient care.

Not applicable (N/A): Procedural step was not indicated or necessary.

Evaluation:

	Peer Evaluation Laboratory Setting	Instructor Evaluation Laboratory Setting	Instructor Evaluation Clinical Setting
Procedural Preparation			
1. Reviews the patient's chart.	S ☐ U ☐ N/A ☐	S ☐ U ☐ N/A ☐	S ☐ U ☐ N/A ☐
2. Verifies the physician's order or the facility's protocol for standard of care.	S ☐ U ☐ N/A ☐	S ☐ U ☐ N/A ☐	S ☐ U ☐ N/A ☐
3. Obtains, cleans, and inspects the appropriate equipment prior to entering the patient's room.	S ☐ U ☐ N/A ☐	S ☐ U ☐ N/A ☐	S ☐ U ☐ N/A ☐
4. Follows PPE requirements, and observes standard precautions for any transmission-based isolation procedure.	S ☐ U ☐ N/A ☐	S ☐ U ☐ N/A ☐	S ☐ U ☐ N/A ☐
5. Identifies the patient using two patient identifiers.	S ☐ U ☐ N/A ☐	S ☐ U ☐ N/A ☐	S ☐ U ☐ N/A ☐
6. Introduces self to the patient and to the family.	S ☐ U ☐ N/A ☐	S ☐ U ☐ N/A ☐	S ☐ U ☐ N/A ☐
7. Explains the procedure to the patient and to the family, and acknowledges the patient's understanding.	S ☐ U ☐ N/A ☐	S ☐ U ☐ N/A ☐	S ☐ U ☐ N/A ☐
8. Performs proper hand hygiene, and puts on gloves, mask, and protective eyewear, as appropriate for the procedure.	S ☐ U ☐ N/A ☐	S ☐ U ☐ N/A ☐	S ☐ U ☐ N/A ☐
Implementation			
1. Places the patient in a comfortable position.	S ☐ U ☐ N/A ☐	S ☐ U ☐ N/A ☐	S ☐ U ☐ N/A ☐
2. Assesses vital signs.	S ☐ U ☐ N/A ☐	S ☐ U ☐ N/A ☐	S ☐ U ☐ N/A ☐
3. Observes for signs and symptoms associated with hypoxemia.	S ☐ U ☐ N/A ☐	S ☐ U ☐ N/A ☐	S ☐ U ☐ N/A ☐
4. Monitors pulse oximetry.	S ☐ U ☐ N/A ☐	S ☐ U ☐ N/A ☐	S ☐ U ☐ N/A ☐
5. Chooses an appropriate oxygen delivery device based on assessment and patient need.	S ☐ U ☐ N/A ☐	S ☐ U ☐ N/A ☐	S ☐ U ☐ N/A ☐

Continued

	Peer Evaluation Laboratory Setting	Instructor Evaluation Laboratory Setting	Instructor Evaluation Clinical Setting
6. Attaches a nasal cannula or mask to the oxygen tube, and attaches the oxygen tube to the oxygen source.	S ☐ U ☐ N/A ☐	S ☐ U ☐ N/A ☐	S ☐ U ☐ N/A ☐
7. Turns on the flow.	S ☐ U ☐ N/A ☐	S ☐ U ☐ N/A ☐	S ☐ U ☐ N/A ☐
8. Applies the oxygen delivery device properly and adjusts to patient's comfort.	S ☐ U ☐ N/A ☐	S ☐ U ☐ N/A ☐	S ☐ U ☐ N/A ☐
9. Allows sufficient slack on the oxygen tube.	S ☐ U ☐ N/A ☐	S ☐ U ☐ N/A ☐	S ☐ U ☐ N/A ☐
10. Adjusts the oxygen flow rate, as needed.	S ☐ U ☐ N/A ☐	S ☐ U ☐ N/A ☐	S ☐ U ☐ N/A ☐
11. Removes the supplies from the patient's room, and cleans the area, as needed.	S ☐ U ☐ N/A ☐	S ☐ U ☐ N/A ☐	S ☐ U ☐ N/A ☐
12. Removes PPE, and performs proper hand hygiene prior to leaving the patient's room.	S ☐ U ☐ N/A ☐	S ☐ U ☐ N/A ☐	S ☐ U ☐ N/A ☐

Evaluation of Procedure

1. Establishes a baseline, or compares with previous measurements.	S ☐ U ☐ N/A ☐	S ☐ U ☐ N/A ☐	S ☐ U ☐ N/A ☐
2. Assesses patient's response to procedure.	S ☐ U ☐ N/A ☐	S ☐ U ☐ N/A ☐	S ☐ U ☐ N/A ☐
3. Develops an appropriate respiratory care plan based on assessment data.	S ☐ U ☐ N/A ☐	S ☐ U ☐ N/A ☐	S ☐ U ☐ N/A ☐
4. Confirms proper functioning of the oxygen delivery device.	S ☐ U ☐ N/A ☐	S ☐ U ☐ N/A ☐	S ☐ U ☐ N/A ☐
5. Considers humidification.	S ☐ U ☐ N/A ☐	S ☐ U ☐ N/A ☐	S ☐ U ☐ N/A ☐
6. Identifies any unexpected outcomes.	S ☐ U ☐ N/A ☐	S ☐ U ☐ N/A ☐	S ☐ U ☐ N/A ☐

Documentation and Reporting

1. Records and reports respiratory assessment findings, method of oxygen delivery, and the patient's response before and during oxygen therapy in the patient's chart.	S ☐ U ☐ N/A ☐	S ☐ U ☐ N/A ☐	S ☐ U ☐ N/A ☐
2. Reports any abnormal findings to the appropriate health care provider.	S ☐ U ☐ N/A ☐	S ☐ U ☐ N/A ☐	S ☐ U ☐ N/A ☐

Comments:

_____

_____

_____

Signatures:

Student _____ Date Passed _____

Instructor (Laboratory Setting) _____ Date Passed _____

Student _____ Date Passed _____

Instructor (Clinical Setting) _____ Date Passed _____

Student _____ Date _____

Instructor (Laboratory Setting) _____ Date _____

Instructor (Clinical Setting) _____ Date _____

Evaluation:

	Peer Evaluation Laboratory Setting			Instructor Evaluation Laboratory Setting			Instructor Evaluation Clinical Setting		
Procedural Preparation									
1. Reviews the patient's chart.	S ☐	U ☐	N/A ☐	S ☐	U ☐	N/A ☐	S ☐	U ☐	N/A ☐
2. Verifies the physician's order or the facility's protocol for standard of care.	S ☐	U ☐	N/A ☐	S ☐	U ☐	N/A ☐	S ☐	U ☐	N/A ☐
3. Obtains, cleans, and inspects the appropriate equipment prior to entering the patient's room.	S ☐	U ☐	N/A ☐	S ☐	U ☐	N/A ☐	S ☐	U ☐	N/A ☐
4. Follows PPE requirements, and observes standard precautions for any transmission-based isolation procedure.	S ☐	U ☐	N/A ☐	S ☐	U ☐	N/A ☐	S ☐	U ☐	N/A ☐
5. Identifies the patient using two patient identifiers.	S ☐	U ☐	N/A ☐	S ☐	U ☐	N/A ☐	S ☐	U ☐	N/A ☐
6. Introduces yourself to the patient and to the family.	S ☐	U ☐	N/A ☐	S ☐	U ☐	N/A ☐	S ☐	U ☐	N/A ☐
7. Explains the procedure to the patient and to the family, and acknowledges the patient's understanding.	S ☐	U ☐	N/A ☐	S ☐	U ☐	N/A ☐	S ☐	U ☐	N/A ☐
8. Performs proper hand hygiene, and puts on gloves, mask, and protective eyewear, as appropriate for the procedure.	S ☐	U ☐	N/A ☐	S ☐	U ☐	N/A ☐	S ☐	U ☐	N/A ☐
Implementation									
1. Places the patient in a comfortable position.	S ☐	U ☐	N/A ☐	S ☐	U ☐	N/A ☐	S ☐	U ☐	N/A ☐
2. Assesses vital signs.	S ☐	U ☐	N/A ☐	S ☐	U ☐	N/A ☐	S ☐	U ☐	N/A ☐
3. Observes for signs and symptoms associated with hypoxemia.	S ☐	U ☐	N/A ☐	S ☐	U ☐	N/A ☐	S ☐	U ☐	N/A ☐
4. Monitors pulse oximetry.	S ☐	U ☐	N/A ☐	S ☐	U ☐	N/A ☐	S ☐	U ☐	N/A ☐
5. Sets up the suction equipment at the patient's bedside, if needed.	S ☐	U ☐	N/A ☐	S ☐	U ☐	N/A ☐	S ☐	U ☐	N/A ☐
6. Observes for patent airway, and removes airway secretions.	S ☐	U ☐	N/A ☐	S ☐	U ☐	N/A ☐	S ☐	U ☐	N/A ☐
7. Attaches a T-tube or tracheostomy collar to the large-bore oxygen tube and to the humidified oxygen source.	S ☐	U ☐	N/A ☐	S ☐	U ☐	N/A ☐	S ☐	U ☐	N/A ☐
8. Adjusts the oxygen flow rate, and adjusts the nebulizer to the proper FIO_2 setting.	S ☐	U ☐	N/A ☐	S ☐	U ☐	N/A ☐	S ☐	U ☐	N/A ☐
9. Attaches the T-tube or tracheostomy collar to the endotracheal or tracheostomy tube.	S ☐	U ☐	N/A ☐	S ☐	U ☐	N/A ☐	S ☐	U ☐	N/A ☐
10. Observes for the T-tube pulling on the endotracheal or tracheostomy tube.	S ☐	U ☐	N/A ☐	S ☐	U ☐	N/A ☐	S ☐	U ☐	N/A ☐
11. Suctions the secretions in the T-tube or tracheostomy collar, if necessary.	S ☐	U ☐	N/A ☐	S ☐	U ☐	N/A ☐	S ☐	U ☐	N/A ☐
12. Removes the supplies from the patient's room, and cleans the area, as needed.	S ☐	U ☐	N/A ☐	S ☐	U ☐	N/A ☐	S ☐	U ☐	N/A ☐

Continued

	Peer Evaluation Laboratory Setting	Instructor Evaluation Laboratory Setting	Instructor Evaluation Clinical Setting
13. Removes PPE, and performs proper hand hygiene prior to leaving the patient's room.	S ☐ U ☐ N/A ☐	S ☐ U ☐ N/A ☐	S ☐ U ☐ N/A ☐

Evaluation of Procedure

1. Establishes a baseline, or compares with previous measurements.	S ☐ U ☐ N/A ☐	S ☐ U ☐ N/A ☐	S ☐ U ☐ N/A ☐
2. Assesses the patient's response to the procedure.	S ☐ U ☐ N/A ☐	S ☐ U ☐ N/A ☐	S ☐ U ☐ N/A ☐
3. Develops an appropriate respiratory care plan based on assessment data.	S ☐ U ☐ N/A ☐	S ☐ U ☐ N/A ☐	S ☐ U ☐ N/A ☐
4. Observes the oxygen tube for accumulation of fluid, and drains the tube correctly.	S ☐ U ☐ N/A ☐	S ☐ U ☐ N/A ☐	S ☐ U ☐ N/A ☐
5. Identifies any unexpected outcomes.	S ☐ U ☐ N/A ☐	S ☐ U ☐ N/A ☐	S ☐ U ☐ N/A ☐

Documentation and Reporting

1. Records and reports respiratory assessment findings, method of oxygen delivery, and the patient's response before and during oxygen therapy in patient's chart.	S ☐ U ☐ N/A ☐	S ☐ U ☐ N/A ☐	S ☐ U ☐ N/A ☐
2. Reports any abnormal findings to the appropriate health care provider.	S ☐ U ☐ N/A ☐	S ☐ U ☐ N/A ☐	S ☐ U ☐ N/A ☐

Comments:

_____

_____

_____

Signatures:

Student _____ Date Passed _____

Instructor (Laboratory Setting) _____ Date Passed _____

Student _____ Date Passed _____

Instructor (Clinical Setting) _____ Date Passed _____

Student _____ Date _____

Instructor (Laboratory Setting) _____ Date _____

Instructor (Clinical Setting) _____ Date _____

Evaluation:

	Peer Evaluation Laboratory Setting			Instructor Evaluation Laboratory Setting			Instructor Evaluation Clinical Setting		
Procedural Preparation									
1. Reviews the patient's chart.	S □	U □	N/A □	S □	U □	N/A □	S □	U □	N/A □
2. Verifies the physician's order or the facility's protocol for standard of care.	S □	U □	N/A □	S □	U □	N/A □	S □	U □	N/A □
3. Obtains, cleans, and inspects the appropriate equipment prior to entering the patient's room.	S □	U □	N/A □	S □	U □	N/A □	S □	U □	N/A □
4. Follows PPE requirements, and observes standard precautions for any transmission-based isolation procedure.	S □	U □	N/A □	S □	U □	N/A □	S □	U □	N/A □
5. Identifies the patient using two patient identifiers.	S □	U □	N/A □	S □	U □	N/A □	S □	U □	N/A □
6. Introduces self to the patient and to the family.	S □	U □	N/A □	S □	U □	N/A □	S □	U □	N/A □
7. Explains the procedure to the patient and to the family, and acknowledges the patient's understanding.	S □	U □	N/A □	S □	U □	N/A □	S □	U □	N/A □
8. Performs proper hand hygiene, and puts on gloves, mask, and protective eyewear, as appropriate for the procedure.	S □	U □	N/A □	S □	U □	N/A □	S □	U □	N/A □
Implementation									
1. Places the patient in a comfortable position	S □	U □	N/A □	S □	U □	N/A □	S □	U □	N/A □
2. Assesses vital signs.	S □	U □	N/A □	S □	U □	N/A □	S □	U □	N/A □
3. Determines the appropriate FIO_2 and flow requirements needed to obtain desired SaO_2 or SpO_2.	S □	U □	N/A □	S □	U □	N/A □	S □	U □	N/A □
4. Attaches the device to a 50-psi gas source(s).	S □	U □	N/A □	S □	U □	N/A □	S □	U □	N/A □
5. For the **air entrainment system** using a mask or tracheostomy collar:									
a. Attaches the device to the flowmeter.	S □	U □	N/A □	S □	U □	N/A □	S □	U □	N/A □
b. Heats, if necessary.	S □	U □	N/A □	S □	U □	N/A □	S □	U □	N/A □
c. Sets to predetermined FIO_2 and flow rate.	S □	U □	N/A □	S □	U □	N/A □	S □	U □	N/A □
d. Ensures proper functioning of the device and aerosol production, if humidified.	S □	U □	N/A □	S □	U □	N/A □	S □	U □	N/A □
e. Places the device on the patient with a mask or a tracheostomy collar.	S □	U □	N/A □	S □	U □	N/A □	S □	U □	N/A □
f. Adjusts FIO_2 and flow to maintain appropriate SpO_2.	S □	U □	N/A □	S □	U □	N/A □	S □	U □	N/A □
g. Adds a water trap to the system, if necessary.	S □	U □	N/A □	S □	U □	N/A □	S □	U □	N/A □
6. For the **Vapotherm system:**									
a. Attaches a disposable patient circuit.	S □	U □	N/A □	S □	U □	N/A □	S □	U □	N/A □
b. Starts up the device.	S □	U □	N/A □	S □	U □	N/A □	S □	U □	N/A □
c. Adjusts the flow.	S □	U □	N/A □	S □	U □	N/A □	S □	U □	N/A □
d. Adjusts the FIO_2.	S □	U □	N/A □	S □	U □	N/A □	S □	U □	N/A □
e. Adjusts the temperature.	S □	U □	N/A □	S □	U □	N/A □	S □	U □	N/A □
f. Connects the system to the patient.	S □	U □	N/A □	S □	U □	N/A □	S □	U □	N/A □

Continued

	Peer Evaluation Laboratory Setting	Instructor Evaluation Laboratory Setting	Instructor Evaluation Clinical Setting
7. For the Fisher and Paykel **Optiflow system:**			
a. Attaches the patient circuit to the high-flow device.	S ☐ U ☐ N/A ☐	S ☐ U ☐ N/A ☐	S ☐ U ☐ N/A ☐
b. Utilizes and warms the appropriate heating device.	S ☐ U ☐ N/A ☐	S ☐ U ☐ N/A ☐	S ☐ U ☐ N/A ☐
c. Connects high-pressure oxygen and air hoses to the wall outlet.	S ☐ U ☐ N/A ☐	S ☐ U ☐ N/A ☐	S ☐ U ☐ N/A ☐
d. Attaches the cannula to the patient:			
i. Sets the flow at 20 to 60 L/min in the adult population, working to meet the patient's inspiratory demand.	S ☐ U ☐ N/A ☐	S ☐ U ☐ N/A ☐	S ☐ U ☐ N/A ☐
ii. Sets the flow at 10 L/min or above in the pediatric patient.	S ☐ U ☐ N/A ☐	S ☐ U ☐ N/A ☐	S ☐ U ☐ N/A ☐
e. Sets FIO_2 to obtain the appropriate SpO_2.	S ☐ U ☐ N/A ☐	S ☐ U ☐ N/A ☐	S ☐ U ☐ N/A ☐
f. Reassesses vital signs.	S ☐ U ☐ N/A ☐	S ☐ U ☐ N/A ☐	S ☐ U ☐ N/A ☐
g. Removes the supplies from the patient's room, and cleans the area, as needed.	S ☐ U ☐ N/A ☐	S ☐ U ☐ N/A ☐	S ☐ U ☐ N/A ☐
h. Removes PPE, and performs proper hand hygiene prior to leaving the patient's room.	S ☐ U ☐ N/A ☐	S ☐ U ☐ N/A ☐	S ☐ U ☐ N/A ☐

Evaluation of Procedure

1. Ensures that the patient is comfortable with the high-flow device.	S ☐ U ☐ N/A ☐	S ☐ U ☐ N/A ☐	S ☐ U ☐ N/A ☐
2. Ensures that the patient's and flow requirements are being met.	S ☐ U ☐ N/A ☐	S ☐ U ☐ N/A ☐	S ☐ U ☐ N/A ☐
3. Develops an appropriate respiratory care plan based on assessment data.	S ☐ U ☐ N/A ☐	S ☐ U ☐ N/A ☐	S ☐ U ☐ N/A ☐
4. Correlates SpO_2 with SaO_2 if arterial blood gas values are available.	S ☐ U ☐ N/A ☐	S ☐ U ☐ N/A ☐	S ☐ U ☐ N/A ☐
5. Identifies any unexpected outcomes	S ☐ U ☐ N/A ☐	S ☐ U ☐ N/A ☐	S ☐ U ☐ N/A ☐

Documentation and Reporting

1. Records findings in the patient's chart.	S ☐ U ☐ N/A ☐	S ☐ U ☐ N/A ☐	S ☐ U ☐ N/A ☐
2. Reports any abnormal findings to the appropriate health care provider.	S ☐ U ☐ N/A ☐	S ☐ U ☐ N/A ☐	S ☐ U ☐ N/A ☐

Comments:

_____

_____

_____

Signatures:

Student _____ Date Passed _____

Instructor (Laboratory Setting) _____ Date Passed _____

Student _____ Date Passed _____

Instructor (Clinical Setting) _____ Date Passed _____

Procedural Assessment 16-1

Student _____ Date _____

Instructor (Laboratory Setting) _____ Date _____

Instructor (Clinical Setting) _____ Date _____

Criteria for assessment success:

The student must obtain all **satisfactory (S)** scores to pass the procedural evaluation. Any **unsatisfactory (U)** scores will result in failure of the procedural assessment.

Scoring:

Satisfactory (S): Procedural step performed correctly with no instructor prompting. Student-initiated correction is acceptable.

Unsatisfactory (U): Procedural step was performed incorrectly, omitted, or performed in a way that compromised patient care.

Not applicable (N/A): Procedural step was not indicated or necessary.

Evaluation:

	Peer Evaluation Laboratory Setting	Instructor Evaluation Laboratory Setting	Instructor Evaluation Clinical Setting
Procedural Preparation			
1. Reviews the patient's chart.	S ☐ U ☐ N/A ☐	S ☐ U ☐ N/A ☐	S ☐ U ☐ N/A ☐
2. Verifies the physician's order or the facility's protocol for standard of care.	S ☐ U ☐ N/A ☐	S ☐ U ☐ N/A ☐	S ☐ U ☐ N/A ☐
3. Obtains, cleans, and inspects the appropriate equipment prior to entering the patient's room.	S ☐ U ☐ N/A ☐	S ☐ U ☐ N/A ☐	S ☐ U ☐ N/A ☐
4. Follows PPE requirements, and observes standard precautions for any transmission-based isolation procedure.	S ☐ U ☐ N/A ☐	S ☐ U ☐ N/A ☐	S ☐ U ☐ N/A ☐
5. Identifies the patient using two patient identifiers.	S ☐ U ☐ N/A ☐	S ☐ U ☐ N/A ☐	S ☐ U ☐ N/A ☐
6. Introduces self to the patient and to the family.	S ☐ U ☐ N/A ☐	S ☐ U ☐ N/A ☐	S ☐ U ☐ N/A ☐
7. Explains the procedure to the patient and to the family, and acknowledges the patient's understanding.	S ☐ U ☐ N/A ☐	S ☐ U ☐ N/A ☐	S ☐ U ☐ N/A ☐
8. Performs proper hand hygiene, and puts on gloves, mask, and protective eyewear, as appropriate for the procedure.	S ☐ U ☐ N/A ☐	S ☐ U ☐ N/A ☐	S ☐ U ☐ N/A ☐
Implementation			
1. Places the patient in the semi-Fowler position, and instructs him or her to breathe normally.	S ☐ U ☐ N/A ☐	S ☐ U ☐ N/A ☐	S ☐ U ☐ N/A ☐
2. Assesses vital signs.	S ☐ U ☐ N/A ☐	S ☐ U ☐ N/A ☐	S ☐ U ☐ N/A ☐
3. Demonstrates how to place the mouthpiece and the hold device.	S ☐ U ☐ N/A ☐	S ☐ U ☐ N/A ☐	S ☐ U ☐ N/A ☐
4. Instructs the patient to inhale slowly and deeply to a maximal inspiration while maintaining a constant flow through the device.	S ☐ U ☐ N/A ☐	S ☐ U ☐ N/A ☐	S ☐ U ☐ N/A ☐

Continued

	Peer Evaluation Laboratory Setting			Instructor Evaluation Laboratory Setting			Instructor Evaluation Clinical Setting		
5. Instructs the patient to hold the breath for 5 to 10 seconds.	S ☐	U ☐	N/A ☐	S ☐	U ☐	N/A ☐	S ☐	U ☐	N/A ☐
6. Instructs the patient to exhale passively through pursed lips (see PA 27-2)	S ☐	U ☐	N/A ☐	S ☐	U ☐	N/A ☐	S ☐	U ☐	N/A ☐
7. Encourages the patient to cough.	S ☐	U ☐	N/A ☐	S ☐	U ☐	N/A ☐	S ☐	U ☐	N/A ☐
8. Advises the patient to perform the maneuver 5 to 10 times per hour while awake.	S ☐	U ☐	N/A ☐	S ☐	U ☐	N/A ☐	S ☐	U ☐	N/A ☐
9. Removes the supplies from the patient's room, and cleans the area, as needed.	S ☐	U ☐	N/A ☐	S ☐	U ☐	N/A ☐	S ☐	U ☐	N/A ☐
10. Removes PPE, and performs proper hand hygiene prior to leaving the patient's room.	S ☐	U ☐	N/A ☐	S ☐	U ☐	N/A ☐	S ☐	U ☐	N/A ☐

Evaluation of Procedure

	Peer Evaluation Laboratory Setting			Instructor Evaluation Laboratory Setting			Instructor Evaluation Clinical Setting		
1. Establishes a baseline, or compares with previous measurements.	S ☐	U ☐	N/A ☐	S ☐	U ☐	N/A ☐	S ☐	U ☐	N/A ☐
2. Assesses the patient's performance of the maneuver, and coaches to improve proficiency with the device.	S ☐	U ☐	N/A ☐	S ☐	U ☐	N/A ☐	S ☐	U ☐	N/A ☐
3. Identifies any unexpected outcomes.	S ☐	U ☐	N/A ☐	S ☐	U ☐	N/A ☐	S ☐	U ☐	N/A ☐
4. Correlates the patient's progress with chest radiographs and blood gas values, if available.	S ☐	U ☐	N/A ☐	S ☐	U ☐	N/A ☐	S ☐	U ☐	N/A ☐

Documentation and Reporting

	Peer Evaluation Laboratory Setting			Instructor Evaluation Laboratory Setting			Instructor Evaluation Clinical Setting		
1. Records the predicted goal volume and the actual volume attained in the patient's chart.	S ☐	U ☐	N/A ☐	S ☐	U ☐	N/A ☐	S ☐	U ☐	N/A ☐
2. Reports any abnormal findings to the appropriate health care provider.	S ☐	U ☐	N/A ☐	S ☐	U ☐	N/A ☐	S ☐	U ☐	N/A ☐

Comments:

_____

_____

_____

Signatures:

Student _____ Date Passed _____

Instructor (Laboratory Setting) _____ Date Passed _____

Student _____ Date Passed _____

Instructor (Clinical Setting) _____ Date Passed _____

Student _____ Date _____

Instructor (Laboratory Setting) _____ Date _____

Instructor (Clinical Setting) _____ Date _____

Criteria for assessment success:

The student must obtain all **satisfactory (S)** scores to pass the procedural evaluation. Any **unsatisfactory (U)** scores will result in failure of the procedural assessment.

Scoring:

Satisfactory (S): Procedural step performed correctly with no instructor prompting. Student-initiated correction is acceptable.

Unsatisfactory (U): Procedural step was performed incorrectly, omitted, or performed in a way that compromised patient care.

Not applicable (N/A): Procedural step was not indicated or necessary.

Evaluation:

	Peer Evaluation Laboratory Setting	Instructor Evaluation Laboratory Setting	Instructor Evaluation Clinical Setting
Procedural Preparation			
1. Reviews the patient's chart.	S ☐ U ☐ N/A ☐	S ☐ U ☐ N/A ☐	S ☐ U ☐ N/A ☐
2. Verifies the physician's order or the facility's protocol for standard of care.	S ☐ U ☐ N/A ☐	S ☐ U ☐ N/A ☐	S ☐ U ☐ N/A ☐
3. Obtains, cleans, and inspects the appropriate equipment prior to entering the patient's room.	S ☐ U ☐ N/A ☐	S ☐ U ☐ N/A ☐	S ☐ U ☐ N/A ☐
4. Follows PPE requirements, and observes standard precautions for any transmission-based isolation procedure.	S ☐ U ☐ N/A ☐	S ☐ U ☐ N/A ☐	S ☐ U ☐ N/A ☐
5. Identifies the patient using two patient identifiers.	S ☐ U ☐ N/A ☐	S ☐ U ☐ N/A ☐	S ☐ U ☐ N/A ☐
6. Introduces yourself to the patient and to the family.	S ☐ U ☐ N/A ☐	S ☐ U ☐ N/A ☐	S ☐ U ☐ N/A ☐
7. Explains the procedure to the patient and to the family, and acknowledges the patient's understanding.	S ☐ U ☐ N/A ☐	S ☐ U ☐ N/A ☐	S ☐ U ☐ N/A ☐
8. Performs proper hand hygiene, and puts on gloves, mask, and protective eyewear, as appropriate for the procedure.	S ☐ U ☐ N/A ☐	S ☐ U ☐ N/A ☐	S ☐ U ☐ N/A ☐
Implementation			
1. Places the patient in the semi-Fowler position, and instructs him or her to breathe normally.	S ☐ U ☐ N/A ☐	S ☐ U ☐ N/A ☐	S ☐ U ☐ N/A ☐
2. Assesses vital signs.	S ☐ U ☐ N/A ☐	S ☐ U ☐ N/A ☐	S ☐ U ☐ N/A ☐
3. Obtains baseline values for inspiratory capacity, expiratory tidal volume, and peak expiratory flow rate.	S ☐ U ☐ N/A ☐	S ☐ U ☐ N/A ☐	S ☐ U ☐ N/A ☐
4. Checks machine sensitivity.	S ☐ U ☐ N/A ☐	S ☐ U ☐ N/A ☐	S ☐ U ☐ N/A ☐
5. Checks the machine and the circuit for leaks.	S ☐ U ☐ N/A ☐	S ☐ U ☐ N/A ☐	S ☐ U ☐ N/A ☐
6. Instructs the patient on how to breathe correctly.	S ☐ U ☐ N/A ☐	S ☐ U ☐ N/A ☐	S ☐ U ☐ N/A ☐

Continued

	Peer Evaluation Laboratory Setting			Instructor Evaluation Laboratory Setting			Instructor Evaluation Clinical Setting		
7. Adjusts the machine as dictated by the patient's ventilatory patterns.	S ☐	U ☐	N/A ☐	S ☐	U ☐	N/A ☐	S ☐	U ☐	N/A ☐
8. Monitors inspiratory capacity, respiratory rate, heart rate, and blood pressure midway through the procedure.	S ☐	U ☐	N/A ☐	S ☐	U ☐	N/A ☐	S ☐	U ☐	N/A ☐
9. Encourages the patient to cough.	S ☐	U ☐	N/A ☐	S ☐	U ☐	N/A ☐	S ☐	U ☐	N/A ☐
10. Reassesses vital signs.	S ☐	U ☐	N/A ☐	S ☐	U ☐	N/A ☐	S ☐	U ☐	N/A ☐
11. Removes the supplies from the patient's room, and cleans the area, as needed.	S ☐	U ☐	N/A ☐	S ☐	U ☐	N/A ☐	S ☐	U ☐	N/A ☐
12. Removes PPE, and performs proper hand hygiene prior to leaving the patient's room.	S ☐	U ☐	N/A ☐	S ☐	U ☐	N/A ☐	S ☐	U ☐	N/A ☐

Evaluation of Procedure

	Peer Evaluation Laboratory Setting			Instructor Evaluation Laboratory Setting			Instructor Evaluation Clinical Setting		
1. Establishes a baseline, or compares with previous measurements.	S ☐	U ☐	N/A ☐	S ☐	U ☐	N/A ☐	S ☐	U ☐	N/A ☐
2. Monitors the effectiveness of therapy.	S ☐	U ☐	N/A ☐	S ☐	U ☐	N/A ☐	S ☐	U ☐	N/A ☐
3. Develops an appropriate respiratory care plan based on assessment data.	S ☐	U ☐	N/A ☐	S ☐	U ☐	N/A ☐	S ☐	U ☐	N/A ☐
4. Returns the patient to the previous oxygen modality.	S ☐	U ☐	N/A ☐	S ☐	U ☐	N/A ☐	S ☐	U ☐	N/A ☐
5. Identifies any unexpected outcomes.	S ☐	U ☐	N/A ☐	S ☐	U ☐	N/A ☐	S ☐	U ☐	N/A ☐

Documentation and Reporting

	Peer Evaluation Laboratory Setting			Instructor Evaluation Laboratory Setting			Instructor Evaluation Clinical Setting		
1. Records findings in the patient's chart.	S ☐	U ☐	N/A ☐	S ☐	U ☐	N/A ☐	S ☐	U ☐	N/A ☐
2. Reports any abnormal findings to the appropriate health care provider.	S ☐	U ☐	N/A ☐	S ☐	U ☐	N/A ☐	S ☐	U ☐	N/A ☐

Comments:

_____

_____

_____

Signatures:

Student _____ Date Passed _____

Instructor (Laboratory Setting) _____ Date Passed _____

Student _____ Date Passed _____

Instructor (Clinical Setting) _____ Date Passed _____

Procedural Assessment 16-3   Administering EzPAP

Student _____ Date _____

Instructor (Laboratory Setting) _____ Date _____

Instructor (Clinical Setting) _____ Date _____

Criteria for assessment success:

The student must obtain all **satisfactory (S)** scores to pass the procedural evaluation. Any **unsatisfactory (U)** scores will result in failure of the procedural assessment.

Scoring:

Satisfactory (S): Procedural step performed correctly with no instructor prompting. Student-initiated correction is acceptable.

Unsatisfactory (U): Procedural step was performed incorrectly, omitted, or performed in a way that compromised patient care.

Not applicable (N/A): Procedural step was not indicated or necessary.

Evaluation:

	Peer Evaluation Laboratory Setting	Instructor Evaluation Laboratory Setting	Instructor Evaluation Clinical Setting
Procedural Preparation			
1. Reviews the patient's chart.	S ☐ U ☐ N/A ☐	S ☐ U ☐ N/A ☐	S ☐ U ☐ N/A ☐
2. Verifies the physician's order or the facility's protocol for standard of care.	S ☐ U ☐ N/A ☐	S ☐ U ☐ N/A ☐	S ☐ U ☐ N/A ☐
3. Obtains, cleans, and inspects the appropriate equipment prior to entering the patient's room.	S ☐ U ☐ N/A ☐	S ☐ U ☐ N/A ☐	S ☐ U ☐ N/A ☐
4. Follows PPE requirements, and observes standard precautions for any transmission-based isolation procedure.	S ☐ U ☐ N/A ☐	S ☐ U ☐ N/A ☐	S ☐ U ☐ N/A ☐
5. Identifies the patient using two patient identifiers.	S ☐ U ☐ N/A ☐	S ☐ U ☐ N/A ☐	S ☐ U ☐ N/A ☐
6. Introduces self to the patient and to the family.	S ☐ U ☐ N/A ☐	S ☐ U ☐ N/A ☐	S ☐ U ☐ N/A ☐
7. Explains the procedure to the patient and to the family, and acknowledges the patient's understanding.	S ☐ U ☐ N/A ☐	S ☐ U ☐ N/A ☐	S ☐ U ☐ N/A ☐
8. Performs proper hand hygiene, and puts on gloves, mask, and protective eyewear, as appropriate for the procedure.	S ☐ U ☐ N/A ☐	S ☐ U ☐ N/A ☐	S ☐ U ☐ N/A ☐
Implementation			
1. Places the patient in the semi-Fowler position.	S ☐ U ☐ N/A ☐	S ☐ U ☐ N/A ☐	S ☐ U ☐ N/A ☐
2. Assesses vital signs.	S ☐ U ☐ N/A ☐	S ☐ U ☐ N/A ☐	S ☐ U ☐ N/A ☐
3. Assembles the unit.	S ☐ U ☐ N/A ☐	S ☐ U ☐ N/A ☐	S ☐ U ☐ N/A ☐
4. Attaches the mouthpiece or face mask to the rounded end of the device.	S ☐ U ☐ N/A ☐	S ☐ U ☐ N/A ☐	S ☐ U ☐ N/A ☐
5. Instructs the patient to relax while performing diaphragmatic breathing (see PA 27-3).	S ☐ U ☐ N/A ☐	S ☐ U ☐ N/A ☐	S ☐ U ☐ N/A ☐
6. Sets the initial flow rate to 5 L/min on the air or oxygen flowmeter.	S ☐ U ☐ N/A ☐	S ☐ U ☐ N/A ☐	S ☐ U ☐ N/A ☐

Continued

	Peer Evaluation Laboratory Setting			Instructor Evaluation Laboratory Setting			Instructor Evaluation Clinical Setting		
7. Attaches the appliance to the patient.	S ☐	U ☐	N/A ☐	S ☐	U ☐	N/A ☐	S ☐	U ☐	N/A ☐
8. Monitors the airway pressure while slowly increasing the flowmeter until the desired expiratory airway pressure is reached (10–20 cmH$_2$O).	S ☐	U ☐	N/A ☐	S ☐	U ☐	N/A ☐	S ☐	U ☐	N/A ☐
9. Instructs the patient to inhale and exhale slowly.	S ☐	U ☐	N/A ☐	S ☐	U ☐	N/A ☐	S ☐	U ☐	N/A ☐
10. Reassesses vital signs.	S ☐	U ☐	N/A ☐	S ☐	U ☐	N/A ☐	S ☐	U ☐	N/A ☐
11. Removes the supplies from the patient's room, and cleans the area, as needed.	S ☐	U ☐	N/A ☐	S ☐	U ☐	N/A ☐	S ☐	U ☐	N/A ☐
12. Removes PPE, and performs proper hand hygiene prior to leaving the patient's room.	S ☐	U ☐	N/A ☐	S ☐	U ☐	N/A ☐	S ☐	U ☐	N/A ☐

Evaluation of Procedure

	Peer Evaluation Laboratory Setting			Instructor Evaluation Laboratory Setting			Instructor Evaluation Clinical Setting		
1. Establishes a baseline, or compares with previous measurements.	S ☐	U ☐	N/A ☐	S ☐	U ☐	N/A ☐	S ☐	U ☐	N/A ☐
2. Assesses the patient's performance of the maneuver, and coaches to improve proficiency with the device.	S ☐	U ☐	N/A ☐	S ☐	U ☐	N/A ☐	S ☐	U ☐	N/A ☐
3. Identifies any unexpected outcomes.	S ☐	U ☐	N/A ☐	S ☐	U ☐	N/A ☐	S ☐	U ☐	N/A ☐
4. Correlates the patient's progress with chest radiographs and blood gas values, if available.	S ☐	U ☐	N/A ☐	S ☐	U ☐	N/A ☐	S ☐	U ☐	N/A ☐

Documentation and Reporting

	Peer Evaluation Laboratory Setting			Instructor Evaluation Laboratory Setting			Instructor Evaluation Clinical Setting		
1. Records the pressure, the flow rates, and the patient's tolerance to the procedure in the patient's chart.	S ☐	U ☐	N/A ☐	S ☐	U ☐	N/A ☐	S ☐	U ☐	N/A ☐
2. Reports any abnormal findings to the appropriate health care provider.	S ☐	U ☐	N/A ☐	S ☐	U ☐	N/A ☐	S ☐	U ☐	N/A ☐

Comments:

_____

_____

_____

Signatures:

Student _____ Date Passed _____

Instructor (Laboratory Setting) _____ Date Passed _____

Student _____ Date Passed _____

Instructor (Clinical Setting) _____ Date Passed _____

Procedural Assessment 16-4 Using the Metaneb system

Student _____ Date _____

Instructor (Laboratory Setting) _____ Date _____

Instructor (Clinical Setting) _____ Date _____

Criteria for assessment success:

The student must obtain all **satisfactory (S)** scores to pass the procedural evaluation. Any **unsatisfactory (U)** scores will result in failure of the procedural assessment.

Scoring:

Satisfactory (S): Procedural step performed correctly with no instructor prompting. Student-initiated correction is acceptable.

Unsatisfactory (U): Procedural step was performed incorrectly, omitted, or performed in a way that compromised patient care.

Not applicable (N/A): Procedural step was not indicated or necessary.

	Peer Evaluation Laboratory Setting	Instructor Evaluation Laboratory Setting	Instructor Evaluation Clinical Setting
Procedural Preparation			
1. Reviews the patient's chart.	S ☐ U ☐ N/A ☐	S ☐ U ☐ N/A ☐	S ☐ U ☐ N/A ☐
2. Verifies the physician's order or the facility's protocol for standard of care.	S ☐ U ☐ N/A ☐	S ☐ U ☐ N/A ☐	S ☐ U ☐ N/A ☐
3. Obtains, cleans, and inspects the appropriate equipment prior to entering the patient's room.	S ☐ U ☐ N/A ☐	S ☐ U ☐ N/A ☐	S ☐ U ☐ N/A ☐
4. Follows PPE requirements, and observes standard precautions for any transmission-based isolation procedure.	S ☐ U ☐ N/A ☐	S ☐ U ☐ N/A ☐	S ☐ U ☐ N/A ☐
5. Identifies the patient using two patient identifiers.	S ☐ U ☐ N/A ☐	S ☐ U ☐ N/A ☐	S ☐ U ☐ N/A ☐
6. Introduces self to the patient and the family.	S ☐ U ☐ N/A ☐	S ☐ U ☐ N/A ☐	S ☐ U ☐ N/A ☐
7. Explains the procedure to the patient and the family, and acknowledges the patient's understanding.	S ☐ U ☐ N/A ☐	S ☐ U ☐ N/A ☐	S ☐ U ☐ N/A ☐
8. Performs proper hand hygiene, and puts on gloves, mask, and protective eyewear, as appropriate for the procedure.	S ☐ U ☐ N/A ☐	S ☐ U ☐ N/A ☐	S ☐ U ☐ N/A ☐
Implementation			
1. Positions the patient upright.	S ☐ U ☐ N/A ☐	S ☐ U ☐ N/A ☐	S ☐ U ☐ N/A ☐
2. Assesses vital signs.	S ☐ U ☐ N/A ☐	S ☐ U ☐ N/A ☐	S ☐ U ☐ N/A ☐
3. Connects the circuit connector to the controller connector port.	S ☐ U ☐ N/A ☐	S ☐ U ☐ N/A ☐	S ☐ U ☐ N/A ☐
4. Fills the nebulizer cup with medications, if applicable.	S ☐ U ☐ N/A ☐	S ☐ U ☐ N/A ☐	S ☐ U ☐ N/A ☐
5. Sets the mode selector to CPEP.	S ☐ U ☐ N/A ☐	S ☐ U ☐ N/A ☐	S ☐ U ☐ N/A ☐
6. Turns the selector ring to the medium resistance setting.	S ☐ U ☐ N/A ☐	S ☐ U ☐ N/A ☐	S ☐ U ☐ N/A ☐
7. Connects the oxygen hose to a 50 psi gas source.	S ☐ U ☐ N/A ☐	S ☐ U ☐ N/A ☐	S ☐ U ☐ N/A ☐
8. Turns master switch on.	S ☐ U ☐ N/A ☐	S ☐ U ☐ N/A ☐	S ☐ U ☐ N/A ☐

Continued

	Peer Evaluation Laboratory Setting			Instructor Evaluation Laboratory Setting			Instructor Evaluation Clinical Setting		
9. Occludes the patient end of the handset and adjusts the CPEP flow until the manometer reads 10 cmH$_2$O.	S ☐	U ☐	N/A ☐	S ☐	U ☐	N/A ☐	S ☐	U ☐	N/A ☐
10. Attaches the mouthpiece or face mask.	S ☐	U ☐	N/A ☐	S ☐	U ☐	N/A ☐	S ☐	U ☐	N/A ☐
11. Encourages slow exhalation.	S ☐	U ☐	N/A ☐	S ☐	U ☐	N/A ☐	S ☐	U ☐	N/A ☐
12. Adjusts the ring selector as applicable for the patient.	S ☐	U ☐	N/A ☐	S ☐	U ☐	N/A ☐	S ☐	U ☐	N/A ☐
13. Continues CPEP for about 2½ minutes.	S ☐	U ☐	N/A ☐	S ☐	U ☐	N/A ☐	S ☐	U ☐	N/A ☐
14. Informs the patient that they are about to feel a pulsating flow of gas.	S ☐	U ☐	N/A ☐	S ☐	U ☐	N/A ☐	S ☐	U ☐	N/A ☐
15. Moves the Higher/Lower switch to the Higher position and changes the mode to CHFO.	S ☐	U ☐	N/A ☐	S ☐	U ☐	N/A ☐	S ☐	U ☐	N/A ☐
16. Encourages slow exhalation.	S ☐	U ☐	N/A ☐	S ☐	U ☐	N/A ☐	S ☐	U ☐	N/A ☐
17. Continues CHFO for about 2½ minutes.	S ☐	U ☐	N/A ☐	S ☐	U ☐	N/A ☐	S ☐	U ☐	N/A ☐
18. Alternates between CPEP and CHFO until therapy is complete.	S ☐	U ☐	N/A ☐	S ☐	U ☐	N/A ☐	S ☐	U ☐	N/A ☐
19. Turns MetaNeb machine off and cleans nebulizer cup.	S ☐	U ☐	N/A ☐	S ☐	U ☐	N/A ☐	S ☐	U ☐	N/A ☐
20. Removes the supplies from the patient's room, and cleans the area, as needed.	S ☐	U ☐	N/A ☐	S ☐	U ☐	N/A ☐	S ☐	U ☐	N/A ☐
21. Removes the PPE, and performs proper hand hygiene prior to leaving the patient's room.	S ☐	U ☐	N/A ☐	S ☐	U ☐	N/A ☐	S ☐	U ☐	N/A ☐

Evaluation of Procedure

1. Establishes a baseline, or compare with previous measurements.	S ☐	U ☐	N/A ☐	S ☐	U ☐	N/A ☐	S ☐	U ☐	N/A ☐
2. Identifies any unexpected outcomes.	S ☐	U ☐	N/A ☐	S ☐	U ☐	N/A ☐	S ☐	U ☐	N/A ☐
3. Correlates the patient's progress with chest radiographs and blood gas values, if available.	S ☐	U ☐	N/A ☐	S ☐	U ☐	N/A ☐	S ☐	U ☐	N/A ☐

Documentation and Reporting

1. Records the settings, medications, and the patient's tolerance to the procedure in the patient's chart.	S ☐	U ☐	N/A ☐	S ☐	U ☐	N/A ☐	S ☐	U ☐	N/A ☐
2. Reports any abnormal findings to the appropriate health care provider.	S ☐	U ☐	N/A ☐	S ☐	U ☐	N/A ☐	S ☐	U ☐	N/A ☐

Comments:

_____

_____

_____

Signatures:

Student _____ Date Passed _____

Instructor (Laboratory Setting) _____ Date Passed _____

Student _____ Date Passed _____

Instructor (Clinical Setting) _____ Date Passed _____

Student _____ Date _____

Instructor (Laboratory Setting) _____ Date _____

Instructor (Clinical Setting) _____ Date _____

Criteria for assessment success:

The student must obtain all **satisfactory (S)** scores to pass the procedural evaluation. Any **unsatisfactory (U)** scores will result in failure of the procedural assessment.

Scoring:

Satisfactory (S): Procedural step performed correctly with no instructor prompting. Student-initiated correction is acceptable.

Unsatisfactory (U): Procedural step was performed incorrectly, omitted, or performed in a way that compromised patient care.

Not applicable (N/A): Procedural step was not indicated or necessary.

Evaluation:

	Peer Evaluation Laboratory Setting	Instructor Evaluation Laboratory Setting	Instructor Evaluation Clinical Setting
Procedural Preparation			
1. Reviews the patient's chart, and identifies the appropriate lobe(s) and segment(s) for drainage.	S ☐ U ☐ N/A ☐	S ☐ U ☐ N/A ☐	S ☐ U ☐ N/A ☐
2. Verifies the physician's order or the facility's protocol for standard of care.	S ☐ U ☐ N/A ☐	S ☐ U ☐ N/A ☐	S ☐ U ☐ N/A ☐
3. Obtains, cleans, and inspects the appropriate equipment prior to entering the patient's room.	S ☐ U ☐ N/A ☐	S ☐ U ☐ N/A ☐	S ☐ U ☐ N/A ☐
4. Follows PPE requirements, and observes standard precautions for any transmission-based isolation procedure.	S ☐ U ☐ N/A ☐	S ☐ U ☐ N/A ☐	S ☐ U ☐ N/A ☐
5. Identifies the patient using two patient identifiers.	S ☐ U ☐ N/A ☐	S ☐ U ☐ N/A ☐	S ☐ U ☐ N/A ☐
6. Introduces self to the patient and to the family.	S ☐ U ☐ N/A ☐	S ☐ U ☐ N/A ☐	S ☐ U ☐ N/A ☐
7. Explains the procedure to the patient and to the family, and acknowledges the patient's understanding.	S ☐ U ☐ N/A ☐	S ☐ U ☐ N/A ☐	S ☐ U ☐ N/A ☐
8. Performs proper hand hygiene, and puts on gloves, mask, and protective eyewear, as appropriate for the procedure.	S ☐ U ☐ N/A ☐	S ☐ U ☐ N/A ☐	S ☐ U ☐ N/A ☐
Implementation			
1. Assesses vital signs.	S ☐ U ☐ N/A ☐	S ☐ U ☐ N/A ☐	S ☐ U ☐ N/A ☐
2. Places the patient in the proper position for drainage.	S ☐ U ☐ N/A ☐	S ☐ U ☐ N/A ☐	S ☐ U ☐ N/A ☐
3. Confirms the patient's comfort in the drainage position.	S ☐ U ☐ N/A ☐	S ☐ U ☐ N/A ☐	S ☐ U ☐ N/A ☐
4. Percusses the patient over the proper segment for 3 to 5 minutes.	S ☐ U ☐ N/A ☐	S ☐ U ☐ N/A ☐	S ☐ U ☐ N/A ☐
5. Instructs the patient to exhale through pursed lips during vibrations.	S ☐ U ☐ N/A ☐	S ☐ U ☐ N/A ☐	S ☐ U ☐ N/A ☐
6. Instructs the patient to cough.	S ☐ U ☐ N/A ☐	S ☐ U ☐ N/A ☐	S ☐ U ☐ N/A ☐

Continued

	Peer Evaluation Laboratory Setting			Instructor Evaluation Laboratory Setting			Instructor Evaluation Clinical Setting		
7. Reassesses vital signs, and continuously observes the patient for any adverse effects or complications during the procedure.	S ☐	U ☐	N/A ☐	S ☐	U ☐	N/A ☐	S ☐	U ☐	N/A ☐
8. Restores the patient to the pretreatment position of comfort.	S ☐	U ☐	N/A ☐	S ☐	U ☐	N/A ☐	S ☐	U ☐	N/A ☐
9. Ensures the patient's stability and comfort.	S ☐	U ☐	N/A ☐	S ☐	U ☐	N/A ☐	S ☐	U ☐	N/A ☐
10. Removes the supplies from the patient's room, and cleans the area, as needed.	S ☐	U ☐	N/A ☐	S ☐	U ☐	N/A ☐	S ☐	U ☐	N/A ☐
11. Removes PPE, and performs proper hand hygiene prior to leaving the patient's room.	S ☐	U ☐	N/A ☐	S ☐	U ☐	N/A ☐	S ☐	U ☐	N/A ☐

Evaluation of Procedure

1. Establishes a baseline, or compares with previous measurements.	S ☐	U ☐	N/A ☐	S ☐	U ☐	N/A ☐	S ☐	U ☐	N/A ☐
2. Develops an appropriate respiratory care plan based on assessment data.	S ☐	U ☐	N/A ☐	S ☐	U ☐	N/A ☐	S ☐	U ☐	N/A ☐
3. Notes any need for oxygen therapy during the procedure.	S ☐	U ☐	N/A ☐	S ☐	U ☐	N/A ☐	S ☐	U ☐	N/A ☐
4. Identifies any unexpected outcomes.	S ☐	U ☐	N/A ☐	S ☐	U ☐	N/A ☐	S ☐	U ☐	N/A ☐

Documentation and Reporting

1. Records findings, including position used, time in position, patient tolerance, and subjective and objective indicators of treatment effectiveness, in the patient's chart.	S ☐	U ☐	N/A ☐	S ☐	U ☐	N/A ☐	S ☐	U ☐	N/A ☐
2. Reports any abnormal findings to the appropriate health care provider.	S ☐	U ☐	N/A ☐	S ☐	U ☐	N/A ☐	S ☐	U ☐	N/A ☐

Comments:

_____

_____

_____

Signatures:

Student _____ Date Passed _____

Instructor (Laboratory Setting) _____ Date Passed _____

Student _____ Date Passed _____

Instructor (Clinical Setting) _____ Date Passed _____

Student _____ Date _____

Instructor (Laboratory Setting) _____ Date _____

Instructor (Clinical Setting) _____ Date _____

Criteria for assessment success:

The student must obtain all **satisfactory (S)** scores to pass the procedural evaluation. Any **unsatisfactory (U)** scores will result in failure of the procedural assessment.

Scoring:

Satisfactory (S): Procedural step performed correctly with no instructor prompting. Student-initiated correction is acceptable.

Unsatisfactory (U): Procedural step was performed incorrectly, omitted, or performed in a way that compromised patient care.

Not applicable (N/A): Procedural step was not indicated or necessary.

Evaluation:

	Peer Evaluation Laboratory Setting	Instructor Evaluation Laboratory Setting	Instructor Evaluation Clinical Setting
Procedural Preparation			
1. Reviews the patient's chart.	S ☐ U ☐ N/A ☐	S ☐ U ☐ N/A ☐	S ☐ U ☐ N/A ☐
2. Verifies the physician's order or the facility's protocol for standard of care.	S ☐ U ☐ N/A ☐	S ☐ U ☐ N/A ☐	S ☐ U ☐ N/A ☐
3. Obtains, cleans, and inspects the appropriate equipment prior to entering the patient's room	S ☐ U ☐ N/A ☐	S ☐ U ☐ N/A ☐	S ☐ U ☐ N/A ☐
4. Follows PPE requirements, and observes standard precautions for any transmission-based isolation procedure.	S ☐ U ☐ N/A ☐	S ☐ U ☐ N/A ☐	S ☐ U ☐ N/A ☐
5. Identifies the patient using two patient identifiers.	S ☐ U ☐ N/A ☐	S ☐ U ☐ N/A ☐	S ☐ U ☐ N/A ☐
6. Introduces self to the patient and to the family.	S ☐ U ☐ N/A ☐	S ☐ U ☐ N/A ☐	S ☐ U ☐ N/A ☐
7. Explains the procedure to the patient and to the family, and acknowledges the patient's understanding.	S ☐ U ☐ N/A ☐	S ☐ U ☐ N/A ☐	S ☐ U ☐ N/A ☐
8. Performs proper hand hygiene, and puts on gloves, mask, and protective eyewear, as appropriate for the procedure.	S ☐ U ☐ N/A ☐	S ☐ U ☐ N/A ☐	S ☐ U ☐ N/A ☐
Implementation			
1. Assesses vital signs.	S ☐ U ☐ N/A ☐	S ☐ U ☐ N/A ☐	S ☐ U ☐ N/A ☐
2. Instructs the patient to assume the sitting position, with one shoulder rotated inward and the head and spine slightly flexed; elevates the head of the bed, if necessary.	S ☐ U ☐ N/A ☐	S ☐ U ☐ N/A ☐	S ☐ U ☐ N/A ☐
3. Instructs the patient to use diaphragmatic breathing techniques.	S ☐ U ☐ N/A ☐	S ☐ U ☐ N/A ☐	S ☐ U ☐ N/A ☐
4. Confirms that the patient can take a deep breath.	S ☐ U ☐ N/A ☐	S ☐ U ☐ N/A ☐	S ☐ U ☐ N/A ☐
5. Instructs the patient to bear down against the glottis, followed by a slight breath-hold, and cough.	S ☐ U ☐ N/A ☐	S ☐ U ☐ N/A ☐	S ☐ U ☐ N/A ☐
6. Supplies tissue for sputum.	S ☐ U ☐ N/A ☐	S ☐ U ☐ N/A ☐	S ☐ U ☐ N/A ☐

Continued

	Peer Evaluation Laboratory Setting			Instructor Evaluation Laboratory Setting			Instructor Evaluation Clinical Setting		
7. Removes the supplies from the patient's room, and cleans the area, as needed.	S ☐	U ☐	N/A ☐	S ☐	U ☐	N/A ☐	S ☐	U ☐	N/A ☐
8. Removes PPE, and performs proper hand hygiene prior to leaving the patient's room.	S ☐	U ☐	N/A ☐	S ☐	U ☐	N/A ☐	S ☐	U ☐	N/A ☐

Evaluation of Procedure

1. Establishes a baseline, or compares with previous measurements.	S ☐	U ☐	N/A ☐	S ☐	U ☐	N/A ☐	S ☐	U ☐	N/A ☐
2. Develops an appropriate respiratory care plan based on assessment data.	S ☐	U ☐	N/A ☐	S ☐	U ☐	N/A ☐	S ☐	U ☐	N/A ☐
3. Evaluates the color, consistency, volume, and odor of sputum.	S ☐	U ☐	N/A ☐	S ☐	U ☐	N/A ☐	S ☐	U ☐	N/A ☐
4. Notes any use of oxygen therapy.	S ☐	U ☐	N/A ☐	S ☐	U ☐	N/A ☐	S ☐	U ☐	N/A ☐
5. Identifies any unexpected outcomes.	S ☐	U ☐	N/A ☐	S ☐	U ☐	N/A ☐	S ☐	U ☐	N/A ☐

Documentation and Reporting

1. Records findings in the patient's chart.	S ☐	U ☐	N/A ☐	S ☐	U ☐	N/A ☐	S ☐	U ☐	N/A ☐
2. Reports any abnormal findings to the appropriate health care provider.	S ☐	U ☐	N/A ☐	S ☐	U ☐	N/A ☐	S ☐	U ☐	N/A ☐

Comments:

_____

_____

_____

Signatures:

Student _____ Date Passed _____

Instructor (Laboratory Setting) _____ Date Passed _____

Student _____ Date Passed _____

Instructor (Clinical Setting) _____ Date Passed _____

Student _____ Date _____

Instructor (Laboratory Setting) _____ Date _____

Instructor (Clinical Setting) _____ Date _____

Criteria for assessment success:

The student must obtain all **satisfactory (S)** scores to pass the procedural evaluation. Any **unsatisfactory (U)** scores will result in failure of the procedural assessment.

Scoring:

Satisfactory (S): Procedural step performed correctly with no instructor prompting. Student-initiated correction is acceptable.

Unsatisfactory (U): Procedural step was performed incorrectly, omitted, or performed in a way that compromised patient care.

Not applicable (N/A): Procedural step was not indicated or necessary.

Evaluation:

	Peer Evaluation Laboratory Setting	Instructor Evaluation Laboratory Setting	Instructor Evaluation Clinical Setting
Procedural Preparation			
1. Reviews the patient's chart.	S ☐ U ☐ N/A ☐	S ☐ U ☐ N/A ☐	S ☐ U ☐ N/A ☐
2. Verifies the physician's order or the facility's protocol for standard of care.	S ☐ U ☐ N/A ☐	S ☐ U ☐ N/A ☐	S ☐ U ☐ N/A ☐
3. Obtains, cleans, and inspects the appropriate equipment prior to entering the patient's room.	S ☐ U ☐ N/A ☐	S ☐ U ☐ N/A ☐	S ☐ U ☐ N/A ☐
4. Follows PPE requirements, and observes standard precautions for any transmission-based isolation procedure.	S ☐ U ☐ N/A ☐	S ☐ U ☐ N/A ☐	S ☐ U ☐ N/A ☐
5. Identifies the patient using two patient identifiers.	S ☐ U ☐ N/A ☐	S ☐ U ☐ N/A ☐	S ☐ U ☐ N/A ☐
6. Introduces self to the patient and to the family.	S ☐ U ☐ N/A ☐	S ☐ U ☐ N/A ☐	S ☐ U ☐ N/A ☐
7. Explains the procedure to the patient and to the family, and acknowledges the patient's understanding.	S ☐ U ☐ N/A ☐	S ☐ U ☐ N/A ☐	S ☐ U ☐ N/A ☐
8. Performs proper hand hygiene, and puts on gloves, mask, and protective eyewear, as appropriate for the procedure.	S ☐ U ☐ N/A ☐	S ☐ U ☐ N/A ☐	S ☐ U ☐ N/A ☐
Implementation			
1. Places the patient in a comfortable position.	S ☐ U ☐ N/A ☐	S ☐ U ☐ N/A ☐	S ☐ U ☐ N/A ☐
2. Assesses vital signs.	S ☐ U ☐ N/A ☐	S ☐ U ☐ N/A ☐	S ☐ U ☐ N/A ☐
3. Instructs the patient to assume the sitting position, with one shoulder rotated inward and the head and spine slightly flexed:			
a. If the patient is unable to do this, elevates the head of the bed.	S ☐ U ☐ N/A ☐	S ☐ U ☐ N/A ☐	S ☐ U ☐ N/A ☐
b. Explains splinting to the postsurgical patient.	S ☐ U ☐ N/A ☐	S ☐ U ☐ N/A ☐	S ☐ U ☐ N/A ☐

Continued

	Peer Evaluation Laboratory Setting	Instructor Evaluation Laboratory Setting	Instructor Evaluation Clinical Setting
4. Confirms that the patient can take a moderate to deep breath.	S ☐ U ☐ N/A ☐	S ☐ U ☐ N/A ☐	S ☐ U ☐ N/A ☐
5. Instructs the patient to take a moderate to deep breath followed by a short breath-hold.	S ☐ U ☐ N/A ☐	S ☐ U ☐ N/A ☐	S ☐ U ☐ N/A ☐
6. Instructs the patient to perform three uninterrupted forced exhalations while saying "huff":			
a. Huff cough #1, with lung deflation	S ☐ U ☐ N/A ☐	S ☐ U ☐ N/A ☐	S ☐ U ☐ N/A ☐
b. Huff cough #2, with further lung deflation	S ☐ U ☐ N/A ☐	S ☐ U ☐ N/A ☐	S ☐ U ☐ N/A ☐
c. Huff cough #3, with still further lung deflation	S ☐ U ☐ N/A ☐	S ☐ U ☐ N/A ☐	S ☐ U ☐ N/A ☐
7. Instructs the patient to take one deep breath in, followed by a single abrupt Huff cough, for final expectoration.	S ☐ U ☐ N/A ☐	S ☐ U ☐ N/A ☐	S ☐ U ☐ N/A ☐
8. Repeats, as necessary, after a brief rest, if clearance is not complete.	S ☐ U ☐ N/A ☐	S ☐ U ☐ N/A ☐	S ☐ U ☐ N/A ☐
9. Instructs the patient to use diaphragmatic breathing techniques following FET.	S ☐ U ☐ N/A ☐	S ☐ U ☐ N/A ☐	S ☐ U ☐ N/A ☐
10. Removes the supplies from the patient's room, and cleans the area, as needed.	S ☐ U ☐ N/A ☐	S ☐ U ☐ N/A ☐	S ☐ U ☐ N/A ☐
11. Removes PPE, and performs proper hand hygiene prior to leaving the patient's room.	S ☐ U ☐ N/A ☐	S ☐ U ☐ N/A ☐	S ☐ U ☐ N/A ☐

Evaluation of Procedure

1. Establishes a baseline, or compares with previous measurements.	S ☐ U ☐ N/A ☐	S ☐ U ☐ N/A ☐	S ☐ U ☐ N/A ☐
2. Develops an appropriate respiratory care plan based on assessment data.	S ☐ U ☐ N/A ☐	S ☐ U ☐ N/A ☐	S ☐ U ☐ N/A ☐
3. Evaluates the color, consistency, volume, and odor of sputum.	S ☐ U ☐ N/A ☐	S ☐ U ☐ N/A ☐	S ☐ U ☐ N/A ☐
4. Notes any use of oxygen therapy.	S ☐ U ☐ N/A ☐	S ☐ U ☐ N/A ☐	S ☐ U ☐ N/A ☐
5. Identifies any unexpected outcomes.	S ☐ U ☐ N/A ☐	S ☐ U ☐ N/A ☐	S ☐ U ☐ N/A ☐

Documentation and Reporting

1. Records findings in the patient's chart.	S ☐ U ☐ N/A ☐	S ☐ U ☐ N/A ☐	S ☐ U ☐ N/A ☐
2. Reports any abnormal findings to the appropriate health care provider.	S ☐ U ☐ N/A ☐	S ☐ U ☐ N/A ☐	S ☐ U ☐ N/A ☐

Comments:

_____

_____

_____

Signatures:

Student _____ Date Passed _____

Instructor (Laboratory Setting) _____ Date Passed _____

Student _____ Date Passed _____

Instructor (Clinical Setting) _____ Date Passed _____

Student _____ Date _____

Instructor (Laboratory Setting) _____ Date _____

Instructor (Clinical Setting) _____ Date _____

Criteria for assessment success:

The student must obtain all **satisfactory (S)** scores to pass the procedural evaluation. Any **unsatisfactory (U)** scores will result in failure of the procedural assessment.

Scoring:

Satisfactory (S): Procedural step performed correctly with no instructor prompting. Student-initiated correction is acceptable.

Unsatisfactory (U): Procedural step was performed incorrectly, omitted, or performed in a way that compromised patient care.

Not applicable (N/A): Procedural step was not indicated or necessary.

Evaluation:

	Peer Evaluation Laboratory Setting	Instructor Evaluation Laboratory Setting	Instructor Evaluation Clinical Setting
Procedural Preparation			
1. Reviews the patient's chart.	S ☐ U ☐ N/A☐	S ☐ U ☐ N/A☐	S ☐ U ☐ N/A☐
2. Verifies the physician's order or the facility's protocol for standard of care.	S ☐ U ☐ N/A☐	S ☐ U ☐ N/A☐	S ☐ U ☐ N/A☐
3. Obtains, cleans, and inspects the appropriate equipment prior to entering the patient's room.	S ☐ U ☐ N/A☐	S ☐ U ☐ N/A☐	S ☐ U ☐ N/A☐
4. Follows PPE requirements, and observes standard precautions for any transmission-based isolation procedure.	S ☐ U ☐ N/A☐	S ☐ U ☐ N/A☐	S ☐ U ☐ N/A☐
5. Identifies the patient using two patient identifiers.	S ☐ U ☐ N/A☐	S ☐ U ☐ N/A☐	S ☐ U ☐ N/A☐
6. Introduces self to the patient and to the family.	S ☐ U ☐ N/A☐	S ☐ U ☐ N/A☐	S ☐ U ☐ N/A☐
7. Explains the procedure to the patient and to the family, and acknowledges the patient's understanding.	S ☐ U ☐ N/A☐	S ☐ U ☐ N/A☐	S ☐ U ☐ N/A☐
8. Performs proper hand hygiene, and puts on gloves, mask, and protective eyewear, as appropriate for the procedure.	S ☐ U ☐ N/A☐	S ☐ U ☐ N/A☐	S ☐ U ☐ N/A☐
Implementation			
1. Places the patient in a comfortable position.	S ☐ U ☐ N/A☐	S ☐ U ☐ N/A☐	S ☐ U ☐ N/A☐
2. Assesses vital signs.	S ☐ U ☐ N/A☐	S ☐ U ☐ N/A☐	S ☐ U ☐ N/A☐
3. Assembles the equipment.	S ☐ U ☐ N/A☐	S ☐ U ☐ N/A☐	S ☐ U ☐ N/A☐
4. Sets the correct pressures: a. Positive pressures from 30 to 50 cmH$_2$O	S ☐ U ☐ N/A☐	S ☐ U ☐ N/A☐	S ☐ U ☐ N/A☐
b. Negative pressures from −30 to −50 cmH$_2$O	S ☐ U ☐ N/A☐	S ☐ U ☐ N/A☐	S ☐ U ☐ N/A☐
5. Sets the correct interval times.	S ☐ U ☐ N/A☐	S ☐ U ☐ N/A☐	S ☐ U ☐ N/A☐

Continued

	Peer Evaluation Laboratory Setting	Instructor Evaluation Laboratory Setting	Instructor Evaluation Clinical Setting
6. Informs the patient about the intended session time and the subsequent period of normal spontaneous or assisted breathing.	S ☐ U ☐ N/A☐	S ☐ U ☐ N/A☐	S ☐ U ☐ N/A☐
7. Repeats the session until secretions are cleared.	S ☐ U ☐ N/A☐	S ☐ U ☐ N/A☐	S ☐ U ☐ N/A☐
8. Reassesses vital signs.	S ☐ U ☐ N/A☐	S ☐ U ☐ N/A☐	S ☐ U ☐ N/A☐
9. Removes the supplies from the patient's room, and cleans the area, as needed.	S ☐ U ☐ N/A☐	S ☐ U ☐ N/A☐	S ☐ U ☐ N/A☐
10. Removes PPE, and performs proper hand hygiene prior to leaving the patient's room.	S ☐ U ☐ N/A☐	S ☐ U ☐ N/A☐	S ☐ U ☐ N/A☐

Evaluation of Procedure

1. Establishes a baseline, or compares with previous measurements.	S ☐ U ☐ N/A☐	S ☐ U ☐ N/A☐	S ☐ U ☐ N/A☐
2. Develops an appropriate respiratory care plan based on assessment data.	S ☐ U ☐ N/A☐	S ☐ U ☐ N/A☐	S ☐ U ☐ N/A☐
3. Notes any use of oxygen therapy.	S ☐ U ☐ N/A☐	S ☐ U ☐ N/A☐	S ☐ U ☐ N/A☐
4. Monitors the patient for any adverse reactions to the procedure.	S ☐ U ☐ N/A☐	S ☐ U ☐ N/A☐	S ☐ U ☐ N/A☐
5. Identifies any unexpected outcomes.	S ☐ U ☐ N/A☐	S ☐ U ☐ N/A☐	S ☐ U ☐ N/A☐

Documentation and Reporting

1. Records findings in the patient's chart.	S ☐ U ☐ N/A☐	S ☐ U ☐ N/A☐	S ☐ U ☐ N/A☐
2. Reports any abnormal findings to the appropriate health care provider.	S ☐ U ☐ N/A☐	S ☐ U ☐ N/A☐	S ☐ U ☐ N/A☐

Comments:

_____

_____

_____

Signatures:

Student _____ Date Passed _____

Instructor (Laboratory Setting) _____ Date Passed _____

Student _____ Date Passed _____

Instructor (Clinical Setting) _____ Date Passed _____

Procedural Assessment 17-5

Implementing positive airway pressure therapy

Student _____ Date _____

Instructor (Laboratory Setting) _____ Date _____

Instructor (Clinical Setting) _____ Date _____

Criteria for assessment success:

The student must obtain all **satisfactory (S)** scores to pass the procedural evaluation. Any **unsatisfactory (U)** scores will result in failure of the procedural assessment.

Scoring:

Satisfactory (S): Procedural step performed correctly with no instructor prompting. Student-initiated correction is acceptable.

Unsatisfactory (U): Procedural step was performed incorrectly, omitted, or performed in a way that compromised patient care.

Not applicable (N/A): Procedural step was not indicated or necessary.

Evaluation:

	Peer Evaluation Laboratory Setting	Instructor Evaluation Laboratory Setting	Instructor Evaluation Clinical Setting
Procedural Preparation			
1. Reviews the patient's chart.	S ☐ U ☐ N/A☐	S ☐ U ☐ N/A☐	S ☐ U ☐ N/A☐
2. Verifies the physician's order or the facility's protocol for standard of care.	S ☐ U ☐ N/A☐	S ☐ U ☐ N/A☐	S ☐ U ☐ N/A☐
3. Obtains, cleans, and inspects the appropriate equipment prior to entering the patient's room.	S ☐ U ☐ N/A☐	S ☐ U ☐ N/A☐	S ☐ U ☐ N/A☐
4. Follows PPE requirements, and observes standard precautions for any transmission-based isolation procedure.	S ☐ U ☐ N/A☐	S ☐ U ☐ N/A☐	S ☐ U ☐ N/A☐
5. Identifies the patient using two patient identifiers.	S ☐ U ☐ N/A☐	S ☐ U ☐ N/A☐	S ☐ U ☐ N/A☐
6. Introduces self to the patient and to the family.	S ☐ U ☐ N/A☐	S ☐ U ☐ N/A☐	S ☐ U ☐ N/A☐
7. Explains the procedure to the patient and to the family, and acknowledges the patient's understanding.	S ☐ U ☐ N/A☐	S ☐ U ☐ N/A☐	S ☐ U ☐ N/A☐
8. Confirms the patient's knowledge of FET.	S ☐ U ☐ N/A☐	S ☐ U ☐ N/A☐	S ☐ U ☐ N/A☐
9. Performs proper hand hygiene, and puts on gloves, mask, and protective eyewear, as appropriate for the procedure.	S ☐ U ☐ N/A☐	S ☐ U ☐ N/A☐	S ☐ U ☐ N/A☐
Implementation			
1. Places the patient in a comfortable position.	S ☐ U ☐ N/A☐	S ☐ U ☐ N/A☐	S ☐ U ☐ N/A☐
2. Assesses vital signs.	S ☐ U ☐ N/A☐	S ☐ U ☐ N/A☐	S ☐ U ☐ N/A☐
3. Brings the equipment to the bedside, provides initial therapy after adjusting the pressure settings to meet the patient's need, and determines treatment pressure (between 10 and 20 cmH₂O).	S ☐ U ☐ N/A☐	S ☐ U ☐ N/A☐	S ☐ U ☐ N/A☐

Continued

	Peer Evaluation Laboratory Setting	Instructor Evaluation Laboratory Setting	Instructor Evaluation Clinical Setting
4. Applies the mask or mouthpiece:			
a. If mask, applies tightly over the mouth and nose; confirms patient comfort.	S ☐ U ☐ N/A☐	S ☐ U ☐ N/A☐	S ☐ U ☐ N/A☐
b. If mouthpiece, instructs the patient to place the lips firmly around it and breathe through the mouth.	S ☐ U ☐ N/A☐	S ☐ U ☐ N/A☐	S ☐ U ☐ N/A☐
5. Instructs the patient as follows:			
a. Take in a larger than normal breath, but do not fill the lungs.	S ☐ U ☐ N/A☐	S ☐ U ☐ N/A☐	S ☐ U ☐ N/A☐
b. Exhale actively, not forcefully, to obtain the treatment pressure.	S ☐ U ☐ N/A☐	S ☐ U ☐ N/A☐	S ☐ U ☐ N/A☐
c. Perform 10 to 20 breaths.	S ☐ U ☐ N/A☐	S ☐ U ☐ N/A☐	S ☐ U ☐ N/A☐
6. Removes the mask or the mouthpiece.	S ☐ U ☐ N/A☐	S ☐ U ☐ N/A☐	S ☐ U ☐ N/A☐
7. Instructs the patient to perform two to three FETs.	S ☐ U ☐ N/A☐	S ☐ U ☐ N/A☐	S ☐ U ☐ N/A☐
8. Repeats the above cycle four to eight times, not exceeding 20 minutes.	S ☐ U ☐ N/A☐	S ☐ U ☐ N/A☐	S ☐ U ☐ N/A☐
9. Reassesses vital signs.	S ☐ U ☐ N/A☐	S ☐ U ☐ N/A☐	S ☐ U ☐ N/A☐
10. Assesses the patient for ability to self-administer the therapy.	S ☐ U ☐ N/A☐	S ☐ U ☐ N/A☐	S ☐ U ☐ N/A☐
11. Removes the supplies from the patient's room, and cleans the area, as needed.	S ☐ U ☐ N/A☐	S ☐ U ☐ N/A☐	S ☐ U ☐ N/A☐
12. Removes PPE, and performs proper hand hygiene prior to leaving the patient's room.	S ☐ U ☐ N/A☐	S ☐ U ☐ N/A☐	S ☐ U ☐ N/A☐

Evaluation of Procedure

1. Establishes a baseline, or compares with previous measurements.	S ☐ U ☐ N/A☐	S ☐ U ☐ N/A☐	S ☐ U ☐ N/A☐
2. Develops an appropriate respiratory care plan based on assessment data.	S ☐ U ☐ N/A☐	S ☐ U ☐ N/A☐	S ☐ U ☐ N/A☐
3. Evaluates for PAP therapy to be used in conjunction with bronchodilator aerosol therapy.	S ☐ U ☐ N/A☐	S ☐ U ☐ N/A☐	S ☐ U ☐ N/A☐
4. Identifies any unexpected outcomes.	S ☐ U ☐ N/A☐	S ☐ U ☐ N/A☐	S ☐ U ☐ N/A☐

Documentation and Reporting

1. Records findings in the patient's chart.	S ☐ U ☐ N/A☐	S ☐ U ☐ N/A☐	S ☐ U ☐ N/A☐
2. Reports any abnormal findings to the appropriate health care provider.	S ☐ U ☐ N/A☐	S ☐ U ☐ N/A☐	S ☐ U ☐ N/A☐

Comments:

_____

_____

_____

Signatures:

Student _____ Date Passed _____

Instructor (Laboratory Setting) _____ Date Passed _____

Student _____ Date Passed _____

Instructor (Clinical Setting) _____ Date Passed _____

Procedural Assessment 17-6

Student _____ Date _____

Instructor (Laboratory Setting) _____ Date _____

Instructor (Clinical Setting) _____ Date _____

Criteria for assessment success:

The student must obtain all **satisfactory (S)** scores to pass the procedural evaluation. Any **unsatisfactory (U)** scores will result in failure of the procedural assessment.

Scoring:

Satisfactory (S): Procedural step performed correctly with no instructor prompting. Student-initiated correction is acceptable.

Unsatisfactory (U): Procedural step was performed incorrectly, omitted, or performed in a way that compromised patient care.

Not applicable (N/A): Procedural step was not indicated or necessary.

Evaluation:

	Peer Evaluation Laboratory Setting	Instructor Evaluation Laboratory Setting	Instructor Evaluation Clinical Setting
Procedural Preparation			
1. Reviews the patient's chart.	S ☐ U ☐ N/A☐	S ☐ U ☐ N/A☐	S ☐ U ☐ N/A☐
2. Verifies the physician's order or the facility's protocol for standard of care.	S ☐ U ☐ N/A☐	S ☐ U ☐ N/A☐	S ☐ U ☐ N/A☐
3. Obtains, cleans, and inspects the appropriate equipment prior to entering the patient's room.	S ☐ U ☐ N/A☐	S ☐ U ☐ N/A☐	S ☐ U ☐ N/A☐
4. Follows PPE requirements, and observes standard precautions for any transmission-based isolation procedure.	S ☐ U ☐ N/A☐	S ☐ U ☐ N/A☐	S ☐ U ☐ N/A☐
5. Identifies the patient using two patient identifiers.	S ☐ U ☐ N/A☐	S ☐ U ☐ N/A☐	S ☐ U ☐ N/A☐
6. Introduces self to the patient and to the family.	S ☐ U ☐ N/A☐	S ☐ U ☐ N/A☐	S ☐ U ☐ N/A☐
7. Explains the procedure to the patient and to the family, and acknowledges the patient's understanding.	S ☐ U ☐ N/A☐	S ☐ U ☐ N/A☐	S ☐ U ☐ N/A☐
8. Performs proper hand hygiene, and puts on gloves, mask, and protective eyewear, as appropriate for the procedure.	S ☐ U ☐ N/A☐	S ☐ U ☐ N/A☐	S ☐ U ☐ N/A☐
Implementation			
1. Places the patient in a comfortable position.	S ☐ U ☐ N/A☐	S ☐ U ☐ N/A☐	S ☐ U ☐ N/A☐
2. Assesses vital signs.	S ☐ U ☐ N/A☐	S ☐ U ☐ N/A☐	S ☐ U ☐ N/A☐
3. Assembles the equipment, plugs it in, and places it near the patient.	S ☐ U ☐ N/A☐	S ☐ U ☐ N/A☐	S ☐ U ☐ N/A☐
4. Places the patient's vest or disposable, single-patient-use, nonstretch vest on the patient.	S ☐ U ☐ N/A☐	S ☐ U ☐ N/A☐	S ☐ U ☐ N/A☐
5. Secures the straps.	S ☐ U ☐ N/A☐	S ☐ U ☐ N/A☐	S ☐ U ☐ N/A☐
6. Sets the controls appropriately.	S ☐ U ☐ N/A☐	S ☐ U ☐ N/A☐	S ☐ U ☐ N/A☐

Continued

	Peer Evaluation Laboratory Setting			Instructor Evaluation Laboratory Setting			Instructor Evaluation Clinical Setting		
7. Informs the patient that therapy will begin.	S ☐	U ☐	N/A☐	S ☐	U ☐	N/A☐	S ☐	U ☐	N/A☐
8. Instructs the patient to pause the therapy to clear secretions.	S ☐	U ☐	N/A☐	S ☐	U ☐	N/A☐	S ☐	U ☐	N/A☐
9. Reassesses vital signs when the therapy is completed.	S ☐	U ☐	N/A☐	S ☐	U ☐	N/A☐	S ☐	U ☐	N/A☐
10. Removes the supplies from the patient's room, and cleans the area, as needed.	S ☐	U ☐	N/A☐	S ☐	U ☐	N/A☐	S ☐	U ☐	N/A☐
11. Removes PPE, and performs proper hand hygiene prior to leaving the patient's room.	S ☐	U ☐	N/A☐	S ☐	U ☐	N/A☐	S ☐	U ☐	N/A☐

Evaluation of Procedure

1. Establishes a baseline, or compares with previous measurements and settings	S ☐	U ☐	N/A☐	S ☐	U ☐	N/A☐	S ☐	U ☐	N/A☐
2. Develops an appropriate respiratory care plan based on assessment data.	S ☐	U ☐	N/A☐	S ☐	U ☐	N/A☐	S ☐	U ☐	N/A☐
3. Notes any use of oxygen or medications during therapy.	S ☐	U ☐	N/A☐	S ☐	U ☐	N/A☐	S ☐	U ☐	N/A☐
4. Identifies any unexpected outcomes.	S ☐	U ☐	N/A☐	S ☐	U ☐	N/A☐	S ☐	U ☐	N/A☐

Documentation and Reporting

1. Records findings in the patient's chart.	S ☐	U ☐	N/A☐	S ☐	U ☐	N/A☐	S ☐	U ☐	N/A☐
2. Reports any abnormal findings to the appropriate health care provider.									

Comments:

_____

_____

_____

Signatures:

Student _____ Date Passed _____

Instructor (Laboratory Setting) _____ Date Passed _____

Student _____ Date Passed _____

Instructor (Clinical Setting) _____ Date Passed _____

Student _____ Date _____

Instructor (Laboratory Setting) _____ Date _____

Instructor (Clinical Setting) _____ Date _____

Criteria for assessment success:
The student must obtain all **satisfactory (S)** scores to pass the procedural evaluation. Any **unsatisfactory (U)** scores will result in failure of the procedural assessment.

Scoring:
Satisfactory (S): Procedural step performed correctly with no instructor prompting. Student-initiated correction is acceptable.
Unsatisfactory (U): Procedural step was performed incorrectly, omitted, or performed in a way that compromised patient care.
Not applicable (N/A): Procedural step was not indicated or necessary.

Evaluation:

	Peer Evaluation Laboratory Setting	Instructor Evaluation Laboratory Setting	Instructor Evaluation Clinical Setting
Procedural Preparation			
1. Reviews the patient's chart.	S ☐ U ☐ N/A☐	S ☐ U ☐ N/A☐	S ☐ U ☐ N/A☐
2. Verifies the physician's order or the facility's protocol for standard of care.	S ☐ U ☐ N/A☐	S ☐ U ☐ N/A☐	S ☐ U ☐ N/A☐
3. Obtains, cleans, and inspects the appropriate equipment prior to entering the patient's room.	S ☐ U ☐ N/A☐	S ☐ U ☐ N/A☐	S ☐ U ☐ N/A☐
4. Follows PPE requirements, and observes standard precautions for any transmission-based isolation procedure.	S ☐ U ☐ N/A☐	S ☐ U ☐ N/A☐	S ☐ U ☐ N/A☐
5. Identifies the patient using two patient identifiers.	S ☐ U ☐ N/A☐	S ☐ U ☐ N/A☐	S ☐ U ☐ N/A☐
6. Introduces self to the patient and to the family.	S ☐ U ☐ N/A☐	S ☐ U ☐ N/A☐	S ☐ U ☐ N/A☐
7. Explains the procedure to the patient and to the family, and acknowledges the patient's understanding.	S ☐ U ☐ N/A☐	S ☐ U ☐ N/A☐	S ☐ U ☐ N/A☐
8. Performs proper hand hygiene, and puts on gloves, mask, and protective eyewear, as appropriate for the procedure.	S ☐ U ☐ N/A☐	S ☐ U ☐ N/A☐	S ☐ U ☐ N/A☐
Implementation			
1. Places the patient in a comfortable position.	S ☐ U ☐ N/A☐	S ☐ U ☐ N/A☐	S ☐ U ☐ N/A☐
2. Assesses vital signs.	S ☐ U ☐ N/A☐	S ☐ U ☐ N/A☐	S ☐ U ☐ N/A☐
3. Selects the appropriate interface.	S ☐ U ☐ N/A☐	S ☐ U ☐ N/A☐	S ☐ U ☐ N/A☐
4. Fills the reservoir with the ordered solution or medication.	S ☐ U ☐ N/A☐	S ☐ U ☐ N/A☐	S ☐ U ☐ N/A☐
5. Turns the device on, and adjusts amplification and frequency to generate sufficient percussion and aerosol.	S ☐ U ☐ N/A☐	S ☐ U ☐ N/A☐	S ☐ U ☐ N/A☐
6. Attaches the device to the patient, and ensures patient comfort.	S ☐ U ☐ N/A☐	S ☐ U ☐ N/A☐	S ☐ U ☐ N/A☐
7. Instructs the patient to cough.	S ☐ U ☐ N/A☐	S ☐ U ☐ N/A☐	S ☐ U ☐ N/A☐

Continued

	Peer Evaluation Laboratory Setting			Instructor Evaluation Laboratory Setting			Instructor Evaluation Clinical Setting		
8. Stops therapy after 20 minutes or after the drug has been completely nebulized.	S ☐	U ☐	N/A☐	S ☐	U ☐	N/A☐	S ☐	U ☐	N/A☐
9. Reassesses vital signs, for efficacy of therapy, and for tolerance.	S ☐	U ☐	N/A☐	S ☐	U ☐	N/A☐	S ☐	U ☐	N/A☐
10. Removes the supplies from the patient's room, and cleans the area, as needed.	S ☐	U ☐	N/A☐	S ☐	U ☐	N/A☐	S ☐	U ☐	N/A☐
11. Removes PPE, and performs proper hand hygiene prior to leaving the patient's room.	S ☐	U ☐	N/A☐	S ☐	U ☐	N/A☐	S ☐	U ☐	N/A☐

Evaluation of Procedure

1. Establishes a baseline, or compares with previous measurements.	S ☐	U ☐	N/A☐	S ☐	U ☐	N/A☐	S ☐	U ☐	N/A☐
2. Develops an appropriate respiratory care plan based on assessment data.	S ☐	U ☐	N/A☐	S ☐	U ☐	N/A☐	S ☐	U ☐	N/A☐
3. Identifies any unexpected outcomes.	S ☐	U ☐	N/A☐	S ☐	U ☐	N/A☐	S ☐	U ☐	N/A☐

Documentation and Reporting

1. Records findings in the patient's chart.	S ☐	U ☐	N/A☐	S ☐	U ☐	N/A☐	S ☐	U ☐	N/A☐
2. Reports any abnormal findings to the appropriate health care provider.	S ☐	U ☐	N/A☐	S ☐	U ☐	N/A☐	S ☐	U ☐	N/A☐

Comments:

_____

_____

_____

Signatures:

Student _____ Date Passed _____

Instructor (Laboratory Setting) _____ Date Passed _____

Student _____ Date Passed _____

Instructor (Clinical Setting) _____ Date Passed _____

Student _____ Date _____

Instructor (Laboratory Setting) _____ Date _____

Instructor (Clinical Setting) _____ Date _____

Criteria for assessment success:

The student must obtain all **satisfactory (S)** scores to pass the procedural evaluation. Any **unsatisfactory (U)** scores will result in failure of the procedural assessment.

Scoring:

Satisfactory (S): Procedural step performed correctly with no instructor prompting. Student-initiated correction is acceptable.

Unsatisfactory (U): Procedural step was performed incorrectly, omitted, or performed in a way that compromised patient care.

Not applicable (N/A): Procedural step was not indicated or necessary.

Evaluation:

	Peer Evaluation Laboratory Setting	Instructor Evaluation Laboratory Setting	Instructor Evaluation Clinical Setting
Procedural Preparation			
1. Reviews the patient's chart.	S ☐ U ☐ N/A ☐	S ☐ U ☐ N/A ☐	S ☐ U ☐ N/A ☐
2. Verifies the physician's order or the facility's protocol for standard of care.	S ☐ U ☐ N/A ☐	S ☐ U ☐ N/A ☐	S ☐ U ☐ N/A ☐
3. Matches the order to the medication administration record (MAR) or electronic MAR (eMAR).	S ☐ U ☐ N/A ☐	S ☐ U ☐ N/A ☐	S ☐ U ☐ N/A ☐
4. Limits distractions during medication preparation.	S ☐ U ☐ N/A ☐	S ☐ U ☐ N/A ☐	S ☐ U ☐ N/A ☐
5. Reads the label on the medication, and compares it with the MAR three times:			
a. Before removing it from supply drawer	S ☐ U ☐ N/A ☐	S ☐ U ☐ N/A ☐	S ☐ U ☐ N/A ☐
b. When placing it in the nebulizer, reservoir device, and metered-dose inhaler (MDI) adapter for endotracheal (ET) tube	S ☐ U ☐ N/A ☐	S ☐ U ☐ N/A ☐	S ☐ U ☐ N/A ☐
c. Just before administering it to the patient	S ☐ U ☐ N/A ☐	S ☐ U ☐ N/A ☐	S ☐ U ☐ N/A ☐
6. Uses aseptic technique when preparing medication.	S ☐ U ☐ N/A ☐	S ☐ U ☐ N/A ☐	S ☐ U ☐ N/A ☐
7. Ensures compatibility if mixing medications for simultaneous delivery.	S ☐ U ☐ N/A ☐	S ☐ U ☐ N/A ☐	S ☐ U ☐ N/A ☐
8. Does not use medication if the label is illegible or the container is unmarked.	S ☐ U ☐ N/A ☐	S ☐ U ☐ N/A ☐	S ☐ U ☐ N/A ☐
9. Follows PPE requirements, and observes standard precautions for any transmission-based isolation procedure.	S ☐ U ☐ N/A ☐	S ☐ U ☐ N/A ☐	S ☐ U ☐ N/A ☐
10. Identifies the patient using two patient identifiers.	S ☐ U ☐ N/A ☐	S ☐ U ☐ N/A ☐	S ☐ U ☐ N/A ☐
11. Introduces self to the patient and to the family.	S ☐ U ☐ N/A ☐	S ☐ U ☐ N/A ☐	S ☐ U ☐ N/A ☐
12. Explains the procedure to the patient and to the family, and acknowledges the patient's understanding.	S ☐ U ☐ N/A ☐	S ☐ U ☐ N/A ☐	S ☐ U ☐ N/A ☐

Continued

	Peer Evaluation Laboratory Setting			Instructor Evaluation Laboratory Setting			Instructor Evaluation Clinical Setting		
13. Performs proper hand hygiene, and puts on gloves, mask, and protective eyewear, as appropriate for the procedure.	S ☐	U ☐	N/A ☐	S ☐	U ☐	N/A ☐	S ☐	U ☐	N/A ☐

Implementation

1. Places the patient in a comfortable position.	S ☐	U ☐	N/A ☐	S ☐	U ☐	N/A ☐	S ☐	U ☐	N/A ☐
2. Assesses vital signs.	S ☐	U ☐	N/A ☐	S ☐	U ☐	N/A ☐	S ☐	U ☐	N/A ☐
3. Follows the six rights of medication administration.	S ☐	U ☐	N/A ☐	S ☐	U ☐	N/A ☐	S ☐	U ☐	N/A ☐
4. Remains with the patient until the medication is gone.	S ☐	U ☐	N/A ☐	S ☐	U ☐	N/A ☐	S ☐	U ☐	N/A ☐
5. Reassesses vital signs.	S ☐	U ☐	N/A ☐	S ☐	U ☐	N/A ☐	S ☐	U ☐	N/A ☐
6. Removes the supplies from the patient's room, and cleans the area, as needed.	S ☐	U ☐	N/A ☐	S ☐	U ☐	N/A ☐	S ☐	U ☐	N/A ☐
7. Removes PPE, and performs proper hand hygiene prior to leaving the patient's room.	S ☐	U ☐	N/A ☐	S ☐	U ☐	N/A ☐	S ☐	U ☐	N/A ☐

Evaluation of Procedure

1. Monitors the patient's response to the medication.	S ☐	U ☐	N/A ☐	S ☐	U ☐	N/A ☐	S ☐	U ☐	N/A ☐
2. Identifies any unexpected outcomes.	S ☐	U ☐	N/A ☐	S ☐	U ☐	N/A ☐	S ☐	U ☐	N/A ☐

Documentation and Reporting

1. Records all the required information in the patient's chart.	S ☐	U ☐	N/A ☐	S ☐	U ☐	N/A ☐	S ☐	U ☐	N/A ☐
2. Documents patient refusal of medication and reason.	S ☐	U ☐	N/A ☐	S ☐	U ☐	N/A ☐	S ☐	U ☐	N/A ☐
3. Reports any adverse medication reactions to the appropriate health care provider.	S ☐	U ☐	N/A ☐	S ☐	U ☐	N/A ☐	S ☐	U ☐	N/A ☐

Comments:

_____

_____

_____

Signatures:

Student _____ Date Passed _____

Instructor (Laboratory Setting) _____ Date Passed _____

Student _____ Date Passed _____

Instructor (Clinical Setting) _____ Date Passed _____

Student _____ Date _____

Instructor (Laboratory Setting) _____ Date _____

Instructor (Clinical Setting) _____ Date _____

Criteria for assessment success:

The student must obtain all **satisfactory (S)** scores to pass the procedural evaluation. Any **unsatisfactory (U)** scores will result in failure of the procedural assessment.

Scoring:

Satisfactory (S): Procedural step performed correctly with no instructor prompting. Student-initiated correction is acceptable.

Unsatisfactory (U): Procedural step was performed incorrectly, omitted, or performed in a way that compromised patient care.

Not applicable (N/A): Procedural step was not indicated or necessary.

Evaluation:

	Peer Evaluation Laboratory Setting	Instructor Evaluation Laboratory Setting	Instructor Evaluation Clinical Setting
Procedural Preparation			
1. Reviews the patient's chart.	S ☐ U ☐ N/A ☐	S ☐ U ☐ N/A ☐	S ☐ U ☐ N/A ☐
2. Verifies the physician's order or the facility's protocol for standard of care.	S ☐ U ☐ N/A ☐	S ☐ U ☐ N/A ☐	S ☐ U ☐ N/A ☐
3. Obtains, cleans, and inspects the appropriate equipment prior to entering the patient's room.	S ☐ U ☐ N/A ☐	S ☐ U ☐ N/A ☐	S ☐ U ☐ N/A ☐
4. Follows PPE requirements, and observes standard precautions for any transmission-based isolation procedure.	S ☐ U ☐ N/A ☐	S ☐ U ☐ N/A ☐	S ☐ U ☐ N/A ☐
5. Identifies the patient using two patient identifiers.	S ☐ U ☐ N/A ☐	S ☐ U ☐ N/A ☐	S ☐ U ☐ N/A ☐
6. Introduces self to the patient and to the family.	S ☐ U ☐ N/A ☐	S ☐ U ☐ N/A ☐	S ☐ U ☐ N/A ☐
7. Explains the procedure to the patient and to the family, and acknowledge the patient's understanding.	S ☐ U ☐ N/A ☐	S ☐ U ☐ N/A ☐	S ☐ U ☐ N/A ☐
8. Performs proper hand hygiene, and puts on gloves, mask, and protective eyewear, as appropriate for the procedure.	S ☐ U ☐ N/A ☐	S ☐ U ☐ N/A ☐	S ☐ U ☐ N/A ☐
Implementation			
1. Places the patient in the upright position.	S ☐ U ☐ N/A ☐	S ☐ U ☐ N/A ☐	S ☐ U ☐ N/A ☐
2. Assesses vital signs.	S ☐ U ☐ N/A ☐	S ☐ U ☐ N/A ☐	S ☐ U ☐ N/A ☐
3. Selects mask or mouthpiece delivery.	S ☐ U ☐ N/A ☐	S ☐ U ☐ N/A ☐	S ☐ U ☐ N/A ☐
4. Places the medication in the nebulizer.	S ☐ U ☐ N/A ☐	S ☐ U ☐ N/A ☐	S ☐ U ☐ N/A ☐
5. Attaches the equipment to the appropriate gas for pneumatic power and proper liter flow.	S ☐ U ☐ N/A ☐	S ☐ U ☐ N/A ☐	S ☐ U ☐ N/A ☐

Continued

	Peer Evaluation Laboratory Setting	Instructor Evaluation Laboratory Setting	Instructor Evaluation Clinical Setting
6. Checks for proper functioning.	S ☐ U ☐ N/A ☐	S ☐ U ☐ N/A ☐	S ☐ U ☐ N/A ☐
7. Coaches the patient to breath slowly through the mouth.	S ☐ U ☐ N/A ☐	S ☐ U ☐ N/A ☐	S ☐ U ☐ N/A ☐
8. Reassesses pulse rate, respiratory rate, and lung sounds half way through the treatment.	S ☐ U ☐ N/A ☐	S ☐ U ☐ N/A ☐	S ☐ U ☐ N/A ☐
9. Continues treatment until the nebulizer sputters.	S ☐ U ☐ N/A ☐	S ☐ U ☐ N/A ☐	S ☐ U ☐ N/A ☐
10. Disconnects the nebulizer from the gas source.			
11. Rinses the nebulizer with sterile water and air-dries it, or discards it, between treatments.	S ☐ U ☐ N/A ☐	S ☐ U ☐ N/A ☐	S ☐ U ☐ N/A ☐
12. Instructs the patient to rinse the mouth following treatment.	S ☐ U ☐ N/A ☐	S ☐ U ☐ N/A ☐	S ☐ U ☐ N/A ☐
13. Reassesses the pulse rate, respiratory rate, and lung sounds following treatment.	S ☐ U ☐ N/A ☐	S ☐ U ☐ N/A ☐	S ☐ U ☐ N/A ☐
14. Removes supplies from the patient's room, and cleans the area, as needed.	S ☐ U ☐ N/A ☐	S ☐ U ☐ N/A ☐	S ☐ U ☐ N/A ☐
15. Removes PPE, and performs proper hand hygiene prior to leaving the patient's room.	S ☐ U ☐ N/A ☐	S ☐ U ☐ N/A ☐	S ☐ U ☐ N/A ☐

Evaluation of Procedure

1. Establishes a baseline, or compares with previous measurements.	S ☐ U ☐ N/A ☐	S ☐ U ☐ N/A ☐	S ☐ U ☐ N/A ☐
2. Reassesses the patient for any adverse response.	S ☐ U ☐ N/A ☐	S ☐ U ☐ N/A ☐	S ☐ U ☐ N/A ☐
3. Discontinues treatment if an adverse reaction occurs.	S ☐ U ☐ N/A ☐	S ☐ U ☐ N/A ☐	S ☐ U ☐ N/A ☐
4. Develops an appropriate respiratory care plan based on assessment data.	S ☐ U ☐ N/A ☐	S ☐ U ☐ N/A ☐	S ☐ U ☐ N/A ☐
5. Identifies any unexpected outcomes.	S ☐ U ☐ N/A ☐	S ☐ U ☐ N/A ☐	S ☐ U ☐ N/A ☐

Documentation and Reporting

1. Records findings in the patient's chart.	S ☐ U ☐ N/A ☐	S ☐ U ☐ N/A ☐	S ☐ U ☐ N/A ☐
2. Reports any abnormal findings to the appropriate health care provider.	S ☐ U ☐ N/A ☐	S ☐ U ☐ N/A ☐	S ☐ U ☐ N/A ☐

Comments:

_____

_____

_____

Signatures:

Student _____ Date Passed _____

Instructor (Laboratory Setting) _____ Date Passed _____

Student _____ Date Passed _____

Instructor (Clinical Setting) _____ Date Passed _____

Procedural Assessment 19-2

Student _____ Date _____

Instructor (Laboratory Setting) _____ Date _____

Instructor (Clinical Setting) _____ Date _____

Scoring:

Satisfactory (S): Procedural step performed correctly with no instructor prompting. Student-initiated correction is acceptable.

Unsatisfactory (U): Procedural step was performed incorrectly, omitted, or performed in a way that compromised patient care.

Not applicable (N/A): Procedural step was not indicated or necessary.

Evaluation:

	Peer Evaluation Laboratory Setting	Instructor Evaluation Laboratory Setting	Instructor Evaluation Clinical Setting
Procedural Preparation			
1. Reviews the patient's chart.	S ☐ U ☐ N/A ☐	S ☐ U ☐ N/A ☐	S ☐ U ☐ N/A ☐
2. Verifies the physician's order or the facility's protocol for standard of care.	S ☐ U ☐ N/A ☐	S ☐ U ☐ N/A ☐	S ☐ U ☐ N/A ☐
3. Obtains, cleans, and inspects the appropriate equipment prior to entering the patient's room.	S ☐ U ☐ N/A ☐	S ☐ U ☐ N/A ☐	S ☐ U ☐ N/A ☐
4. Follows PPE requirements, and observes standard precautions for any transmission-based isolation procedure.	S ☐ U ☐ N/A ☐	S ☐ U ☐ N/A ☐	S ☐ U ☐ N/A ☐
5. Identifies the patient using two patient identifiers.	S ☐ U ☐ N/A ☐	S ☐ U ☐ N/A ☐	S ☐ U ☐ N/A ☐
6. Introduces self to the patient and to the family.	S ☐ U ☐ N/A ☐	S ☐ U ☐ N/A ☐	S ☐ U ☐ N/A ☐
7. Explains the procedure to the patient and to the family, and acknowledges the patient's understanding.	S ☐ U ☐ N/A ☐	S ☐ U ☐ N/A ☐	S ☐ U ☐ N/A ☐
8. Performs proper hand hygiene, and puts on gloves, mask, and protective eyewear, as appropriate for the procedure.	S ☐ U ☐ N/A ☐	S ☐ U ☐ N/A ☐	S ☐ U ☐ N/A ☐
Implementation			
1. Places the patient in the upright position, and instructs him or her to breathe normally.	S ☐ U ☐ N/A ☐	S ☐ U ☐ N/A ☐	S ☐ U ☐ N/A ☐
2. Assesses vital signs.	S ☐ U ☐ N/A ☐	S ☐ U ☐ N/A ☐	S ☐ U ☐ N/A ☐
3. Shakes the pMDI vigorously.	S ☐ U ☐ N/A ☐	S ☐ U ☐ N/A ☐	S ☐ U ☐ N/A ☐
4. Before the first use of a new pMDI, and when the pMDI has not been used for several days, primes the pMDI by pointing it into the air (away from people) and actuates it.	S ☐ U ☐ N/A ☐	S ☐ U ☐ N/A ☐	S ☐ U ☐ N/A ☐
5. Assembles the apparatus, and uncaps the mouthpiece, ensuring no loose objects are present in the device.	S ☐ U ☐ N/A ☐	S ☐ U ☐ N/A ☐	S ☐ U ☐ N/A ☐
6. Instructs patient in using an open-mouth technique. For the open-mouth technique	S ☐ U ☐ N/A ☐	S ☐ U ☐ N/A ☐	S ☐ U ☐ N/A ☐

Continued

	Peer Evaluation Laboratory Setting			Instructor Evaluation Laboratory Setting			Instructor Evaluation Clinical Setting		
7. Instructs patient in using an closed-mouth technique.	S □	U □	N/A □	S □	U □	N/A □	S □	U □	N/A □
8. Instructs patient in using a reservoir device.	S □	U □	N/A □	S □	U □	N/A □	S □	U □	N/A □
9. Instructs the patient to hold the breath up to, but no longer than, 10 seconds and relax and breathe normally.	S □	U □	N/A □	S □	U □	N/A □	S □	U □	N/A □
10. Instructs the patient to wait 1 minute between puffs.	S □	U □	N/A □	S □	U □	N/A □	S □	U □	N/A □
11. Disassembles the apparatus, and recaps the mouthpiece.	S □	U □	N/A □	S □	U □	N/A □	S □	U □	N/A □
12. Reassesses vital signs.	S □	U □	N/A □	S □	U □	N/A □	S □	U □	N/A □
13. Removes the supplies from the patient's room, and cleans the area, as needed.	S □	U □	N/A □	S □	U □	N/A □	S □	U □	N/A □
14. Removes PPE, and performs proper hand hygiene prior to leaving the patient's room.	S □	U □	N/A □	S □	U □	N/A □	S □	U □	N/A □

Evaluation of Procedure

1. Has patient demonstrate the use of the pMDI.	S □	U □	N/A □	S □	U □	N/A □	S □	U □	N/A □
2. Evaluates the patient for any side effects of the medication.	S □	U □	N/A □	S □	U □	N/A □	S □	U □	N/A □
3. Identifies any unexpected outcomes.	S □	U □	N/A □	S □	U □	N/A □	S □	U □	N/A □

Documentation and Reporting

1. Records the times used and the dose in the patient's chart.	S □	U □	N/A □	S □	U □	N/A □	S □	U □	N/A □
2. Reports any abnormal findings to the appropriate health care provider.	S □	U □	N/A □	S □	U □	N/A □	S □	U □	N/A □

Comments:

_____

_____

_____

Signatures:

Student _____ Date Passed _____

Instructor (Laboratory Setting) _____ Date Passed _____

Student _____ Date Passed _____

Instructor (Clinical Setting) _____ Date Passed _____

Student _____ Date _____

Instructor (Laboratory Setting) _____ Date _____

Instructor (Clinical Setting) _____ Date _____

Criteria for assessment success:

The student must obtain all **satisfactory (S)** scores to pass the procedural evaluation. Any **unsatisfactory (U)** scores will result in failure of the procedural assessment.

Scoring:

Satisfactory (S): Procedural step performed correctly with no instructor prompting. Student-initiated correction is acceptable.

Unsatisfactory (U): Procedural step was performed incorrectly, omitted, or performed in a way that compromised patient care.

Not applicable (N/A): Procedural step was not indicated or necessary.

Evaluation:

	Peer Evaluation Laboratory Setting	Instructor Evaluation Laboratory Setting	Instructor Evaluation Clinical Setting
Procedural Preparation			
1. Reviews the patient's chart.	S ☐ U ☐ N/A ☐	S ☐ U ☐ N/A ☐	S ☐ U ☐ N/A ☐
2. Verifies the physician's order or the facility's protocol for standard of care.	S ☐ U ☐ N/A ☐	S ☐ U ☐ N/A ☐	S ☐ U ☐ N/A ☐
3. Obtains, cleans, and inspects the appropriate equipment prior to entering the patient's room.	S ☐ U ☐ N/A ☐	S ☐ U ☐ N/A ☐	S ☐ U ☐ N/A ☐
4. Follows PPE requirements, and observes standard precautions for any transmission-based isolation procedure.	S ☐ U ☐ N/A ☐	S ☐ U ☐ N/A ☐	S ☐ U ☐ N/A ☐
5. Identifies the patient using two patient identifiers.	S ☐ U ☐ N/A ☐	S ☐ U ☐ N/A ☐	S ☐ U ☐ N/A ☐
6. Introduces self to the patient and to the family.	S ☐ U ☐ N/A ☐	S ☐ U ☐ N/A ☐	S ☐ U ☐ N/A ☐
7. Explains the procedure to the patient and to the family, and acknowledges the patient's understanding.	S ☐ U ☐ N/A ☐	S ☐ U ☐ N/A ☐	S ☐ U ☐ N/A ☐
8. Performs proper hand hygiene, and puts on gloves, mask, and protective eyewear, as appropriate for the procedure.	S ☐ U ☐ N/A ☐	S ☐ U ☐ N/A ☐	S ☐ U ☐ N/A ☐
Implementation			
1. Places the patient in the upright position, and instructs him or her to breathe normally.	S ☐ U ☐ N/A ☐	S ☐ U ☐ N/A ☐	S ☐ U ☐ N/A ☐
2. Assesses vital signs.	S ☐ U ☐ N/A ☐	S ☐ U ☐ N/A ☐	S ☐ U ☐ N/A ☐
3. Loads a dose while keeping the device upright.	S ☐ U ☐ N/A ☐	S ☐ U ☐ N/A ☐	S ☐ U ☐ N/A ☐
4. Instructs the patient to exhale slowly and completely.	S ☐ U ☐ N/A ☐	S ☐ U ☐ N/A ☐	S ☐ U ☐ N/A ☐

Continued

	Peer Evaluation Laboratory Setting			Instructor Evaluation Laboratory Setting			Instructor Evaluation Clinical Setting		
5. Instructs the patient to seal the lips around the mouthpiece and inhale deeply and forcefully.	S ☐	U ☐	N/A ☐	S ☐	U ☐	N/A ☐	S ☐	U ☐	N/A ☐
6. Instructs the patient to repeat the process until the dose is completely delivered.	S ☐	U ☐	N/A ☐	S ☐	U ☐	N/A ☐	S ☐	U ☐	N/A ☐
7. Instructs the patient to rinse the mouth out once the treatment is completed.	S ☐	U ☐	N/A ☐	S ☐	U ☐	N/A ☐	S ☐	U ☐	N/A ☐
8. Reassesses vital signs.	S ☐	U ☐	N/A ☐	S ☐	U ☐	N/A ☐	S ☐	U ☐	N/A ☐
9. Removes the supplies from the patient's room, and cleans the area, as needed.	S ☐	U ☐	N/A ☐	S ☐	U ☐	N/A ☐	S ☐	U ☐	N/A ☐
10. Removes PPE, and performs proper hand hygiene prior to leaving the patient's room.	S ☐	U ☐	N/A ☐	S ☐	U ☐	N/A ☐	S ☐	U ☐	N/A ☐

Evaluation of Procedure

1. Has the patient demonstrate the use of the DPI during the next scheduled treatment.	S ☐	U ☐	N/A ☐	S ☐	U ☐	N/A ☐	S ☐	U ☐	N/A ☐
2. Evaluates the patient for any side effects of the medication.	S ☐	U ☐	N/A ☐	S ☐	U ☐	N/A ☐	S ☐	U ☐	N/A ☐
3. Identifies any unexpected outcomes.	S ☐	U ☐	N/A ☐	S ☐	U ☐	N/A ☐	S ☐	U ☐	N/A ☐

Documentation and Reporting

1. Records the times used and the dose in the patient's chart.	S ☐	U ☐	N/A ☐	S ☐	U ☐	N/A ☐	S ☐	U ☐	N/A ☐
2. Reports any abnormal findings to the appropriate health care provider.	S ☐	U ☐	N/A ☐	S ☐	U ☐	N/A ☐	S ☐	U ☐	N/A ☐

Comments:

_____

_____

_____

Signatures:

Student _____ Date Passed _____

Instructor (Laboratory Setting) _____ Date Passed _____

Student _____ Date Passed _____

Instructor (Clinical Setting) _____ Date Passed _____

Student _____ Date _____

Instructor (Laboratory Setting) _____ Date _____

Instructor (Clinical Setting) _____ Date _____

Criteria for assessment success:

The student must obtain all **satisfactory (S)** scores to pass the procedural evaluation. Any **unsatisfactory (U)** scores will result in failure of the procedural assessment.

Scoring:

Satisfactory (S): Procedural step performed correctly with no instructor prompting. Student-initiated correction is acceptable.

Unsatisfactory (U): Procedural step was performed incorrectly, omitted, or performed in a way that compromised patient care.

Not applicable (N/A): Procedural step was not indicated or necessary.

Evaluation:

	Peer Evaluation Laboratory Setting	Instructor Evaluation Laboratory Setting	Instructor Evaluation Clinical Setting
Procedural Preparation			
1. Reviews the patient's chart.	S ☐ U ☐ N/A ☐	S ☐ U ☐ N/A ☐	S ☐ U ☐ N/A ☐
2. Verifies the physician's order or the facility's protocol for standard of care.	S ☐ U ☐ N/A ☐	S ☐ U ☐ N/A ☐	S ☐ U ☐ N/A ☐
3. Obtains, cleans, and inspects the appropriate equipment prior to entering the patient's room.	S ☐ U ☐ N/A ☐	S ☐ U ☐ N/A ☐	S ☐ U ☐ N/A ☐
4. Follows PPE requirements, and observes standard precautions for any transmission-based isolation procedure.	S ☐ U ☐ N/A ☐	S ☐ U ☐ N/A ☐	S ☐ U ☐ N/A ☐
5. Identifies the patient using two patient identifiers.	S ☐ U ☐ N/A ☐	S ☐ U ☐ N/A ☐	S ☐ U ☐ N/A ☐
6. Introduces self to the patient and to the family.	S ☐ U ☐ N/A ☐	S ☐ U ☐ N/A ☐	S ☐ U ☐ N/A ☐
7. Explains the procedure to the patient and to the family, and acknowledges the patient's understanding.	S ☐ U ☐ N/A ☐	S ☐ U ☐ N/A ☐	S ☐ U ☐ N/A ☐
8. Performs proper hand hygiene, and puts on gloves, mask, and protective eyewear, as appropriate for the procedure.	S ☐ U ☐ N/A ☐	S ☐ U ☐ N/A ☐	S ☐ U ☐ N/A ☐
Implementation			
1. Places the patient in a comfortable position, and instructs him or her to breathe normally.	S ☐ U ☐ N/A ☐	S ☐ U ☐ N/A ☐	S ☐ U ☐ N/A ☐
2. Assesses vital signs.	S ☐ U ☐ N/A ☐	S ☐ U ☐ N/A ☐	S ☐ U ☐ N/A ☐
3. Instructs patient. For first-time use of Combivent Respimat.	S ☐ U ☐ N/A ☐	S ☐ U ☐ N/A ☐	S ☐ U ☐ N/A ☐
4. Instructs patient. For priming the Combivent Respimat.	S ☐ U ☐ N/A ☐	S ☐ U ☐ N/A ☐	S ☐ U ☐ N/A ☐
5. Instructs patient. For daily use of Combivent Respimat.	S ☐ U ☐ N/A ☐	S ☐ U ☐ N/A ☐	S ☐ U ☐ N/A ☐

Continued

	Peer Evaluation Laboratory Setting			Instructor Evaluation Laboratory Setting			Instructor Evaluation Clinical Setting		
6. Removes the supplies from the patient's room, and cleans the area, as needed.	S ☐	U ☐	N/A ☐	S ☐	U ☐	N/A ☐	S ☐	U ☐	N/A ☐
7. Removes PPE, and performs proper hand hygiene prior to leaving the patient's room.	S ☐	U ☐	N/A ☐	S ☐	U ☐	N/A ☐	S ☐	U ☐	N/A ☐

Evaluation of Procedure

1. Establishes a baseline, or compares with previous measurements.	S ☐	U ☐	N/A ☐	S ☐	U ☐	N/A ☐	S ☐	U ☐	N/A ☐
2. Develops an appropriate respiratory care plan based on assessment data.	S ☐	U ☐	N/A ☐	S ☐	U ☐	N/A ☐	S ☐	U ☐	N/A ☐
3. Identifies any unexpected outcomes.	S ☐	U ☐	N/A ☐	S ☐	U ☐	N/A ☐	S ☐	U ☐	N/A ☐

Documentation and Reporting

1. Records findings in the patient's chart.	S ☐	U ☐	N/A ☐	S ☐	U ☐	N/A ☐	S ☐	U ☐	N/A ☐
2. Reports any abnormal findings to the appropriate health care provider.	S ☐	U ☐	N/A ☐	S ☐	U ☐	N/A ☐	S ☐	U ☐	N/A ☐

Comments:

_____

_____

_____

Signatures:

Student _____ Date Passed _____

Instructor (Laboratory Setting) _____ Date Passed _____

Student _____ Date Passed _____

Instructor (Clinical Setting) _____ Date Passed _____

Student _____ Date _____

Instructor (Laboratory Setting) _____ Date _____

Instructor (Clinical Setting) _____ Date _____

Criteria for assessment success:

The student must obtain all **satisfactory (S)** scores to pass the procedural evaluation. Any **unsatisfactory (U)** scores will result in failure of the procedural assessment.

Scoring:

Satisfactory (S): Procedural step performed correctly with no instructor prompting. Student-initiated correction is acceptable.

Unsatisfactory (U): Procedural step was performed incorrectly, omitted, or performed in a way that compromised patient care.

Not applicable (N/A): Procedural step was not indicated or necessary.

Evaluation:

	Peer Evaluation Laboratory Setting	Instructor Evaluation Laboratory Setting	Instructor Evaluation Clinical Setting
Procedural Preparation			
1. Cleans the exterior surface of the ventilator per the manufacturer's instructions.	S ☐ U ☐ N/A ☐	S ☐ U ☐ N/A ☐	S ☐ U ☐ N/A ☐
2. Attaches the appropriate inspiratory and expiratory filters.	S ☐ U ☐ N/A ☐	S ☐ U ☐ N/A ☐	S ☐ U ☐ N/A ☐
3. Attaches a clean ventilator tubing circuit to the ventilator.	S ☐ U ☐ N/A ☐	S ☐ U ☐ N/A ☐	S ☐ U ☐ N/A ☐
4. Connects the ventilator to the compressed oxygen and air outlets.	S ☐ U ☐ N/A ☐	S ☐ U ☐ N/A ☐	S ☐ U ☐ N/A ☐
5. Plugs the ventilator into the appropriate electrical outlet.	S ☐ U ☐ N/A ☐	S ☐ U ☐ N/A ☐	S ☐ U ☐ N/A ☐
Implementation			
1. Follows the ventilator manufacturer's instructions to initiate the ventilator diagnostic process.	S ☐ U ☐ N/A ☐	S ☐ U ☐ N/A ☐	S ☐ U ☐ N/A ☐
2. Follows the ventilator instructions to complete the diagnostic process.	S ☐ U ☐ N/A ☐	S ☐ U ☐ N/A ☐	S ☐ U ☐ N/A ☐
3. Keeps the ventilator covered until use.	S ☐ U ☐ N/A ☐	S ☐ U ☐ N/A ☐	S ☐ U ☐ N/A ☐
Evaluation of Procedure			
1. Establishes that all pressure tests have been completed successfully.	S ☐ U ☐ N/A ☐	S ☐ U ☐ N/A ☐	S ☐ U ☐ N/A ☐
2. Establishes that all flow tests have been completed successfully.	S ☐ U ☐ N/A ☐	S ☐ U ☐ N/A ☐	S ☐ U ☐ N/A ☐
3. Establishes that all volume tests have been completed successfully.	S ☐ U ☐ N/A ☐	S ☐ U ☐ N/A ☐	S ☐ U ☐ N/A ☐
4. Establishes that all tubing compliance tests have been completed successfully.	S ☐ U ☐ N/A ☐	S ☐ U ☐ N/A ☐	S ☐ U ☐ N/A ☐

Continued

	Peer Evaluation Laboratory Setting			Instructor Evaluation Laboratory Setting			Instructor Evaluation Clinical Setting		
5. Establishes that all oxygen sensor tests have been completed successfully.	S ☐	U ☐	N/A ☐	S ☐	U ☐	N/A ☐	S ☐	U ☐	N/A ☐
6. Establishes that all leak tests have been completed successfully.	S ☐	U ☐	N/A ☐	S ☐	U ☐	N/A ☐	S ☐	U ☐	N/A ☐
Documentation and Reporting									
1. Records successful tests in the appropriate log and on the ventilator.	S ☐	U ☐	N/A ☐	S ☐	U ☐	N/A ☐	S ☐	U ☐	N/A ☐
2. Reports failure to the appropriate health care provider.	S ☐	U ☐	N/A ☐	S ☐	U ☐	N/A ☐	S ☐	U ☐	N/A ☐

Comments:

_____

_____

_____

Signatures:

Student _____ Date Passed _____

Instructor (Laboratory Setting) _____ Date Passed _____

Student _____ Date Passed _____

Instructor (Clinical Setting) _____ Date Passed _____

Procedural Assessment 20-2   Wave form analysis

Student _____ Date _____

Instructor (Laboratory Setting) _____ Date _____

Instructor (Clinical Setting) _____ Date _____

Criteria for assessment success:

The student must obtain all **satisfactory (S)** scores to pass the procedural evaluation. Any **unsatisfactory (U)** scores will result in failure of the procedural assessment.

Scoring:

Satisfactory (S): Procedural step performed correctly with no instructor prompting. Student-initiated correction is acceptable.

Unsatisfactory (U): Procedural step was performed incorrectly, omitted, or performed in a way that compromised patient care.

Not applicable (N/A): Procedural step was not indicated or necessary.

Evaluation:

	Peer Evaluation Laboratory Setting	Instructor Evaluation Laboratory Setting	Instructor Evaluation Clinical Setting
Procedural Preparation			
1. Reviews the patient's chart.	S ☐ U ☐ N/A ☐	S ☐ U ☐ N/A ☐	S ☐ U ☐ N/A ☐
2. Verifies the physician's order or the facility's protocol for standard of care.	S ☐ U ☐ N/A ☐	S ☐ U ☐ N/A ☐	S ☐ U ☐ N/A ☐
3. Obtains, cleans, and inspects the appropriate equipment prior to entering the patient's room.	S ☐ U ☐ N/A ☐	S ☐ U ☐ N/A ☐	S ☐ U ☐ N/A ☐
4. Follows PPE requirements, and observes standard precautions for any transmission based isolation procedure.	S ☐ U ☐ N/A ☐	S ☐ U ☐ N/A ☐	S ☐ U ☐ N/A ☐
5. Identifies the patient using two patient identifiers.	S ☐ U ☐ N/A ☐	S ☐ U ☐ N/A ☐	S ☐ U ☐ N/A ☐
6. Introduces self to the patient and to the family.	S ☐ U ☐ N/A ☐	S ☐ U ☐ N/A ☐	S ☐ U ☐ N/A ☐
7. Explains the procedure to the patient and to the family, and acknowledges the patient's understanding.	S ☐ U ☐ N/A ☐	S ☐ U ☐ N/A ☐	S ☐ U ☐ N/A ☐
8. Performs proper hand hygiene, and puts on gloves, mask, and protective eyewear, as appropriate for the procedure.	S ☐ U ☐ N/A ☐	S ☐ U ☐ N/A ☐	S ☐ U ☐ N/A ☐
Implementation			
1. Identifies the desired wave form for analysis:			
a. Pressure-time	S ☐ U ☐ N/A ☐	S ☐ U ☐ N/A ☐	S ☐ U ☐ N/A ☐
b. Flow-time	S ☐ U ☐ N/A ☐	S ☐ U ☐ N/A ☐	S ☐ U ☐ N/A ☐
c. Volume-time	S ☐ U ☐ N/A ☐	S ☐ U ☐ N/A ☐	S ☐ U ☐ N/A ☐
2. Analyzes the wave form for:			
a. Changes in resistance	S ☐ U ☐ N/A ☐	S ☐ U ☐ N/A ☐	S ☐ U ☐ N/A ☐
b. Leaks	S ☐ U ☐ N/A ☐	S ☐ U ☐ N/A ☐	S ☐ U ☐ N/A ☐
c. Air trapping	S ☐ U ☐ N/A ☐	S ☐ U ☐ N/A ☐	S ☐ U ☐ N/A ☐
d. Inadequate inspiratory flow	S ☐ U ☐ N/A ☐	S ☐ U ☐ N/A ☐	S ☐ U ☐ N/A ☐

Continued

	Peer Evaluation Laboratory Setting			Instructor Evaluation Laboratory Setting			Instructor Evaluation Clinical Setting		
3. Calculates static compliance, if applicable for the mode.	S ☐	U ☐	N/A ☐	S ☐	U ☐	N/A ☐	S ☐	U ☐	N/A ☐
4. Adjusts the ventilator per protocols and as needed.	S ☐	U ☐	N/A ☐	S ☐	U ☐	N/A ☐	S ☐	U ☐	N/A ☐
5. Removes PPE, and performs proper hand hygiene prior to leaving the patient's room.	S ☐	U ☐	N/A ☐	S ☐	U ☐	N/A ☐	S ☐	U ☐	N/A ☐
Evaluation of Procedure									
1. Establishes a baseline, or compares with previous wave form analyses.	S ☐	U ☐	N/A ☐	S ☐	U ☐	N/A ☐	S ☐	U ☐	N/A ☐
2. Develops an appropriate respiratory care plan based on assessment data.	S ☐	U ☐	N/A ☐	S ☐	U ☐	N/A ☐	S ☐	U ☐	N/A ☐
3. Identifies any unexpected outcomes.	S ☐	U ☐	N/A ☐	S ☐	U ☐	N/A ☐	S ☐	U ☐	N/A ☐
Documentation and Reporting									
1. Records changes and findings in the patient's chart or on the ventilator flow sheet.	S ☐	U ☐	N/A ☐	S ☐	U ☐	N/A ☐	S ☐	U ☐	N/A ☐

Comments:

_____

_____

_____

Signatures:

Student _____ Date Passed _____

Instructor (Laboratory Setting) _____ Date Passed _____

Student _____ Date Passed _____

Instructor (Clinical Setting) _____ Date Passed _____

Student _____ Date _____

Instructor (Laboratory Setting) _____ Date _____

Instructor (Clinical Setting) _____ Date _____

Criteria for assessment success:

The student must obtain all **satisfactory (S)** scores to pass the procedural evaluation. Any **unsatisfactory (U)** scores will result in failure of the procedural assessment.

Scoring:

Satisfactory (S): Procedural step performed correctly with no instructor prompting. Student-initiated correction is acceptable.

Unsatisfactory (U): Procedural step was performed incorrectly, omitted, or performed in a way that compromised patient care.

Not applicable (N/A): Procedural step was not indicated or necessary.

Evaluation:

	Peer Evaluation Laboratory Setting	Instructor Evaluation Laboratory Setting	Instructor Evaluation Clinical Setting
Procedural Preparation			
1. Reviews the patient's chart.	S ☐ U ☐ N/A ☐	S ☐ U ☐ N/A ☐	S ☐ U ☐ N/A ☐
2. Verifies the physician's order or the facility's protocol for standard of care.	S ☐ U ☐ N/A ☐	S ☐ U ☐ N/A ☐	S ☐ U ☐ N/A ☐
3. Obtains, cleans, and inspects the appropriate equipment prior to entering the patient's room.	S ☐ U ☐ N/A ☐	S ☐ U ☐ N/A ☐	S ☐ U ☐ N/A ☐
4. Follows PPE requirements, and observes standard precautions for any transmission-based isolation procedure.	S ☐ U ☐ N/A ☐	S ☐ U ☐ N/A ☐	S ☐ U ☐ N/A ☐
5. Identifies the patient using two patient identifiers.	S ☐ U ☐ N/A ☐	S ☐ U ☐ N/A ☐	S ☐ U ☐ N/A ☐
6. Introduces self to the patient and to the family.	S ☐ U ☐ N/A ☐	S ☐ U ☐ N/A ☐	S ☐ U ☐ N/A ☐
7. Explains the procedure to the patient and to the family, and acknowledges the patient's understanding.	S ☐ U ☐ N/A ☐	S ☐ U ☐ N/A ☐	S ☐ U ☐ N/A ☐
8. Performs proper hand hygiene, and puts on gloves, mask, and protective eyewear, as appropriate for the procedure.	S ☐ U ☐ N/A ☐	S ☐ U ☐ N/A ☐	S ☐ U ☐ N/A ☐
Implementation			
1. Places the patient in a comfortable position.	S ☐ U ☐ N/A ☐	S ☐ U ☐ N/A ☐	S ☐ U ☐ N/A ☐
2. Assesses vital signs.	S ☐ U ☐ N/A ☐	S ☐ U ☐ N/A ☐	S ☐ U ☐ N/A ☐
3. Determines the noninvasive interface for use with CPAP or BiPAP.	S ☐ U ☐ N/A ☐	S ☐ U ☐ N/A ☐	S ☐ U ☐ N/A ☐
4. Ensures proper fit of interface to prevent excessive leaks.	S ☐ U ☐ N/A ☐	S ☐ U ☐ N/A ☐	S ☐ U ☐ N/A ☐

Continued

	Peer Evaluation Laboratory Setting	Instructor Evaluation Laboratory Setting	Instructor Evaluation Clinical Setting
5. Assembles the circuit, and plugs in, attaches to the gas source(s), and tests the device. **For CPAP**			
a. Selects the CPAP mode, or other vendor-specific name.	S ☐ U ☐ N/A ☐	S ☐ U ☐ N/A ☐	S ☐ U ☐ N/A ☐
b. Selects the appropriate CPAP level.	S ☐ U ☐ N/A ☐	S ☐ U ☐ N/A ☐	S ☐ U ☐ N/A ☐
c. Selects the appropriate FiO_2 level.	S ☐ U ☐ N/A ☐	S ☐ U ☐ N/A ☐	S ☐ U ☐ N/A ☐
For BiPAP			
d. Selects the BiPAP levels.	S ☐ U ☐ N/A ☐	S ☐ U ☐ N/A ☐	S ☐ U ☐ N/A ☐
e. Selects any additional BiPAP options.	S ☐ U ☐ N/A ☐	S ☐ U ☐ N/A ☐	S ☐ U ☐ N/A ☐
f. Selects the appropriate FIO_2 level.	S ☐ U ☐ N/A ☐	S ☐ U ☐ N/A ☐	S ☐ U ☐ N/A ☐
6. Connects the device to the patient, and readjusts the interface, as needed, to prevent leaks.	S ☐ U ☐ N/A ☐	S ☐ U ☐ N/A ☐	S ☐ U ☐ N/A ☐
7. Reassesses vital signs, and monitors the patient.	S ☐ U ☐ N/A ☐	S ☐ U ☐ N/A ☐	S ☐ U ☐ N/A ☐
8. Removes the supplies from the patient's room, and cleans the area, as needed.	S ☐ U ☐ N/A ☐	S ☐ U ☐ N/A ☐	S ☐ U ☐ N/A ☐
9. Removes the PPE, and performs proper hand hygiene prior to leaving the patient's room.	S ☐ U ☐ N/A ☐	S ☐ U ☐ N/A ☐	S ☐ U ☐ N/A ☐

Evaluation of Procedure

1. Establishes a baseline, or compares with previous measurements.	S ☐ U ☐ N/A ☐	S ☐ U ☐ N/A ☐	S ☐ U ☐ N/A ☐
2. Develops an appropriate respiratory care plan based on assessment data.	S ☐ U ☐ N/A ☐	S ☐ U ☐ N/A ☐	S ☐ U ☐ N/A ☐
3. Obtains arterial blood gas values, and obtains an order for chest radiography, if indicated.	S ☐ U ☐ N/A ☐	S ☐ U ☐ N/A ☐	S ☐ U ☐ N/A ☐
4. Identifies any unexpected outcomes.	S ☐ U ☐ N/A ☐	S ☐ U ☐ N/A ☐	S ☐ U ☐ N/A ☐

Documentation and Reporting

1. Records findings in the patient's chart.	S ☐ U ☐ N/A ☐	S ☐ U ☐ N/A ☐	S ☐ U ☐ N/A ☐
2. Reports any abnormal findings to the appropriate health care provider.	S ☐ U ☐ N/A ☐	S ☐ U ☐ N/A ☐	S ☐ U ☐ N/A ☐

Comments:

_____

_____

_____

Signatures:

Student _____ Date Passed _____

Instructor (Laboratory Setting) _____ Date Passed _____

Student _____ Date Passed _____

Instructor (Clinical Setting) _____ Date Passed _____

Student _____ Date _____

Instructor _____ Date _____

Location _____ Date _____

Criteria for assessment success:

The student must obtain all **satisfactory (S)** scores to pass the procedural evaluation. Any **unsatisfactory (U)** scores will result in failure of the procedural assessment.

Scoring:

Satisfactory (S): Procedural step performed correctly with no instructor prompting. Student-initiated correction is acceptable.

Unsatisfactory (U): Procedural step was performed incorrectly, omitted, or performed in a way that compromised patient care.

Not applicable (N/A): Procedural step was not indicated or necessary.

Evaluation:

	Peer Evaluation Laboratory Setting	Instructor Evaluation Laboratory Setting	Instructor Evaluation Clinical Setting
Procedural Preparation			
1. Reviews the patient's chart for patient's current vital signs and ventilator settings.	S ☐ U ☐ N/A ☐	S ☐ U ☐ N/A ☐	S ☐ U ☐ N/A ☐
2. Reviews the patient's most recent blood gas or SpO$_2$ values.	S ☐ U ☐ N/A ☐	S ☐ U ☐ N/A ☐	S ☐ U ☐ N/A ☐
3. Reviews the most recent chest radiograph.	S ☐ U ☐ N/A ☐	S ☐ U ☐ N/A ☐	S ☐ U ☐ N/A ☐
4. Identifies the current sedation medications.	S ☐ U ☐ N/A ☐	S ☐ U ☐ N/A ☐	S ☐ U ☐ N/A ☐
5. Verifies the physician's order or the facility's protocol for standard of care.	S ☐ U ☐ N/A ☐	S ☐ U ☐ N/A ☐	S ☐ U ☐ N/A ☐
6. Obtains, cleans, and inspects the appropriate equipment prior to entering the patient's room.	S ☐ U ☐ N/A ☐	S ☐ U ☐ N/A ☐	S ☐ U ☐ N/A ☐
7. Follows PPE requirements, and observes standard precautions for any transmission-based isolation procedure.	S ☐ U ☐ N/A ☐	S ☐ U ☐ N/A ☐	S ☐ U ☐ N/A ☐
8. Identifies the patient using two patient identifiers.	S ☐ U ☐ N/A ☐	S ☐ U ☐ N/A ☐	S ☐ U ☐ N/A ☐
9. Introduces self to the patient and to the family.	S ☐ U ☐ N/A ☐	S ☐ U ☐ N/A ☐	S ☐ U ☐ N/A ☐
10. Explains the procedure to the patient and to the family, and acknowledges the patient's understanding.	S ☐ U ☐ N/A ☐	S ☐ U ☐ N/A ☐	S ☐ U ☐ N/A ☐
11. Performs proper hand hygiene, and puts on gloves, mask, and protective eyewear, as appropriate for the procedure.	S ☐ U ☐ N/A ☐	S ☐ U ☐ N/A ☐	S ☐ U ☐ N/A ☐
Implementation			
1. Performs the patient assessment before conducting the ventilator assessment.	S ☐ U ☐ N/A ☐	S ☐ U ☐ N/A ☐	S ☐ U ☐ N/A ☐
2. Examines appearance, comfort, and ventilator synchrony.	S ☐ U ☐ N/A ☐	S ☐ U ☐ N/A ☐	S ☐ U ☐ N/A ☐

Continued

	Peer Evaluation Laboratory Setting			Instructor Evaluation Laboratory Setting			Instructor Evaluation Clinical Setting		
3. Confirms stabilization of the interface device.	S ☐	U ☐	N/A ☐	S ☐	U ☐	N/A ☐	S ☐	U ☐	N/A ☐
4. Assesses breath sounds; suctions, if indicated.	S ☐	U ☐	N/A ☐	S ☐	U ☐	N/A ☐	S ☐	U ☐	N/A ☐
5. Observes chest-rise.	S ☐	U ☐	N/A ☐	S ☐	U ☐	N/A ☐	S ☐	U ☐	N/A ☐
6. Evaluates the chest tubes.	S ☐	U ☐	N/A ☐	S ☐	U ☐	N/A ☐	S ☐	U ☐	N/A ☐
7. Palpates the peripheral pulses.	S ☐	U ☐	N/A ☐	S ☐	U ☐	N/A ☐	S ☐	U ☐	N/A ☐
8. Inspects the indwelling catheter(s).	S ☐	U ☐	N/A ☐	S ☐	U ☐	N/A ☐	S ☐	U ☐	N/A ☐
9. Elevates the head of the bed to at least 30 degrees.	S ☐	U ☐	N/A ☐	S ☐	U ☐	N/A ☐	S ☐	U ☐	N/A ☐
10. Performs oral care.	S ☐	U ☐	N/A ☐	S ☐	U ☐	N/A ☐	S ☐	U ☐	N/A ☐
11. Assesses the ventilator function and settings.	S ☐	U ☐	N/A ☐	S ☐	U ☐	N/A ☐	S ☐	U ☐	N/A ☐
12. Ensures that the manual ventilation device and the suction equipment are available at the patient's bedside.	S ☐	U ☐	N/A ☐	S ☐	U ☐	N/A ☐	S ☐	U ☐	N/A ☐
13. Removes the supplies from the patient's room, and cleans the area, as needed.	S ☐	U ☐	N/A ☐	S ☐	U ☐	N/A ☐	S ☐	U ☐	N/A ☐
14. Removes PPE, and performs proper hand hygiene prior to leaving the patient's room.	S ☐	U ☐	N/A ☐	S ☐	U ☐	N/A ☐	S ☐	U ☐	N/A ☐

Evaluation of Procedure

1. Establishes a baseline, or compares with previous measurements.	S ☐	U ☐	N/A ☐	S ☐	U ☐	N/A ☐	S ☐	U ☐	N/A ☐
2. Develops an appropriate respiratory careplan based on assessment data.	S ☐	U ☐	N/A ☐	S ☐	U ☐	N/A ☐	S ☐	U ☐	N/A ☐
3. Corrects any problems.	S ☐	U ☐	N/A ☐	S ☐	U ☐	N/A ☐	S ☐	U ☐	N/A ☐
4. Considers discontinuation of noninvasive ventilation, if indicated.	S ☐	U ☐	N/A ☐	S ☐	U ☐	N/A ☐	S ☐	U ☐	N/A ☐
5. Identifies any unexpected outcomes.	S ☐	U ☐	N/A ☐	S ☐	U ☐	N/A ☐	S ☐	U ☐	N/A ☐
6. Considers mechanical ventilation, if indicated.	S ☐	U ☐	N/A ☐	S ☐	U ☐	N/A ☐	S ☐	U ☐	N/A ☐

Documentation and Reporting

1. Records findings in the patient's chart.	S ☐	U ☐	N/A ☐	S ☐	U ☐	N/A ☐	S ☐	U ☐	N/A ☐
2. Reports any abnormal findings to the appropriate health care provider.	S ☐	U ☐	N/A ☐	S ☐	U ☐	N/A ☐	S ☐	U ☐	N/A ☐

Comments:

_____

_____

Signatures:

Student _____ Date Passed _____

Instructor (Laboratory Setting) _____ Date Passed _____

Student _____ Date Passed _____

Instructor (Clinical Setting) _____ Date Passed _____

Procedural Assessment 22-1

Initiation of invasive mechanical ventilation

Student _____ Date _____

Instructor (Laboratory Setting) _____ Date _____

Instructor (Clinical Setting) _____ Date _____

Criteria for assessment success:

The student must obtain all **satisfactory (S)** scores to pass the procedural evaluation. Any **unsatisfactory (U)** scores will result in failure of the procedural assessment.

Scoring:

Satisfactory (S): Procedural step performed correctly with no instructor prompting. Student-initiated correction is acceptable.

Unsatisfactory (U): Procedural step was performed incorrectly, omitted, or performed in a way that compromised patient care.

Not applicable (N/A): Procedural step was not indicated or necessary.

Evaluation:

	Peer Evaluation Laboratory Setting	Instructor Evaluation Laboratory Setting	Instructor Evaluation Clinical Setting
Procedural Preparation			
1. Reviews the patient's chart.	S ☐ U ☐ N/A ☐	S ☐ U ☐ N/A ☐	S ☐ U ☐ N/A ☐
2. Verifies the physician's order or the facility's protocol for standard of care.	S ☐ U ☐ N/A ☐	S ☐ U ☐ N/A ☐	S ☐ U ☐ N/A ☐
3. Obtains, cleans, and inspects the appropriate equipment prior to entering the patient's room.	S ☐ U ☐ N/A ☐	S ☐ U ☐ N/A ☐	S ☐ U ☐ N/A ☐
4. Follows PPE requirements, and observes standard precautions for any transmission-based isolation procedure.	S ☐ U ☐ N/A ☐	S ☐ U ☐ N/A ☐	S ☐ U ☐ N/A ☐
5. Identifies the patient using two patient identifiers.	S ☐ U ☐ N/A ☐	S ☐ U ☐ N/A ☐	S ☐ U ☐ N/A ☐
6. Introduces self to the patient and to the family.	S ☐ U ☐ N/A ☐	S ☐ U ☐ N/A ☐	S ☐ U ☐ N/A ☐
7. Explains the procedure to the patient and to the family, and acknowledges the patient's understanding.	S ☐ U ☐ N/A ☐	S ☐ U ☐ N/A ☐	S ☐ U ☐ N/A ☐
8. Performs proper hand hygiene, and puts on gloves, mask, and protective eyewear, as appropriate for the procedure.	S ☐ U ☐ N/A ☐	S ☐ U ☐ N/A ☐	S ☐ U ☐ N/A ☐
Implementation			
1. Assesses vital signs.	S ☐ U ☐ N/A ☐	S ☐ U ☐ N/A ☐	S ☐ U ☐ N/A ☐
2. Establishes and implements the appropriate settings, or executes the physician's orders for the following setup decisions:			
a. Type and method of artificial airway	S ☐ U ☐ N/A ☐	S ☐ U ☐ N/A ☐	S ☐ U ☐ N/A ☐
b. Partial versus full support	S ☐ U ☐ N/A ☐	S ☐ U ☐ N/A ☐	S ☐ U ☐ N/A ☐
c. Mode of ventilation	S ☐ U ☐ N/A ☐	S ☐ U ☐ N/A ☐	S ☐ U ☐ N/A ☐
3. Establishes and implements the appropriate settings, or executes the physician's orders for the following ventilatory values:			
a. Trigger method and sensitivity	S ☐ U ☐ N/A ☐	S ☐ U ☐ N/A ☐	S ☐ U ☐ N/A ☐
b. Tidal volume or pressure level	S ☐ U ☐ N/A ☐	S ☐ U ☐ N/A ☐	S ☐ U ☐ N/A ☐

Continued

	Peer Evaluation Laboratory Setting			Instructor Evaluation Laboratory Setting			Instructor Evaluation Clinical Setting		
c. Frequency	S ☐	U ☐	N/A ☐	S ☐	U ☐	N/A ☐	S ☐	U ☐	N/A ☐
d. Inspiratory flow, inspiratory time, expiratory time, or I : E ratio	S ☐	U ☐	N/A ☐	S ☐	U ☐	N/A ☐	S ☐	U ☐	N/A ☐
e. Inspiratory flow waveform	S ☐	U ☐	N/A ☐	S ☐	U ☐	N/A ☐	S ☐	U ☐	N/A ☐
f. FIO_2	S ☐	U ☐	N/A ☐	S ☐	U ☐	N/A ☐	S ☐	U ☐	N/A ☐
g. PEEP or CPAP	S ☐	U ☐	N/A ☐	S ☐	U ☐	N/A ☐	S ☐	U ☐	N/A ☐
4. Attaches the patient to the ventilator.	S ☐	U ☐	N/A ☐	S ☐	U ☐	N/A ☐	S ☐	U ☐	N/A ☐
5. Performs initial assessment of ventilatory support:									
a. Inspection, palpation, and auscultation	S ☐	U ☐	N/A ☐	S ☐	U ☐	N/A ☐	S ☐	U ☐	N/A ☐
b. Position of artificial airway and cuff pressure	S ☐	U ☐	N/A ☐	S ☐	U ☐	N/A ☐	S ☐	U ☐	N/A ☐
c. Pulse, blood pressure, oximetry, and ECG	S ☐	U ☐	N/A ☐	S ☐	U ☐	N/A ☐	S ☐	U ☐	N/A ☐
d. Patient–ventilatory system breathing circuit, humidifier, and ventilator settings	S ☐	U ☐	N/A ☐	S ☐	U ☐	N/A ☐	S ☐	U ☐	N/A ☐
6. Establishes and implements the appropriate settings, for alarms and backup values	S ☐	U ☐	N/A ☐	S ☐	U ☐	N/A ☐	S ☐	U ☐	N/A ☐
7. Allows enough slack on the circuit so that the artificial airway remains secure.	S ☐	U ☐	N/A ☐	S ☐	U ☐	N/A ☐	S ☐	U ☐	N/A ☐
8. Confirms placement of or places the manual ventilation device at the patient's bedside.	S ☐	U ☐	N/A ☐	S ☐	U ☐	N/A ☐	S ☐	U ☐	N/A ☐
9. Removes the supplies from the patient's room, and cleans the area, as needed.	S ☐	U ☐	N/A ☐	S ☐	U ☐	N/A ☐	S ☐	U ☐	N/A ☐
10. Removes PPE, and performs proper hand hygiene prior to leaving the patient's room.	S ☐	U ☐	N/A ☐	S ☐	U ☐	N/A ☐	S ☐	U ☐	N/A ☐

Evaluation of Procedure

1. Establishes a baseline, or compares with previous measurements:									
a. Obtains ABG values, and confirms that chest radiography has been ordered.	S ☐	U ☐	N/A ☐	S ☐	U ☐	N/A ☐	S ☐	U ☐	N/A ☐
b. Evaluates the radiograph when it becomes available.	S ☐	U ☐	N/A ☐	S ☐	U ☐	N/A ☐	S ☐	U ☐	N/A ☐
2. Develops an appropriate respiratory care plan based on assessment data.	S ☐	U ☐	N/A ☐	S ☐	U ☐	N/A ☐	S ☐	U ☐	N/A ☐
3. Identifies any unexpected outcomes.	S ☐	U ☐	N/A ☐	S ☐	U ☐	N/A ☐	S ☐	U ☐	N/A ☐

Documentation and Reporting

1. Records findings in the patient's chart.	S ☐	U ☐	N/A ☐	S ☐	U ☐	N/A ☐	S ☐	U ☐	N/A ☐
2. Reports any abnormal findings to the appropriate health care provider.	S ☐	U ☐	N/A ☐	S ☐	U ☐	N/A ☐	S ☐	U ☐	N/A ☐

Comments:

_____

_____

_____

Signatures:

Student _____ Date Passed _____

Instructor (Laboratory Setting) _____ Date Passed _____

Student _____ Date Passed _____

Instructor (Clinical Setting) _____ Date Passed _____

Procedural Assessment 22-2

Assessing a patient-ventilator system

Student _____ Date _____

Instructor (Laboratory Setting) _____ Date _____

Instructor (Clinical Setting) _____ Date _____

Criteria for assessment success:

The student must obtain all **satisfactory (S)** scores to pass the procedural evaluation. Any **unsatisfactory (U)** scores will result in failure of the procedural assessment.

Scoring:

Satisfactory (S): Procedural step performed correctly with no instructor prompting. Student-initiated correction is acceptable.

Unsatisfactory (U): Procedural step was performed incorrectly, omitted, or performed in a way that compromised patient care.

Not applicable (N/A): Procedural step was not indicated or necessary.

Evaluation:

	Peer Evaluation Laboratory Setting	Instructor Evaluation Laboratory Setting	Instructor Evaluation Clinical Setting
Procedural Preparation			
1. Reviews the patient's chart for the patient's current vital signs and ventilator settings.	S ☐ U ☐ N/A ☐	S ☐ U ☐ N/A ☐	S ☐ U ☐ N/A ☐
2. Reviews the patient's most recent ABG or SpO_2 values.	S ☐ U ☐ N/A ☐	S ☐ U ☐ N/A ☐	S ☐ U ☐ N/A ☐
3. Reviews the most recent chest radiograph.	S ☐ U ☐ N/A ☐	S ☐ U ☐ N/A ☐	S ☐ U ☐ N/A ☐
4. Identifies the current sedation medications.	S ☐ U ☐ N/A ☐	S ☐ U ☐ N/A ☐	S ☐ U ☐ N/A ☐
5. Verifies the physician's order or the facility's protocol for standard of care.	S ☐ U ☐ N/A ☐	S ☐ U ☐ N/A ☐	S ☐ U ☐ N/A ☐
6. Obtains, cleans, and inspects the appropriate equipment prior to entering the patient's room.	S ☐ U ☐ N/A ☐	S ☐ U ☐ N/A ☐	S ☐ U ☐ N/A ☐
7. Identifies the patient using two patient identifiers.	S ☐ U ☐ N/A ☐	S ☐ U ☐ N/A ☐	S ☐ U ☐ N/A ☐
8. Follows PPE requirements, and observes standard precautions for any transmission-based isolation procedure.	S ☐ U ☐ N/A ☐	S ☐ U ☐ N/A ☐	S ☐ U ☐ N/A ☐
9. Introduces self to the patient and to the family.	S ☐ U ☐ N/A ☐	S ☐ U ☐ N/A ☐	S ☐ U ☐ N/A ☐
10. Explains the procedure to the patient and to the family, and acknowledges the patient's understanding.	S ☐ U ☐ N/A ☐	S ☐ U ☐ N/A ☐	S ☐ U ☐ N/A ☐
11. Performs proper hand hygiene, and puts on gloves, mask, and protective eyewear, as appropriate for the procedure.	S ☐ U ☐ N/A ☐	S ☐ U ☐ N/A ☐	S ☐ U ☐ N/A ☐
Implementation			
1. Approaches the patient before approaching the ventilator.	S ☐ U ☐ N/A ☐	S ☐ U ☐ N/A ☐	S ☐ U ☐ N/A ☐
2. Performs patient assessment.	S ☐ U ☐ N/A ☐	S ☐ U ☐ N/A ☐	S ☐ U ☐ N/A ☐

Continued

	Peer Evaluation Laboratory Setting			Instructor Evaluation Laboratory Setting			Instructor Evaluation Clinical Setting		
3. Assesses ventilator functions and settings: C_S	S ☐	U ☐	N/A ☐	S ☐	U ☐	N/A ☐	S ☐	U ☐	N/A ☐
4. Ensures that the manual ventilation device and the suction equipment are available at the patient's bedside.	S ☐	U ☐	N/A ☐	S ☐	U ☐	N/A ☐	S ☐	U ☐	N/A ☐
5. Ensures that replacement tracheostomy tubes are available at the patient's bedside.	S ☐	U ☐	N/A ☐	S ☐	U ☐	N/A ☐	S ☐	U ☐	N/A ☐
6. Removes the supplies from the patient's room, and cleans the area, as needed.	S ☐	U ☐	N/A ☐	S ☐	U ☐	N/A ☐	S ☐	U ☐	N/A ☐
7. Removes PPE, and performs proper hand hygiene prior to leaving the patient's room.	S ☐	U ☐	N/A ☐	S ☐	U ☐	N/A ☐	S ☐	U ☐	N/A ☐

Evaluation of Procedure

	Peer Evaluation Laboratory Setting			Instructor Evaluation Laboratory Setting			Instructor Evaluation Clinical Setting		
1. Establishes a baseline, or compares with previous measurements.	S ☐	U ☐	N/A ☐	S ☐	U ☐	N/A ☐	S ☐	U ☐	N/A ☐
2. Develops an appropriate respiratory diagnosis based on assessment data.	S ☐	U ☐	N/A ☐	S ☐	U ☐	N/A ☐	S ☐	U ☐	N/A ☐
3. Ensures that lung protective therapy is in place.	S ☐	U ☐	N/A ☐	S ☐	U ☐	N/A ☐	S ☐	U ☐	N/A ☐
4. Considers mode change, discontinuation of mechanical ventilation, or weaning.	S ☐	U ☐	N/A ☐	S ☐	U ☐	N/A ☐	S ☐	U ☐	N/A ☐
5. Identifies any unexpected outcomes.	S ☐	U ☐	N/A ☐	S ☐	U ☐	N/A ☐	S ☐	U ☐	N/A ☐

Documentation and Reporting

	Peer Evaluation Laboratory Setting			Instructor Evaluation Laboratory Setting			Instructor Evaluation Clinical Setting		
1. Records findings in the patient's chart.	S ☐	U ☐	N/A ☐	S ☐	U ☐	N/A ☐	S ☐	U ☐	N/A ☐
2. Reports any abnormal findings to the appropriate health care provider.	S ☐	U ☐	N/A ☐	S ☐	U ☐	N/A ☐	S ☐	U ☐	N/A ☐

Comments:

_____

_____

_____

Signatures:

Student _____ Date Passed _____

Instructor (Laboratory Setting) _____ Date Passed _____

Student _____ Date Passed _____

Instructor (Clinical Setting) _____ Date Passed _____

Student _____ Date _____

Instructor (Laboratory Setting) _____ Date _____

Instructor (Clinical Setting) _____ Date _____

Criteria for assessment success:

The student must obtain all **satisfactory (S)** scores to pass the procedural evaluation. Any **unsatisfactory (U)** scores will result in failure of the procedural assessment.

Scoring:

Satisfactory (S): Procedural step performed correctly with no instructor prompting. Student-initiated correction is acceptable.

Unsatisfactory (U): Procedural step was performed incorrectly, omitted, or performed in a way that compromised patient care.

Not applicable (N/A): Procedural step was not indicated or necessary.

Evaluation:

	Peer Evaluation Laboratory Setting	Instructor Evaluation Laboratory Setting	Instructor Evaluation Clinical Setting
Procedural Preparation			
1. Reviews the patient's chart.	S ☐ U ☐ N/A ☐	S ☐ U ☐ N/A ☐	S ☐ U ☐ N/A ☐
2. Verifies the physician's order or the facility's protocol for standard of care.	S ☐ U ☐ N/A ☐	S ☐ U ☐ N/A ☐	S ☐ U ☐ N/A ☐
3. Obtains, cleans, and inspects the appropriate equipment prior to entering the patient's room.	S ☐ U ☐ N/A ☐	S ☐ U ☐ N/A ☐	S ☐ U ☐ N/A ☐
4. Follows PPE requirements, and observes standard precautions for any transmission-based isolation procedure.	S ☐ U ☐ N/A ☐	S ☐ U ☐ N/A ☐	S ☐ U ☐ N/A ☐
5. Identifies the patient using two patient identifiers.	S ☐ U ☐ N/A ☐	S ☐ U ☐ N/A ☐	S ☐ U ☐ N/A ☐
6. Introduces self to the patient and to the family.	S ☐ U ☐ N/A ☐	S ☐ U ☐ N/A ☐	S ☐ U ☐ N/A ☐
7. Explains the procedure to the patient and to the family, and acknowledges the patient's understanding.	S ☐ U ☐ N/A ☐	S ☐ U ☐ N/A ☐	S ☐ U ☐ N/A ☐
8. Performs proper hand hygiene, and puts on gloves, mask, and protective eyewear, as appropriate for the procedure.	S ☐ U ☐ N/A ☐	S ☐ U ☐ N/A ☐	S ☐ U ☐ N/A ☐
Implementation			
1. Performs a patient–ventilator system assessment (see PA 22-2).	S ☐ U ☐ N/A ☐	S ☐ U ☐ N/A ☐	S ☐ U ☐ N/A ☐
2. Identifies PIP.	S ☐ U ☐ N/A ☐	S ☐ U ☐ N/A ☐	S ☐ U ☐ N/A ☐
3. Identifies exhaled V_T	S ☐ U ☐ N/A ☐	S ☐ U ☐ N/A ☐	S ☐ U ☐ N/A ☐
4. Identifies PEEP.	S ☐ U ☐ N/A ☐	S ☐ U ☐ N/A ☐	S ☐ U ☐ N/A ☐
5. Identifies auto-PEEP.	S ☐ U ☐ N/A ☐	S ☐ U ☐ N/A ☐	S ☐ U ☐ N/A ☐
6. Identifies total PEEP (PEEP + auto-PEEP).	S ☐ U ☐ N/A ☐	S ☐ U ☐ N/A ☐	S ☐ U ☐ N/A ☐

Continued

	Peer Evaluation Laboratory Setting			Instructor Evaluation Laboratory Setting			Instructor Evaluation Clinical Setting		
7. To calculate (C_D):									
a. Subtracts total PEEP from PIP.	S ☐	U ☐	N/A ☐	S ☐	U ☐	N/A ☐	S ☐	U ☐	N/A ☐
b. Divides exhaled tidal volume by the number obtained in step 7a.	S ☐	U ☐	N/A ☐	S ☐	U ☐	N/A ☐	S ☐	U ☐	N/A ☐
c. Reports C_D in mL/cmH$_2$O.	S ☐	U ☐	N/A ☐	S ☐	U ☐	N/A ☐	S ☐	U ☐	N/A ☐
8. To calculate C_S:									
a. Observes several ventilator respiratory cycles.	S ☐	U ☐	N/A ☐	S ☐	U ☐	N/A ☐	S ☐	U ☐	N/A ☐
b. Performs an inspiratory hold maneuver to obtain plateau pressure.	S ☐	U ☐	N/A ☐	S ☐	U ☐	N/A ☐	S ☐	U ☐	N/A ☐
c. Subtracts total PEEP from plateau pressure.	S ☐	U ☐	N/A ☐	S ☐	U ☐	N/A ☐	S ☐	U ☐	N/A ☐
d. Divides exhaled tidal volume by the number obtained in 8c.	S ☐	U ☐	N/A ☐	S ☐	U ☐	N/A ☐	S ☐	U ☐	N/A ☐
e. Reports C_S in mL/cmH$_2$O.	S ☐	U ☐	N/A ☐	S ☐	U ☐	N/A ☐	S ☐	U ☐	N/A ☐
9. Removes the supplies from the patient's room, and cleans the area, as needed.	S ☐	U ☐	N/A ☐	S ☐	U ☐	N/A ☐	S ☐	U ☐	N/A ☐
10. Removes PPE, and performs proper hand hygiene prior to leaving the patient's room.	S ☐	U ☐	N/A ☐	S ☐	U ☐	N/A ☐	S ☐	U ☐	N/A ☐

Evaluation of Procedure

1. Establishes a baseline, or compares with previous measurements.	S ☐	U ☐	N/A ☐	S ☐	U ☐	N/A ☐	S ☐	U ☐	N/A ☐
2. Develops an appropriate respiratory care plan based on assessment data.	S ☐	U ☐	N/A ☐	S ☐	U ☐	N/A ☐	S ☐	U ☐	N/A ☐
3. Notes any increasing FIO$_2$ requirements.	S ☐	U ☐	N/A ☐	S ☐	U ☐	N/A ☐	S ☐	U ☐	N/A ☐
4. Observes trends in the C_D and C_S, and uses the findings to determine improvement or deterioration of the underlying disease process.	S ☐	U ☐	N/A ☐	S ☐	U ☐	N/A ☐	S ☐	U ☐	N/A ☐
5. Identifies any unexpected outcomes.	S ☐	U ☐	N/A ☐	S ☐	U ☐	N/A ☐	S ☐	U ☐	N/A ☐

Documentation and Reporting

1. Records findings in the patient's chart.	S ☐	U ☐	N/A ☐	S ☐	U ☐	N/A ☐	S ☐	U ☐	N/A ☐
2. Reports any abnormal findings to the appropriate health care provider.	S ☐	U ☐	N/A ☐	S ☐	U ☐	N/A ☐	S ☐	U ☐	N/A ☐

Comments:

_____

_____

_____

Signatures:

Student _____ Date Passed _____

Instructor (Laboratory Setting) _____ Date Passed _____

Student _____ Date Passed _____

Instructor (Clinical Setting) _____ Date Passed _____

Procedural Assessment 23-1 Monitoring oxygenation

Student _____ Date _____

Instructor (Laboratory Setting) _____ Date _____

Instructor (Clinical Setting) _____ Date _____

Criteria for assessment success:

The student must obtain all **satisfactory (S)** scores to pass the procedural evaluation. Any **unsatisfactory (U)** scores will result in failure of the procedural assessment.

Scoring:

Satisfactory (S): Procedural step performed correctly with no instructor prompting. Student-initiated correction is acceptable.

Unsatisfactory (U): Procedural step was performed incorrectly, omitted, or performed in a way that compromised patient care.

Not applicable (N/A): Procedural step was not indicated or necessary.

Evaluation:

	Peer Evaluation Laboratory Setting	Instructor Evaluation Laboratory Setting	Instructor Evaluation Clinical Setting
Procedural Preparation			
1. Reviews the patient's chart.	S ☐ U ☐ N/A ☐	S ☐ U ☐ N/A ☐	S ☐ U ☐ N/A ☐
2. Verifies the physician's order or the facility's protocol for standard of care.	S ☐ U ☐ N/A ☐	S ☐ U ☐ N/A ☐	S ☐ U ☐ N/A ☐
3. Obtains, cleans, and inspects the appropriate equipment prior to entering the patient's room.	S ☐ U ☐ N/A ☐	S ☐ U ☐ N/A ☐	S ☐ U ☐ N/A ☐
4. Follows PPE requirements, and observes standard precautions for any transmission-based isolation procedure.	S ☐ U ☐ N/A ☐	S ☐ U ☐ N/A ☐	S ☐ U ☐ N/A ☐
5. Identifies the patient using two patient identifiers.	S ☐ U ☐ N/A ☐	S ☐ U ☐ N/A ☐	S ☐ U ☐ N/A ☐
6. Introduces self to the patient and to the family.	S ☐ U ☐ N/A ☐	S ☐ U ☐ N/A ☐	S ☐ U ☐ N/A ☐
7. Explains the procedure to the patient and to the family, and acknowledges the patient's understanding.	S ☐ U ☐ N/A ☐	S ☐ U ☐ N/A ☐	S ☐ U ☐ N/A ☐
8. Performs proper hand hygiene, and puts on gloves, mask, and protective eyewear, as appropriate for the procedure.	S ☐ U ☐ N/A ☐	S ☐ U ☐ N/A ☐	S ☐ U ☐ N/A ☐
Implementation			
1. Assesses vital signs.	S ☐ U ☐ N/A ☐	S ☐ U ☐ N/A ☐	S ☐ U ☐ N/A ☐
2. Observes for signs and symptoms of inadequate oxygenation.	S ☐ U ☐ N/A ☐	S ☐ U ☐ N/A ☐	S ☐ U ☐ N/A ☐
3. Calculates oxygen consumption ($\dot{V}O_2$).	S ☐ U ☐ N/A ☐	S ☐ U ☐ N/A ☐	S ☐ U ☐ N/A ☐
4. Calculates the alveolar–arterial oxygen tension difference [$P(A\text{-}a)O_2$].	S ☐ U ☐ N/A ☐	S ☐ U ☐ N/A ☐	S ☐ U ☐ N/A ☐
5. Calculates the P/F ratio.	S ☐ U ☐ N/A ☐	S ☐ U ☐ N/A ☐	S ☐ U ☐ N/A ☐

Continued

	Peer Evaluation Laboratory Setting			Instructor Evaluation Laboratory Setting			Instructor Evaluation Clinical Setting		
6. Calculates the oxygenation index (OI).	S ☐	U ☐	N/A ☐	S ☐	U ☐	N/A ☐	S ☐	U ☐	N/A ☐
7. Removes the supplies from the patient's room, and cleans the area, as needed.	S ☐	U ☐	N/A ☐	S ☐	U ☐	N/A ☐	S ☐	U ☐	N/A ☐
8. Removes PPE, and performs proper hand hygiene prior to leaving the patient's room.	S ☐	U ☐	N/A ☐	S ☐	U ☐	N/A ☐	S ☐	U ☐	N/A ☐
Evaluation of Procedure									
1. Establishes a baseline, or compares with previous measurements.	S ☐	U ☐	N/A ☐	S ☐	U ☐	N/A ☐	S ☐	U ☐	N/A ☐
2. Observes the trends in the oxygenation indices.	S ☐	U ☐	N/A ☐	S ☐	U ☐	N/A ☐	S ☐	U ☐	N/A ☐
3. Develops an appropriate respiratory care plan based on assessment data.	S ☐	U ☐	N/A ☐	S ☐	U ☐	N/A ☐	S ☐	U ☐	N/A ☐
4. Identifies any unexpected outcomes.	S ☐	U ☐	N/A ☐	S ☐	U ☐	N/A ☐	S ☐	U ☐	N/A ☐
5. Lowers the FIO_2, when indicated.	S ☐	U ☐	N/A ☐	S ☐	U ☐	N/A ☐	S ☐	U ☐	N/A ☐
Documentation and Reporting									
1. Records findings in the patient's chart.	S ☐	U ☐	N/A ☐	S ☐	U ☐	N/A ☐	S ☐	U ☐	N/A ☐
2. Reports any abnormal findings to the appropriate health care provider.	S ☐	U ☐	N/A ☐	S ☐	U ☐	N/A ☐	S ☐	U ☐	N/A ☐

Comments:

_____

_____

_____

Signatures:

Student _____ Date Passed _____

Instructor (Laboratory Setting) _____ Date Passed _____

Student _____ Date Passed _____

Instructor (Clinical Setting) _____ Date Passed _____

Procedural Assessment 23-2 — Monitoring ventilation

Student _____ Date _____

Instructor (Laboratory Setting) _____ Date _____

Instructor (Clinical Setting) _____ Date _____

Criteria for assessment success:

The student must obtain all **satisfactory (S)** scores to pass the procedural evaluation. Any **unsatisfactory (U)** scores will result in failure of the procedural assessment.

Scoring:

Satisfactory (S): Procedural step performed correctly with no instructor prompting. Student-initiated correction is acceptable.

Unsatisfactory (U): Procedural step was performed incorrectly, omitted, or performed in a way that compromised patient care.

Not applicable (N/A): Procedural step was not indicated or necessary.

Evaluation:

	Peer Evaluation Laboratory Setting	Instructor Evaluation Laboratory Setting	Instructor Evaluation Clinical Setting
Procedural Preparation			
1. Reviews the patient's chart.	S ☐ U ☐ N/A ☐	S ☐ U ☐ N/A ☐	S ☐ U ☐ N/A ☐
2. Verifies the physician's order or the facility's protocol for standard of care.	S ☐ U ☐ N/A ☐	S ☐ U ☐ N/A ☐	S ☐ U ☐ N/A ☐
3. Obtains, cleans, and inspects the appropriate equipment prior to entering the patient's room.	S ☐ U ☐ N/A ☐	S ☐ U ☐ N/A ☐	S ☐ U ☐ N/A ☐
4. Follows PPE requirements, and observes standard precautions for any transmission-based isolation procedure.	S ☐ U ☐ N/A ☐	S ☐ U ☐ N/A ☐	S ☐ U ☐ N/A ☐
5. Identifies the patient using two patient identifiers.	S ☐ U ☐ N/A ☐	S ☐ U ☐ N/A ☐	S ☐ U ☐ N/A ☐
6. Introduces self to the patient and to the family.	S ☐ U ☐ N/A ☐	S ☐ U ☐ N/A ☐	S ☐ U ☐ N/A ☐
7. Explains the procedure to the patient and to the family, and acknowledges the patient's understanding.	S ☐ U ☐ N/A ☐	S ☐ U ☐ N/A ☐	S ☐ U ☐ N/A ☐
8. Performs proper hand hygiene, and puts on gloves, mask, and protective eyewear, as appropriate for the procedure.	S ☐ U ☐ N/A ☐	S ☐ U ☐ N/A ☐	S ☐ U ☐ N/A ☐
Implementation			
1. Assesses vital signs.	S ☐ U ☐ N/A ☐	S ☐ U ☐ N/A ☐	S ☐ U ☐ N/A ☐
2. Observes for signs and symptoms of inadequate ventilation.	S ☐ U ☐ N/A ☐	S ☐ U ☐ N/A ☐	S ☐ U ☐ N/A ☐
3. Calculates the V_D/V_T.	S ☐ U ☐ N/A ☐	S ☐ U ☐ N/A ☐	S ☐ U ☐ N/A ☐
4. Calculates minute ventilation.	S ☐ U ☐ N/A ☐	S ☐ U ☐ N/A ☐	S ☐ U ☐ N/A ☐
5. Compares inspired tidal volume versus expired tidal volume.	S ☐ U ☐ N/A ☐	S ☐ U ☐ N/A ☐	S ☐ U ☐ N/A ☐

Continued

	Peer Evaluation Laboratory Setting			Instructor Evaluation Laboratory Setting			Instructor Evaluation Clinical Setting		
6. Removes the supplies from the patient's room, and cleans the area, as needed.	S □	U □	N/A □	S □	U □	N/A □	S □	U □	N/A □
7. Removes PPE, and performs proper hand hygiene prior to leaving the patient's room.	S □	U □	N/A □	S □	U □	N/A □	S □	U □	N/A □

Evaluation of Procedure

1. Establishes a baseline, or compares with previous measurements.	S □	U □	N/A □	S □	U □	N/A □	S □	U □	N/A □
2. Observes trends in ventilation adequacies.	S □	U □	N/A □	S □	U □	N/A □	S □	U □	N/A □
3. Develops an appropriate respiratory care plan based on assessment data.	S □	U □	N/A □	S □	U □	N/A □	S □	U □	N/A □
4. Identifies any unexpected outcomes.	S □	U □	N/A □	S □	U □	N/A □	S □	U □	N/A □
5. Lowers the fractional inspired oxygen (FIO_2) level, when indicated.	S □	U □	N/A □	S □	U □	N/A □	S □	U □	N/A □

Documentation and Reporting

1. Records findings in the patient's chart.	S □	U □	N/A □	S □	U □	N/A □	S □	U □	N/A □
2. Reports any abnormal findings to the appropriate health care provider.	S □	U □	N/A □	S □	U □	N/A □	S □	U □	N/A □

Comments:

_____

_____

_____

Signatures:

Student _____ Date Passed _____

Instructor (Laboratory Setting) _____ Date Passed _____

Student _____ Date Passed _____

Instructor (Clinical Setting) _____ Date Passed _____

Student _____ Date _____

Instructor (Laboratory Setting) _____ Date _____

Instructor (Clinical Setting) _____ Date _____

Criteria for assessment success:

The student must obtain all **satisfactory (S)** scores to pass the procedural evaluation. Any **unsatisfactory (U)** scores will result in failure of the procedural assessment.

Scoring:

Satisfactory (S): Procedural step performed correctly with no instructor prompting. Student-initiated correction is acceptable.

Unsatisfactory (U): Procedural step was performed incorrectly, omitted, or performed in a way that compromised patient care.

Not applicable (N/A): Procedural step was not indicated or necessary.

Evaluation:

	Peer Evaluation Laboratory Setting	Instructor Evaluation Laboratory Setting	Instructor Evaluation Clinical Setting
Procedural Preparation			
1. Reviews the patient's chart.	S ☐ U ☐ N/A ☐	S ☐ U ☐ N/A ☐	S ☐ U ☐ N/A ☐
2. Identifies possible factors that preclude the use of a recruitment maneuver and discusses the clinical situation with the appropriate supervising health care provider.	S ☐ U ☐ N/A ☐	S ☐ U ☐ N/A ☐	S ☐ U ☐ N/A ☐
3. Verifies the physician's order or the facility's protocol for standard of care.	S ☐ U ☐ N/A ☐	S ☐ U ☐ N/A ☐	S ☐ U ☐ N/A ☐
4. Follows personal protective equipment (PPE) requirements, and observes standard precautions for any transmission-based isolation procedure.	S ☐ U ☐ N/A ☐	S ☐ U ☐ N/A ☐	S ☐ U ☐ N/A ☐
5. Identifies the patient using two patient identifiers.	S ☐ U ☐ N/A ☐	S ☐ U ☐ N/A ☐	S ☐ U ☐ N/A ☐
6. Introduces self to the patient and to the family.	S ☐ U ☐ N/A ☐	S ☐ U ☐ N/A ☐	S ☐ U ☐ N/A ☐
7. Explains the procedure to the patient and to the family, and acknowledges the patient's understanding.	S ☐ U ☐ N/A ☐	S ☐ U ☐ N/A ☐	S ☐ U ☐ N/A ☐
8. Performs proper hand hygiene, and puts on gloves, mask, and protective eyewear, as appropriate for the procedure.	S ☐ U ☐ N/A ☐	S ☐ U ☐ N/A ☐	S ☐ U ☐ N/A ☐
Implementation			
1. Positions the patient.	S ☐ U ☐ N/A ☐	S ☐ U ☐ N/A ☐	S ☐ U ☐ N/A ☐
2. Discusses with the bedside nurse that the recruitment maneuver is about to begin.	S ☐ U ☐ N/A ☐	S ☐ U ☐ N/A ☐	S ☐ U ☐ N/A ☐
3. Assesses vital signs.	S ☐ U ☐ N/A ☐	S ☐ U ☐ N/A ☐	S ☐ U ☐ N/A ☐
4. Ensures that the patient is relaxed and comfortable, allowing ventilator-delivered control breaths.	S ☐ U ☐ N/A ☐	S ☐ U ☐ N/A ☐	S ☐ U ☐ N/A ☐
5. Documents baseline vital signs, SpO_2, E_TCO_2, if available.	S ☐ U ☐ N/A ☐	S ☐ U ☐ N/A ☐	S ☐ U ☐ N/A ☐
6. Changes the ventilator mode to "Pressure Control."	S ☐ U ☐ N/A ☐	S ☐ U ☐ N/A ☐	S ☐ U ☐ N/A ☐

Continued

	Peer Evaluation Laboratory Setting			Instructor Evaluation Laboratory Setting			Instructor Evaluation Clinical Setting		
7. Ensures that the tidal volumes are similar to baseline and are adequate.	S ☐	U ☐	N/A ☐	S ☐	U ☐	N/A ☐	S ☐	U ☐	N/A ☐
8. Engages available documentation for recording changes in compliance, tidal volume, and ventilatory pressures during the maneuver.	S ☐	U ☐	N/A ☐	S ☐	U ☐	N/A ☐	S ☐	U ☐	N/A ☐
9. Records baseline compliance, exhaled tidal volume, and ventilator pressures.	S ☐	U ☐	N/A ☐	S ☐	U ☐	N/A ☐	S ☐	U ☐	N/A ☐
10. While maintaining a consistent ΔP, increases PEEP by 2 cmH_2O.	S ☐	U ☐	N/A ☐	S ☐	U ☐	N/A ☐	S ☐	U ☐	N/A ☐
11. After 1 minute, records compliance, tidal volume, and ventilator pressures.	S ☐	U ☐	N/A ☐	S ☐	U ☐	N/A ☐	S ☐	U ☐	N/A ☐
12. Ensures that patient comfort, hemodynamics, and oxygenation are acceptable.	S ☐	U ☐	N/A ☐	S ☐	U ☐	N/A ☐	S ☐	U ☐	N/A ☐
13. If increase in PEEP results in tidal volumes greater than 10 mL/kg, reduces ΔP by 2 cmH_2O	S ☐	U ☐	N/A ☐	S ☐	U ☐	N/A ☐	S ☐	U ☐	N/A ☐
14. If a discrete increase in PEEP results in a large improvement in compliance or tidal volume, records the pressure at which this occurs as the "opening pressure."	S ☐	U ☐	N/A ☐	S ☐	U ☐	N/A ☐	S ☐	U ☐	N/A ☐
15. Repeats PEEP increase every minute until compliance does not increase or decrease.	S ☐	U ☐	N/A ☐	S ☐	U ☐	N/A ☐	S ☐	U ☐	N/A ☐
16. Records this PEEP level as the PEEP where "full recruitment" is achieved.	S ☐	U ☐	N/A ☐	S ☐	U ☐	N/A ☐	S ☐	U ☐	N/A ☐
17. Decreases PEEP by 2 cmH_2O every minute until "derecruitment" occurs.	S ☐	U ☐	N/A ☐	S ☐	U ☐	N/A ☐	S ☐	U ☐	N/A ☐
18. Records the pressure at which the drop occurred as the "closing pressure."	S ☐	U ☐	N/A ☐	S ☐	U ☐	N/A ☐	S ☐	U ☐	N/A ☐
19. Increases PEEP again by 2 cmH_2O every minute up to full recruitment pressure, and drops by 2 cmH_2O every minute to PEEP of 2 cmH_2O above closing pressure.	S ☐	U ☐	N/A ☐	S ☐	U ☐	N/A ☐	S ☐	U ☐	N/A ☐
20. Records this pressure as "optimal PEEP."	S ☐	U ☐	N/A ☐	S ☐	U ☐	N/A ☐	S ☐	U ☐	N/A ☐
21. Reassesses vital signs.	S ☐	U ☐	N/A ☐	S ☐	U ☐	N/A ☐	S ☐	U ☐	N/A ☐
22. Removes the supplies from the patient's room, and cleans the area, as needed.	S ☐	U ☐	N/A ☐	S ☐	U ☐	N/A ☐	S ☐	U ☐	N/A ☐
23. Removes PPE, and performs proper hand hygiene prior to leaving the patient's room.	S ☐	U ☐	N/A ☐	S ☐	U ☐	N/A ☐	S ☐	U ☐	N/A ☐

Evaluation of Procedure

1. Establishes a baseline, or compares with previous measurements.	S ☐	U ☐	N/A ☐	S ☐	U ☐	N/A ☐	S ☐	U ☐	N/A ☐
2. Develops an appropriate respiratory care plan based on assessment data.	S ☐	U ☐	N/A ☐	S ☐	U ☐	N/A ☐	S ☐	U ☐	N/A ☐
3. Identifies any unexpected outcomes.	S ☐	U ☐	N/A ☐	S ☐	U ☐	N/A ☐	S ☐	U ☐	N/A ☐
4. Correlates findings with changes in patient oxygenation, ventilation, and other vital signs.	S ☐	U ☐	N/A ☐	S ☐	U ☐	N/A ☐	S ☐	U ☐	N/A ☐

Documentation and Reporting

1. Records the final ventilator settings, if available.	S ☐	U ☐	N/A ☐	S ☐	U ☐	N/A ☐	S ☐	U ☐	N/A ☐
2. Reports any abnormal findings to the appropriate health care provider.	S ☐	U ☐	N/A ☐	S ☐	U ☐	N/A ☐	S ☐	U ☐	N/A ☐

Comments:

_____

_____

_____

Signatures:

Student _____ Date Passed _____

Instructor (Laboratory Setting) _____ Date Passed _____

Student _____ Date Passed _____

Instructor (Clinical Setting) _____ Date Passed _____

Comments:

Signatures

Student	Date Passed
Instructor (Laboratory Setting)	Date Passed
Student	Date Passed
Instructor (Clinical Setting)	Date Passed

Student _____ Date _____

Instructor (Laboratory Setting) _____ Date _____

Instructor (Clinical Setting) _____ Date _____

Criteria for assessment success:

Student must obtain all **satisfactory (S)** scores in order to pass the procedural evaluation. Any **unsatisfactory (U)** scores will result in failure of the procedural assessment.

Scoring:

Satisfactory (S): Procedural step performed correctly with no instructor prompting. Student-initiated correction is acceptable.

Unsatisfactory (U): Procedural step was performed incorrectly, omitted, or performed in a way that compromised patient care.

Not applicable (N/A): Procedural step was not indicated or necessary.

Evaluation:

	Peer Evaluation Laboratory Setting	Instructor Evaluation Laboratory Setting	Instructor Evaluation Clinical Setting
Procedural Preparation			
1. Reviews the patient's chart.	S ☐ U ☐ N/A ☐	S ☐ U ☐ N/A ☐	S ☐ U ☐ N/A ☐
2. Verifies the physician's order or the facility's protocol for standard of care.	S ☐ U ☐ N/A ☐	S ☐ U ☐ N/A ☐	S ☐ U ☐ N/A ☐
3. Obtains, cleans, and inspects the appropriate equipment prior to entering the patient's room.	S ☐ U ☐ N/A ☐	S ☐ U ☐ N/A ☐	S ☐ U ☐ N/A ☐
4. Follows PPE requirements, and observes standard precautions for any transmission-based isolation procedure.	S ☐ U ☐ N/A ☐	S ☐ U ☐ N/A ☐	S ☐ U ☐ N/A ☐
5. Identifies the patient using two patient identifiers.	S ☐ U ☐ N/A ☐	S ☐ U ☐ N/A ☐	S ☐ U ☐ N/A ☐
6. Introduces self to the patient and to the family.	S ☐ U ☐ N/A ☐	S ☐ U ☐ N/A ☐	S ☐ U ☐ N/A ☐
7. Explains the procedure to the patient and to the family, and acknowledges the patient's understanding.	S ☐ U ☐ N/A ☐	S ☐ U ☐ N/A ☐	S ☐ U ☐ N/A ☐
8. Performs proper hand hygiene, and puts on gloves, mask, and protective eyewear, as appropriate for the procedure.	S ☐ U ☐ N/A ☐	S ☐ U ☐ N/A ☐	S ☐ U ☐ N/A ☐
Implementation			
1. Places the patient in a comfortable position, and instructs him or her to breathe normally.	S ☐ U ☐ N/A ☐	S ☐ U ☐ N/A ☐	S ☐ U ☐ N/A ☐
2. Assesses vital signs continuously throughout procedure, reassures patient as necessary	S ☐ U ☐ N/A ☐	S ☐ U ☐ N/A ☐	S ☐ U ☐ N/A ☐
3. Opens chest tube insertion tray with sterile technique	S ☐ U ☐ N/A ☐	S ☐ U ☐ N/A ☐	S ☐ U ☐ N/A ☐
4. Assists with preparation of the equipment and insertion site.	S ☐ U ☐ N/A ☐	S ☐ U ☐ N/A ☐	S ☐ U ☐ N/A ☐
5. Following insertion, connects chest tube to the closed chest drainage system (CDS).	S ☐ U ☐ N/A ☐	S ☐ U ☐ N/A ☐	S ☐ U ☐ N/A ☐

Continued

	Peer Evaluation Laboratory Setting			Instructor Evaluation Laboratory Setting			Instructor Evaluation Clinical Setting		
6. Checks CDS for rise and fall of the water column and applies ordered amount of suction.	S ☐	U ☐	N/A ☐	S ☐	U ☐	N/A ☐	S ☐	U ☐	N/A ☐
7. Assists with suturing and applies occlusive dressing.	S ☐	U ☐	N/A ☐	S ☐	U ☐	N/A ☐	S ☐	U ☐	N/A ☐
8. Secures all connection points to the drainage system.	S ☐	U ☐	N/A ☐	S ☐	U ☐	N/A ☐	S ☐	U ☐	N/A ☐
9. Secures the tube below the dressing to the patient's skin.	S ☐	U ☐	N/A ☐	S ☐	U ☐	N/A ☐	S ☐	U ☐	N/A ☐
10. Reassesses vital signs.	S ☐	U ☐	N/A ☐	S ☐	U ☐	N/A ☐	S ☐	U ☐	N/A ☐
11. Removes the supplies from the patient's room, and cleans the area, as needed.	S ☐	U ☐	N/A ☐	S ☐	U ☐	N/A ☐	S ☐	U ☐	N/A ☐
12. Removes PPE, and performs proper hand hygiene prior to leaving the patient's room.	S ☐	U ☐	N/A ☐	S ☐	U ☐	N/A ☐	S ☐	U ☐	N/A ☐

Evaluation of Procedure

1. Ensures chest x-ray is ordered to confirm tube placement.	S ☐	U ☐	N/A ☐	S ☐	U ☐	N/A ☐	S ☐	U ☐	N/A ☐
2. Assesses patient for pain at insertion site.	S ☐	U ☐	N/A ☐	S ☐	U ☐	N/A ☐	S ☐	U ☐	N/A ☐
3. Ensures vital signs are assessed every 1 to 4 hours, or per protocols.	S ☐	U ☐	N/A ☐	S ☐	U ☐	N/A ☐	S ☐	U ☐	N/A ☐
4. Develops appropriate respiratory care plan based on assessment data.	S ☐	U ☐	N/A ☐	S ☐	U ☐	N/A ☐	S ☐	U ☐	N/A ☐
5. Identifies any unexpected outcomes.	S ☐	U ☐	N/A ☐	S ☐	U ☐	N/A ☐	S ☐	U ☐	N/A ☐

Documentation and Reporting

1. Records vital signs during and after procedure in patient's chart.	S ☐	U ☐	N/A ☐	S ☐	U ☐	N/A ☐	S ☐	U ☐	N/A ☐
2. Reports any abnormal findings to the appropriate health care provider.	S ☐	U ☐	N/A ☐	S ☐	U ☐	N/A ☐	S ☐	U ☐	N/A ☐

Comments:

_____

_____

_____

Signatures:

Student _____ Date Passed _____

Instructor (Laboratory Setting) _____ Date Passed _____

Student _____ Date Passed _____

Instructor (Clinical Setting) _____ Date Passed _____

Procedural Assessment 23-5

Student _____ Date _____

Instructor (Laboratory Setting) _____ Date _____

Instructor (Clinical Setting) _____ Date _____

Criteria for assessment success:

The student must obtain all **satisfactory (S)** scores to pass the procedural evaluation. Any **unsatisfactory (U)** scores will result in failure of the procedural assessment.

Scoring:

Satisfactory (S): Procedural step performed correctly with no instructor prompting. Student-initiated correction is acceptable.

Unsatisfactory (U): Procedural step was performed incorrectly, omitted, or performed in a way that compromised patient care.

Not applicable (N/A): Procedural step was not indicated or necessary.

Evaluation:

	Peer Evaluation Laboratory Setting	Instructor Evaluation Laboratory Setting	Instructor Evaluation Clinical Setting
Procedural Preparation			
1. Reviews the patient's chart.	S ☐ U ☐ N/A ☐	S ☐ U ☐ N/A ☐	S ☐ U ☐ N/A ☐
2. Verifies the physician's order or the facility's protocol for standard of care.	S ☐ U ☐ N/A ☐	S ☐ U ☐ N/A ☐	S ☐ U ☐ N/A ☐
3. Obtains, cleans, and inspects the appropriate equipment prior to entering the patient's room.	S ☐ U ☐ N/A ☐	S ☐ U ☐ N/A ☐	S ☐ U ☐ N/A ☐
4. Follows PPE requirements, and observes standard precautions for any transmission-based isolation procedure.	S ☐ U ☐ N/A ☐	S ☐ U ☐ N/A ☐	S ☐ U ☐ N/A ☐
5. Identifies the patient using two patient identifiers.	S ☐ U ☐ N/A ☐	S ☐ U ☐ N/A ☐	S ☐ U ☐ N/A ☐
6. Introduces self to the patient and to the family.	S ☐ U ☐ N/A ☐	S ☐ U ☐ N/A ☐	S ☐ U ☐ N/A ☐
7. Explains the procedure to the patient and to the family, and acknowledges the patient's understanding.	S ☐ U ☐ N/A ☐	S ☐ U ☐ N/A ☐	S ☐ U ☐ N/A ☐
8. Performs proper hand hygiene, and puts on gloves, mask, and protective eyewear, as appropriate for the procedure.	S ☐ U ☐ N/A ☐	S ☐ U ☐ N/A ☐	S ☐ U ☐ N/A ☐
Implementation			
1. Following placement, assesses vital signs per protocol or as follows:			
a. Every 15 min 2 times	S ☐ U ☐ N/A ☐	S ☐ U ☐ N/A ☐	S ☐ U ☐ N/A ☐
b. Every 30 min 1 time	S ☐ U ☐ N/A ☐	S ☐ U ☐ N/A ☐	S ☐ U ☐ N/A ☐
c. Every 1 hour for 4 hours after insertion	S ☐ U ☐ N/A ☐	S ☐ U ☐ N/A ☐	S ☐ U ☐ N/A ☐
d. Reassesses every 2 to 4 hours after insertion	S ☐ U ☐ N/A ☐	S ☐ U ☐ N/A ☐	S ☐ U ☐ N/A ☐
2. Monitors the amount and type of drainage.	S ☐ U ☐ N/A ☐	S ☐ U ☐ N/A ☐	S ☐ U ☐ N/A ☐
3. Assesses the patient and the system for leaks.	S ☐ U ☐ N/A ☐	S ☐ U ☐ N/A ☐	S ☐ U ☐ N/A ☐
4. Maintains and checks the chest tubes for patency.	S ☐ U ☐ N/A ☐	S ☐ U ☐ N/A ☐	S ☐ U ☐ N/A ☐

Continued

	Peer Evaluation Laboratory Setting			Instructor Evaluation Laboratory Setting			Instructor Evaluation Clinical Setting		
5. Assesses the insertion site and adjacent skin.	S ☐	U ☐	N/A ☐	S ☐	U ☐	N/A ☐	S ☐	U ☐	N/A ☐
6. Removes the supplies from the patient's room, and cleans the area, as needed.	S ☐	U ☐	N/A ☐	S ☐	U ☐	N/A ☐	S ☐	U ☐	N/A ☐
7. Removes PPE, and performs proper hand hygiene prior to leaving the patient's room.	S ☐	U ☐	N/A ☐	S ☐	U ☐	N/A ☐	S ☐	U ☐	N/A ☐

Evaluation of Procedure

1. Establishes a baseline, or compares with previous measurements.	S ☐	U ☐	N/A ☐	S ☐	U ☐	N/A ☐	S ☐	U ☐	N/A ☐
2. Develops an appropriate respiratory care plan based on assessment data.	S ☐	U ☐	N/A ☐	S ☐	U ☐	N/A ☐	S ☐	U ☐	N/A ☐
3. Identifies any unexpected outcomes.	S ☐	U ☐	N/A ☐	S ☐	U ☐	N/A ☐	S ☐	U ☐	N/A ☐

Documentation and Reporting

1. Records findings in the patient's chart.	S ☐	U ☐	N/A ☐	S ☐	U ☐	N/A ☐	S ☐	U ☐	N/A ☐
2. Reports any abnormal findings to the appropriate health care provider.	S ☐	U ☐	N/A ☐	S ☐	U ☐	N/A ☐	S ☐	U ☐	N/A ☐

Comments:

_____

_____

_____

Signatures:

Student _____ Date Passed _____

Instructor (Laboratory Setting) _____ Date Passed _____

Student _____ Date Passed _____

Instructor (Clinical Setting) _____ Date Passed _____

Procedural Assessment 24-1

Venipuncture

Student _____ Date _____

Instructor (Laboratory Setting) _____ Date _____

Instructor (Clinical Setting) _____ Date _____

Criteria for assessment success:

The student must obtain all **satisfactory (S)** scores to pass the procedural evaluation. Any **unsatisfactory (U)** scores will result in failure of the procedural assessment.

Scoring:

Satisfactory (S): Procedural step performed correctly with no instructor prompting. Student-initiated correction is acceptable.

Unsatisfactory (U): Procedural step was performed incorrectly, omitted, or performed in a way that compromised patient care.

Not applicable (N/A): Procedural step was not indicated or necessary.

Evaluation:

	Peer Evaluation Laboratory Setting	Instructor Evaluation Laboratory Setting	Instructor Evaluation Clinical Setting
Procedural Preparation			
1. Reviews the patient's chart.	S ☐ U ☐ N/A ☐	S ☐ U ☐ N/A ☐	S ☐ U ☐ N/A ☐
2. Verifies the physician's order or the facility's protocol for standard of care.	S ☐ U ☐ N/A ☐	S ☐ U ☐ N/A ☐	S ☐ U ☐ N/A ☐
3. Obtains, cleans, and inspects the appropriate equipment prior to entering the patient's room.	S ☐ U ☐ N/A ☐	S ☐ U ☐ N/A ☐	S ☐ U ☐ N/A ☐
4. Follows PPE requirements, and observes standard precautions for any transmission-based isolation procedure.	S ☐ U ☐ N/A ☐	S ☐ U ☐ N/A ☐	S ☐ U ☐ N/A ☐
5. Identifies the patient using two patient identifiers.	S ☐ U ☐ N/A ☐	S ☐ U ☐ N/A ☐	S ☐ U ☐ N/A ☐
6. Introduces self to the patient and to the family.	S ☐ U ☐ N/A ☐	S ☐ U ☐ N/A ☐	S ☐ U ☐ N/A ☐
7. Explains the procedure to the patient and to the family, and acknowledges the patient's understanding.	S ☐ U ☐ N/A ☐	S ☐ U ☐ N/A ☐	S ☐ U ☐ N/A ☐
8. Performs proper hand hygiene, and puts on gloves, mask, and protective eyewear, as appropriate for the procedure.	S ☐ U ☐ N/A ☐	S ☐ U ☐ N/A ☐	S ☐ U ☐ N/A ☐
Implementation			
1. Places the patient in a comfortable position.	S ☐ U ☐ N/A ☐	S ☐ U ☐ N/A ☐	S ☐ U ☐ N/A ☐
2. Prepares the equipment needed at the bedside.	S ☐ U ☐ N/A ☐	S ☐ U ☐ N/A ☐	S ☐ U ☐ N/A ☐
3. Assesses vital signs.	S ☐ U ☐ N/A ☐	S ☐ U ☐ N/A ☐	S ☐ U ☐ N/A ☐
4. Ensures adequate lighting.	S ☐ U ☐ N/A ☐	S ☐ U ☐ N/A ☐	S ☐ U ☐ N/A ☐
5. Chooses the appropriate site for venipuncture.	S ☐ U ☐ N/A ☐	S ☐ U ☐ N/A ☐	S ☐ U ☐ N/A ☐

Continued

	Peer Evaluation Laboratory Setting	Instructor Evaluation Laboratory Setting	Instructor Evaluation Clinical Setting
6. Applies tourniquet above the selected site, and gently palpated the vein with a finger.	S ☐ U ☐ N/A ☐	S ☐ U ☐ N/A ☐	S ☐ U ☐ N/A ☐
7. Instructs the patient to clench the fist and performs venipuncture using one of the following methods. a. Syringe the needle or butterfly method or b. Vacutainer method	S ☐ U ☐ N/A ☐ S ☐ U ☐ N/A ☐	S ☐ U ☐ N/A ☐ S ☐ U ☐ N/A ☐	S ☐ U ☐ N/A ☐ S ☐ U ☐ N/A ☐
8. Applies gauze with tape over the puncture site.	S ☐ U ☐ N/A ☐	S ☐ U ☐ N/A ☐	S ☐ U ☐ N/A ☐
9. Checks the tubes, and wipes with alcohol, if necessary.	S ☐ U ☐ N/A ☐	S ☐ U ☐ N/A ☐	S ☐ U ☐ N/A ☐
10. Assists the patient to a comfortable position, if previously moved.	S ☐ U ☐ N/A ☐	S ☐ U ☐ N/A ☐	S ☐ U ☐ N/A ☐
11. Labels every tube with patient information, Date and time the specimen was collected, and the initials of the person who collected it.	S ☐ U ☐ N/A ☐	S ☐ U ☐ N/A ☐	S ☐ U ☐ N/A ☐
12. Disposes of all used supplies and soiled equipment.	S ☐ U ☐ N/A ☐	S ☐ U ☐ N/A ☐	S ☐ U ☐ N/A ☐
13. Removes unused supplies from the patient's room, and cleans the area, as needed.	S ☐ U ☐ N/A ☐	S ☐ U ☐ N/A ☐	S ☐ U ☐ N/A ☐
14. Removes PPE, and performs proper hand hygiene prior to leaving the patient's room.	S ☐ U ☐ N/A ☐	S ☐ U ☐ N/A ☐	S ☐ U ☐ N/A ☐
15. Bags and transports the tubes to the laboratory, according to the facility's protocols.	S ☐ U ☐ N/A ☐	S ☐ U ☐ N/A ☐	S ☐ U ☐ N/A ☐

Evaluation of Procedure

1. Reassesses the venipuncture site.	S ☐ U ☐ N/A ☐	S ☐ U ☐ N/A ☐	S ☐ U ☐ N/A ☐
2. Establishes a baseline, or reviews laboratory data.	S ☐ U ☐ N/A ☐	S ☐ U ☐ N/A ☐	S ☐ U ☐ N/A ☐
3. Develops an appropriate respiratory care plan based on assessment data.	S ☐ U ☐ N/A ☐	S ☐ U ☐ N/A ☐	S ☐ U ☐ N/A ☐
4. Identifies any unexpected outcomes.	S ☐ U ☐ N/A ☐	S ☐ U ☐ N/A ☐	S ☐ U ☐ N/A ☐

Documentation and Reporting

1. Records the data related to the venipuncture sampling in the patient's chart.	S ☐ U ☐ N/A ☐	S ☐ U ☐ N/A ☐	S ☐ U ☐ N/A ☐
2. Reports any "stat" critical values to the appropriate health care provider.	S ☐ U ☐ N/A ☐	S ☐ U ☐ N/A ☐	S ☐ U ☐ N/A ☐

Comments:

_____

_____

_____

Signatures:

Student _____ Date Passed _____

Instructor (Laboratory Setting) _____ Date Passed _____

Student _____ Date Passed _____

Instructor (Clinical Setting) _____ Date Passed _____

Procedural Assessment 24-2

Interpreting basic laboratory values

Student _____ Date _____

Instructor (Laboratory Setting) _____ Date _____

Instructor (Clinical Setting) _____ Date _____

Criteria for assessment success:

The student must obtain all **satisfactory (S)** scores to pass the procedural evaluation. Any **unsatisfactory (U)** scores will result in failure of the procedural assessment.

Scoring:

Satisfactory (S): Procedural step performed correctly with no instructor prompting. Student-initiated correction is acceptable.

Unsatisfactory (U): Procedural step was performed incorrectly, omitted, or performed in a way that compromised patient care.

Not applicable (N/A): Procedural step was not indicated or necessary.

Evaluation:

	Peer Evaluation Laboratory Setting	Instructor Evaluation Laboratory Setting	Instructor Evaluation Clinical Setting
Procedural Preparation			
1. Reviews the patient's chart.	S ☐ U ☐ N/A ☐	S ☐ U ☐ N/A ☐	S ☐ U ☐ N/A ☐
2. Identifies the laboratory values for interpretation that relate to the respiratory status of the patient.	S ☐ U ☐ N/A ☐	S ☐ U ☐ N/A ☐	S ☐ U ☐ N/A ☐
Implementation			
1. Evaluates the complete blood cell count.	S ☐ U ☐ N/A ☐	S ☐ U ☐ N/A ☐	S ☐ U ☐ N/A ☐
2. Evaluates the basic or comprehensive metabolic panel.	S ☐ U ☐ N/A ☐	S ☐ U ☐ N/A ☐	S ☐ U ☐ N/A ☐
3. Evaluates the enzyme tests.	S ☐ U ☐ N/A ☐	S ☐ U ☐ N/A ☐	S ☐ U ☐ N/A ☐
4. Evaluates the coagulation studies.	S ☐ U ☐ N/A ☐	S ☐ U ☐ N/A ☐	S ☐ U ☐ N/A ☐
Evaluation of Procedure			
1. Identifies any critical test values	S ☐ U ☐ N/A ☐	S ☐ U ☐ N/A ☐	S ☐ U ☐ N/A ☐
2. Develops an appropriate respiratory care plan based on laboratory data.	S ☐ U ☐ N/A ☐	S ☐ U ☐ N/A ☐	S ☐ U ☐ N/A ☐
Documentation and Reporting			
1. Reports the critical test values immediately to the appropriate health care provider.	S ☐ U ☐ N/A ☐	S ☐ U ☐ N/A ☐	S ☐ U ☐ N/A ☐

Comments:

_____

_____

_____

Signatures:

Student _____ Date Passed _____

Instructor (Laboratory Setting) _____ Date Passed _____

Student _____ Date Passed _____

Instructor (Clinical Setting) _____ Date Passed _____

Procedural Assessment 24-3

Student _____ Date _____

Instructor (Laboratory Setting) _____ Date _____

Instructor (Clinical Setting) _____ Date _____

Criteria for assessment success:

The student must obtain all **satisfactory (S)** scores to pass the procedural evaluation. Any **unsatisfactory (U)** scores will result in failure of the procedural assessment.

Scoring:

Satisfactory (S): Procedural step performed correctly with no instructor prompting. Student-initiated correction is acceptable.

Unsatisfactory (U): Procedural step was performed incorrectly, omitted, or performed in a way that compromised patient care.

Not applicable (N/A): Procedural step was not indicated or necessary.

Evaluation:

	Peer Evaluation Laboratory Setting			Instructor Evaluation Laboratory Setting			Instructor Evaluation Clinical Setting		
Procedural Preparation									
1. Reviews the patient's chart.	S ☐	U ☐	N/A ☐	S ☐	U ☐	N/A ☐	S ☐	U ☐	N/A ☐
2. Verifies the physician's order or the facility's protocol for standard of care.	S ☐	U ☐	N/A ☐	S ☐	U ☐	N/A ☐	S ☐	U ☐	N/A ☐
3. Obtains, cleans, and inspects the appropriate equipment prior to entering the patient's room.	S ☐	U ☐	N/A ☐	S ☐	U ☐	N/A ☐	S ☐	U ☐	N/A ☐
4. Follows PPE requirements, and observes standard precautions for any transmission-based isolation procedure.	S ☐	U ☐	N/A ☐	S ☐	U ☐	N/A ☐	S ☐	U ☐	N/A ☐
5. Identifies the patient using two patient identifiers.	S ☐	U ☐	N/A ☐	S ☐	U ☐	N/A ☐	S ☐	U ☐	N/A ☐
6. Introduces self to the patient and to the family.	S ☐	U ☐	N/A ☐	S ☐	U ☐	N/A ☐	S ☐	U ☐	N/A ☐
7. Explains the procedure to the patient and to the family, and acknowledges the patient's understanding.	S ☐	U ☐	N/A ☐	S ☐	U ☐	N/A ☐	S ☐	U ☐	N/A ☐
8. Performs proper hand hygiene, and puts on gloves, mask, and protective eyewear, as appropriate for the procedure.	S ☐	U ☐	N/A ☐	S ☐	U ☐	N/A ☐	S ☐	U ☐	N/A ☐
Implementation									
1. Places the patient in a comfortable position.	S ☐	U ☐	N/A ☐	S ☐	U ☐	N/A ☐	S ☐	U ☐	N/A ☐
2. Assesses vital signs.	S ☐	U ☐	N/A ☐	S ☐	U ☐	N/A ☐	S ☐	U ☐	N/A ☐
3. Ensures adequate lighting.	S ☐	U ☐	N/A ☐	S ☐	U ☐	N/A ☐	S ☐	U ☐	N/A ☐
4. Organizes the equipment at the bedside table.	S ☐	U ☐	N/A ☐	S ☐	U ☐	N/A ☐	S ☐	U ☐	N/A ☐
5. Prepares the infusion tube for the solution.	S ☐	U ☐	N/A ☐	S ☐	U ☐	N/A ☐	S ☐	U ☐	N/A ☐
6. Prepares a heparin or normal saline lock for infusion.	S ☐	U ☐	N/A ☐	S ☐	U ☐	N/A ☐	S ☐	U ☐	N/A ☐

Continued

	Peer Evaluation Laboratory Setting			Instructor Evaluation Laboratory Setting			Instructor Evaluation Clinical Setting		
7. Applies face shield and mask, if indicated.	S ☐	U ☐	N/A ☐	S ☐	U ☐	N/A ☐	S ☐	U ☐	N/A ☐
8. Identifies accessible vein, and applies tourniquet over the gown sleeve 3 to 4 inches above the selected insertion site.	S ☐	U ☐	N/A ☐	S ☐	U ☐	N/A ☐	S ☐	U ☐	N/A ☐
9. Selects an appropriate well-dilated vein for IV insertion.	S ☐	U ☐	N/A ☐	S ☐	U ☐	N/A ☐	S ☐	U ☐	N/A ☐
10. Cleanses the site with appropriate antiseptic in a circular pattern.	S ☐	U ☐	N/A ☐	S ☐	U ☐	N/A ☐	S ☐	U ☐	N/A ☐
11. Performs venipuncture.	S ☐	U ☐	N/A ☐	S ☐	U ☐	N/A ☐	S ☐	U ☐	N/A ☐
12. Observes the flash of blood, lowers the needle until almost flush with skin, and advances the catheter approximately one eighth to one quarter of an inch.	S ☐	U ☐	N/A ☐	S ☐	U ☐	N/A ☐	S ☐	U ☐	N/A ☐
13. Continues to hold skin taut, and advances the catheter until the hub rests at the insertion site; snaps back the needle or withdraws the needle by using the appropriate technique for specific ONC IV safety device.	S ☐	U ☐	N/A ☐	S ☐	U ☐	N/A ☐	S ☐	U ☐	N/A ☐
14. Stabilizes the catheter with one hand while removing the needle, and releases the tourniquet with the other hand.	S ☐	U ☐	N/A ☐	S ☐	U ☐	N/A ☐	S ☐	U ☐	N/A ☐
15. Connects the end of the infusion tube set of heparin or saline lock adapter to the end of catheter.	S ☐	U ☐	N/A ☐	S ☐	U ☐	N/A ☐	S ☐	U ☐	N/A ☐
16. Flushes the injection cap of the saline lock, if needed.	S ☐	U ☐	N/A ☐	S ☐	U ☐	N/A ☐	S ☐	U ☐	N/A ☐
17. Slides the clamp open slowly to begin infusion.	S ☐	U ☐	N/A ☐	S ☐	U ☐	N/A ☐	S ☐	U ☐	N/A ☐
18. Secures the catheter following the agency's protocol.	S ☐	U ☐	N/A ☐	S ☐	U ☐	N/A ☐	S ☐	U ☐	N/A ☐
19. Observes the site for any swelling or infiltration.	S ☐	U ☐	N/A ☐	S ☐	U ☐	N/A ☐	S ☐	U ☐	N/A ☐
20. Applies sterile dressing over the site.	S ☐	U ☐	N/A ☐	S ☐	U ☐	N/A ☐	S ☐	U ☐	N/A ☐
21. Secures the tube.	S ☐	U ☐	N/A ☐	S ☐	U ☐	N/A ☐	S ☐	U ☐	N/A ☐
22. Rechecks the IV line for flow, or sets to KVO ("keep vein open").	S ☐	U ☐	N/A ☐	S ☐	U ☐	N/A ☐	S ☐	U ☐	N/A ☐
23. Disposes of the sharps in the appropriate container.	S ☐	U ☐	N/A ☐	S ☐	U ☐	N/A ☐	S ☐	U ☐	N/A ☐
24. Removes the supplies from the patient's room, and cleans the area, as needed.	S ☐	U ☐	N/A ☐	S ☐	U ☐	N/A ☐	S ☐	U ☐	N/A ☐
25. Removes PPE, and performs proper hand hygiene prior to leaving the patient's room.	S ☐	U ☐	N/A ☐	S ☐	U ☐	N/A ☐	S ☐	U ☐	N/A ☐

Evaluation of Procedure

	Peer Evaluation Laboratory Setting			Instructor Evaluation Laboratory Setting			Instructor Evaluation Clinical Setting		
1. Advises the patient on how to move around with the IV line in place.	S ☐	U ☐	N/A ☐	S ☐	U ☐	N/A ☐	S ☐	U ☐	N/A ☐
2. Observes the patient's response to IV therapy.	S ☐	U ☐	N/A ☐	S ☐	U ☐	N/A ☐	S ☐	U ☐	N/A ☐
3. Identifies any unexpected outcomes.	S ☐	U ☐	N/A ☐	S ☐	U ☐	N/A ☐	S ☐	U ☐	N/A ☐

	Peer Evaluation Laboratory Setting	Instructor Evaluation Laboratory Setting	Instructor Evaluation Clinical Setting
Documentation and Reporting			
1. Records IV insertion and information about the infusion and the insertion site.	S ☐ U ☐ N/A ☐	S ☐ U ☐ N/A ☐	S ☐ U ☐ N/A ☐
2. Documents use of ultrasonography during IV line placement.	S ☐ U ☐ N/A ☐	S ☐ U ☐ N/A ☐	S ☐ U ☐ N/A ☐
3. Reports any abnormal findings to the appropriate health care provider.	S ☐ U ☐ N/A ☐	S ☐ U ☐ N/A ☐	S ☐ U ☐ N/A ☐

Comments:

_____

_____

_____

Signatures:

Student _____ Date Passed _____

Instructor (Laboratory Setting) _____ Date Passed _____

Student _____ Date Passed _____

Instructor (Clinical Setting) _____ Date Passed _____

Procedural Assessment 24-4

Student _____ Date _____

Instructor (Laboratory Setting) _____ Date _____

Instructor (Clinical Setting) _____ Date _____

Criteria for assessment success:

The student must obtain all **satisfactory (S)** scores to pass the procedural evaluation. Any **unsatisfactory (U)** scores will result in failure of the procedural assessment.

Scoring:

Satisfactory (S): Procedural step performed correctly with no instructor prompting. Student-initiated correction is acceptable.

Unsatisfactory (U): Procedural step was performed incorrectly, omitted, or performed in a way that compromised patient care.

Not applicable (N/A): Procedural step was not indicated or necessary.

Evaluation:

	Peer Evaluation Laboratory Setting	Instructor Evaluation Laboratory Setting	Instructor Evaluation Clinical Setting
Procedural Preparation			
1. Reviews the patient's chart.	S ☐ U ☐ N/A ☐	S ☐ U ☐ N/A ☐	S ☐ U ☐ N/A ☐
2. Verifies the physician's order or the facility's protocol for standard of care.	S ☐ U ☐ N/A ☐	S ☐ U ☐ N/A ☐	S ☐ U ☐ N/A ☐
3. Obtains, cleans, and inspects the appropriate equipment prior to entering the patient's room.	S ☐ U ☐ N/A ☐	S ☐ U ☐ N/A ☐	S ☐ U ☐ N/A ☐
4. Follows PPE requirements, and observes standard precautions for any transmission-based isolation procedure.	S ☐ U ☐ N/A ☐	S ☐ U ☐ N/A ☐	S ☐ U ☐ N/A ☐
5. Identifies the patient using two patient identifiers.	S ☐ U ☐ N/A ☐	S ☐ U ☐ N/A ☐	S ☐ U ☐ N/A ☐
6. Introduces self to the patient and to the family.	S ☐ U ☐ N/A ☐	S ☐ U ☐ N/A ☐	S ☐ U ☐ N/A ☐
7. Explains the procedure to the patient and to the family, and acknowledges the patient's understanding.	S ☐ U ☐ N/A ☐	S ☐ U ☐ N/A ☐	S ☐ U ☐ N/A ☐
8. Performs proper hand hygiene, and puts on gloves, mask, and protective eyewear, as appropriate for the procedure.	S ☐ U ☐ N/A ☐	S ☐ U ☐ N/A ☐	S ☐ U ☐ N/A ☐
Implementation			
1. Places the patient in a comfortable position.	S ☐ U ☐ N/A ☐	S ☐ U ☐ N/A ☐	S ☐ U ☐ N/A ☐
2. Turns the IV tubing roller clamp to the "off" position.	S ☐ U ☐ N/A ☐	S ☐ U ☐ N/A ☐	S ☐ U ☐ N/A ☐
3. Removes the IV site dressing carefully, and removes the tape securing the catheter gently.	S ☐ U ☐ N/A ☐	S ☐ U ☐ N/A ☐	S ☐ U ☐ N/A ☐
4. Cleanses the site with an appropriate antiseptic, and allows it to dry.	S ☐ U ☐ N/A ☐	S ☐ U ☐ N/A ☐	S ☐ U ☐ N/A ☐

Continued

	Peer Evaluation Laboratory Setting			Instructor Evaluation Laboratory Setting			Instructor Evaluation Clinical Setting		
5. Places sterile gauze over the site, and withdraws the catheter completely.	S ☐	U ☐	N/A ☐	S ☐	U ☐	N/A ☐	S ☐	U ☐	N/A ☐
6. Applies pressure to the site for 2 to 3 minutes, according to the patient's medical or medication history.	S ☐	U ☐	N/A ☐	S ☐	U ☐	N/A ☐	S ☐	U ☐	N/A ☐
7. Inspects the catheter for intactness and the tip for integrity.	S ☐	U ☐	N/A ☐	S ☐	U ☐	N/A ☐	S ☐	U ☐	N/A ☐
8. Applies a clean folded gauze dressing over the site, and secures it with tape.	S ☐	U ☐	N/A ☐	S ☐	U ☐	N/A ☐	S ☐	U ☐	N/A ☐
9. Discards the used IV catheter and IV supplies in the appropriate container.	S ☐	U ☐	N/A ☐	S ☐	U ☐	N/A ☐	S ☐	U ☐	N/A ☐
10. Removes the supplies from the patient's room, and cleans the area, as needed.	S ☐	U ☐	N/A ☐	S ☐	U ☐	N/A ☐	S ☐	U ☐	N/A ☐
11. Removes PPE, and performs proper hand hygiene prior to leaving the patient's room.	S ☐	U ☐	N/A ☐	S ☐	U ☐	N/A ☐	S ☐	U ☐	N/A ☐

Evaluation of Procedure

1. Observes the site for evidence of bleeding, redness, pain, drainage, or swelling.	S ☐	U ☐	N/A ☐	S ☐	U ☐	N/A ☐	S ☐	U ☐	N/A ☐
2. Identifies any unexpected outcomes.	S ☐	U ☐	N/A ☐	S ☐	U ☐	N/A ☐	S ☐	U ☐	N/A ☐

Documentation and Reporting

1. Records findings in the patient's chart.	S ☐	U ☐	N/A ☐	S ☐	U ☐	N/A ☐	S ☐	U ☐	N/A ☐
2. Reports any abnormal findings to the appropriate health care provider.	S ☐	U ☐	N/A ☐	S ☐	U ☐	N/A ☐	S ☐	U ☐	N/A ☐

Comments:

_____

_____

_____

Signatures:

Student _____ Date Passed _____

Instructor (Laboratory Setting) _____ Date Passed _____

Student _____ Date Passed _____

Instructor (Clinical Setting) _____ Date Passed _____

Student _____ Date _____

Instructor _____ Date _____

Location _____ Date _____

Criteria for assessment success:

The student must obtain all satisfactory (S) scores to pass the procedural evaluation. Any unsatisfactory (U) scores will result in failure of the procedural assessment.

Scoring:

Satisfactory (S): Procedural step performed correctly with no instructor prompting. Student-initiated correction is acceptable.

Unsatisfactory (U): Procedural step was performed incorrectly, omitted, or performed in a way that compromised patient care.

Not applicable (N/A): Procedural step was not indicated or necessary.

Evaluation:

	Peer Evaluation Laboratory Setting			Instructor Evaluation Laboratory Setting			Instructor Evaluation Clinical Setting		
Procedural Preparation									
1. Reviews the patient's chart.	S ☐	U ☐	N/A ☐	S ☐	U ☐	N/A ☐	S ☐	U ☐	N/A ☐
2. Verifies the physician's order or the facility's protocol for standard of care.	S ☐	U ☐	N/A ☐	S ☐	U ☐	N/A ☐	S ☐	U ☐	N/A ☐
3. Checks the chart for the presence of the consent form.	S ☐	U ☐	N/A ☐	S ☐	U ☐	N/A ☐	S ☐	U ☐	N/A ☐
4. Obtains, cleans, and inspects the appropriate equipment prior to entering the patient's room.	S ☐	U ☐	N/A ☐	S ☐	U ☐	N/A ☐	S ☐	U ☐	N/A ☐
5. Follows PPE requirements, and observes standard precautions for any transmission-based isolation procedure.	S ☐	U ☐	N/A ☐	S ☐	U ☐	N/A ☐	S ☐	U ☐	N/A ☐
6. Identifies the patient using two patient identifiers.	S ☐	U ☐	N/A ☐	S ☐	U ☐	N/A ☐	S ☐	U ☐	N/A ☐
7. Introduces self to the patient and to the family.	S ☐	U ☐	N/A ☐	S ☐	U ☐	N/A ☐	S ☐	U ☐	N/A ☐
8. Explains the procedure to the patient and to the family, and acknowledges the patient's understanding.	S ☐	U ☐	N/A ☐	S ☐	U ☐	N/A ☐	S ☐	U ☐	N/A ☐
9. Performs proper hand hygiene, and puts on gloves, mask, and protective eyewear, as appropriate for the procedure.	S ☐	U ☐	N/A ☐	S ☐	U ☐	N/A ☐	S ☐	U ☐	N/A ☐
Implementation									
1. Places the patient in a comfortable position.	S ☐	U ☐	N/A ☐	S ☐	U ☐	N/A ☐	S ☐	U ☐	N/A ☐
2. Assesses vital signs, and checks for pacers, filters, and tunneled catheters.	S ☐	U ☐	N/A ☐	S ☐	U ☐	N/A ☐	S ☐	U ☐	N/A ☐
3. Performs vein assessment, and chooses the site.	S ☐	U ☐	N/A ☐	S ☐	U ☐	N/A ☐	S ☐	U ☐	N/A ☐
4. Washes the insertion area with soap and water, and discards used supplies; removes gloves.	S ☐	U ☐	N/A ☐	S ☐	U ☐	N/A ☐	S ☐	U ☐	N/A ☐
5. Measures and makes note of the required catheter length.	S ☐	U ☐	N/A ☐	S ☐	U ☐	N/A ☐	S ☐	U ☐	N/A ☐

Continued

	Peer Evaluation Laboratory Setting			Instructor Evaluation Laboratory Setting			Instructor Evaluation Clinical Setting		
6. Positions a tourniquet high on the patient's arm, but does not constrict blood flow.	S ☐	U ☐	N/A ☐	S ☐	U ☐	N/A ☐	S ☐	U ☐	N/A ☐
7. Opens the PICC line insertion kit, and places it on sterile field.	S ☐	U ☐	N/A ☐	S ☐	U ☐	N/A ☐	S ☐	U ☐	N/A ☐
8. Applies sterile gown and gloves.	S ☐	U ☐	N/A ☐	S ☐	U ☐	N/A ☐	S ☐	U ☐	N/A ☐
9. Fills a 10-mL syringe with normal saline.	S ☐	U ☐	N/A ☐	S ☐	U ☐	N/A ☐	S ☐	U ☐	N/A ☐
10. Adds the injection port to the extension tube, and primes it with normal saline, leaving the syringe attached.	S ☐	U ☐	N/A ☐	S ☐	U ☐	N/A ☐	S ☐	U ☐	N/A ☐
11. Utilizes ultrasonography to identify the appropriate vessel.	S ☐	U ☐	N/A ☐	S ☐	U ☐	N/A ☐	S ☐	U ☐	N/A ☐
12. Prepares the site with 2% chlorhexidine.	S ☐	U ☐	N/A ☐	S ☐	U ☐	N/A ☐	S ☐	U ☐	N/A ☐
13. Removes and discards gloves.	S ☐	U ☐	N/A ☐	S ☐	U ☐	N/A ☐	S ☐	U ☐	N/A ☐
14. Applies the tourniquet.	S ☐	U ☐	N/A ☐	S ☐	U ☐	N/A ☐	S ☐	U ☐	N/A ☐
15. Applies a new pair of sterile gloves.	S ☐	U ☐	N/A ☐	S ☐	U ☐	N/A ☐	S ☐	U ☐	N/A ☐
16. Places the patient in a 15- to 25-degree Trendelenburg position (if not contraindicated).	S ☐	U ☐	N/A ☐	S ☐	U ☐	N/A ☐	S ☐	U ☐	N/A ☐
17. Places sterile drapes over the prepped area.	S ☐	U ☐	N/A ☐	S ☐	U ☐	N/A ☐	S ☐	U ☐	N/A ☐
18. Utilizes ultrasonography to identify landmarks, and administers local anesthesia.	S ☐	U ☐	N/A ☐	S ☐	U ☐	N/A ☐	S ☐	U ☐	N/A ☐
19. Advances the insertion needle into the vein.	S ☐	U ☐	N/A ☐	S ☐	U ☐	N/A ☐	S ☐	U ☐	N/A ☐
20. Performs the modified Seldinger technique.	S ☐	U ☐	N/A ☐	S ☐	U ☐	N/A ☐	S ☐	U ☐	N/A ☐
21. Releases the tourniquet, and instructs the patient to drop the chin to the chest.	S ☐	U ☐	N/A ☐	S ☐	U ☐	N/A ☐	S ☐	U ☐	N/A ☐
22. Advances the remainder of the catheter while monitoring the patient's heart rate and rhythm.	S ☐	U ☐	N/A ☐	S ☐	U ☐	N/A ☐	S ☐	U ☐	N/A ☐
23. Instructs the patient to turn the head away from the insertion site.	S ☐	U ☐	N/A ☐	S ☐	U ☐	N/A ☐	S ☐	U ☐	N/A ☐
24. Pulls the introducer from the insertion site, and removes it.	S ☐	U ☐	N/A ☐	S ☐	U ☐	N/A ☐	S ☐	U ☐	N/A ☐
25. Applies pressure cap, secures the line, and applies antimicrobial patch and dressing.	S ☐	U ☐	N/A ☐	S ☐	U ☐	N/A ☐	S ☐	U ☐	N/A ☐
26. Reassesses vital signs.	S ☐	U ☐	N/A ☐	S ☐	U ☐	N/A ☐	S ☐	U ☐	N/A ☐
27. Removes the supplies from the patient's room, and cleans the area, as needed.	S ☐	U ☐	N/A ☐	S ☐	U ☐	N/A ☐	S ☐	U ☐	N/A ☐
28. Removes PPE, and performs proper hand hygiene prior to leaving the patient's room.	S ☐	U ☐	N/A ☐	S ☐	U ☐	N/A ☐	S ☐	U ☐	N/A ☐

Evaluation of Procedure

	Peer Evaluation Laboratory Setting			Instructor Evaluation Laboratory Setting			Instructor Evaluation Clinical Setting		
1. Orders a postinsertion radiograph to confirm placement.	S ☐	U ☐	N/A ☐	S ☐	U ☐	N/A ☐	S ☐	U ☐	N/A ☐
2. Monitors the patient for complications.	S ☐	U ☐	N/A ☐	S ☐	U ☐	N/A ☐	S ☐	U ☐	N/A ☐
3. Identifies any unexpected outcomes.	S ☐	U ☐	N/A ☐	S ☐	U ☐	N/A ☐	S ☐	U ☐	N/A ☐

Documentation and Reporting

	Peer Evaluation Laboratory Setting			Instructor Evaluation Laboratory Setting			Instructor Evaluation Clinical Setting		
1. Records findings in the patient's chart.	S ☐	U ☐	N/A ☐	S ☐	U ☐	N/A ☐	S ☐	U ☐	N/A ☐
2. Reports any abnormal findings to the appropriate health care provider.	S ☐	U ☐	N/A ☐	S ☐	U ☐	N/A ☐	S ☐	U ☐	N/A ☐

Comments:

_____

_____

_____

Signatures:

Student _____   Date Passed _____

Instructor (Laboratory Setting) _____   Date Passed _____

Student _____   Date Passed _____

Instructor (Clinical Setting) _____   Date Passed _____

Comments:

_____

_____

_____

Signatures:

Student _____ Date Passed _____

Instructor (Laboratory Setting) _____ Date Passed _____

Student _____ Date Passed _____

Instructor (Clinical Setting) _____ Date Passed _____

Student _____ Date _____

Instructor (Laboratory Setting) _____ Date _____

Instructor (Clinical Setting) _____ Date _____

Criteria for assessment success:

The student must obtain all **satisfactory (S)** scores to pass the procedural evaluation. Any **unsatisfactory (U)** scores will result in failure of the procedural assessment.

Scoring:

Satisfactory (S): Procedural step performed correctly with no instructor prompting. Student-initiated correction is acceptable.

Unsatisfactory (U): Procedural step was performed incorrectly, omitted, or performed in a way that compromised patient care.

Not applicable (N/A): Procedural step was not indicated or necessary.

Evaluation:

	Peer Evaluation Laboratory Setting	Instructor Evaluation Laboratory Setting	Instructor Evaluation Clinical Setting
Procedural Preparation			
1. Reviews the patient's chart.	S ☐ U ☐ N/A ☐	S ☐ U ☐ N/A ☐	S ☐ U ☐ N/A ☐
2. Verifies the physician's order or the facility's protocol for standard of care.	S ☐ U ☐ N/A ☐	S ☐ U ☐ N/A ☐	S ☐ U ☐ N/A ☐
3. Obtains, cleans, and inspects the appropriate equipment prior to entering the patient's room.	S ☐ U ☐ N/A ☐	S ☐ U ☐ N/A ☐	S ☐ U ☐ N/A ☐
4. Follows PPE requirements, and observes standard precautions for any transmission-based isolation procedure.	S ☐ U ☐ N/A ☐	S ☐ U ☐ N/A ☐	S ☐ U ☐ N/A ☐
5. Identifies the patient using two patient identifiers.	S ☐ U ☐ N/A ☐	S ☐ U ☐ N/A ☐	S ☐ U ☐ N/A ☐
6. Introduces self to the patient and to the family.	S ☐ U ☐ N/A ☐	S ☐ U ☐ N/A ☐	S ☐ U ☐ N/A ☐
7. Explains the procedure to the patient and to the family, and acknowledges the patient's understanding.	S ☐ U ☐ N/A ☐	S ☐ U ☐ N/A ☐	S ☐ U ☐ N/A ☐
8. Performs proper hand hygiene, and puts on gloves, mask, and protective eyewear, as appropriate for the procedure.	S ☐ U ☐ N/A ☐	S ☐ U ☐ N/A ☐	S ☐ U ☐ N/A ☐
Implementation			
1. Places the patient in a comfortable position.	S ☐ U ☐ N/A ☐	S ☐ U ☐ N/A ☐	S ☐ U ☐ N/A ☐
2. Assesses vital signs.	S ☐ U ☐ N/A ☐	S ☐ U ☐ N/A ☐	S ☐ U ☐ N/A ☐
3. Assesses the patient for SBT readiness.	S ☐ U ☐ N/A ☐	S ☐ U ☐ N/A ☐	S ☐ U ☐ N/A ☐
4. Records the patient's baseline values.	S ☐ U ☐ N/A ☐	S ☐ U ☐ N/A ☐	S ☐ U ☐ N/A ☐
5. Advises the patient about when the SBT will commence.	S ☐ U ☐ N/A ☐	S ☐ U ☐ N/A ☐	S ☐ U ☐ N/A ☐
6. Changes the ventilator to the spontaneous mode with zero PSV and zero CPAP.	S ☐ U ☐ N/A ☐	S ☐ U ☐ N/A ☐	S ☐ U ☐ N/A ☐

Continued

	Peer Evaluation Laboratory Setting			Instructor Evaluation Laboratory Setting			Instructor Evaluation Clinical Setting		
7. Maintains the fractional inspired oxygen (FiO_2) that the patient is receiving on mechanical ventilation.	S ☐	U ☐	N/A ☐	S ☐	U ☐	N/A ☐	S ☐	U ☐	N/A ☐
8. Monitors and records the SBT start data.	S ☐	U ☐	N/A ☐	S ☐	U ☐	N/A ☐	S ☐	U ☐	N/A ☐
9. Considers extubation if the patient tolerated SBT for 30 to 120 minutes.	S ☐	U ☐	N/A ☐	S ☐	U ☐	N/A ☐	S ☐	U ☐	N/A ☐
10. Identifies SBT failing criteria and reestablishes previous ventilator settings.	S ☐	U ☐	N/A ☐	S ☐	U ☐	N/A ☐	S ☐	U ☐	N/A ☐
11. Reassesses vital signs at the end of the SBT.	S ☐	U ☐	N/A ☐	S ☐	U ☐	N/A ☐	S ☐	U ☐	N/A ☐
12. Removes the supplies from the patient's room, and cleans the area, as needed.	S ☐	U ☐	N/A ☐	S ☐	U ☐	N/A ☐	S ☐	U ☐	N/A ☐
13. Removes PPE, and performs proper hand hygiene prior to leaving the patient's room.	S ☐	U ☐	N/A ☐	S ☐	U ☐	N/A ☐	S ☐	U ☐	N/A ☐

Evaluation of Procedure

	Peer Evaluation Laboratory Setting			Instructor Evaluation Laboratory Setting			Instructor Evaluation Clinical Setting		
1. Establishes a baseline, or compares with previous SBT attempts.	S ☐	U ☐	N/A ☐	S ☐	U ☐	N/A ☐	S ☐	U ☐	N/A ☐
2. Develops an appropriate respiratory care plan based on SBT data.	S ☐	U ☐	N/A ☐	S ☐	U ☐	N/A ☐	S ☐	U ☐	N/A ☐
3. Repeats the SBT over multiple days, as needed or per protocol.	S ☐	U ☐	N/A ☐	S ☐	U ☐	N/A ☐	S ☐	U ☐	N/A ☐
4. Identifies any unexpected outcomes.	S ☐	U ☐	N/A ☐	S ☐	U ☐	N/A ☐	S ☐	U ☐	N/A ☐

Documentation and Reporting

	Peer Evaluation Laboratory Setting			Instructor Evaluation Laboratory Setting			Instructor Evaluation Clinical Setting		
1. Records findings in the patient's chart.	S ☐	U ☐	N/A ☐	S ☐	U ☐	N/A ☐	S ☐	U ☐	N/A ☐
2. Notifies the physician of SBT results.	S ☐	U ☐	N/A ☐	S ☐	U ☐	N/A ☐	S ☐	U ☐	N/A ☐
3. Reports any abnormal findings to the appropriate health care provider.	S ☐	U ☐	N/A ☐	S ☐	U ☐	N/A ☐	S ☐	U ☐	N/A ☐

Comments:

_____

_____

_____

Signatures:

Student _____ Date Passed _____

Instructor (Laboratory Setting) _____ Date Passed _____

Student _____ Date Passed _____

Instructor (Clinical Setting) _____ Date Passed _____

Procedural Assessment 25-2   Weaning process

Student _____ Date _____

Instructor (Laboratory Setting) _____ Date _____

Instructor (Clinical Setting) _____ Date _____

Criteria for assessment success:

The student must obtain all **satisfactory (S)** scores to pass the procedural evaluation. Any **unsatisfactory (U)** scores will result in failure of the procedural assessment.

Scoring:

Satisfactory (S): Procedural step performed correctly with no instructor prompting. Student-initiated correction is acceptable.

Unsatisfactory (U): Procedural step was performed incorrectly, omitted, or performed in a way that compromised patient care.

Not applicable (N/A): Procedural step was not indicated or necessary.

Evaluation:

	Peer Evaluation Laboratory Setting	Instructor Evaluation Laboratory Setting	Instructor Evaluation Clinical Setting
Procedural Preparation			
1. Reviews the patient's chart.	S ☐ U ☐ N/A ☐	S ☐ U ☐ N/A ☐	S ☐ U ☐ N/A ☐
2. Verifies the physician's order or the facility's protocol for standard of care.	S ☐ U ☐ N/A ☐	S ☐ U ☐ N/A ☐	S ☐ U ☐ N/A ☐
3. Obtains, cleans, and inspects the appropriate equipment prior to entering the patient's room.	S ☐ U ☐ N/A ☐	S ☐ U ☐ N/A ☐	S ☐ U ☐ N/A ☐
4. Follows PPE requirements, and observes standard precautions for any transmission-based isolation procedure.	S ☐ U ☐ N/A ☐	S ☐ U ☐ N/A ☐	S ☐ U ☐ N/A ☐
5. Identifies the patient using two patient identifiers.	S ☐ U ☐ N/A ☐	S ☐ U ☐ N/A ☐	S ☐ U ☐ N/A ☐
6. Introduces self to the patient and to the family.	S ☐ U ☐ N/A ☐	S ☐ U ☐ N/A ☐	S ☐ U ☐ N/A ☐
7. Explains the procedure to the patient and to the family, and acknowledges the patient's understanding.	S ☐ U ☐ N/A ☐	S ☐ U ☐ N/A ☐	S ☐ U ☐ N/A ☐
8. Performs proper hand hygiene, and puts on gloves, mask, and protective eyewear, as appropriate for the procedure.	S ☐ U ☐ N/A ☐	S ☐ U ☐ N/A ☐	S ☐ U ☐ N/A ☐
Implementation			
1. Places the patient in a comfortable position.	S ☐ U ☐ N/A ☐	S ☐ U ☐ N/A ☐	S ☐ U ☐ N/A ☐
2. Assesses vital signs.	S ☐ U ☐ N/A ☐	S ☐ U ☐ N/A ☐	S ☐ U ☐ N/A ☐
3. Informs the patient that he or she will feel different from how it was when on full support and to breathe normally.	S ☐ U ☐ N/A ☐	S ☐ U ☐ N/A ☐	S ☐ U ☐ N/A ☐

Continued

	Peer Evaluation Laboratory Setting	Instructor Evaluation Laboratory Setting	Instructor Evaluation Clinical Setting
4. Determines the weaning process mode:			
a. Gradually lengthening SBTs via the mechanical ventilator or with a T-piece alternating with mechanical ventilatory support.	S ☐ U ☐ N/A ☐	S ☐ U ☐ N/A ☐	S ☐ U ☐ N/A ☐
b. Pressure support method.	S ☐ U ☐ N/A ☐	S ☐ U ☐ N/A ☐	S ☐ U ☐ N/A ☐
c. SIMV method.	S ☐ U ☐ N/A ☐	S ☐ U ☐ N/A ☐	S ☐ U ☐ N/A ☐
5. Monitors patient data.	S ☐ U ☐ N/A ☐	S ☐ U ☐ N/A ☐	S ☐ U ☐ N/A ☐
6. Places the patient back on stable, nonfatiguing ventilator settings.	S ☐ U ☐ N/A ☐	S ☐ U ☐ N/A ☐	S ☐ U ☐ N/A ☐
7. Performs a patient–ventilator system assessment following the weaning process.	S ☐ U ☐ N/A ☐	S ☐ U ☐ N/A ☐	S ☐ U ☐ N/A ☐
8. Removes the supplies from the patient's room, and cleans the area, as needed.	S ☐ U ☐ N/A ☐	S ☐ U ☐ N/A ☐	S ☐ U ☐ N/A ☐
9. Removes PPE, and performs proper hand hygiene prior to leaving the patient's room.	S ☐ U ☐ N/A ☐	S ☐ U ☐ N/A ☐	S ☐ U ☐ N/A ☐

Evaluation of Procedure

1. Establishes a baseline, or compares with previous weaning attempts.	S ☐ U ☐ N/A ☐	S ☐ U ☐ N/A ☐	S ☐ U ☐ N/A ☐
2. Develops an appropriate respiratory care plan based on assessment data.	S ☐ U ☐ N/A ☐	S ☐ U ☐ N/A ☐	S ☐ U ☐ N/A ☐
3. Identifies any unexpected outcomes.	S ☐ U ☐ N/A ☐	S ☐ U ☐ N/A ☐	S ☐ U ☐ N/A ☐

Documentation and Reporting

1. Records the procedure in the patient's chart.	S ☐ U ☐ N/A ☐	S ☐ U ☐ N/A ☐	S ☐ U ☐ N/A ☐
2. Notifies the physician of weaning results.	S ☐ U ☐ N/A ☐	S ☐ U ☐ N/A ☐	S ☐ U ☐ N/A ☐
3. Reports any abnormal findings to the appropriate health care provider.	S ☐ U ☐ N/A ☐	S ☐ U ☐ N/A ☐	S ☐ U ☐ N/A ☐

Comments:

_____

_____

_____

Signatures:

Student _____ Date Passed _____

Instructor (Laboratory Setting) _____ Date Passed _____

Student _____ Date Passed _____

Instructor (Clinical Setting) _____ Date Passed _____

Procedural Assessment 25-3   Terminal weaning

Student _____ Date _____

Instructor (Laboratory Setting) _____ Date _____

Instructor (Clinical Setting) _____ Date _____

Criteria for assessment success:

The student must obtain all **satisfactory (S)** scores to pass the procedural evaluation. Any **unsatisfactory (U)** scores will result in failure of the procedural assessment.

Scoring:

Satisfactory (S): Procedural step performed correctly with no instructor prompting. Student-initiated correction is acceptable.

Unsatisfactory (U): Procedural step was performed incorrectly, omitted, or performed in a way that compromised patient care.

Not applicable (N/A): Procedural step was not indicated or necessary.

Evaluation:

	Peer Evaluation Laboratory Setting	Instructor Evaluation Laboratory Setting	Instructor Evaluation Clinical Setting
Procedural Preparation			
1. Reviews the patient's chart.	S ☐ U ☐ N/A ☐	S ☐ U ☐ N/A ☐	S ☐ U ☐ N/A ☐
2. Verifies the physician's order or the facility's protocol for standard of care.	S ☐ U ☐ N/A ☐	S ☐ U ☐ N/A ☐	S ☐ U ☐ N/A ☐
3. Obtains, cleans, and inspects the appropriate equipment prior to entering the patient's room.	S ☐ U ☐ N/A ☐	S ☐ U ☐ N/A ☐	S ☐ U ☐ N/A ☐
4. Follows PPE requirements, and observes standard precautions for any transmission-based isolation procedure.	S ☐ U ☐ N/A ☐	S ☐ U ☐ N/A ☐	S ☐ U ☐ N/A ☐
5. Identifies the patient using two patient identifiers.	S ☐ U ☐ N/A ☐	S ☐ U ☐ N/A ☐	S ☐ U ☐ N/A ☐
6. Introduces self to the patient and to the family.	S ☐ U ☐ N/A ☐	S ☐ U ☐ N/A ☐	S ☐ U ☐ N/A ☐
7. Explains the procedure to the patient and to the family, and acknowledges the patient's understanding.	S ☐ U ☐ N/A ☐	S ☐ U ☐ N/A ☐	S ☐ U ☐ N/A ☐
8. Performs proper hand hygiene, and puts on gloves, mask, and protective eyewear, as appropriate for the procedure.	S ☐ U ☐ N/A ☐	S ☐ U ☐ N/A ☐	S ☐ U ☐ N/A ☐
Implementation			
1. Places the patient in a comfortable position.	S ☐ U ☐ N/A ☐	S ☐ U ☐ N/A ☐	S ☐ U ☐ N/A ☐
2. Assesses vital signs.	S ☐ U ☐ N/A ☐	S ☐ U ☐ N/A ☐	S ☐ U ☐ N/A ☐
3. Ensures that all key health care team members are present.	S ☐ U ☐ N/A ☐	S ☐ U ☐ N/A ☐	S ☐ U ☐ N/A ☐
4. Ensures that all key family members are present.	S ☐ U ☐ N/A ☐	S ☐ U ☐ N/A ☐	S ☐ U ☐ N/A ☐
5. Prepares the patient and the family for what to expect.	S ☐ U ☐ N/A ☐	S ☐ U ☐ N/A ☐	S ☐ U ☐ N/A ☐
6. Silences all ventilator alarms.	S ☐ U ☐ N/A ☐	S ☐ U ☐ N/A ☐	S ☐ U ☐ N/A ☐

Continued

	Peer Evaluation Laboratory Setting			Instructor Evaluation Laboratory Setting			Instructor Evaluation Clinical Setting		
7. Withdraws ventilatory support.	S ☐	U ☐	N/A ☐	S ☐	U ☐	N/A ☐	S ☐	U ☐	N/A ☐
8. Provides oxygen therapy, as ordered or per protocol.	S ☐	U ☐	N/A ☐	S ☐	U ☐	N/A ☐	S ☐	U ☐	N/A ☐
9. Reassesses vital signs only as necessary to ensure patient comfort.	S ☐	U ☐	N/A ☐	S ☐	U ☐	N/A ☐	S ☐	U ☐	N/A ☐
10. Provides time for the patient and the family to be alone, if indicated.	S ☐	U ☐	N/A ☐	S ☐	U ☐	N/A ☐	S ☐	U ☐	N/A ☐
11. Removes the supplies from the patient's room, and cleans the area, as needed.	S ☐	U ☐	N/A ☐	S ☐	U ☐	N/A ☐	S ☐	U ☐	N/A ☐
12. Removes PPE, and performs proper hand hygiene prior to leaving the patient's room.	S ☐	U ☐	N/A ☐	S ☐	U ☐	N/A ☐	S ☐	U ☐	N/A ☐

Evaluation of Procedure

	Peer Evaluation Laboratory Setting			Instructor Evaluation Laboratory Setting			Instructor Evaluation Clinical Setting		
1. Notes any use of oxygen therapy.	S ☐	U ☐	N/A ☐	S ☐	U ☐	N/A ☐	S ☐	U ☐	N/A ☐
2. Identifies any unexpected outcomes.	S ☐	U ☐	N/A ☐	S ☐	U ☐	N/A ☐	S ☐	U ☐	N/A ☐
3. Ensures patient comfort.	S ☐	U ☐	N/A ☐	S ☐	U ☐	N/A ☐	S ☐	U ☐	N/A ☐

Documentation and Reporting

	Peer Evaluation Laboratory Setting			Instructor Evaluation Laboratory Setting			Instructor Evaluation Clinical Setting		
1. Records findings in the patient's chart.	S ☐	U ☐	N/A ☐	S ☐	U ☐	N/A ☐	S ☐	U ☐	N/A ☐
2. Reports any abnormal findings to the appropriate health care provider.	S ☐	U ☐	N/A ☐	S ☐	U ☐	N/A ☐	S ☐	U ☐	N/A ☐

Comments:

_____

_____

_____

Signatures:

Student _____   Date Passed _____

Instructor (Laboratory Setting) _____   Date Passed _____

Student _____   Date Passed _____

Instructor (Clinical Setting) _____   Date Passed _____

Procedural Assessment 26-1

Student _____ Date _____

Instructor (Laboratory Setting) _____ Date _____

Instructor (Clinical Setting) _____ Date _____

Criteria for assessment success:

The student must obtain all **satisfactory (S)** scores to pass the procedural evaluation. Any **unsatisfactory (U)** scores will result in failure of the procedural assessment.

Scoring:

Satisfactory (S): Procedural step performed correctly with no instructor prompting. Student-initiated correction is acceptable.

Unsatisfactory (U): Procedural step was performed incorrectly, omitted, or performed in a way that compromised patient care.

Not applicable (N/A): Procedural step was not indicated or necessary.

Evaluation:

	Peer Evaluation Laboratory Setting	Instructor Evaluation Laboratory Setting	Instructor Evaluation Clinical Setting
Procedural Preparation			
1. Reviews the patient's chart.	S ☐ U ☐ N/A ☐	S ☐ U ☐ N/A ☐	S ☐ U ☐ N/A ☐
2. Verifies the physician's order or the facility's protocol for standard of care.	S ☐ U ☐ N/A ☐	S ☐ U ☐ N/A ☐	S ☐ U ☐ N/A ☐
3. Obtains, cleans, and inspects the appropriate equipment prior to entering the patient's room.	S ☐ U ☐ N/A ☐	S ☐ U ☐ N/A ☐	S ☐ U ☐ N/A ☐
4. Follows PPE requirements, and observes standard precautions for any transmission-based isolation procedure.	S ☐ U ☐ N/A ☐	S ☐ U ☐ N/A ☐	S ☐ U ☐ N/A ☐
5. Identifies the patient using two patient identifiers.	S ☐ U ☐ N/A ☐	S ☐ U ☐ N/A ☐	S ☐ U ☐ N/A ☐
6. Introduces self to the patient and to the family.	S ☐ U ☐ N/A ☐	S ☐ U ☐ N/A ☐	S ☐ U ☐ N/A ☐
7. Explains the procedure to the patient and to the family, and acknowledges the patient's understanding.	S ☐ U ☐ N/A ☐	S ☐ U ☐ N/A ☐	S ☐ U ☐ N/A ☐
8. Performs proper hand hygiene, and puts on gloves, mask, and protective eyewear, as appropriate for the procedure.	S ☐ U ☐ N/A ☐	S ☐ U ☐ N/A ☐	S ☐ U ☐ N/A ☐
Implementation			
1. Places the patient in a comfortable position.	S ☐ U ☐ N/A ☐	S ☐ U ☐ N/A ☐	S ☐ U ☐ N/A ☐
2. Assesses vital signs.	S ☐ U ☐ N/A ☐	S ☐ U ☐ N/A ☐	S ☐ U ☐ N/A ☐
3. Assesses the upper airway for abnormalities.	S ☐ U ☐ N/A ☐	S ☐ U ☐ N/A ☐	S ☐ U ☐ N/A ☐
4. Obtains the interface and securing devices.	S ☐ U ☐ N/A ☐	S ☐ U ☐ N/A ☐	S ☐ U ☐ N/A ☐

Continued

	Peer Evaluation Laboratory Setting			Instructor Evaluation Laboratory Setting			Instructor Evaluation Clinical Setting		
5. Establishes and implements the appropriate settings, or executes the physician's orders:									
a. CPAP level	S ☐	U ☐	N/A ☐	S ☐	U ☐	N/A ☐	S ☐	U ☐	N/A ☐
b. IPAP and EPAP levels (if ordered)	S ☐	U ☐	N/A ☐	S ☐	U ☐	N/A ☐	S ☐	U ☐	N/A ☐
c. Rate (If ordered)	S ☐	U ☐	N/A ☐	S ☐	U ☐	N/A ☐	S ☐	U ☐	N/A ☐
d. FiO_2	S ☐	U ☐	N/A ☐	S ☐	U ☐	N/A ☐	S ☐	U ☐	N/A ☐
6. Applies and secures the device to the patient.	S ☐	U ☐	N/A ☐	S ☐	U ☐	N/A ☐	S ☐	U ☐	N/A ☐
7. Ensures suitable fit and minimal leak.	S ☐	U ☐	N/A ☐	S ☐	U ☐	N/A ☐	S ☐	U ☐	N/A ☐
8. Ensures patient comfort.	S ☐	U ☐	N/A ☐	S ☐	U ☐	N/A ☐	S ☐	U ☐	N/A ☐
9. Reassesses vital signs.	S ☐	U ☐	N/A ☐	S ☐	U ☐	N/A ☐	S ☐	U ☐	N/A ☐
10. Sets the alarms appropriately.	S ☐	U ☐	N/A ☐	S ☐	U ☐	N/A ☐	S ☐	U ☐	N/A ☐
11. Sets up the noninvasive monitors.	S ☐	U ☐	N/A ☐	S ☐	U ☐	N/A ☐	S ☐	U ☐	N/A ☐
12. Removes the supplies from the patient's room, and cleans the area, as needed.	S ☐	U ☐	N/A ☐	S ☐	U ☐	N/A ☐	S ☐	U ☐	N/A ☐
13. Removes PPE, and performs proper hand hygiene prior to leaving the patient's room.	S ☐	U ☐	N/A ☐	S ☐	U ☐	N/A ☐	S ☐	U ☐	N/A ☐

Evaluation of Procedure

	Peer Evaluation Laboratory Setting			Instructor Evaluation Laboratory Setting			Instructor Evaluation Clinical Setting		
1. Establishes a baseline, or compares with previous measurements.	S ☐	U ☐	N/A ☐	S ☐	U ☐	N/A ☐	S ☐	U ☐	N/A ☐
2. Develops an appropriate respiratory care plan based on assessment data.	S ☐	U ☐	N/A ☐	S ☐	U ☐	N/A ☐	S ☐	U ☐	N/A ☐
3. Identifies any unexpected outcomes.	S ☐	U ☐	N/A ☐	S ☐	U ☐	N/A ☐	S ☐	U ☐	N/A ☐

Documentation and Reporting

	Peer Evaluation Laboratory Setting			Instructor Evaluation Laboratory Setting			Instructor Evaluation Clinical Setting		
1. Records findings in the patient's chart.	S ☐	U ☐	N/A ☐	S ☐	U ☐	N/A ☐	S ☐	U ☐	N/A ☐
2. Reports any abnormal findings to the appropriate health care provider.	S ☐	U ☐	N/A ☐	S ☐	U ☐	N/A ☐	S ☐	U ☐	N/A ☐

Comments:

_____

_____

_____

Signatures:

Student _____ Date Passed _____

Instructor (Laboratory Setting) _____ Date Passed _____

Student _____ Date Passed _____

Instructor (Clinical Setting) _____ Date Passed _____

Student _____ Date _____

Instructor _____ Date _____

Location _____ Date _____

Criteria for assessment success:

The student must obtain all **satisfactory (S)** scores to pass the procedural evaluation. Any **unsatisfactory (U)** scores will result in failure of the procedural assessment.

Scoring:

Satisfactory (S): Procedural step performed correctly with no instructor prompting. Student-initiated correction is acceptable.

Unsatisfactory (U): Procedural step was performed incorrectly, omitted, or performed in a way that compromised patient care.

Not applicable (N/A): Procedural step was not indicated or necessary.

Evaluation:

	Peer Evaluation Laboratory Setting	Instructor Evaluation Laboratory Setting	Instructor Evaluation Clinical Setting
Procedural Preparation			
1. Reviews the patient's chart for the patient's current vital signs and NIV settings.	S ☐ U ☐ N/A ☐	S ☐ U ☐ N/A ☐	S ☐ U ☐ N/A ☐
2. Reviews the patient's most recent blood gas or SpO$_2$ values.	S ☐ U ☐ N/A ☐	S ☐ U ☐ N/A ☐	S ☐ U ☐ N/A ☐
3. Reviews the most recent chest radiograph.	S ☐ U ☐ N/A ☐	S ☐ U ☐ N/A ☐	S ☐ U ☐ N/A ☐
4. Identifies the current sedation medications.	S ☐ U ☐ N/A ☐	S ☐ U ☐ N/A ☐	S ☐ U ☐ N/A ☐
5. Verifies the physician's order or the facility's protocol for standard of care.	S ☐ U ☐ N/A ☐	S ☐ U ☐ N/A ☐	S ☐ U ☐ N/A ☐
6. Obtains, cleans, and inspects the appropriate equipment prior to entering the patient's room.	S ☐ U ☐ N/A ☐	S ☐ U ☐ N/A ☐	S ☐ U ☐ N/A ☐
7. Follows PPE requirements, and observes standard precautions for any transmission-based isolation procedure.	S ☐ U ☐ N/A ☐	S ☐ U ☐ N/A ☐	S ☐ U ☐ N/A ☐
8. Identifies the patient using two patient identifiers.	S ☐ U ☐ N/A ☐	S ☐ U ☐ N/A ☐	S ☐ U ☐ N/A ☐
9. Introduces self to the patient and to the family.	S ☐ U ☐ N/A ☐	S ☐ U ☐ N/A ☐	S ☐ U ☐ N/A ☐
10. Explains the procedure to the patient and to the family, and acknowledges the patient's understanding.	S ☐ U ☐ N/A ☐	S ☐ U ☐ N/A ☐	S ☐ U ☐ N/A ☐
11. Performs proper hand hygiene, and puts on gloves, mask, and protective eyewear, as appropriate for the procedure.	S ☐ U ☐ N/A ☐	S ☐ U ☐ N/A ☐	S ☐ U ☐ N/A ☐
Implementation			
1. Approaches the patient before approaching the CPAP generator.	S ☐ U ☐ N/A ☐	S ☐ U ☐ N/A ☐	S ☐ U ☐ N/A ☐
2. Assesses the patient.	S ☐ U ☐ N/A ☐	S ☐ U ☐ N/A ☐	S ☐ U ☐ N/A ☐
3. Assesses NIV generator function and settings.	S ☐ U ☐ N/A ☐	S ☐ U ☐ N/A ☐	S ☐ U ☐ N/A ☐

Continued

	Peer Evaluation Laboratory Setting			Instructor Evaluation Laboratory Setting			Instructor Evaluation Clinical Setting		
4. Ensures that the manual ventilation device and the suction equipment are available at the patient's bedside.	S ☐	U ☐	N/A ☐	S ☐	U ☐	N/A ☐	S ☐	U ☐	N/A ☐
5. Removes the supplies from the patient's room, and cleans the area, as needed.	S ☐	U ☐	N/A ☐	S ☐	U ☐	N/A ☐	S ☐	U ☐	N/A ☐
6. Removes PPE, and performs proper hand hygiene prior to leaving the patient's room.	S ☐	U ☐	N/A ☐	S ☐	U ☐	N/A ☐	S ☐	U ☐	N/A ☐

Evaluation of Procedure

1. Establishes a baseline, or compares with previous measurements.	S ☐	U ☐	N/A ☐	S ☐	U ☐	N/A ☐	S ☐	U ☐	N/A ☐
2. Develops an appropriate respiratory care plan based on assessment data.	S ☐	U ☐	N/A ☐	S ☐	U ☐	N/A ☐	S ☐	U ☐	N/A ☐
3. Identifies any unexpected outcomes.	S ☐	U ☐	N/A ☐	S ☐	U ☐	N/A ☐	S ☐	U ☐	N/A ☐

Documentation and Reporting

1. Records findings in the patient's chart.	S ☐	U ☐	N/A ☐	S ☐	U ☐	N/A ☐	S ☐	U ☐	N/A ☐
2. Reports any abnormal findings to the appropriate health care provider.	S ☐	U ☐	N/A ☐	S ☐	U ☐	N/A ☐	S ☐	U ☐	N/A ☐

Comments:

_____

_____

_____

Signatures:

Student _____ Date Passed _____

Instructor _____ Date Passed _____

Student _____ Date _____

Instructor (Laboratory Setting) _____ Date _____

Instructor (Clinical Setting) _____ Date _____

Criteria for assessment success:

The student must obtain all **satisfactory (S)** scores to pass the procedural evaluation. Any **unsatisfactory (U)** scores will result in failure of the procedural assessment.

Scoring:

Satisfactory (S): Procedural step performed correctly with no instructor prompting. Student-initiated correction is acceptable.

Unsatisfactory (U): Procedural step was performed incorrectly, omitted, or performed in a way that compromised patient care.

Not applicable (N/A): Procedural step was not indicated or necessary.

Evaluation:

	Peer Evaluation Laboratory Setting	Instructor Evaluation Laboratory Setting	Instructor Evaluation Clinical Setting
Procedural Preparation			
1. Reviews the patient's chart.	S ☐ U ☐ N/A ☐	S ☐ U ☐ N/A ☐	S ☐ U ☐ N/A ☐
2. Verifies the physician's order or the facility's protocol for standard of care.	S ☐ U ☐ N/A ☐	S ☐ U ☐ N/A ☐	S ☐ U ☐ N/A ☐
3. Obtains, cleans, and inspects the appropriate equipment prior to entering the patient's room.	S ☐ U ☐ N/A ☐	S ☐ U ☐ N/A ☐	S ☐ U ☐ N/A ☐
4. Follows PPE requirements, and observes standard precautions for any transmission-based isolation procedure.	S ☐ U ☐ N/A ☐	S ☐ U ☐ N/A ☐	S ☐ U ☐ N/A ☐
5. Identifies the patient using two patient identifiers.	S ☐ U ☐ N/A ☐	S ☐ U ☐ N/A ☐	S ☐ U ☐ N/A ☐
6. Introduces self to the patient and to the family.	S ☐ U ☐ N/A ☐	S ☐ U ☐ N/A ☐	S ☐ U ☐ N/A ☐
7. Explains the procedure to the patient and to the family, and acknowledges the patient's understanding.	S ☐ U ☐ N/A ☐	S ☐ U ☐ N/A ☐	S ☐ U ☐ N/A ☐
8. Performs proper hand hygiene, and puts on gloves, mask, and protective eyewear, as appropriate for the procedure.	S ☐ U ☐ N/A ☐	S ☐ U ☐ N/A ☐	S ☐ U ☐ N/A ☐
Implementation			
1. Places the patient in a comfortable position.	S ☐ U ☐ N/A ☐	S ☐ U ☐ N/A ☐	S ☐ U ☐ N/A ☐
2. Assesses vital signs.	S ☐ U ☐ N/A ☐	S ☐ U ☐ N/A ☐	S ☐ U ☐ N/A ☐
3. Establishes an airway: a. Ensures, or consults on, the proper tube size for the procedure.	S ☐ U ☐ N/A ☐	S ☐ U ☐ N/A ☐	S ☐ U ☐ N/A ☐
b. Ensures proper depth of tube placement.	S ☐ U ☐ N/A ☐	S ☐ U ☐ N/A ☐	S ☐ U ☐ N/A ☐
c. Assists or performs the tube securing procedure.	S ☐ U ☐ N/A ☐	S ☐ U ☐ N/A ☐	S ☐ U ☐ N/A ☐

Continued

	Peer Evaluation Laboratory Setting			Instructor Evaluation Laboratory Setting			Instructor Evaluation Clinical Setting		
4. Establishes and implements the appropriate settings, or executes the physician's orders:									
a. Mode	S ☐	U ☐	N/A ☐	S ☐	U ☐	N/A ☐	S ☐	U ☐	N/A ☐
b. Tidal volume or inspiratory pressure	S ☐	U ☐	N/A ☐	S ☐	U ☐	N/A ☐	S ☐	U ☐	N/A ☐
c. Frequency	S ☐	U ☐	N/A ☐	S ☐	U ☐	N/A ☐	S ☐	U ☐	N/A ☐
d. Inspiratory time	S ☐	U ☐	N/A ☐	S ☐	U ☐	N/A ☐	S ☐	U ☐	N/A ☐
e. Inspiratory rise time	S ☐	U ☐	N/A ☐	S ☐	U ☐	N/A ☐	S ☐	U ☐	N/A ☐
f. Flow pattern	S ☐	U ☐	N/A ☐	S ☐	U ☐	N/A ☐	S ☐	U ☐	N/A ☐
g. PEEP level	S ☐	U ☐	N/A ☐	S ☐	U ☐	N/A ☐	S ☐	U ☐	N/A ☐
h. FiO_2	S ☐	U ☐	N/A ☐	S ☐	U ☐	N/A ☐	S ☐	U ☐	N/A ☐
i. Pressure support	S ☐	U ☐	N/A ☐	S ☐	U ☐	N/A ☐	S ☐	U ☐	N/A ☐
j. Inspiratory cycle off % or ventilator-specific equivalent	S ☐	U ☐	N/A ☐	S ☐	U ☐	N/A ☐	S ☐	U ☐	N/A ☐
k. Trigger	S ☐	U ☐	N/A ☐	S ☐	U ☐	N/A ☐	S ☐	U ☐	N/A ☐
5. Reassesses vital signs.	S ☐	U ☐	N/A ☐	S ☐	U ☐	N/A ☐	S ☐	U ☐	N/A ☐
6. Sets the alarms appropriately.	S ☐	U ☐	N/A ☐	S ☐	U ☐	N/A ☐	S ☐	U ☐	N/A ☐
7. Removes the supplies from the patient's room, and cleans the area, as needed.	S ☐	U ☐	N/A ☐	S ☐	U ☐	N/A ☐	S ☐	U ☐	N/A ☐
8. Removes PPE, and performs proper hand hygiene prior to leaving the patient's room.	S ☐	U ☐	N/A ☐	S ☐	U ☐	N/A ☐	S ☐	U ☐	N/A ☐

Evaluation of Procedure

1. Establishes a baseline, or compares with previous measurements.	S ☐	U ☐	N/A ☐	S ☐	U ☐	N/A ☐	S ☐	U ☐	N/A ☐
2. Develops an appropriate respiratory care plan based on assessment data.	S ☐	U ☐	N/A ☐	S ☐	U ☐	N/A ☐	S ☐	U ☐	N/A ☐
3. Identifies any unexpected outcomes.	S ☐	U ☐	N/A ☐	S ☐	U ☐	N/A ☐	S ☐	U ☐	N/A ☐

Documentation and Reporting

1. Records findings in the patient's chart.	S ☐	U ☐	N/A ☐	S ☐	U ☐	N/A ☐	S ☐	U ☐	N/A ☐
2. Reports any abnormal findings to the appropriate health care provider.	S ☐	U ☐	N/A ☐	S ☐	U ☐	N/A ☐	S ☐	U ☐	N/A ☐

Comments:

_____

_____

_____

_____

Signatures:

Student _____ Date Passed _____

Instructor (Laboratory Setting) _____ Date Passed _____

Student _____ Date Passed _____

Instructor (Clinical Setting) _____ Date Passed _____

Procedural Assessment 26-4

Student _____ Date _____

Instructor _____ Date _____

Location _____ Date _____

Criteria for assessment success:

The student must obtain all **satisfactory (S)** scores to pass the procedural evaluation. Any **unsatisfactory (U)** scores will result in failure of the procedural assessment.

Scoring:

Satisfactory (S): Procedural step performed correctly with no instructor prompting. Student-initiated correction is acceptable.

Unsatisfactory (U): Procedural step was performed incorrectly, omitted, or performed in a way that compromised patient care.

Not applicable (N/A): Procedural step was not indicated or necessary.

Evaluation:

	Peer Evaluation Laboratory Setting	Instructor Evaluation Laboratory Setting	Instructor Evaluation Clinical Setting
Procedural Preparation			
1. Reviews the patient chart for the patient's current vital signs and ventilator settings.	S ☐ U ☐ N/A ☐	S ☐ U ☐ N/A ☐	S ☐ U ☐ N/A ☐
2. Reviews the patient's most recent ABG or SpO$_2$ values.	S ☐ U ☐ N/A ☐	S ☐ U ☐ N/A ☐	S ☐ U ☐ N/A ☐
3. Reviews the patient's most recent chest radiograph.	S ☐ U ☐ N/A ☐	S ☐ U ☐ N/A ☐	S ☐ U ☐ N/A ☐
4. Identifies the current sedation medications.	S ☐ U ☐ N/A ☐	S ☐ U ☐ N/A ☐	S ☐ U ☐ N/A ☐
5. Verifies the physician's order or the facility's protocol for standard of care.	S ☐ U ☐ N/A ☐	S ☐ U ☐ N/A ☐	S ☐ U ☐ N/A ☐
6. Obtains, cleans, and inspects the appropriate equipment prior to entering the patient's room.	S ☐ U ☐ N/A ☐	S ☐ U ☐ N/A ☐	S ☐ U ☐ N/A ☐
7. Follows PPE requirements, and observes standard precautions for any transmission-based isolation procedure.	S ☐ U ☐ N/A ☐	S ☐ U ☐ N/A ☐	S ☐ U ☐ N/A ☐
8. Identifies the patient using two patient identifiers.	S ☐ U ☐ N/A ☐	S ☐ U ☐ N/A ☐	S ☐ U ☐ N/A ☐
9. Introduces self to the patient and to the family.	S ☐ U ☐ N/A ☐	S ☐ U ☐ N/A ☐	S ☐ U ☐ N/A ☐
10. Explains the procedure to the patient and to the family, and acknowledges the patient's understanding.	S ☐ U ☐ N/A ☐	S ☐ U ☐ N/A ☐	S ☐ U ☐ N/A ☐
11. Performs proper hand hygiene, and puts on gloves, mask, and protective eyewear, as appropriate for the procedure.	S ☐ U ☐ N/A ☐	S ☐ U ☐ N/A ☐	S ☐ U ☐ N/A ☐
Implementation			
1. Approaches and assesses the patient before assessing ventilator functions and settings.	S ☐ U ☐ N/A ☐	S ☐ U ☐ N/A ☐	S ☐ U ☐ N/A ☐
2. Assesses the patient.	S ☐ U ☐ N/A ☐	S ☐ U ☐ N/A ☐	S ☐ U ☐ N/A ☐
3. Assesses the ventilator function and settings.	S ☐ U ☐ N/A ☐	S ☐ U ☐ N/A ☐	S ☐ U ☐ N/A ☐

Continued

	Peer Evaluation Laboratory Setting			Instructor Evaluation Laboratory Setting			Instructor Evaluation Clinical Setting		
4. Ensures that the manual ventilation device and the suction equipment are available at the patient's bedside.	S ☐	U ☐	N/A ☐	S ☐	U ☐	N/A ☐	S ☐	U ☐	N/A ☐
5. Ensures that replacement tracheostomy tubes are available at the patient's bedside.	S ☐	U ☐	N/A ☐	S ☐	U ☐	N/A ☐	S ☐	U ☐	N/A ☐
6. Removes the supplies from the patient's room, and cleans the area, as needed.	S ☐	U ☐	N/A ☐	S ☐	U ☐	N/A ☐	S ☐	U ☐	N/A ☐
7. Removes PPE, and performs proper hand hygiene prior to leaving the patient's room.	S ☐	U ☐	N/A ☐	S ☐	U ☐	N/A ☐	S ☐	U ☐	N/A ☐

Evaluation of Procedure

	Peer Evaluation Laboratory Setting			Instructor Evaluation Laboratory Setting			Instructor Evaluation Clinical Setting		
1. Establishes a baseline, or compares with previous measurements.	S ☐	U ☐	N/A ☐	S ☐	U ☐	N/A ☐	S ☐	U ☐	N/A ☐
2. Develops an appropriate respiratory care plan based on assessment data.	S ☐	U ☐	N/A ☐	S ☐	U ☐	N/A ☐	S ☐	U ☐	N/A ☐
3. Ensures that lung protective therapy is in place.	S ☐	U ☐	N/A ☐	S ☐	U ☐	N/A ☐	S ☐	U ☐	N/A ☐
4. Considers discontinuation of mechanical ventilation or weaning.	S ☐	U ☐	N/A ☐	S ☐	U ☐	N/A ☐	S ☐	U ☐	N/A ☐
5. Identifies any unexpected outcomes.	S ☐	U ☐	N/A ☐	S ☐	U ☐	N/A ☐	S ☐	U ☐	N/A ☐

Documentation and Reporting

	Peer Evaluation Laboratory Setting			Instructor Evaluation Laboratory Setting			Instructor Evaluation Clinical Setting		
1. Records findings in the patient's chart.	S ☐	U ☐	N/A ☐	S ☐	U ☐	N/A ☐	S ☐	U ☐	N/A ☐
2. Reports any abnormal findings to the appropriate health care provider.	S ☐	U ☐	N/A ☐	S ☐	U ☐	N/A ☐	S ☐	U ☐	N/A ☐

Comments:

_____

_____

_____

Signatures:

Student _____ Date Passed _____

Instructor _____ Date Passed _____

Procedural Assessment 26-5

Initiating high-frequency ventilation

Student _____ Date _____

Instructor (Laboratory Setting) _____ Date _____

Instructor (Clinical Setting) _____ Date _____

Criteria for assessment success:

The student must obtain all **satisfactory (S)** scores to pass the procedural evaluation. Any **unsatisfactory (U)** scores will result in failure of the procedural assessment.

Scoring:

Satisfactory (S): Procedural step performed correctly with no instructor prompting. Student-initiated correction is acceptable.

Unsatisfactory (U): Procedural step was performed incorrectly, omitted, or performed in a way that compromised patient care.

Not applicable (N/A): Procedural step was not indicated or necessary.

Evaluation:

	Peer Evaluation Laboratory Setting	Instructor Evaluation Laboratory Setting	Instructor Evaluation Clinical Setting
Procedural Preparation			
1. Reviews the patient's chart.	S ☐ U ☐ N/A ☐	S ☐ U ☐ N/A ☐	S ☐ U ☐ N/A ☐
2. Verifies the physician's order or the facility's protocol for standard of care.	S ☐ U ☐ N/A ☐	S ☐ U ☐ N/A ☐	S ☐ U ☐ N/A ☐
3. Obtains, cleans, and inspects the appropriate equipment prior to entering the patient's room.	S ☐ U ☐ N/A ☐	S ☐ U ☐ N/A ☐	S ☐ U ☐ N/A ☐
4. Follows PPE requirements, and observes standard precautions for any transmission-based isolation procedure.	S ☐ U ☐ N/A ☐	S ☐ U ☐ N/A ☐	S ☐ U ☐ N/A ☐
5. Identifies the patient using two patient identifiers.	S ☐ U ☐ N/A ☐	S ☐ U ☐ N/A ☐	S ☐ U ☐ N/A ☐
6. Introduces self to the patient and to the family.	S ☐ U ☐ N/A ☐	S ☐ U ☐ N/A ☐	S ☐ U ☐ N/A ☐
7. Explains the procedure to the patient and to the family, and acknowledges the patient's understanding.	S ☐ U ☐ N/A ☐	S ☐ U ☐ N/A ☐	S ☐ U ☐ N/A ☐
8. Performs proper hand hygiene, and puts on gloves, mask, and protective eyewear, as appropriate for the procedure.	S ☐ U ☐ N/A ☐	S ☐ U ☐ N/A ☐	S ☐ U ☐ N/A ☐
Implementation			
1. Positions the patient.	S ☐ U ☐ N/A ☐	S ☐ U ☐ N/A ☐	S ☐ U ☐ N/A ☐
2. Assesses baseline data: ventilatory, oxygenation and circulatory status.	S ☐ U ☐ N/A ☐	S ☐ U ☐ N/A ☐	S ☐ U ☐ N/A ☐
3. Ensures patency of the endotracheal tube.	S ☐ U ☐ N/A ☐	S ☐ U ☐ N/A ☐	S ☐ U ☐ N/A ☐
4. Suctions the patient, if needed.	S ☐ U ☐ N/A ☐	S ☐ U ☐ N/A ☐	S ☐ U ☐ N/A ☐
5. Performs a recruitment maneuver of 35 to 40 cmH$_2$O for 30 to 40 seconds.	S ☐ U ☐ N/A ☐	S ☐ U ☐ N/A ☐	S ☐ U ☐ N/A ☐

Continued

	Peer Evaluation Laboratory Setting	Instructor Evaluation Laboratory Setting	Instructor Evaluation Clinical Setting
6. Establishes and implements the appropriate settings, or executes the physician's orders:			
For oscillation:			
a. Mean airway pressure	S ☐ U ☐ N/A ☐	S ☐ U ☐ N/A ☐	S ☐ U ☐ N/A ☐
b. Frequency	S ☐ U ☐ N/A ☐	S ☐ U ☐ N/A ☐	S ☐ U ☐ N/A ☐
c. Fractional inspired oxygen (FiO_2)	S ☐ U ☐ N/A ☐	S ☐ U ☐ N/A ☐	S ☐ U ☐ N/A ☐
d. Amplitude ΔP	S ☐ U ☐ N/A ☐	S ☐ U ☐ N/A ☐	S ☐ U ☐ N/A ☐
e. Inspiratory time %	S ☐ U ☐ N/A ☐	S ☐ U ☐ N/A ☐	S ☐ U ☐ N/A ☐
f. Bias flow	S ☐ U ☐ N/A ☐	S ☐ U ☐ N/A ☐	S ☐ U ☐ N/A ☐
For jet ventilation:			
a. MAP and PEEP	S ☐ U ☐ N/A ☐	S ☐ U ☐ N/A ☐	S ☐ U ☐ N/A ☐
b. Rate of jet ventilator	S ☐ U ☐ N/A ☐	S ☐ U ☐ N/A ☐	S ☐ U ☐ N/A ☐
c. HFV on-time	S ☐ U ☐ N/A ☐	S ☐ U ☐ N/A ☐	S ☐ U ☐ N/A ☐
d. HFV PIP	S ☐ U ☐ N/A ☐	S ☐ U ☐ N/A ☐	S ☐ U ☐ N/A ☐
e. Rate of conventional ventilator	S ☐ U ☐ N/A ☐	S ☐ U ☐ N/A ☐	S ☐ U ☐ N/A ☐
f. Settings for conventional mechanical ventilator breaths	S ☐ U ☐ N/A ☐	S ☐ U ☐ N/A ☐	S ☐ U ☐ N/A ☐
g. FiO_2	S ☐ U ☐ N/A ☐	S ☐ U ☐ N/A ☐	S ☐ U ☐ N/A ☐
h. Servo pressure and MAP	S ☐ U ☐ N/A ☐	S ☐ U ☐ N/A ☐	S ☐ U ☐ N/A ☐
7. Reassesses vital signs.	S ☐ U ☐ N/A ☐	S ☐ U ☐ N/A ☐	S ☐ U ☐ N/A ☐
8. Sets the alarms appropriately.	S ☐ U ☐ N/A ☐	S ☐ U ☐ N/A ☐	S ☐ U ☐ N/A ☐
9. Removes the supplies from the patient's room, and cleans the area, as needed.	S ☐ U ☐ N/A ☐	S ☐ U ☐ N/A ☐	S ☐ U ☐ N/A ☐
10. Removes PPE, and performs proper hand hygiene prior to leaving the patient's room.	S ☐ U ☐ N/A ☐	S ☐ U ☐ N/A ☐	S ☐ U ☐ N/A ☐

Evaluation of Procedure

1. Establishes a baseline, or compares with previous measurements.	S ☐ U ☐ N/A ☐	S ☐ U ☐ N/A ☐	S ☐ U ☐ N/A ☐
2. Develops an appropriate respiratory care plan based on assessment data.	S ☐ U ☐ N/A ☐	S ☐ U ☐ N/A ☐	S ☐ U ☐ N/A ☐
3. Considers adding inhaled pulmonary vasodilator therapy.	S ☐ U ☐ N/A ☐	S ☐ U ☐ N/A ☐	S ☐ U ☐ N/A ☐
4. Identifies any unexpected outcomes.	S ☐ U ☐ N/A ☐	S ☐ U ☐ N/A ☐	S ☐ U ☐ N/A ☐

Documentation and Reporting

1. Records findings in the patient's chart.	S ☐ U ☐ N/A ☐	S ☐ U ☐ N/A ☐	S ☐ U ☐ N/A ☐
2. Reports any abnormal findings to the appropriate health care provider.	S ☐ U ☐ N/A ☐	S ☐ U ☐ N/A ☐	S ☐ U ☐ N/A ☐

Comments:

_____

_____

_____

Signatures:

Student _____ Date Passed _____

Instructor (Laboratory Setting) _____ Date Passed _____

Student _____ Date Passed _____

Instructor (Clinical Setting) _____ Date Passed _____

Student _____ Date _____

Instructor _____ Date _____

Location _____ Date _____

Criteria for assessment success:

The student must obtain all satisfactory (S) scores to pass the procedural evaluation. Any unsatisfactory (U) scores will result in failure of the procedural assessment.

Scoring:

Satisfactory (S): Procedural step performed correctly with no instructor prompting. Student-initiated correction is acceptable.

Unsatisfactory (U): Procedural step was performed incorrectly, omitted, or performed in a way that compromised patient care.

Not applicable (N/A): Procedural step was not indicated or necessary.

Evaluation:

	Peer Evaluation Laboratory Setting	Instructor Evaluation Laboratory Setting	Instructor Evaluation Clinical Setting
Procedural Preparation			
1. Reviews the patient's chart.	S ☐ U ☐ N/A ☐	S ☐ U ☐ N/A ☐	S ☐ U ☐ N/A ☐
2. Verifies the physician's order or the facility's protocol for standard of care.	S ☐ U ☐ N/A ☐	S ☐ U ☐ N/A ☐	S ☐ U ☐ N/A ☐
3. Obtains, cleans, and inspects the appropriate equipment.	S ☐ U ☐ N/A ☐	S ☐ U ☐ N/A ☐	S ☐ U ☐ N/A ☐
4. Follows PPE requirements, and observes standard precautions for any transmission-based isolation procedure.	S ☐ U ☐ N/A ☐	S ☐ U ☐ N/A ☐	S ☐ U ☐ N/A ☐
5. Identifies the patient using two patient identifiers.	S ☐ U ☐ N/A ☐	S ☐ U ☐ N/A ☐	S ☐ U ☐ N/A ☐
6. Introduces self to the patient and to the family.	S ☐ U ☐ N/A ☐	S ☐ U ☐ N/A ☐	S ☐ U ☐ N/A ☐
7. Explains the procedure to the patient and to the family, and acknowledges the patient's understanding.	S ☐ U ☐ N/A ☐	S ☐ U ☐ N/A ☐	S ☐ U ☐ N/A ☐
8. Performs proper hand hygiene, and puts on gloves.	S ☐ U ☐ N/A ☐	S ☐ U ☐ N/A ☐	S ☐ U ☐ N/A ☐
9. Confirms that the patient is wearing comfortable clothing and appropriate shoes for walking.	S ☐ U ☐ N/A ☐	S ☐ U ☐ N/A ☐	S ☐ U ☐ N/A ☐
10. Advises the patient to use the usual walking aids during the test.	S ☐ U ☐ N/A ☐	S ☐ U ☐ N/A ☐	S ☐ U ☐ N/A ☐
11. Confirms that the patient has not exercised vigorously within 2 hours of beginning the test.	S ☐ U ☐ N/A ☐	S ☐ U ☐ N/A ☐	S ☐ U ☐ N/A ☐
12. Ensures that the patient has sat at rest in a chair located near the starting position for at least 10 minutes prior to the test.	S ☐ U ☐ N/A ☐	S ☐ U ☐ N/A ☐	S ☐ U ☐ N/A ☐
Implementation			
1. Places the patient in a comfortable position, and instructs him or her to breathe normally.	S ☐ U ☐ N/A ☐	S ☐ U ☐ N/A ☐	S ☐ U ☐ N/A ☐
2. Applies the pulse oximeter on the patient's finger, and uses a carry strap for the device.	S ☐ U ☐ N/A ☐	S ☐ U ☐ N/A ☐	S ☐ U ☐ N/A ☐

Continued

	Peer Evaluation Laboratory Setting			Instructor Evaluation Laboratory Setting			Instructor Evaluation Clinical Setting		
3. Adjusts the pulse oximeter to "continuously read."	S ☐	U ☐	N/A ☐	S ☐	U ☐	N/A ☐	S ☐	U ☐	N/A ☐
4. Prepares the clipboard with the documentation.	S ☐	U ☐	N/A ☐	S ☐	U ☐	N/A ☐	S ☐	U ☐	N/A ☐
5. Assesses 0 minute stats.	S ☐	U ☐	N/A ☐	S ☐	U ☐	N/A ☐	S ☐	U ☐	N/A ☐
6. Sets the timer to 6 minutes.	S ☐	U ☐	N/A ☐	S ☐	U ☐	N/A ☐	S ☐	U ☐	N/A ☐
7. Places the cone at the starting point, and readies a cone to mark where the patient ends the test.	S ☐	U ☐	N/A ☐	S ☐	U ☐	N/A ☐	S ☐	U ☐	N/A ☐
8. Shows and explains the Borg scale and pain level scale to the patient before the test.	S ☐	U ☐	N/A ☐	S ☐	U ☐	N/A ☐	S ☐	U ☐	N/A ☐
9. Explains the objective of the test to the patient.	S ☐	U ☐	N/A ☐	S ☐	U ☐	N/A ☐	S ☐	U ☐	N/A ☐
10. Demonstrates the test by walking one lap of the track or a premeasured distance for the patient.	S ☐	U ☐	N/A ☐	S ☐	U ☐	N/A ☐	S ☐	U ☐	N/A ☐
11. Instructs the patient on how to perform the test, and explains that he or she will.	S ☐	U ☐	N/A ☐	S ☐	U ☐	N/A ☐	S ☐	U ☐	N/A ☐
12. Instructs the patient to begin the test.	S ☐	U ☐	N/A ☐	S ☐	U ☐	N/A ☐	S ☐	U ☐	N/A ☐
13. Updates the patient after the first minute and every minute thereafter.	S ☐	U ☐	N/A ☐	S ☐	U ☐	N/A ☐	S ☐	U ☐	N/A ☐
14. Assesses the 3-minute stats.	S ☐	U ☐	N/A ☐	S ☐	U ☐	N/A ☐	S ☐	U ☐	N/A ☐
15. Instructs the patient to sit in the chair and assesses the 6-minute stats.	S ☐	U ☐	N/A ☐	S ☐	U ☐	N/A ☐	S ☐	U ☐	N/A ☐
16. Removes the supplies from the patient's room, and cleans the area, as needed.	S ☐	U ☐	N/A ☐	S ☐	U ☐	N/A ☐	S ☐	U ☐	N/A ☐
17. Removes PPE, and performs proper hand hygiene.	S ☐	U ☐	N/A ☐	S ☐	U ☐	N/A ☐	S ☐	U ☐	N/A ☐

Evaluation of Procedure

1. Establishes a baseline, and compares with 0-, 3-, and 6-minute measurements.	S ☐	U ☐	N/A ☐	S ☐	U ☐	N/A ☐	S ☐	U ☐	N/A ☐
2. Develops an appropriate respiratory care plan based on assessment data.	S ☐	U ☐	N/A ☐	S ☐	U ☐	N/A ☐	S ☐	U ☐	N/A ☐
3. Identifies any unexpected outcomes.	S ☐	U ☐	N/A ☐	S ☐	U ☐	N/A ☐	S ☐	U ☐	N/A ☐
4. Trends the test over several pulmonary rehab sessions.	S ☐	U ☐	N/A ☐	S ☐	U ☐	N/A ☐	S ☐	U ☐	N/A ☐

Documentation and Reporting

1. Records findings in the patient's chart.	S ☐	U ☐	N/A ☐	S ☐	U ☐	N/A ☐	S ☐	U ☐	N/A ☐
2. Records the number of laps the patient completed.	S ☐	U ☐	N/A ☐	S ☐	U ☐	N/A ☐	S ☐	U ☐	N/A ☐
3. Reports any abnormal findings to the appropriate health care provider.	S ☐	U ☐	N/A ☐	S ☐	U ☐	N/A ☐	S ☐	U ☐	N/A ☐

Comments:

_____

_____

_____

Signatures:

Student _____   Date Passed _____

Instructor _____   Date Passed _____

Procedural Assessment 27-2

Student _____ Date _____

Instructor (Laboratory Setting) _____ Date _____

Instructor (Clinical Setting) _____ Date _____

Criteria for assessment success:

The student must obtain all **satisfactory (S)** scores to pass the procedural evaluation. Any **unsatisfactory (U)** scores will result in failure of the procedural assessment.

Scoring:

Satisfactory (S): Procedural step performed correctly with no instructor prompting. Student-initiated correction is acceptable.

Unsatisfactory (U): Procedural step was performed incorrectly, omitted, or performed in a way that compromised patient care.

Not applicable (N/A): Procedural step was not indicated or necessary.

Evaluation:

	Peer Evaluation Laboratory Setting	Instructor Evaluation Laboratory Setting	Instructor Evaluation Clinical Setting
Procedural Preparation			
1. Reviews the patient's chart.	S ☐ U ☐ N/A ☐	S ☐ U ☐ N/A ☐	S ☐ U ☐ N/A ☐
2. Verifies the physician's order or the facility's protocol for standard of care.	S ☐ U ☐ N/A ☐	S ☐ U ☐ N/A ☐	S ☐ U ☐ N/A ☐
3. Follows PPE requirements, and observes standard precautions for any transmission-based isolation procedure.	S ☐ U ☐ N/A ☐	S ☐ U ☐ N/A ☐	S ☐ U ☐ N/A ☐
4. Identifies the patient using two patient identifiers.	S ☐ U ☐ N/A ☐	S ☐ U ☐ N/A ☐	S ☐ U ☐ N/A ☐
5. Introduces self to the patient and to the family.	S ☐ U ☐ N/A ☐	S ☐ U ☐ N/A ☐	S ☐ U ☐ N/A ☐
6. Explains the procedure to the patient and to the family, and acknowledges the patient's understanding.	S ☐ U ☐ N/A ☐	S ☐ U ☐ N/A ☐	S ☐ U ☐ N/A ☐
7. Performs proper hand hygiene, and puts on gloves, mask, and protective eyewear, as appropriate for the procedure.	S ☐ U ☐ N/A ☐	S ☐ U ☐ N/A ☐	S ☐ U ☐ N/A ☐
Implementation			
1. Places the patient in a comfortable position, and instructs him or her to breathe normally.	S ☐ U ☐ N/A ☐	S ☐ U ☐ N/A ☐	S ☐ U ☐ N/A ☐
2. Assesses vital signs.	S ☐ U ☐ N/A ☐	S ☐ U ☐ N/A ☐	S ☐ U ☐ N/A ☐
3. Instructs the patient to close the mouth and inhale slowly and deeply through the nose.	S ☐ U ☐ N/A ☐	S ☐ U ☐ N/A ☐	S ☐ U ☐ N/A ☐
4. Instructs the patient to exhale though pursed lips, as in whistling.	S ☐ U ☐ N/A ☐	S ☐ U ☐ N/A ☐	S ☐ U ☐ N/A ☐
5. Instructs the patient to prolong the exhalation to twice the length of inspiration.	S ☐ U ☐ N/A ☐	S ☐ U ☐ N/A ☐	S ☐ U ☐ N/A ☐

Continued

	Peer Evaluation Laboratory Setting			Instructor Evaluation Laboratory Setting			Instructor Evaluation Clinical Setting		
6. Instructs the patient to practice PLB during an activity.	S ☐	U ☐	N/A ☐	S ☐	U ☐	N/A ☐	S ☐	U ☐	N/A ☐
7. Instructs the patient to practice exhaling during the most strenuous part of a task.	S ☐	U ☐	N/A ☐	S ☐	U ☐	N/A ☐	S ☐	U ☐	N/A ☐
8. Removes PPE, and performs proper hand hygiene.	S ☐	U ☐	N/A ☐	S ☐	U ☐	N/A ☐	S ☐	U ☐	N/A ☐

Evaluation of Procedure

1. Develops an appropriate respiratory care plan based on assessment data.	S ☐	U ☐	N/A ☐	S ☐	U ☐	N/A ☐	S ☐	U ☐	N/A ☐
2. Notes any use of oxygen therapy.	S ☐	U ☐	N/A ☐	S ☐	U ☐	N/A ☐	S ☐	U ☐	N/A ☐
3. Evaluates the patient's ability to demonstrate the procedure.	S ☐	U ☐	N/A ☐	S ☐	U ☐	N/A ☐	S ☐	U ☐	N/A ☐
4. Identifies any unexpected outcomes.	S ☐	U ☐	N/A ☐	S ☐	U ☐	N/A ☐	S ☐	U ☐	N/A ☐

Documentation and Reporting

1. Records findings in the patient's chart.	S ☐	U ☐	N/A ☐	S ☐	U ☐	N/A ☐	S ☐	U ☐	N/A ☐
2. Reports any abnormal findings to the appropriate health care provider.	S ☐	U ☐	N/A ☐	S ☐	U ☐	N/A ☐	S ☐	U ☐	N/A ☐

Comments:

_____

_____

_____

Signatures:

Student _____ Date Passed _____

Instructor (Laboratory Setting) _____ Date Passed _____

Student _____ Date Passed _____

Instructor (Clinical Setting) _____ Date Passed _____

Student _____ Date _____

Instructor (Laboratory Setting) _____ Date _____

Instructor (Clinical Setting) _____ Date _____

Criteria for assessment success:

The student must obtain all **satisfactory (S)** scores to pass the procedural evaluation. Any **unsatisfactory (U)** scores will result in failure of the procedural assessment.

Scoring:

Satisfactory (S): Procedural step performed correctly with no instructor prompting. Student-initiated correction is acceptable.

Unsatisfactory (U): Procedural step was performed incorrectly, omitted, or performed in a way that compromised patient care.

Not applicable (N/A): Procedural step was not indicated or necessary.

Evaluation:

	Peer Evaluation Laboratory Setting	Instructor Evaluation Laboratory Setting	Instructor Evaluation Clinical Setting
Procedural Preparation			
1. Reviews the patient's chart.	S ☐ U ☐ N/A ☐	S ☐ U ☐ N/A ☐	S ☐ U ☐ N/A ☐
2. Verifies the physician's order or the facility's protocol for standard of care.	S ☐ U ☐ N/A ☐	S ☐ U ☐ N/A ☐	S ☐ U ☐ N/A ☐
3. Follows PPE requirements, and observes standard precautions for any transmission-based isolation procedure.	S ☐ U ☐ N/A ☐	S ☐ U ☐ N/A ☐	S ☐ U ☐ N/A ☐
4. Identifies the patient using two patient identifiers.	S ☐ U ☐ N/A ☐	S ☐ U ☐ N/A ☐	S ☐ U ☐ N/A ☐
5. Introduces self to the patient and to the family.	S ☐ U ☐ N/A ☐	S ☐ U ☐ N/A ☐	S ☐ U ☐ N/A ☐
6. Explains the procedure to the patient and to the family, and acknowledges the patient's understanding.	S ☐ U ☐ N/A ☐	S ☐ U ☐ N/A ☐	S ☐ U ☐ N/A ☐
7. Performs proper hand hygiene, and puts on gloves, mask, and protective eyewear, as appropriate for the procedure.	S ☐ U ☐ N/A ☐	S ☐ U ☐ N/A ☐	S ☐ U ☐ N/A ☐
Implementation			
1. Places the patient in a comfortable position, and instructs him or her to breathe normally.	S ☐ U ☐ N/A ☐	S ☐ U ☐ N/A ☐	S ☐ U ☐ N/A ☐
2. Assesses vital signs, and obtains a baseline pulse oximetry reading.	S ☐ U ☐ N/A ☐	S ☐ U ☐ N/A ☐	S ☐ U ☐ N/A ☐
3. Instructs the patient to place one hand on the abdomen just below the rib cage and the other hand on the chest.	S ☐ U ☐ N/A ☐	S ☐ U ☐ N/A ☐	S ☐ U ☐ N/A ☐
4. Instructs the patient to observe the rise and fall of the abdominal wall during inspiration and expiration.	S ☐ U ☐ N/A ☐	S ☐ U ☐ N/A ☐	S ☐ U ☐ N/A ☐
5. Explains the relationship between the abdominal wall and the diaphragm.	S ☐ U ☐ N/A ☐	S ☐ U ☐ N/A ☐	S ☐ U ☐ N/A ☐

Continued

	Peer Evaluation Laboratory Setting			Instructor Evaluation Laboratory Setting			Instructor Evaluation Clinical Setting		
6. Instructs the patient to perform diaphragmatic breathing in conjunction with pursed-lip breathing.	S ☐	U ☐	N/A ☐	S ☐	U ☐	N/A ☐	S ☐	U ☐	N/A ☐
7. Coaches the patient to keep the upper chest movement to the minimum.	S ☐	U ☐	N/A ☐	S ☐	U ☐	N/A ☐	S ☐	U ☐	N/A ☐
8. If diaphragmatic movement is not satisfactory, gently pushes in on the patient's abdomen during exhalation to get the desired response.	S ☐	U ☐	N/A ☐	S ☐	U ☐	N/A ☐	S ☐	U ☐	N/A ☐
9. Removes PPE, and performs proper hand hygiene.	S ☐	U ☐	N/A ☐	S ☐	U ☐	N/A ☐	S ☐	U ☐	N/A ☐

Evaluation of Procedure

1. Develops an appropriate respiratory care plan based on assessment data.	S ☐	U ☐	N/A ☐	S ☐	U ☐	N/A ☐	S ☐	U ☐	N/A ☐
2. Notes any use of oxygen therapy.	S ☐	U ☐	N/A ☐	S ☐	U ☐	N/A ☐	S ☐	U ☐	N/A ☐
3. Identifies any unexpected outcomes.	S ☐	U ☐	N/A ☐	S ☐	U ☐	N/A ☐	S ☐	U ☐	N/A ☐
4. Corrects any paradoxical movement.	S ☐	U ☐	N/A ☐	S ☐	U ☐	N/A ☐	S ☐	U ☐	N/A ☐

Documentation and Reporting

1. Records findings in the patient's chart.	S ☐	U ☐	N/A ☐	S ☐	U ☐	N/A ☐	S ☐	U ☐	N/A ☐
2. Reports any abnormal findings to the appropriate health care provider.	S ☐	U ☐	N/A ☐	S ☐	U ☐	N/A ☐	S ☐	U ☐	N/A ☐

Comments:

_____

_____

_____

Signatures:

Student _____ Date Passed _____

Instructor (Laboratory Setting) _____ Date Passed _____

Student _____ Date Passed _____

Instructor (Clinical Setting) _____ Date Passed _____

Student _____ Date _____

Instructor (Laboratory Setting) _____ Date _____

Instructor (Clinical Setting) _____ Date _____

Criteria for assessment success:

The student must obtain all **satisfactory (S)** scores to pass the procedural evaluation. Any **unsatisfactory (U)** scores will result in failure of the procedural assessment.

Scoring:

Satisfactory (S): Procedural step performed correctly with no instructor prompting. Student-initiated correction is acceptable.

Unsatisfactory (U): Procedural step was performed incorrectly, omitted, or performed in a way that compromised patient care.

Not applicable (N/A): Procedural step was not indicated or necessary.

Evaluation:

	Peer Evaluation Laboratory Setting	Instructor Evaluation Laboratory Setting	Instructor Evaluation Clinical Setting
Procedural Preparation			
1. Reviews the patient's chart.	S ☐ U ☐ N/A ☐	S ☐ U ☐ N/A ☐	S ☐ U ☐ N/A ☐
2. Verifies the physician's order or the facility's protocol for standard of care.	S ☐ U ☐ N/A ☐	S ☐ U ☐ N/A ☐	S ☐ U ☐ N/A ☐
3. Obtains, cleans, and inspects the appropriate equipment.	S ☐ U ☐ N/A ☐	S ☐ U ☐ N/A ☐	S ☐ U ☐ N/A ☐
4. Follows PPE requirements, and observes standard precautions for any transmission-based isolation procedure.	S ☐ U ☐ N/A ☐	S ☐ U ☐ N/A ☐	S ☐ U ☐ N/A ☐
5. Identifies the patient using two patient identifiers.	S ☐ U ☐ N/A ☐	S ☐ U ☐ N/A ☐	S ☐ U ☐ N/A ☐
6. Introduces self to the patient and to the family.	S ☐ U ☐ N/A ☐	S ☐ U ☐ N/A ☐	S ☐ U ☐ N/A ☐
7. Explains the procedure to the patient and to the family, and acknowledges the patient's understanding.	S ☐ U ☐ N/A ☐	S ☐ U ☐ N/A ☐	S ☐ U ☐ N/A ☐
8. Performs proper hand hygiene, and puts on gloves, mask, and protective eyewear, as appropriate for the procedure.	S ☐ U ☐ N/A ☐	S ☐ U ☐ N/A ☐	S ☐ U ☐ N/A ☐
Implementation			
1. Places the patient in a comfortable position, and instructs him or her to breathe normally.	S ☐ U ☐ N/A ☐	S ☐ U ☐ N/A ☐	S ☐ U ☐ N/A ☐
2. Assesses vital signs.	S ☐ U ☐ N/A ☐	S ☐ U ☐ N/A ☐	S ☐ U ☐ N/A ☐
3. Brings the NIF meter and the IMT to the patient.	S ☐ U ☐ N/A ☐	S ☐ U ☐ N/A ☐	S ☐ U ☐ N/A ☐
4. Using the NIF meter, instructs the patient to generate the strongest negative pressure possible with one breath. Repeat the test two more times, making the best effort.	S ☐ U ☐ N/A ☐	S ☐ U ☐ N/A ☐	S ☐ U ☐ N/A ☐
5. Calculates one third of the best effort.	S ☐ U ☐ N/A ☐	S ☐ U ☐ N/A ☐	S ☐ U ☐ N/A ☐

Continued

	Peer Evaluation Laboratory Setting			Instructor Evaluation Laboratory Setting			Instructor Evaluation Clinical Setting		
6. Sets the IMT device to generate a slightly greater effort than one third of the best effort.	S ☐	U ☐	N/A ☐	S ☐	U ☐	N/A ☐	S ☐	U ☐	N/A ☐
7. Explains to the patient that he or she will feel resistance to breathing only on inspiration.	S ☐	U ☐	N/A ☐	S ☐	U ☐	N/A ☐	S ☐	U ☐	N/A ☐
8. Informs the patient that 30 minutes per session, per day at least 5 days per week, is the goal.	S ☐	U ☐	N/A ☐	S ☐	U ☐	N/A ☐	S ☐	U ☐	N/A ☐
9. If the patient is unable to complete 30 minutes, advises the patient to break it into two 15-minute sessions.	S ☐	U ☐	N/A ☐	S ☐	U ☐	N/A ☐	S ☐	U ☐	N/A ☐
10. Instructs the patient to cough.	S ☐	U ☐	N/A ☐	S ☐	U ☐	N/A ☐	S ☐	U ☐	N/A ☐
11. Reassesses vital signs.	S ☐	U ☐	N/A ☐	S ☐	U ☐	N/A ☐	S ☐	U ☐	N/A ☐
12. Removes the supplies used, and cleans the area, as needed.	S ☐	U ☐	N/A ☐	S ☐	U ☐	N/A ☐	S ☐	U ☐	N/A ☐
13. Removes PPE, and performs proper hand hygiene prior to leaving the patient's room.	S ☐	U ☐	N/A ☐	S ☐	U ☐	N/A ☐	S ☐	U ☐	N/A ☐

Evaluation of Procedure

1. Establishes a baseline, or compares with previous measurements.	S ☐	U ☐	N/A ☐	S ☐	U ☐	N/A ☐	S ☐	U ☐	N/A ☐
2. Develops an appropriate respiratory care plan based on assessment data.	S ☐	U ☐	N/A ☐	S ☐	U ☐	N/A ☐	S ☐	U ☐	N/A ☐
3. Notes any use of oxygen therapy.	S ☐	U ☐	N/A ☐	S ☐	U ☐	N/A ☐	S ☐	U ☐	N/A ☐
4. Identifies any unexpected outcomes.	S ☐	U ☐	N/A ☐	S ☐	U ☐	N/A ☐	S ☐	U ☐	N/A ☐

Documentation and Reporting

1. Records findings in the patient's chart.	S ☐	U ☐	N/A ☐	S ☐	U ☐	N/A ☐	S ☐	U ☐	N/A ☐
2. Documents the NIF meter value and the starting IMT setting.	S ☐	U ☐	N/A ☐	S ☐	U ☐	N/A ☐	S ☐	U ☐	N/A ☐
3. Documents the patient's ability to perform the therapy and any coaching needed.	S ☐	U ☐	N/A ☐	S ☐	U ☐	N/A ☐	S ☐	U ☐	N/A ☐
4. Reports any abnormal findings to the appropriate health care provider.	S ☐	U ☐	N/A ☐	S ☐	U ☐	N/A ☐	S ☐	U ☐	N/A ☐

Comments:

_____

_____

_____

Signatures:

Student _____ Date Passed _____

Instructor (Laboratory Setting) _____ Date Passed _____

Student _____ Date Passed _____

Instructor (Clinical Setting) _____ Date Passed _____

Procedural Assessment 27-5

Teaching active cycle of breathing technique

Student _____ Date _____

Instructor (Laboratory Setting) _____ Date _____

Instructor (Clinical Setting) _____ Date _____

Criteria for assessment success:

The student must obtain all **satisfactory (S)** scores to pass the procedural evaluation. Any **unsatisfactory (U)** scores will result in failure of the procedural assessment.

Scoring:

Satisfactory (S): Procedural step performed correctly with no instructor prompting. Student-initiated correction is acceptable.

Unsatisfactory (U): Procedural step was performed incorrectly, omitted, or performed in a way that compromised patient care.

Not applicable (N/A): Procedural step was not indicated or necessary.

Evaluation:

	Peer Evaluation Laboratory Setting	Instructor Evaluation Laboratory Setting	Instructor Evaluation Clinical Setting
Procedural Preparation			
1. Reviews the patient's chart.	S ☐ U ☐ N/A ☐	S ☐ U ☐ N/A ☐	S ☐ U ☐ N/A ☐
2. Verifies the physician's order or the facility's protocol for standard of care.	S ☐ U ☐ N/A ☐	S ☐ U ☐ N/A ☐	S ☐ U ☐ N/A ☐
3. Follows PPE requirements, and observes standard precautions for any transmission-based isolation procedure.	S ☐ U ☐ N/A ☐	S ☐ U ☐ N/A ☐	S ☐ U ☐ N/A ☐
4. Identifies the patient using two patient identifiers.	S ☐ U ☐ N/A ☐	S ☐ U ☐ N/A ☐	S ☐ U ☐ N/A ☐
5. Introduces self to the patient and to the family.	S ☐ U ☐ N/A ☐	S ☐ U ☐ N/A ☐	S ☐ U ☐ N/A ☐
6. Explains the procedure to the patient and to the family, and acknowledges the patient's understanding.	S ☐ U ☐ N/A ☐	S ☐ U ☐ N/A ☐	S ☐ U ☐ N/A ☐
7. Performs proper hand hygiene, and puts on gloves.	S ☐ U ☐ N/A ☐	S ☐ U ☐ N/A ☐	S ☐ U ☐ N/A ☐
Implementation			
1. Places the patient in a comfortable position, and instructs him or her to breathe normally.	S ☐ U ☐ N/A ☐	S ☐ U ☐ N/A ☐	S ☐ U ☐ N/A ☐
2. Assesses vital signs.	S ☐ U ☐ N/A ☐	S ☐ U ☐ N/A ☐	S ☐ U ☐ N/A ☐
3. Instructs the patient to relax and control the breathing using diaphragmatic breathing.	S ☐ U ☐ N/A ☐	S ☐ U ☐ N/A ☐	S ☐ U ☐ N/A ☐
4. Instructs the patient to perform three or four thoracic expansion exercises: a. Instructs patient to take deep inhalation and relaxed exhalation.	S ☐ U ☐ N/A ☐	S ☐ U ☐ N/A ☐	S ☐ U ☐ N/A ☐
b. Informs the patient that this may be accompanied by percussion, vibration, or compression.	S ☐ U ☐ N/A ☐	S ☐ U ☐ N/A ☐	S ☐ U ☐ N/A ☐
5. Instructs the patient to perform three or four thoracic expansion exercises again.	S ☐ U ☐ N/A ☐	S ☐ U ☐ N/A ☐	S ☐ U ☐ N/A ☐

Continued

	Peer Evaluation Laboratory Setting			Instructor Evaluation Laboratory Setting			Instructor Evaluation Clinical Setting		
6. Instructs the patient to perform one or two forced expiratory techniques.	S ☐	U ☐	N/A ☐	S ☐	U ☐	N/A ☐	S ☐	U ☐	N/A ☐
7. Instructs the patient to again perform three or four thoracic expansion exercises.	S ☐	U ☐	N/A ☐	S ☐	U ☐	N/A ☐	S ☐	U ☐	N/A ☐
8. Removes PPE, and performs proper hand hygiene prior to leaving the patient's room.	S ☐	U ☐	N/A ☐	S ☐	U ☐	N/A ☐	S ☐	U ☐	N/A ☐

Evaluation of Procedure

1. Develops an appropriate respiratory care plan based on assessment data.	S ☐	U ☐	N/A ☐	S ☐	U ☐	N/A ☐	S ☐	U ☐	N/A ☐
2. Evaluates the color, consistency, volume, and odor of sputum.	S ☐	U ☐	N/A ☐	S ☐	U ☐	N/A ☐	S ☐	U ☐	N/A ☐
3. Notes any use of oxygen therapy.	S ☐	U ☐	N/A ☐	S ☐	U ☐	N/A ☐	S ☐	U ☐	N/A ☐
4. Identifies any unexpected outcomes.	S ☐	U ☐	N/A ☐	S ☐	U ☐	N/A ☐	S ☐	U ☐	N/A ☐

Documentation and Reporting

1. Records findings in the patient's chart.	S ☐	U ☐	N/A ☐	S ☐	U ☐	N/A ☐	S ☐	U ☐	N/A ☐
2. Reports any abnormal findings to the appropriate health care provider.	S ☐	U ☐	N/A ☐	S ☐	U ☐	N/A ☐	S ☐	U ☐	N/A ☐

Comments:

_____

_____

_____

Signatures:

Student _____ Date Passed _____

Instructor (Laboratory Setting) _____ Date Passed _____

Student _____ Date Passed _____

Instructor (Clinical Setting) _____ Date Passed _____

Procedural Assessment 27-6   Autogenic drainage

Student _____ Date _____

Instructor (Laboratory Setting) _____ Date _____

Instructor (Clinical Setting) _____ Date _____

Criteria for assessment success:

The student must obtain all **satisfactory (S)** scores to pass the procedural evaluation. Any **unsatisfactory (U)** scores will result in failure of the procedural assessment.

Scoring:

Satisfactory (S): Procedural step performed correctly with no instructor prompting. Student-initiated correction is acceptable.

Unsatisfactory (U): Procedural step was performed incorrectly, omitted, or performed in a way that compromised patient care.

Not applicable (N/A): Procedural step was not indicated or necessary.

Evaluation:

	Peer Evaluation Laboratory Setting	Instructor Evaluation Laboratory Setting	Instructor Evaluation Clinical Setting
Procedural Preparation			
1. Reviews the patient's chart.	S ☐ U ☐ N/A ☐	S ☐ U ☐ N/A ☐	S ☐ U ☐ N/A ☐
2. Verifies the physician's order or the facility's protocol for standard of care.	S ☐ U ☐ N/A ☐	S ☐ U ☐ N/A ☐	S ☐ U ☐ N/A ☐
3. Follows PPE requirements, and observes standard precautions for any transmission-based isolation procedure.	S ☐ U ☐ N/A ☐	S ☐ U ☐ N/A ☐	S ☐ U ☐ N/A ☐
4. Identifies the patient using two patient identifiers.	S ☐ U ☐ N/A ☐	S ☐ U ☐ N/A ☐	S ☐ U ☐ N/A ☐
5. Introduces self to the patient and to the family.	S ☐ U ☐ N/A ☐	S ☐ U ☐ N/A ☐	S ☐ U ☐ N/A ☐
6. Explains the procedure to the patient and to the family, and acknowledges the patient's understanding.	S ☐ U ☐ N/A ☐	S ☐ U ☐ N/A ☐	S ☐ U ☐ N/A ☐
7. Performs proper hand hygiene, and puts on gloves, mask, and protective eyewear, as appropriate for the procedure.	S ☐ U ☐ N/A ☐	S ☐ U ☐ N/A ☐	S ☐ U ☐ N/A ☐
Implementation			
1. Places the patient in a comfortable position, and instructs him or her to breathe normally.	S ☐ U ☐ N/A ☐	S ☐ U ☐ N/A ☐	S ☐ U ☐ N/A ☐
2. Assesses vital signs.	S ☐ U ☐ N/A ☐	S ☐ U ☐ N/A ☐	S ☐ U ☐ N/A ☐
3. Instructs the patient to use diaphragmatic breathing during the three phases of AD:			
a. Full inspiratory capacity maneuver, followed by low-lung-volume breathing	S ☐ U ☐ N/A ☐	S ☐ U ☐ N/A ☐	S ☐ U ☐ N/A ☐
b. Breathing at low to middle lung volumes	S ☐ U ☐ N/A ☐	S ☐ U ☐ N/A ☐	S ☐ U ☐ N/A ☐
c. Breathing at increasing lung volumes readying mucus for expulsion	S ☐ U ☐ N/A ☐	S ☐ U ☐ N/A ☐	S ☐ U ☐ N/A ☐

Continued

	Peer Evaluation Laboratory Setting			Instructor Evaluation Laboratory Setting			Instructor Evaluation Clinical Setting		
4. Instructs the patient to perform forced expiratory technique once all three phases have been completed.	S ☐	U ☐	N/A ☐	S ☐	U ☐	N/A ☐	S ☐	U ☐	N/A ☐
5. Repeat steps 3 and 4 until all mucous is removed.	S ☐	U ☐	N/A ☐	S ☐	U ☐	N/A ☐	S ☐	U ☐	N/A ☐
6. Removes PPE, and performs proper hand hygiene.	S ☐	U ☐	N/A ☐	S ☐	U ☐	N/A ☐	S ☐	U ☐	N/A ☐
Evaluation of Procedure									
1. Develops an appropriate respiratory care plan based on assessment data.	S ☐	U ☐	N/A ☐	S ☐	U ☐	N/A ☐	S ☐	U ☐	N/A ☐
2. Evaluates the color, consistency, volume, and odor of sputum.	S ☐	U ☐	N/A ☐	S ☐	U ☐	N/A ☐	S ☐	U ☐	N/A ☐
3. Notes any use of oxygen therapy.	S ☐	U ☐	N/A ☐	S ☐	U ☐	N/A ☐	S ☐	U ☐	N/A ☐
4. Identifies any unexpected outcomes.	S ☐	U ☐	N/A ☐	S ☐	U ☐	N/A ☐	S ☐	U ☐	N/A ☐
Documentation and Reporting									
1. Records findings in the patient's chart.	S ☐	U ☐	N/A ☐	S ☐	U ☐	N/A ☐	S ☐	U ☐	N/A ☐
2. Reports any abnormal findings to the appropriate health care provider.	S ☐	U ☐	N/A ☐	S ☐	U ☐	N/A ☐	S ☐	U ☐	N/A ☐

Comments:

_____

_____

_____

Signatures:

Student _____ Date Passed _____

Instructor (Laboratory Setting) _____ Date Passed _____

Student _____ Date Passed _____

Instructor (Clinical Setting) _____ Date Passed _____

Procedural Assessment 28-1

Assessing the polysomnography patient

Student _____ Date _____

Instructor (Laboratory Setting) _____ Date _____

Instructor (Clinical Setting) _____ Date _____

Criteria for assessment success:

The student must obtain all **satisfactory (S)** scores to pass the procedural evaluation. Any **unsatisfactory (U)** scores will result in failure of the procedural assessment.

Scoring:

Satisfactory (S): Procedural step performed correctly with no instructor prompting. Student-initiated correction is acceptable.

Unsatisfactory (U): Procedural step was performed incorrectly, omitted, or performed in a way that compromised patient care.

Not applicable (N/A): Procedural step was not indicated or necessary.

Evaluation:

	Peer Evaluation Laboratory Setting	Instructor Evaluation Laboratory Setting	Instructor Evaluation Clinical Setting
Procedural Preparation			
1. Reviews the patient's chart.	S ☐ U ☐ N/A ☐	S ☐ U ☐ N/A ☐	S ☐ U ☐ N/A ☐
2. Verifies the physician's order or the facility's protocol for standard of care and appropriate study type.	S ☐ U ☐ N/A ☐	S ☐ U ☐ N/A ☐	S ☐ U ☐ N/A ☐
3. Identifies the patient using two patient identifiers.	S ☐ U ☐ N/A ☐	S ☐ U ☐ N/A ☐	S ☐ U ☐ N/A ☐
4. Follows the facility's protocol for patient interaction, and introduces self to the patient and the family.	S ☐ U ☐ N/A ☐	S ☐ U ☐ N/A ☐	S ☐ U ☐ N/A ☐
Implementation			
1. Obtains patient history for medication allergies and substance allergies	S ☐ U ☐ N/A ☐	S ☐ U ☐ N/A ☐	S ☐ U ☐ N/A ☐
2. Asks the patient to verbally describe the reason he or she has come to the sleep lab, and expectations of the testing procedure and potential treatments to be accomplished during the study.	S ☐ U ☐ N/A ☐	S ☐ U ☐ N/A ☐	S ☐ U ☐ N/A ☐
3. Determines if the patient has had issues with claustrophobia.	S ☐ U ☐ N/A ☐	S ☐ U ☐ N/A ☐	S ☐ U ☐ N/A ☐
4. Determines if the patient has special physical needs to be addressed prior to the start of the procedure.	S ☐ U ☐ N/A ☐	S ☐ U ☐ N/A ☐	S ☐ U ☐ N/A ☐
5. Instructs the patient to complete a presleep questionnaire.	S ☐ U ☐ N/A ☐	S ☐ U ☐ N/A ☐	S ☐ U ☐ N/A ☐
6. Reviews the completed presleep questionnaire with the patient to ensure accuracy.	S ☐ U ☐ N/A ☐	S ☐ U ☐ N/A ☐	S ☐ U ☐ N/A ☐
7. Determines any comorbidities that may be of concern during the procedure (i.e., cardiovascular abnormalities, diabetes, seizures, neuromuscular disorders, pulmonary disease, etc.).	S ☐ U ☐ N/A ☐	S ☐ U ☐ N/A ☐	S ☐ U ☐ N/A ☐

Continued

	Peer Evaluation Laboratory Setting			Instructor Evaluation Laboratory Setting			Instructor Evaluation Clinical Setting		
8. Obtains written permission from the patient to monitor, record, and acquire video during the procedure and to treat breathing-related sleep disorders diagnosed in the sleep laboratory.	S ☐	U ☐	N/A ☐	S ☐	U ☐	N/A ☐	S ☐	U ☐	N/A ☐

Evaluation of Procedure

1. Establishes patient rapport, and gains patient confidence.	S ☐	U ☐	N/A ☐	S ☐	U ☐	N/A ☐	S ☐	U ☐	N/A ☐
2. Develops an appropriate sleep related breathing treatment plan based on assessment data.	S ☐	U ☐	N/A ☐	S ☐	U ☐	N/A ☐	S ☐	U ☐	N/A ☐
3. Identifies any unexpected testing outcomes.	S ☐	U ☐	N/A ☐	S ☐	U ☐	N/A ☐	S ☐	U ☐	N/A ☐

Documentation and Reporting

1. Records the PSG findings in the patient's chart.	S ☐	U ☐	N/A ☐	S ☐	U ☐	N/A ☐	S ☐	U ☐	N/A ☐
2. Reports any abnormal findings to the appropriate health care provider.	S ☐	U ☐	N/A ☐	S ☐	U ☐	N/A ☐	S ☐	U ☐	N/A ☐
3. Informs the patient about the poststudy follow-up process.	S ☐	U ☐	N/A ☐	S ☐	U ☐	N/A ☐	S ☐	U ☐	N/A ☐

Comments:

_____

_____

_____

Signatures:

Student _____ Date Passed _____

Instructor (Laboratory Setting) _____ Date Passed _____

Student _____ Date Passed _____

Instructor (Clinical Setting) _____ Date Passed _____

Procedural Assessment 28-2

Educating the polysomnography patient

Student _____ Date _____

Instructor (Laboratory Setting) _____ Date _____

Instructor (Clinical Setting) _____ Date _____

Criteria for assessment success:

The student must obtain all **satisfactory (S)** scores to pass the procedural evaluation. Any **unsatisfactory (U)** scores will result in failure of the procedural assessment.

Scoring:

Satisfactory (S): Procedural step performed correctly with no instructor prompting. Student-initiated correction is acceptable.

Unsatisfactory (U): Procedural step was performed incorrectly, omitted, or performed in a way that compromised patient care.

Not applicable (N/A): Procedural step was not indicated or necessary.

Evaluation:

	Peer Evaluation Laboratory Setting	Instructor Evaluation Laboratory Setting	Instructor Evaluation Clinical Setting
Procedural Preparation			
1. Reviews the patient's chart.	S ☐ U ☐ N/A ☐	S ☐ U ☐ N/A ☐	S ☐ U ☐ N/A ☐
2. Verifies the physician's order or the facility's protocol for standard of care and for the appropriate study type.	S ☐ U ☐ N/A ☐	S ☐ U ☐ N/A ☐	S ☐ U ☐ N/A ☐
Implementation			
1. Clearly explains the reason for PSG testing to the patient, making sure that he or she understands.	S ☐ U ☐ N/A ☐	S ☐ U ☐ N/A ☐	S ☐ U ☐ N/A ☐
2. Explains the process of ancillary monitoring device application.	S ☐ U ☐ N/A ☐	S ☐ U ☐ N/A ☐	S ☐ U ☐ N/A ☐
3. Educates the patient about sleep-disordered breathing and PAP treatment	S ☐ U ☐ N/A ☐	S ☐ U ☐ N/A ☐	S ☐ U ☐ N/A ☐
4. Discusses PAP therapy to include the acclimation process, equipment orientation, and benefits of PAP therapy (see "PAP Therapy").	S ☐ U ☐ N/A ☐	S ☐ U ☐ N/A ☐	S ☐ U ☐ N/A ☐
5. Answers all patient questions and concerns before proceeding with testing to ensure the patient's comfort and compliance with the procedure.	S ☐ U ☐ N/A ☐	S ☐ U ☐ N/A ☐	S ☐ U ☐ N/A ☐
Evaluation of Procedure			
1. Establishes patient confidence.	S ☐ U ☐ N/A ☐	S ☐ U ☐ N/A ☐	S ☐ U ☐ N/A ☐
2. Determines patient competence.	S ☐ U ☐ N/A ☐	S ☐ U ☐ N/A ☐	S ☐ U ☐ N/A ☐
3. Develops an appropriate care plan based on the patient's response to education.	S ☐ U ☐ N/A ☐	S ☐ U ☐ N/A ☐	S ☐ U ☐ N/A ☐
4. Identifies any unexpected outcomes.	S ☐ U ☐ N/A ☐	S ☐ U ☐ N/A ☐	S ☐ U ☐ N/A ☐
Documentation and Reporting			
1. Records patient education in the patient's chart.	S ☐ U ☐ N/A ☐	S ☐ U ☐ N/A ☐	S ☐ U ☐ N/A ☐

Continued

Comments:

_____

_____

_____

Signatures:

Student _____ Date Passed _____

Instructor (Laboratory Setting) _____ Date Passed _____

Student _____ Date Passed _____

Instructor (Clinical Setting) _____ Date Passed _____

»» **Procedural Assessment 28-3**

**Introducing and fitting
the positive airway
pressure interface**

Student _____ Date _____

Instructor (Laboratory Setting) _____ Date _____

Instructor (Clinical Setting) _____ Date _____

Criteria for assessment success:

The student must obtain all **satisfactory (S)** scores to pass the procedural evaluation. Any **unsatisfactory (U)** scores will result in failure of the procedural assessment.

Scoring:

Satisfactory (S): Procedural step performed correctly with no instructor prompting. Student-initiated correction is acceptable.

Unsatisfactory (U): Procedural step was performed incorrectly, omitted, or performed in a way that compromised patient care.

Not applicable (N/A): Procedural step was not indicated or necessary.

Evaluation:

	Peer Evaluation Laboratory Setting	Instructor Evaluation Laboratory Setting	Instructor Evaluation Clinical Setting
Procedural Preparation			
1. Reviews the patient's chart.	S ☐ U ☐ N/A ☐	S ☐ U ☐ N/A ☐	S ☐ U ☐ N/A ☐
2. Verifies the physician's order or the facility's protocol for standard of care.	S ☐ U ☐ N/A ☐	S ☐ U ☐ N/A ☐	S ☐ U ☐ N/A ☐
3. Obtains, cleans, and inspects the appropriate equipment prior to entering the patient's room.	S ☐ U ☐ N/A ☐	S ☐ U ☐ N/A ☐	S ☐ U ☐ N/A ☐
4. Identifies the patient using two patient identifiers.	S ☐ U ☐ N/A ☐	S ☐ U ☐ N/A ☐	S ☐ U ☐ N/A ☐
5. Introduces self to the patient and to the family.	S ☐ U ☐ N/A ☐	S ☐ U ☐ N/A ☐	S ☐ U ☐ N/A ☐
6. Explains the procedure to the patient and to the family, and acknowledges the patient's understanding.	S ☐ U ☐ N/A ☐	S ☐ U ☐ N/A ☐	S ☐ U ☐ N/A ☐
7. Performs proper hand hygiene, and puts on gloves.	S ☐ U ☐ N/A ☐	S ☐ U ☐ N/A ☐	S ☐ U ☐ N/A ☐
Implementation			
1. Provides a detailed explanation of the devices used for PAP therapy	S ☐ U ☐ N/A ☐	S ☐ U ☐ N/A ☐	S ☐ U ☐ N/A ☐
2. Presents multiple options of interfaces (masks) to the patient.	S ☐ U ☐ N/A ☐	S ☐ U ☐ N/A ☐	S ☐ U ☐ N/A ☐
3. Provides explanations for the pros and cons of each interface device.	S ☐ U ☐ N/A ☐	S ☐ U ☐ N/A ☐	S ☐ U ☐ N/A ☐
4. Asks the patient to choose the most comfortable interface, and ensures that the appropriate size and fit have been selected for the patient.	S ☐ U ☐ N/A ☐	S ☐ U ☐ N/A ☐	S ☐ U ☐ N/A ☐
5. Demonstrates understanding of PAP interfaces.	S ☐ U ☐ N/A ☐	S ☐ U ☐ N/A ☐	S ☐ U ☐ N/A ☐
6. Instructs the patient to sit comfortably on the side of the bed.	S ☐ U ☐ N/A ☐	S ☐ U ☐ N/A ☐	S ☐ U ☐ N/A ☐
7. Explains the concept of PAP and how the device will assist with breathing during the night.	S ☐ U ☐ N/A ☐	S ☐ U ☐ N/A ☐	S ☐ U ☐ N/A ☐
8. Instructs the patient to breathe normally in and out through the nose.	S ☐ U ☐ N/A ☐	S ☐ U ☐ N/A ☐	S ☐ U ☐ N/A ☐

Continued

	Peer Evaluation Laboratory Setting	Instructor Evaluation Laboratory Setting	Instructor Evaluation Clinical Setting
9. Assists the patient with applying the interface and headgear.	S ☐ U ☐ N/A ☐	S ☐ U ☐ N/A ☐	S ☐ U ☐ N/A ☐
10. Introduces PAP at 4 cmH₂O pressure	S ☐ U ☐ N/A ☐	S ☐ U ☐ N/A ☐	S ☐ U ☐ N/A ☐
11. Reassures and supports the patient.	S ☐ U ☐ N/A ☐	S ☐ U ☐ N/A ☐	S ☐ U ☐ N/A ☐
12. Assesses for leak(s) around the edges of the interface, and makes adjustments, as needed.	S ☐ U ☐ N/A ☐	S ☐ U ☐ N/A ☐	S ☐ U ☐ N/A ☐
13. Uses the minimal amount of headgear tension to maintain an adequate interface seal.	S ☐ U ☐ N/A ☐	S ☐ U ☐ N/A ☐	S ☐ U ☐ N/A ☐
14. Adjusts the interface if the measured leak is unacceptable, or changes the interface if adequate seal cannot be maintained.	S ☐ U ☐ N/A ☐	S ☐ U ☐ N/A ☐	S ☐ U ☐ N/A ☐
15. Instructs the patient to lie down in the supine position.	S ☐ U ☐ N/A ☐	S ☐ U ☐ N/A ☐	S ☐ U ☐ N/A ☐
16. Assures the patient that PAP will be initiated only if indicated by findings on polysomnogram.	S ☐ U ☐ N/A ☐	S ☐ U ☐ N/A ☐	S ☐ U ☐ N/A ☐
17. Determines patient tolerance of interface and PAP pressure by allowing time to acclimate to any changes with interface or position.	S ☐ U ☐ N/A ☐	S ☐ U ☐ N/A ☐	S ☐ U ☐ N/A ☐
18. Removes the supplies from the patient's room, and cleans the area, as needed.	S ☐ U ☐ N/A ☐	S ☐ U ☐ N/A ☐	S ☐ U ☐ N/A ☐
19. Performs proper hand hygiene prior to leaving the patient's room.	S ☐ U ☐ N/A ☐	S ☐ U ☐ N/A ☐	S ☐ U ☐ N/A ☐

Evaluation of Procedure

1. Establishes patient confidence.	S ☐ U ☐ N/A ☐	S ☐ U ☐ N/A ☐	S ☐ U ☐ N/A ☐
2. Develops an appropriate care plan based on the patient's response to PAP.	S ☐ U ☐ N/A ☐	S ☐ U ☐ N/A ☐	S ☐ U ☐ N/A ☐
3. Identifies any unexpected outcomes.	S ☐ U ☐ N/A ☐	S ☐ U ☐ N/A ☐	S ☐ U ☐ N/A ☐

Documentation and Reporting

1. Records the PAP acclimation process in the patient's chart.	S ☐ U ☐ N/A ☐	S ☐ U ☐ N/A ☐	S ☐ U ☐ N/A ☐
2. Documents the preferred PAP interface used during the acclimation period.	S ☐ U ☐ N/A ☐	S ☐ U ☐ N/A ☐	S ☐ U ☐ N/A ☐
3. Notes patient concerns or apprehension about PAP therapy.	S ☐ U ☐ N/A ☐	S ☐ U ☐ N/A ☐	S ☐ U ☐ N/A ☐
4. Identifies and documents any expected outcomes.	S ☐ U ☐ N/A ☐	S ☐ U ☐ N/A ☐	S ☐ U ☐ N/A ☐

Comments:

_____

_____

Signatures:

Student _____ Date Passed _____

Instructor (Laboratory Setting) _____ Date Passed _____

Student _____ Date Passed _____

Instructor (Clinical Setting) _____ Date Passed _____

Student _____ Date _____

Instructor (Laboratory Setting) _____ Date _____

Instructor (Clinical Setting) _____ Date _____

Criteria for assessment success:

The student must obtain all **satisfactory (S)** scores to pass the procedural evaluation. Any **unsatisfactory (U)** scores will result in failure of the procedural assessment.

Scoring:

Satisfactory (S): Procedural step performed correctly with no instructor prompting. Student-initiated correction is acceptable.

Unsatisfactory (U): Procedural step was performed incorrectly, omitted, or performed in a way that compromised patient care.

Not applicable (N/A): Procedural step was not indicated or necessary.

Evaluation:

	Peer Evaluation Laboratory Setting	Instructor Evaluation Laboratory Setting	Instructor Evaluation Clinical Setting
Procedural Preparation			
1. Obtains, cleans, and inspects appropriate equipment.	S ☐ U ☐ N/A ☐	S ☐ U ☐ N/A ☐	S ☐ U ☐ N/A ☐
2. Identifies the patient using two patient identifiers.	S ☐ U ☐ N/A ☐	S ☐ U ☐ N/A ☐	S ☐ U ☐ N/A ☐
3. Introduces self to the patient and to the family.	S ☐ U ☐ N/A ☐	S ☐ U ☐ N/A ☐	S ☐ U ☐ N/A ☐
4. Explains the procedure to the patient and to the family, and acknowledges the patient's understanding.	S ☐ U ☐ N/A ☐	S ☐ U ☐ N/A ☐	S ☐ U ☐ N/A ☐
5. Performs proper hand hygiene, and puts on gloves.	S ☐ U ☐ N/A ☐	S ☐ U ☐ N/A ☐	S ☐ U ☐ N/A ☐
Implementation			
1. Demonstrates accurate EEG electrode placement using the International 10-20 Electrode Placement System. a. Correctly measures and identifies the EEG sites.	S ☐ U ☐ N/A ☐	S ☐ U ☐ N/A ☐	S ☐ U ☐ N/A ☐
2. Prepares each electrode site to ensure quality, artifact-free tracings.	S ☐ U ☐ N/A ☐	S ☐ U ☐ N/A ☐	S ☐ U ☐ N/A ☐
3. Applies the appropriate electrode to the site with electrode paste. a. Glues the electrode in place with collodian and gauze.	S ☐ U ☐ N/A ☐	S ☐ U ☐ N/A ☐	S ☐ U ☐ N/A ☐
b. Applies EOG electrodes using an offset pattern.	S ☐ U ☐ N/A ☐	S ☐ U ☐ N/A ☐	S ☐ U ☐ N/A ☐
c. Applies chin EMG electrodes	S ☐ U ☐ N/A ☐	S ☐ U ☐ N/A ☐	S ☐ U ☐ N/A ☐
d. Applies leg EMG electrodes.	S ☐ U ☐ N/A ☐	S ☐ U ☐ N/A ☐	S ☐ U ☐ N/A ☐
e. Applies ECG electrodes, and displays lead II on the monitor.	S ☐ U ☐ N/A ☐	S ☐ U ☐ N/A ☐	S ☐ U ☐ N/A ☐
4. Appropriately places the airflow thermistor and pressure transducer.	S ☐ U ☐ N/A ☐	S ☐ U ☐ N/A ☐	S ☐ U ☐ N/A ☐
5. Applies the snoring microphone for recording snoring.	S ☐ U ☐ N/A ☐	S ☐ U ☐ N/A ☐	S ☐ U ☐ N/A ☐
6. Applies the effort belts.	S ☐ U ☐ N/A ☐	S ☐ U ☐ N/A ☐	S ☐ U ☐ N/A ☐

Continued

	Peer Evaluation Laboratory Setting			Instructor Evaluation Laboratory Setting			Instructor Evaluation Clinical Setting		
7. Applies the pulse oximeter securely.	S ☐	U ☐	N/A ☐	S ☐	U ☐	N/A ☐	S ☐	U ☐	N/A ☐
8. Securely affixes electrode wires to allow freedom of movement for the patient.	S ☐	U ☐	N/A ☐	S ☐	U ☐	N/A ☐	S ☐	U ☐	N/A ☐

Evaluation of Procedure

	Peer Evaluation Laboratory Setting			Instructor Evaluation Laboratory Setting			Instructor Evaluation Clinical Setting		
1. Obtains clear, artifact-free signals during polysomnography.	S ☐	U ☐	N/A ☐	S ☐	U ☐	N/A ☐	S ☐	U ☐	N/A ☐
2. Demonstrates full understanding of the International 10-20 System.	S ☐	U ☐	N/A ☐	S ☐	U ☐	N/A ☐	S ☐	U ☐	N/A ☐
3. Verbalizes understanding of nomenclature used in the 10-20 System	S ☐	U ☐	N/A ☐	S ☐	U ☐	N/A ☐	S ☐	U ☐	N/A ☐
4. Identifies the four skull landmarks correctly.	S ☐	U ☐	N/A ☐	S ☐	U ☐	N/A ☐	S ☐	U ☐	N/A ☐
5. Uses precise measurements for electrode placement.	S ☐	U ☐	N/A ☐	S ☐	U ☐	N/A ☐	S ☐	U ☐	N/A ☐
6. Follows the correct sequence of measurement.	S ☐	U ☐	N/A ☐	S ☐	U ☐	N/A ☐	S ☐	U ☐	N/A ☐
7. Correctly identifies the EEG site necessary for polysomnography.	S ☐	U ☐	N/A ☐	S ☐	U ☐	N/A ☐	S ☐	U ☐	N/A ☐
8. Follows the recommended electrode site preparation.	S ☐	U ☐	N/A ☐	S ☐	U ☐	N/A ☐	S ☐	U ☐	N/A ☐
9. Applies the appropriate amount of electrode paste to the scalp with each EEG electrode.	S ☐	U ☐	N/A ☐	S ☐	U ☐	N/A ☐	S ☐	U ☐	N/A ☐
10. Demonstrates proper sequence of electrode application and demonstrates appropriate caution when using collodian.	S ☐	U ☐	N/A ☐	S ☐	U ☐	N/A ☐	S ☐	U ☐	N/A ☐

Documentation and Reporting

	Peer Evaluation Laboratory Setting			Instructor Evaluation Laboratory Setting			Instructor Evaluation Clinical Setting		
1. Records the PSG recording data in the patient's chart.	S ☐	U ☐	N/A ☐	S ☐	U ☐	N/A ☐	S ☐	U ☐	N/A ☐

Comments:

_____

_____

_____

Signatures:

Student _____ Date Passed _____

Instructor (Laboratory Setting) _____ Date Passed _____

Student _____ Date Passed _____

Instructor (Clinical Setting) _____ Date Passed _____

Student _____ Date _____

Instructor (Laboratory Setting) _____ Date _____

Instructor (Clinical Setting) _____ Date _____

Criteria for assessment success:

The student must obtain all **satisfactory (S)** scores to pass the procedural evaluation. Any **unsatisfactory (U)** scores will result in failure of the procedural assessment.

Scoring:

Satisfactory (S): Procedural step performed correctly with no instructor prompting. Student-initiated correction is acceptable.

Unsatisfactory (U): Procedural step was performed incorrectly, omitted, or performed in a way that compromised patient care.

Not applicable (N/A): Procedural step was not indicated or necessary.

Evaluation:

	Peer Evaluation Laboratory Setting	Instructor Evaluation Laboratory Setting	Instructor Evaluation Clinical Setting
Procedural Preparation			
1. Prepares the patient for bedtime.	S ☐ U ☐ N/A ☐	S ☐ U ☐ N/A ☐	S ☐ U ☐ N/A ☐
2. Assists the patient to bed and to a comfortable supine position.	S ☐ U ☐ N/A ☐	S ☐ U ☐ N/A ☐	S ☐ U ☐ N/A ☐
3. Explains the process of calibration or biocalibration to the patient.	S ☐ U ☐ N/A ☐	S ☐ U ☐ N/A ☐	S ☐ U ☐ N/A ☐
4. Selects the appropriate testing protocol (i.e., split-night, titration, MSLT, MWT).	S ☐ U ☐ N/A ☐	S ☐ U ☐ N/A ☐	S ☐ U ☐ N/A ☐
Implementation			
1. Performs amplifier and montage calibration, confirming all signals from the amplifier are responding correctly.	S ☐ U ☐ N/A ☐	S ☐ U ☐ N/A ☐	S ☐ U ☐ N/A ☐
2. Asks the patient to perform biocalibration immediately before the "lights out" command.	S ☐ U ☐ N/A ☐	S ☐ U ☐ N/A ☐	S ☐ U ☐ N/A ☐
3. Ensures that all signals obtained are clean and artifact free and that all ancillary devices are working properly.	S ☐ U ☐ N/A ☐	S ☐ U ☐ N/A ☐	S ☐ U ☐ N/A ☐
4. Instructs the patient to get comfortable, close the eyes, and try to go to sleep.	S ☐ U ☐ N/A ☐	S ☐ U ☐ N/A ☐	S ☐ U ☐ N/A ☐
5. Marks the beginning of the procedure in the record.	S ☐ U ☐ N/A ☐	S ☐ U ☐ N/A ☐	S ☐ U ☐ N/A ☐
6. Documents physiologic data at 30-minute intervals.	S ☐ U ☐ N/A ☐	S ☐ U ☐ N/A ☐	S ☐ U ☐ N/A ☐
7. Documents body position changes, interventions, or disruption in monitoring clearly in the record.	S ☐ U ☐ N/A ☐	S ☐ U ☐ N/A ☐	S ☐ U ☐ N/A ☐
8. Documents ending of the testing period with the "lights on" tag.	S ☐ U ☐ N/A ☐	S ☐ U ☐ N/A ☐	S ☐ U ☐ N/A ☐
9. Performs montage calibrations to verify signal integrity.	S ☐ U ☐ N/A ☐	S ☐ U ☐ N/A ☐	S ☐ U ☐ N/A ☐

Continued

	Peer Evaluation Laboratory Setting			Instructor Evaluation Laboratory Setting			Instructor Evaluation Clinical Setting		

Evaluation of Procedure

	Peer Evaluation Laboratory Setting			Instructor Evaluation Laboratory Setting			Instructor Evaluation Clinical Setting		
1. Adjusts monitoring devices, as needed, to obtain artifact-free signals.	S ☐	U ☐	N/A ☐	S ☐	U ☐	N/A ☐	S ☐	U ☐	N/A ☐
2. Documents maneuvers performed during biocalibration.	S ☐	U ☐	N/A ☐	S ☐	U ☐	N/A ☐	S ☐	U ☐	N/A ☐
3. Documents the data obtained at the required intervals during the procedure.	S ☐	U ☐	N/A ☐	S ☐	U ☐	N/A ☐	S ☐	U ☐	N/A ☐
4. Documents the pertinent data, when needed, between the regular charting intervals.	S ☐	U ☐	N/A ☐	S ☐	U ☐	N/A ☐	S ☐	U ☐	N/A ☐
5. Ends the recording interval with the "lights on" tag.	S ☐	U ☐	N/A ☐	S ☐	U ☐	N/A ☐	S ☐	U ☐	N/A ☐
6. Performs amplifier calibration at the end of the testing period to verify signal integrity.	S ☐	U ☐	N/A ☐	S ☐	U ☐	N/A ☐	S ☐	U ☐	N/A ☐

Documentation and Reporting

	Peer Evaluation Laboratory Setting			Instructor Evaluation Laboratory Setting			Instructor Evaluation Clinical Setting		
1. Documents each biocalibration maneuver in the polysomnographic record.	S ☐	U ☐	N/A ☐	S ☐	U ☐	N/A ☐	S ☐	U ☐	N/A ☐
2. Obtains clear, artifact-free signals during polysomnography.	S ☐	U ☐	N/A ☐	S ☐	U ☐	N/A ☐	S ☐	U ☐	N/A ☐
3. Records the data obtained at the required intervals during the procedure.	S ☐	U ☐	N/A ☐	S ☐	U ☐	N/A ☐	S ☐	U ☐	N/A ☐
4. Ensures that the PSG event tags are present to allow for data assessment.	S ☐	U ☐	N/A ☐	S ☐	U ☐	N/A ☐	S ☐	U ☐	N/A ☐

Comments:

_____

_____

_____

Signatures:

Student _____ Date Passed _____

Instructor (Laboratory Setting) _____ Date Passed _____

Student _____ Date Passed _____

Instructor (Clinical Setting) _____ Date Passed _____

Procedural Assessment 28-6

Student _____ Date _____

Instructor (Laboratory Setting) _____ Date _____

Instructor (Clinical Setting) _____ Date _____

Criteria for assessment success:

The student must obtain all **satisfactory (S)** scores to pass the procedural evaluation. Any **unsatisfactory (U)** scores will result in failure of the procedural assessment.

Scoring:

Satisfactory (S): Procedural step performed correctly with no instructor prompting. Student-initiated correction is acceptable.

Unsatisfactory (U): Procedural step was performed incorrectly, omitted, or performed in a way that compromised patient care.

Not applicable (N/A): Procedural step was not indicated or necessary.

Evaluation:

	Peer Evaluation Laboratory Setting	Instructor Evaluation Laboratory Setting	Instructor Evaluation Clinical Setting
Procedural Preparation			
1. Reviews the patient's chart.	S ☐ U ☐ N/A ☐	S ☐ U ☐ N/A ☐	S ☐ U ☐ N/A ☐
Implementation			
1. Performs initial passes through the polysomnogram to score sleep stages according to the AASM guidelines.	S ☐ U ☐ N/A ☐	S ☐ U ☐ N/A ☐	S ☐ U ☐ N/A ☐
2. Performs a second pass through the record to score sleep-related breathing events according to the AASM guidelines.	S ☐ U ☐ N/A ☐	S ☐ U ☐ N/A ☐	S ☐ U ☐ N/A ☐
3. Performs additional passes through the record, as needed, for cardiac events, and limb movements and other event-related arousals, according to the AASM guidelines.	S ☐ U ☐ N/A ☐	S ☐ U ☐ N/A ☐	S ☐ U ☐ N/A ☐
4. Demonstrates understanding of sleep architecture.	S ☐ U ☐ N/A ☐	S ☐ U ☐ N/A ☐	S ☐ U ☐ N/A ☐
Evaluation of Procedure			
1. Identifies sleep onset.	S ☐ U ☐ N/A ☐	S ☐ U ☐ N/A ☐	S ☐ U ☐ N/A ☐
2. Identifies changes in sleep stages.	S ☐ U ☐ N/A ☐	S ☐ U ☐ N/A ☐	S ☐ U ☐ N/A ☐
3. Identifies arousals.	S ☐ U ☐ N/A ☐	S ☐ U ☐ N/A ☐	S ☐ U ☐ N/A ☐
4. Identifies sleep-related breathing events.	S ☐ U ☐ N/A ☐	S ☐ U ☐ N/A ☐	S ☐ U ☐ N/A ☐
5. Identifies cardiac arrhythmias.	S ☐ U ☐ N/A ☐	S ☐ U ☐ N/A ☐	S ☐ U ☐ N/A ☐
6. Identifies abnormal limb and other movements during sleep.	S ☐ U ☐ N/A ☐	S ☐ U ☐ N/A ☐	S ☐ U ☐ N/A ☐
7. Differentiate between abnormal events and artifact.	S ☐ U ☐ N/A ☐	S ☐ U ☐ N/A ☐	S ☐ U ☐ N/A ☐
8. Calculates sleep latency.	S ☐ U ☐ N/A ☐	S ☐ U ☐ N/A ☐	S ☐ U ☐ N/A ☐
9. Calculates rapid eye movement (REM) latency.	S ☐ U ☐ N/A ☐	S ☐ U ☐ N/A ☐	S ☐ U ☐ N/A ☐

Continued

	Peer Evaluation Laboratory Setting			Instructor Evaluation Laboratory Setting			Instructor Evaluation Clinical Setting		
10. Calculates apnea–hypopnea index (AHI).	S ☐	U ☐	N/A ☐	S ☐	U ☐	N/A ☐	S ☐	U ☐	N/A ☐
11. Calculates respiratory disturbance index (RDI).	S ☐	U ☐	N/A ☐	S ☐	U ☐	N/A ☐	S ☐	U ☐	N/A ☐
12. Identifies source of sleep arousals	S ☐	U ☐	N/A ☐	S ☐	U ☐	N/A ☐	S ☐	U ☐	N/A ☐

Documentation and Reporting

1. Records patient information in the patient's chart.	S ☐	U ☐	N/A ☐	S ☐	U ☐	N/A ☐	S ☐	U ☐	N/A ☐

Comments:

_____

_____

_____

Signatures:

Student _____ Date Passed _____

Instructor (Laboratory Setting) _____ Date Passed _____

Student _____ Date Passed _____

Instructor (Clinical Setting) _____ Date Passed _____

Procedural Assessment 29-1   Discharge planning

Student _____ Date _____

Instructor (Laboratory Setting) _____ Date _____

Instructor (Clinical Setting) _____ Date _____

Criteria for assessment success:

The student must obtain all **satisfactory (S)** scores to pass the procedural evaluation. Any **unsatisfactory (U)** scores will result in failure of the procedural assessment.

Scoring:

Satisfactory (S): Procedural step performed correctly with no instructor prompting. Student-initiated correction is acceptable.

Unsatisfactory (U): Procedural step was performed incorrectly, omitted, or performed in a way that compromised patient care.

Not applicable (N/A): Procedural step was not indicated or necessary.

Evaluation:

	Peer Evaluation Laboratory Setting	Instructor Evaluation Laboratory Setting	Instructor Evaluation Clinical Setting
Procedural Preparation			
1. Reviews the patient's chart.	S ☐ U ☐ N/A ☐	S ☐ U ☐ N/A ☐	S ☐ U ☐ N/A ☐
2. Verifies the transfer order to an alternative setting.	S ☐ U ☐ N/A ☐	S ☐ U ☐ N/A ☐	S ☐ U ☐ N/A ☐
3. Assesses the patient and the family members for need for teaching.	S ☐ U ☐ N/A ☐	S ☐ U ☐ N/A ☐	S ☐ U ☐ N/A ☐
4. Collaborates with the physician and staff in other disciplines about the patient's need for referral for home health care services provided by an extended care facility.	S ☐ U ☐ N/A ☐	S ☐ U ☐ N/A ☐	S ☐ U ☐ N/A ☐
Implementation			
1. Performs patient evaluation, including the following:			
a. Assesses the patient's medical condition.	S ☐ U ☐ N/A ☐	S ☐ U ☐ N/A ☐	S ☐ U ☐ N/A ☐
b. Evaluates the psychosocial condition of the patient and the family.	S ☐ U ☐ N/A ☐	S ☐ U ☐ N/A ☐	S ☐ U ☐ N/A ☐
c. Determines the respiratory and ventilatory support required.	S ☐ U ☐ N/A ☐	S ☐ U ☐ N/A ☐	S ☐ U ☐ N/A ☐
d. Assesses for the patient's physical and functional ability to perform activities of daily living.	S ☐ U ☐ N/A ☐	S ☐ U ☐ N/A ☐	S ☐ U ☐ N/A ☐
e. Sets up goals of care.	S ☐ U ☐ N/A ☐	S ☐ U ☐ N/A ☐	S ☐ U ☐ N/A ☐
2. Performs a site evaluation for continuing care, including the following:			
a. Determines the number of personnel required.	S ☐ U ☐ N/A ☐	S ☐ U ☐ N/A ☐	S ☐ U ☐ N/A ☐
b. Evaluates the physical environment's safety and suitability.	S ☐ U ☐ N/A ☐	S ☐ U ☐ N/A ☐	S ☐ U ☐ N/A ☐
c. Establishes the equipment and supplies needed.	S ☐ U ☐ N/A ☐	S ☐ U ☐ N/A ☐	S ☐ U ☐ N/A ☐
d. Evaluates financial resources.	S ☐ U ☐ N/A ☐	S ☐ U ☐ N/A ☐	S ☐ U ☐ N/A ☐

Continued

	Peer Evaluation Laboratory Setting			Instructor Evaluation Laboratory Setting			Instructor Evaluation Clinical Setting		
3. Develops a multidisciplinary plan of care based on the patient's needs and goals, including the following:									
a. Plans for integration into the community.	S ☐	U ☐	N/A ☐	S ☐	U ☐	N/A ☐	S ☐	U ☐	N/A ☐
b. Plans for the administration of medications.	S ☐	U ☐	N/A ☐	S ☐	U ☐	N/A ☐	S ☐	U ☐	N/A ☐
c. Determines patient self-care, when appropriate.	S ☐	U ☐	N/A ☐	S ☐	U ☐	N/A ☐	S ☐	U ☐	N/A ☐
d. Establishes a method for ongoing assessment of outcomes.	S ☐	U ☐	N/A ☐	S ☐	U ☐	N/A ☐	S ☐	U ☐	N/A ☐
e. Determines the roles and responsibilities of the team members for daily care management.	S ☐	U ☐	N/A ☐	S ☐	U ☐	N/A ☐	S ☐	U ☐	N/A ☐
f. Sets up a method to assess the growth and development of pediatric patients.	S ☐	U ☐	N/A ☐	S ☐	U ☐	N/A ☐	S ☐	U ☐	N/A ☐
g. Establishes a documented mechanism for securing and training additional caregivers.	S ☐	U ☐	N/A ☐	S ☐	U ☐	N/A ☐	S ☐	U ☐	N/A ☐
h. Establishes a mechanism for communication among all of the health care team members.	S ☐	U ☐	N/A ☐	S ☐	U ☐	N/A ☐	S ☐	U ☐	N/A ☐
i. Sets up an alternative emergency and contingency plan.	S ☐	U ☐	N/A ☐	S ☐	U ☐	N/A ☐	S ☐	U ☐	N/A ☐
j. Sets up follow-up plans.	S ☐	U ☐	N/A ☐	S ☐	U ☐	N/A ☐	S ☐	U ☐	N/A ☐
k. Plans for the use, maintenance, and troubleshooting of equipment.	S ☐	U ☐	N/A ☐	S ☐	U ☐	N/A ☐	S ☐	U ☐	N/A ☐
l. Establishes the time for implementation.	S ☐	U ☐	N/A ☐	S ☐	U ☐	N/A ☐	S ☐	U ☐	N/A ☐

Evaluation of Procedure

1. Ensures that the discharge plan meets the patient's goals.	S ☐	U ☐	N/A ☐	S ☐	U ☐	N/A ☐	S ☐	U ☐	N/A ☐
2. Evaluates any readmissions following discharge plan failure.	S ☐	U ☐	N/A ☐	S ☐	U ☐	N/A ☐	S ☐	U ☐	N/A ☐
3. Ensures that a discharge plan coordinator monitors the patient following discharge.	S ☐	U ☐	N/A ☐	S ☐	U ☐	N/A ☐	S ☐	U ☐	N/A ☐
4. Modifies the plan according to the patient's goals.	S ☐	U ☐	N/A ☐	S ☐	U ☐	N/A ☐	S ☐	U ☐	N/A ☐

Documentation and Reporting

1. Assesses progress, and conducts a follow-up.	S ☐	U ☐	N/A ☐	S ☐	U ☐	N/A ☐	S ☐	U ☐	N/A ☐
2. Communicates with other disciplines involved in patient care.	S ☐	U ☐	N/A ☐	S ☐	U ☐	N/A ☐	S ☐	U ☐	N/A ☐
3. Documents all findings.	S ☐	U ☐	N/A ☐	S ☐	U ☐	N/A ☐	S ☐	U ☐	N/A ☐

Comments:

_____

_____

_____

Signatures:

Student _____ Date Passed _____

Instructor (Laboratory Setting) _____ Date Passed _____

Student _____ Date Passed _____

Instructor (Clinical Setting) _____ Date Passed _____

Student _____ Date _____

Instructor (Laboratory Setting) _____ Date _____

Instructor (Clinical Setting) _____ Date _____

Criteria for assessment success:

The student must obtain all **satisfactory (S)** scores to pass the procedural evaluation. Any **unsatisfactory (U)** scores will result in failure of the procedural assessment.

Scoring:

Satisfactory (S): Procedural step performed correctly with no instructor prompting. Student-initiated correction is acceptable.

Unsatisfactory (U): Procedural step was performed incorrectly, omitted, or performed in a way that compromised patient care.

Not applicable (N/A): Procedural step was not indicated or necessary.

Evaluation:

	Peer Evaluation Laboratory Setting	Instructor Evaluation Laboratory Setting	Instructor Evaluation Clinical Setting
Procedural Preparation			
1. Reviews the patient's chart.	S ☐ U ☐ N/A ☐	S ☐ U ☐ N/A ☐	S ☐ U ☐ N/A ☐
2. Assesses the patient's home environment for availability of adequate electrical power for the oxygen concentrator.	S ☐ U ☐ N/A ☐	S ☐ U ☐ N/A ☐	S ☐ U ☐ N/A ☐
3. Assesses the patient's or the caregiver's knowledge of oxygen therapy and ability to recognize signs and symptoms of hypoxia.	S ☐ U ☐ N/A ☐	S ☐ U ☐ N/A ☐	S ☐ U ☐ N/A ☐
4. Determines the availability of readily available resource for assistance with home oxygen systems.	S ☐ U ☐ N/A ☐	S ☐ U ☐ N/A ☐	S ☐ U ☐ N/A ☐
5. Determines the presence of a backup system in the event of a power failure.	S ☐ U ☐ N/A ☐	S ☐ U ☐ N/A ☐	S ☐ U ☐ N/A ☐
6. Identifies the patient using two patient identifiers.	S ☐ U ☐ N/A ☐	S ☐ U ☐ N/A ☐	S ☐ U ☐ N/A ☐
7. Introduces self to the patient and the family.	S ☐ U ☐ N/A ☐	S ☐ U ☐ N/A ☐	S ☐ U ☐ N/A ☐
8. Explains the procedure to the patient or the family.	S ☐ U ☐ N/A ☐	S ☐ U ☐ N/A ☐	S ☐ U ☐ N/A ☐
9. Performs proper hand hygiene.	S ☐ U ☐ N/A ☐	S ☐ U ☐ N/A ☐	S ☐ U ☐ N/A ☐
Implementation			
1. Selects the setting in the home where patient is more likely to use oxygen.	S ☐ U ☐ N/A ☐	S ☐ U ☐ N/A ☐	S ☐ U ☐ N/A ☐
2. Places the oxygen delivery system in a safe place in the home.	S ☐ U ☐ N/A ☐	S ☐ U ☐ N/A ☐	S ☐ U ☐ N/A ☐
3. Discusses safety measures and proper storage.	S ☐ U ☐ N/A ☐	S ☐ U ☐ N/A ☐	S ☐ U ☐ N/A ☐

Continued

	Peer Evaluation Laboratory Setting			Instructor Evaluation Laboratory Setting			Instructor Evaluation Clinical Setting		
4. Demonstrates the steps for preparation and completion of oxygen therapy.									
a. Compressed oxygen system:	S ☐	U ☐	N/A ☐	S ☐	U ☐	N/A ☐	S ☐	U ☐	N/A ☐
b. Oxygen concentrator system:	S ☐	U ☐	N/A ☐	S ☐	U ☐	N/A ☐	S ☐	U ☐	N/A ☐
c. Liquid oxygen system:	S ☐	U ☐	N/A ☐	S ☐	U ☐	N/A ☐	S ☐	U ☐	N/A ☐
5. Connects the oxygen delivery device to the oxygen delivery system.	S ☐	U ☐	N/A ☐	S ☐	U ☐	N/A ☐	S ☐	U ☐	N/A ☐
6. Adjusts the liter flow, and places the device on the patient.	S ☐	U ☐	N/A ☐	S ☐	U ☐	N/A ☐	S ☐	U ☐	N/A ☐
7. Performs hand hygiene.	S ☐	U ☐	N/A ☐	S ☐	U ☐	N/A ☐	S ☐	U ☐	N/A ☐
8. Instructs the patient or the caregiver not to change the oxygen flow rate.	S ☐	U ☐	N/A ☐	S ☐	U ☐	N/A ☐	S ☐	U ☐	N/A ☐
9. Instructs the patient to place a "No Smoking—Oxygen in Use" sign at each entrance to the home.	S ☐	U ☐	N/A ☐	S ☐	U ☐	N/A ☐	S ☐	U ☐	N/A ☐
10. Provides and discusses the written materials regarding the system.	S ☐	U ☐	N/A ☐	S ☐	U ☐	N/A ☐	S ☐	U ☐	N/A ☐
11. Instructs the patient or the caregiver on how to recognize the signs and symptoms of hypoxia and upper respiratory infection and when to notify the physician.	S ☐	U ☐	N/A ☐	S ☐	U ☐	N/A ☐	S ☐	U ☐	N/A ☐
12. Discusses the emergency plan for dealing with respiratory distress, power failure, or a natural disaster.	S ☐	U ☐	N/A ☐	S ☐	U ☐	N/A ☐	S ☐	U ☐	N/A ☐
13. Provides instructions with regard to activating 9-1-1.	S ☐	U ☐	N/A ☐	S ☐	U ☐	N/A ☐	S ☐	U ☐	N/A ☐

Evaluation of Procedure

1. Monitors the oxygen delivery rate.	S ☐	U ☐	N/A ☐	S ☐	U ☐	N/A ☐	S ☐	U ☐	N/A ☐
2. Evaluates the patient's or the caregiver's ability to administer oxygen therapy.	S ☐	U ☐	N/A ☐	S ☐	U ☐	N/A ☐	S ☐	U ☐	N/A ☐
3. Evaluates any problem with oxygen delivery at home.	S ☐	U ☐	N/A ☐	S ☐	U ☐	N/A ☐	S ☐	U ☐	N/A ☐
4. Has the patient or the caregiver verbalize safety guidelines and emergency plans.	S ☐	U ☐	N/A ☐	S ☐	U ☐	N/A ☐	S ☐	U ☐	N/A ☐
5. Identifies unexpected outcomes.	S ☐	U ☐	N/A ☐	S ☐	U ☐	N/A ☐	S ☐	U ☐	N/A ☐

Documentation and Reporting

1. Records the teaching plan, and documents the patient's learning.	S ☐	U ☐	N/A ☐	S ☐	U ☐	N/A ☐	S ☐	U ☐	N/A ☐

Comments:

_____

_____

_____

Signatures:

Student _____ Date Passed _____

Instructor (Laboratory Setting) _____ Date Passed _____

Student _____ Date Passed _____

Instructor (Clinical Setting) _____ Date Passed _____

Student _____ Date _____

Instructor (Laboratory Setting) _____ Date _____

Instructor (Clinical Setting) _____ Date _____

Criteria for assessment success:

The student must obtain all **satisfactory (S)** scores to pass the procedural evaluation. Any **unsatisfactory (U)** scores will result in failure of the procedural assessment.

Scoring:

Satisfactory (S): Procedural step performed correctly with no instructor prompting. Student-initiated correction is acceptable.

Unsatisfactory (U): Procedural step was performed incorrectly, omitted, or performed in a way that compromised patient care.

Not applicable (N/A): Procedural step was not indicated or necessary.

Evaluation:

	Peer Evaluation Laboratory Setting	Instructor Evaluation Laboratory Setting	Instructor Evaluation Clinical Setting
Procedural Preparation			
1. Reviews the patient's chart.	S ☐ U ☐ N/A ☐	S ☐ U ☐ N/A ☐	S ☐ U ☐ N/A ☐
2. Verifies the physician's order or the facility's protocol for standard of care.	S ☐ U ☐ N/A ☐	S ☐ U ☐ N/A ☐	S ☐ U ☐ N/A ☐
3. Obtains, cleans, and inspects the appropriate equipment prior to entering the patient's room.	S ☐ U ☐ N/A ☐	S ☐ U ☐ N/A ☐	S ☐ U ☐ N/A ☐
4. Follows PPE requirements, and observes standard precautions for any transmission-based isolation procedure.	S ☐ U ☐ N/A ☐	S ☐ U ☐ N/A ☐	S ☐ U ☐ N/A ☐
5. Identifies the patient using two patient identifiers.	S ☐ U ☐ N/A ☐	S ☐ U ☐ N/A ☐	S ☐ U ☐ N/A ☐
6. Introduces self to the patient and to the family.	S ☐ U ☐ N/A ☐	S ☐ U ☐ N/A ☐	S ☐ U ☐ N/A ☐
7. Explains the procedure to the patient and to the family, and acknowledges the patient's understanding.	S ☐ U ☐ N/A ☐	S ☐ U ☐ N/A ☐	S ☐ U ☐ N/A ☐
8. Performs proper hand hygiene, and puts on gloves, mask, and protective eyewear, as appropriate for the procedure.	S ☐ U ☐ N/A ☐	S ☐ U ☐ N/A ☐	S ☐ U ☐ N/A ☐
Implementation			
1. Demonstrates necessary infection control procedures to the patient, the family, or the caregiver.	S ☐ U ☐ N/A ☐	S ☐ U ☐ N/A ☐	S ☐ U ☐ N/A ☐
2. Assesses vital signs.	S ☐ U ☐ N/A ☐	S ☐ U ☐ N/A ☐	S ☐ U ☐ N/A ☐
3. Instructs the family or the caregiver on the basic assessment to determine patient tolerance or distress.	S ☐ U ☐ N/A ☐	S ☐ U ☐ N/A ☐	S ☐ U ☐ N/A ☐
4. Evaluates and ensures airway patency.	S ☐ U ☐ N/A ☐	S ☐ U ☐ N/A ☐	S ☐ U ☐ N/A ☐

Continued

	Peer Evaluation Laboratory Setting	Instructor Evaluation Laboratory Setting	Instructor Evaluation Clinical Setting
5. Instructs the caregiver while performing the following tasks:			
a. Sets the initial vent settings according to protocol or the physician's orders.	S ☐ U ☐ N/A ☐	S ☐ U ☐ N/A ☐	S ☐ U ☐ N/A ☐
b. Sets the alarms.	S ☐ U ☐ N/A ☐	S ☐ U ☐ N/A ☐	S ☐ U ☐ N/A ☐
c. Checks all the accessory equipment.	S ☐ U ☐ N/A ☐	S ☐ U ☐ N/A ☐	S ☐ U ☐ N/A ☐
d. Charges the battery pack.	S ☐ U ☐ N/A ☐	S ☐ U ☐ N/A ☐	S ☐ U ☐ N/A ☐
e. Troubleshoots any problems.	S ☐ U ☐ N/A ☐	S ☐ U ☐ N/A ☐	S ☐ U ☐ N/A ☐
f. Cleans or disinfects any equipment, as needed, based on the manufacturer's specifications.	S ☐ U ☐ N/A ☐	S ☐ U ☐ N/A ☐	S ☐ U ☐ N/A ☐
6. Removes the supplies from the patient's room, and cleans the area, as needed.	S ☐ U ☐ N/A ☐	S ☐ U ☐ N/A ☐	S ☐ U ☐ N/A ☐
7. Removes PPE, and performs proper hand hygiene prior to leaving the patient's room.	S ☐ U ☐ N/A ☐	S ☐ U ☐ N/A ☐	S ☐ U ☐ N/A ☐

Evaluation of Procedure

	Peer Evaluation Laboratory Setting	Instructor Evaluation Laboratory Setting	Instructor Evaluation Clinical Setting
1. Establishes a baseline, or compares with previous measurements.	S ☐ U ☐ N/A ☐	S ☐ U ☐ N/A ☐	S ☐ U ☐ N/A ☐
2. Evaluates the emergency plan.	S ☐ U ☐ N/A ☐	S ☐ U ☐ N/A ☐	S ☐ U ☐ N/A ☐
3. Develops an appropriate respiratory care plan based on assessment data.	S ☐ U ☐ N/A ☐	S ☐ U ☐ N/A ☐	S ☐ U ☐ N/A ☐
4. Identifies the need for any ventilatory setting changes:			
a. Contacts the physician for change orders, or follows protocols.	S ☐ U ☐ N/A ☐	S ☐ U ☐ N/A ☐	S ☐ U ☐ N/A ☐
5. Identifies any unexpected outcomes.	S ☐ U ☐ N/A ☐	S ☐ U ☐ N/A ☐	S ☐ U ☐ N/A ☐

Documentation and Reporting

	Peer Evaluation Laboratory Setting	Instructor Evaluation Laboratory Setting	Instructor Evaluation Clinical Setting
1. Records findings in the patient's chart.	S ☐ U ☐ N/A ☐	S ☐ U ☐ N/A ☐	S ☐ U ☐ N/A ☐
2. Reports any abnormal findings to the appropriate health care provider.	S ☐ U ☐ N/A ☐	S ☐ U ☐ N/A ☐	S ☐ U ☐ N/A ☐

Comments:

_____

_____

_____

Signatures:

Student _____ Date Passed _____

Instructor (Laboratory Setting) _____ Date Passed _____

Student _____ Date Passed _____

Instructor (Clinical Setting) _____ Date Passed _____

Student _____ Date _____

Instructor (Laboratory Setting) _____ Date _____

Instructor (Clinical Setting) _____ Date _____

Criteria for assessment success:

The student must obtain all **satisfactory (S)** scores to pass the procedural evaluation. Any **unsatisfactory (U)** scores will result in failure of the procedural assessment.

Scoring:

Satisfactory (S): Procedural step performed correctly with no instructor prompting. Student-initiated correction is acceptable.

Unsatisfactory (U): Procedural step was performed incorrectly, omitted, or performed in a way that compromised patient care.

Not applicable (N/A): Procedural step was not indicated or necessary.

Evaluation:

	Peer Evaluation Laboratory Setting	Instructor Evaluation Laboratory Setting	Instructor Evaluation Clinical Setting
Procedural Preparation			
1. Reviews the patient's chart.	S ☐ U ☐ N/A ☐	S ☐ U ☐ N/A ☐	S ☐ U ☐ N/A ☐
2. Verifies the physician's order or the facility's protocol for standard of care.	S ☐ U ☐ N/A ☐	S ☐ U ☐ N/A ☐	S ☐ U ☐ N/A ☐
3. Obtains, cleans, and inspects the appropriate equipment prior to entering the patient's room.	S ☐ U ☐ N/A ☐	S ☐ U ☐ N/A ☐	S ☐ U ☐ N/A ☐
4. Follows PPE requirements, and observes standard precautions for any transmission-based isolation procedure.	S ☐ U ☐ N/A ☐	S ☐ U ☐ N/A ☐	S ☐ U ☐ N/A ☐
5. Identifies the patient using two patient identifiers.	S ☐ U ☐ N/A ☐	S ☐ U ☐ N/A ☐	S ☐ U ☐ N/A ☐
6. Introduces self to the patient and to the family.	S ☐ U ☐ N/A ☐	S ☐ U ☐ N/A ☐	S ☐ U ☐ N/A ☐
7. Explains the procedure to the patient and to the family, and acknowledge the patient's understanding.	S ☐ U ☐ N/A ☐	S ☐ U ☐ N/A ☐	S ☐ U ☐ N/A ☐
8. Assesses the patient's or caregiver's ability to perform tracheostomy care and suctioning.	S ☐ U ☐ N/A ☐	S ☐ U ☐ N/A ☐	S ☐ U ☐ N/A ☐
9. Performs proper hand hygiene, and puts on gloves, mask, and protective eyewear, as appropriate for the procedure.	S ☐ U ☐ N/A ☐	S ☐ U ☐ N/A ☐	S ☐ U ☐ N/A ☐
Implementation			
1. Places the patient in a comfortable position.	S ☐ U ☐ N/A ☐	S ☐ U ☐ N/A ☐	S ☐ U ☐ N/A ☐
2. Assesses vital signs.	S ☐ U ☐ N/A ☐	S ☐ U ☐ N/A ☐	S ☐ U ☐ N/A ☐
3. For suctioning: a. Puts on sterile gloves. b. Instructs, demonstrates, and observes the steps of aseptic preparation and technique for suctioning tracheostomy tube.	S ☐ U ☐ N/A ☐ S ☐ U ☐ N/A ☐	S ☐ U ☐ N/A ☐ S ☐ U ☐ N/A ☐	S ☐ U ☐ N/A ☐ S ☐ U ☐ N/A ☐

Continued

	Peer Evaluation Laboratory Setting			Instructor Evaluation Laboratory Setting			Instructor Evaluation Clinical Setting		
c. Preoxygenates the patient, if he or she is receiving supplemental oxygen.	S ☐	U ☐	N/A ☐	S ☐	U ☐	N/A ☐	S ☐	U ☐	N/A ☐
d. Instructs, demonstrates, and observes nasal and oral suctioning to be done as needed.	S ☐	U ☐	N/A ☐	S ☐	U ☐	N/A ☐	S ☐	U ☐	N/A ☐
e. Instructs the patient to take three deep breaths.	S ☐	U ☐	N/A ☐	S ☐	U ☐	N/A ☐	S ☐	U ☐	N/A ☐
f. Instructs, demonstrates, and observes disconnection and disposal of the suction catheter.	S ☐	U ☐	N/A ☐	S ☐	U ☐	N/A ☐	S ☐	U ☐	N/A ☐
4. For tracheostomy care:									
a. Instructs, demonstrates, and observes the tracheostomy care technique.	S ☐	U ☐	N/A ☐	S ☐	U ☐	N/A ☐	S ☐	U ☐	N/A ☐
b. Instructs, demonstrates, and observes proper disposal of any used equipment in the appropriate container.	S ☐	U ☐	N/A ☐	S ☐	U ☐	N/A ☐	S ☐	U ☐	N/A ☐
c. Instructs, demonstrates, and observes proper disinfection of any reusable equipment.	S ☐	U ☐	N/A ☐	S ☐	U ☐	N/A ☐	S ☐	U ☐	N/A ☐
5. Guides the caregiver during each step.	S ☐	U ☐	N/A ☐	S ☐	U ☐	N/A ☐	S ☐	U ☐	N/A ☐
6. Removes the supplies from the patient's room, and cleans the area, as needed.	S ☐	U ☐	N/A ☐	S ☐	U ☐	N/A ☐	S ☐	U ☐	N/A ☐
7. Removes PPE, and performs proper hand hygiene prior to leaving the patient's room.	S ☐	U ☐	N/A ☐	S ☐	U ☐	N/A ☐	S ☐	U ☐	N/A ☐

Evaluation of Procedure

	Peer Evaluation Laboratory Setting			Instructor Evaluation Laboratory Setting			Instructor Evaluation Clinical Setting		
1. Instructs the patient or the caregiver to state the signs and symptoms of complications from the procedure.	S ☐	U ☐	N/A ☐	S ☐	U ☐	N/A ☐	S ☐	U ☐	N/A ☐
2. Observes the patient or the caregiver demonstrating proper techniques independently.	S ☐	U ☐	N/A ☐	S ☐	U ☐	N/A ☐	S ☐	U ☐	N/A ☐
3. Instructs the patient or the caregiver about the steps to take in an emergency situation.	S ☐	U ☐	N/A ☐	S ☐	U ☐	N/A ☐	S ☐	U ☐	N/A ☐

Documentation and Reporting

	Peer Evaluation Laboratory Setting			Instructor Evaluation Laboratory Setting			Instructor Evaluation Clinical Setting		
1. Records the instructions and skills demonstrated and the correctness of self-care or care delivered by the caregiver.	S ☐	U ☐	N/A ☐	S ☐	U ☐	N/A ☐	S ☐	U ☐	N/A ☐
2. Reports any abnormal findings to the appropriate health care provider.	S ☐	U ☐	N/A ☐	S ☐	U ☐	N/A ☐	S ☐	U ☐	N/A ☐

Comments:

_____

_____

_____

Signatures:

Student _____ Date Passed _____

Instructor (Laboratory Setting) _____ Date Passed _____

Student _____ Date Passed _____

Instructor (Clinical Setting) _____ Date Passed _____

Glossary

A

Acidemia A state in which arterial blood is more acidic than normal (pH < 7.35).

Acidosis Nonrespiratory processes resulting in acidemia.

Active cycle breathing technique Airway clearance strategy consisting of repeated cycles of breathing control and thoracic expansion, followed by the forced expiratory technique.

Adventitious lung sounds Abnormal lung sounds superimposed on the basic underlying breath sounds.

Aerosol Suspension of solid or liquid particles in a gas.

Aerosol therapy The delivery of sterile water or hypotonic, isotonic, or hypertonic saline aerosols.

Air bronchograms Lucent tubular shadows running through areas of consolidation.

Air trapping An abnormal retention of air in the lungs making it difficult to exhale completely.

Algorithms Predetermined group of directions to solve a problem in a finite number of steps.

Alkalemia Combining form meaning a decreased hydrogen ion concentration in the blood; as applied to arterial blood, denotes pH >7.45.

Alkalosis Nonrespiratory processes resulting in alkalemia.

Allen's test Most common technique to determine the adequacy of ulnar circulation.

Alternative settings A location outside of the hospital setting.

Alveolar and arterial oxygen tension difference Difference between the alveolar and arterial PO_2, usually about 5 to 10 mm Hg when breathing room air.

Ambulation The process of helping a bed ridden patient to begin to sit up, stand, and walk around on his or her own.

American Standard Safety System (ASSS) Specifications adopted in the United States and Canada for threaded high-pressure connections between compressed gas cylinders and their attachments.

Arterial blood gas A blood test that is performed using blood from an artery.

Arterial line A thin catheter inserted into an artery, also called an *art-line*.

Artifact Anything such as a substance, structure, or piece of data or information that is artificially made and may be extraneous, irrelevant, or unwanted. In radiologic imaging, spurious electronic signals may appear as an artifact in an image with as much strength as the signals produced by real objects, thereby confusing the radiologist and the results of any examination.

Atelectasis Abnormal collapse of distal lung parenchyma.

Augment To make something greater by adding to it; increase.

Autogenic drainage Modification of directed coughing, beginning with low-lung-volume breathing, inspiratory breath holds, and controlled exhalation and progressing to increased inspired volumes and expiratory flows.

Auto-PEEP Abnormal and usually undetected residual pressure above atmospheric remaining in the alveoli at end-exhalation due to dynamic air trapping. Also called *intrinsic PEEP.*

B

Bag mask A hand-held device used to provide positive pressure ventilation to a patient who is not breathing or who is breathing inadequately.

Baseline pressure The pressure from which inspiration begins and at which expiration ends during mechanical ventilation; also known as *expiratory pressure*. Normal baseline pressure is atmospheric. Positive pressures can be applied to increase the baseline above atmospheric.

Basic metabolic panel A set of eight blood chemistry tests that provide key information regarding fluid and electrolyte status, kidney function, blood sugar levels, and response to various medications and other medical therapies.

Bilevel positive airway pressure (BiPAP) Spontaneous breath mode of ventilatory support, which allows separate regulation of the inspiratory and expiratory pressures.

Bipolar leads A record obtained with two electrodes placed on different regions of the body, each electrode contributing significantly to the record, bipolar leads have one positive and one negative pole; for example, a standard limb lead.

Borg scale Validated scale used by patients to quantify the severity of their dyspnea.

Bronchoscopy Process of passing a bronchoscope into the airways for diagnostic testing, therapeutic purposes, or both.

C

Capnography Process of obtaining a tracing of the proportion of carbon dioxide in expired air using a capnograph.

Cephalization Refers to the increased visualization of pulmonary blood vessels on the chest radiograph in the nondependent regions of the lung; often a sign of left heart failure.

Certified Respiratory Therapist (CRT) A respiratory therapist who has successfully completed the technician (entry-level) certification examination of the NBRC.

Characteristics of medical gases Features that help distinguish a medical gas.

Chest physical therapy (CPT) Collection of therapeutic techniques designed to aid clearance of secretion, improve ventilation, and enhance the conditioning of the respiratory muscles; includes positioning techniques, chest percussion and vibration, directed coughing, and various breathing and conditioning exercises.

Clinical Practice Guidelines (CPGs) Evidence-based research that provides the basis for sound clinical practice and recommendations. (www.rcjournal.com/cpgs)

Clinical Simulation Examination (CSE) An examination for the advanced credentialing of respiratory therapists in the United States.

Cohorting Grouping individuals who share a common characteristic, for example, members of the same age or the same sex, or individuals sharing a common infection.

Combivent Respimat A single inhaler that provides a slow-moving mist containing two different medicines, ipratropium bromide and albuterol (Boehringer-Ingleheim, Ridgefield, CT).

Co-morbidities A concomitant but unrelated pathologic or disease process.

Complete blood cell count (CBC) A determination of the number of red and white blood cells per cubic millimeter of blood. CBC is one of the most routinely performed tests in a clinical laboratory and one of the most valuable screening and diagnostic techniques.

Comprehensive metabolic panel A panel of 14 blood tests that serves as an initial broad medical screening tool.

Compressed oxygen Oxygen that is compressed and stored in cylinders under several thousands of pounds of pressure.

Condensation Change of state from gas to liquid, as with water vapor condensation.

Contact precautions Safeguards designed to reduce the risk of transmission of epidemiologically important microorganisms by direct or indirect contact.

Contagion A disease-producing agent.

Continuing Respiratory Care Education (CRCE) Specific learning activities for the purpose of documenting attendance at a designated seminar or course of instruction.

Continuous positive airway pressure (CPAP) Method of ventilatory support whereby the patient breathes spontaneously without mechanical assistance against threshold resistance, with pressure above atmospheric pressure at the airway throughout breathing.

Credentials A proof of qualification, competence, or authority issued to an individual by a third party.

Curriculum vitae (CV) A summary of one's education, professional history, and job qualifications, as for a prospective employer.

D

Dead space-to-tidal volume ratio Percentage of the tidal volume that does not participate in gas exchange, usually about 30% to 35%.

Decannulation The removal of a cannula or tube that may have been inserted during a surgical procedure.

Defibrillation Termination of ventricular fibrillation by delivering a direct electric countershock to the patient's precordium.

Delta P (ΔP) Also called *driving pressure*; the pressure that drives a fluid, or gas, from one point to another.

Depolarization Reduction of a membrane potential to a less negative value; in cardiac fibers, this results in the release of calcium ions into the myofibrils and activates the contractile process.

Diameter-Index Safety System (DISS) Specifications established to prevent accidental interchange of low-pressure (less than 200 psig) medical gas connectors. The DISS is used in respiratory care to connect equipment to a low-pressure gas source.

Diaphragmatic breathing Breathing that is done by focusing on contracting the diaphragm; air enters the lungs, and the belly expands during this type of breathing. This deep breathing is marked by expansion of the abdomen, rather than the chest, when breathing.

Differential diagnosis Systematic diagnostic method used to identify the presence of a diagnosis where multiple alternatives are possible.

Discharge planning An assessment of an inpatient's medical condition for the purpose of arranging for appropriate continuing care upon leaving the facility.

Disinfection The process of destroying at least the vegetative phase of pathogenic microorganisms by physical or chemical means.

Driving pressure A basic, compelling urge.

Drug administration phase Identifies drug dosage forms and routes of adminstration.

Dry-powder inhaler A device that delivers medication to the lungs in the form of a dry powder.

Dynamic compliance The compliance of the lung at any given time during actual movement of air.

E

Electrode A device attached to skin on certain parts of a patient's body during electrocardiography (ECG).

End expiratory flow The flow (or speed) of air coming out of the lung.

End expiratory pressure The pressure at the end of the expiratory phase, measured relative to atmospheric pressure. The location of the pressure must be specified but is usually the airway opening.

End-diastolic volume (EDV) Volume of blood remaining in the left ventricle after the ventricle has contracted.

Erythrocytes Red blood cells.

Evidence-based medicine The meticulous, explicit, and judicious use of current best evidence in making decisions about the care of individual patients.

Expiratory reserve volume (ERV) Total amount of gas that can be exhaled from the lung following a quiet exhalation.

Extubation The process of withdrawing a tube from an orifice or cavity of the body.

F

Flow-oriented device Measures flow to achieve result.

Fomites Nonliving material such as bed linens or equipment, which may transmit pathogenic organisms to a person who comes into contact with the object.

Forced expiratory flow between 25% and 75% ($FEF_{25\%-75\%}$) Measure of the average expiratory flow during the middle half of the forced vital capacity.

Forced expiratory technique Modification of the normal cough sequence designed to facilitate clearance of bronchial secretions while minimizing the likelihood of bronchiolar collapse.

Forced expired volume in 1 second (FEV_1) Maximum volume of gas that the patient can exhale during the first second of the forced vital capacity maneuver.

Forced expired volume in 1 second-to-vital capacity ratio (FEV_1/FVC) Percent of the measured forced vital capacity that can be exhaled in 1 second.

Forced vital capacity (FVC) Maximum volume of gas that the subject can exhale as forcefully and as quickly as possible.

Fractional distillation Process of separating the components of a liquid mixture according to their boiling points via the application of heat; the primary commercial process used to produce oxygen.

Full ventilatory support Ventilatory support modes in which the ventilator provides all the minute ventilation requirements of the patient.

Functional residual capacity (FRC) Total amount of gas left in the lungs after a resting expiration.

G

Gradient Change in the value of a quantity (as temperature, pressure, or concentration) with change in a given variable and especially per unit distance in a specified direction.

H

Health care–associated infections (HAIs) Infections that patients get while receiving treatment for medical or surgical conditions.

Health Insurance Portability and Accountability Act (HIPAA) An act that was passed by Congress in 1996 and does the following: provides the ability to transfer and continue health insurance coverage for millions of American workers and their families when they change or lose their jobs; reduces health care fraud and abuse; mandates industry-wide standards for health care information on electronic billing and other processes; and requires the protection and confidential handling of protected health information.

Hematology Branch of medicine involved in the study of blood morphology, physiology, and pathology.

Hematoma A localized collection of blood outside the blood vessels, also called a *bruise*.

High-frequency jet ventilation (HFJV) Ventilatory support provided at rates significantly higher than normal breathing frequencies.

High-frequency oscillatory ventilation (HFOV) Uses rates into the thousands, up to about 4000 cycles per minute. HFOV ventilators use either a small piston or a device similar to a stereo speaker, both of which deliver gas in a "to-and-fro" motion, pushing gas in during inspiration and drawing gas out during exhalation.

High-flow systems Oxygen therapy equipment that supplies inspired gases at a consistent preset oxygen concentration.

Humidifier Device that adds molecular water to gas.

Hypoxemia Abnormal deficiency of oxygen in arterial blood.

Hypoxia Abnormal condition in which the oxygen available to body cells is inadequate to meet their metabolic needs.

I

Incentive spirometry (IS) The process of encouraging the bed-ridden patient to take deep breaths to avoid atelectasis; most often done with the use of an incentive spirometer that provides feedback to the patient when a predetermined lung volume is reached during an inspiratory breath.

Incident An occurrence of an action or situation.

Infiltrates Fluid that passes through body tissues.

Injectate Material that is injected.

Inspiratory capacity (IC) Maximum amount of air that can be inhaled from the resting end-expiratory level or FRC; the sum of the tidal volume and inspiratory reserve volume.

Inspiratory muscle trainer A device designed to strengthen respiratory muscles through the use of resistance during the inspiratory effort.

Inspiratory reserve volume (IRV) Maximum volume of air that can be inhaled following a normal quiet inspiration.

Inspissated (of a fluid) Thickened or hardened through the absorption or evaporation of the liquid portion, as can occur with respiratory secretion when the upper airway is bypassed.

Intensive care unit (ICU) A special department of a hospital or health care facility that treats patients with the most severe and life-threatening illnesses and injuries and those requiring constant, close monitoring and support from specialist equipment and medication to maintain normal bodily functions, also known as *critical care unit (CCU)*.

Interfaces Devices used to deliver respiratory therapies, commonly used when referring to oxygen delivery devices.

Intermittent positive pressure breathing (IPPB) Application of positive pressure breaths to a patient for a relatively short period (10 to 20 minutes).

Intubation Passage of a tube into a body aperture; commonly refers to the insertion of an endotracheal tube within the trachea.

Invasive Characterized by a tendency to spread or infiltrate; also refers to the use of diagnostic or therapeutic methods requiring access to the inside of the body.

Isovolumetric Of, relating to, or characterized by unchanging volume; *especially* relating to or being an early phase of ventricular systole, in which the cardiac muscle exerts increasing pressure on the contents of the ventricle without significant change in the muscle fiber length and the ventricular volume remains constant.

K

Keep vein open (KVO) A slow drip rate providing enough fluid flow to keep the end of the catheter from clotting off; equal to approximately 8 to 15 drops per minute.

Kerley B lines Thin lines seen near the pleural edge on a chest radiograph as a result of increased pulmonary capillary pressures.

L

Leukocytes White blood cells, part of the formed elements of the circulating blood system.

Licensure A restricted practice requiring a license, which gives a permission to practice; in the case of respiratory care, licensing is granted through a professional body or a licensing board composed of advanced practitioners who oversee the applications for licenses.

Liquid oxygen A bluish translucent liquid obtained by compressing gaseous oxygen and then cooling it below its boiling point.

Long-term acute care hospital (LTACH) A health care facility specializing in treating patients requiring extended hospitalization.

Low-flow systems Variable performance oxygen therapy device that delivers oxygen at a flow that provides only a portion of the patient's inspired gas needs. Also called *variable performance system*.

Lumen The bore of a tube (as of a hollow needle or catheter).

M

Mean airway pressure Average pressure applied to the airway.

Modified Seldinger technique A medical technique for inserting catheters into blood vessels.

N

Noninvasive ventilation (NIV) Mechanical ventilation performed without intubation or tracheostomy, usually with mask ventilation.

Noninvasive Pertaining to a diagnostic or therapeutic technique that does not require skin to be broken or a cavity or organ of the body to be entered; for example, obtaining a blood pressure reading by auscultation with a stethoscope and sphygmomanometer.

O

Obstructive pulmonary disease Any respiratory disease characterized by decreased airway size and increased airway secretions.

Oscillation Back-and-forth motion; vibration or the effects of mechanical or electrical vibration.

Over-the-needle IV catheter (ONC) A large-bore sharp needle housed within an indwelling stylet, inside a thin-walled plastic tube.

Oxygen concentrator A device providing oxygen therapy to a patient at minimally to substantially higher concentrations than available in ambient air.

Oxygen consumption An expression of the rate at which oxygen is used by tissues, usually given in microliters of oxygen consumed in 1 hour by 1 milligram dry weight of tissue.

P

PaO_2/FiO_2 ratio Also called the *P/F ratio*; the ratio of arterial oxygen concentration to the fraction of inspired oxygen.

Partial ventilatory support Modes of ventilatory support in which the patient must contribute to the total minute volume with spontaneous breathing.

Peak airway pressure The highest pressure achieved during inspiration on positive pressure ventilation; also called *peak pressure* and *peak inspiratory pressure*.

Peak inspiratory flow Uppermost inspiratory flow rate.

PEEP of best compliance or optimal PEEP Generally correlates with the point where alveolar de-recruitment does not occur.

Peer-reviewed literature Work that has been evaluated by one or more people with competence similar to that of the producers of the work; peer review methods are used to maintain standards of quality, improve performance, and provide credibility.

Peripherally inserted central catheter (PICC) A form of intravenous access that can be used for a prolonged period.

Pertinent negative Absence of a sign or symptom that helps substantiate or identify a patient's condition.

Pertinent positive Presence of a sign or symptom that helps substantiate or identify a patient's condition.

Pharmacodynamic phase Mechanisms of drug action that cause effects on the body.

Pharmacokinetic phase Time, course, and disposition of a drug in the body.

Physiologic shunt Percentage of the cardiac output that does not participate in gas exchange in the lung.

Picture Archive Communication Systems (PACS) A medical imaging technology that provides economical storage of, and convenient access to, images from multiple modalities.

Pin-Index Safety System (PISS) Part of the American standard safety system, these specifications apply only to the valve outlets of small cylinders, up to and including size E, which use a yoke-type connection.

Plateau pressure Pressure in the patient's airway during mechanical ventilation resulting from the application of an end-inspiratory hold. This is equal to the average peak alveolar pressure.

Point-of-care testing Analysis at the bedside, as opposed to conventional laboratory testing.

Positive end-expiratory pressure (PEEP) Application and maintenance of pressure above atmospheric pressure at the airway throughout the expiratory phase of positive-pressure mechanical ventilation.

Postural drainage, percussion, and vibration (PDPV) Postural drainage pertains to placing the body in a position that allows mucus to drain from the smaller airways into the main airway with gravity. Percussion is a repetitive tapping on the designated position. Vibration is the placement of hands along the ribs in the direction of the expiratory movement of the chest. A small rapid vibration (tremor) and slight pressure are applied during exhalation to accentuate this phase of the respiratory cycle.

Precordial leads Electrodes that are placed directly on the chest during electrocardiography (V_1, V_2, V_3, V_4, V_5 and V_6).

Pressure control ventilation Mode of ventilatory support in which mandatory support breaths are delivered to the patient at a set inspiratory pressure.

Pressurized metered-dose inhaler A device that delivers a specific amount of medication to the lungs, in the form of a short burst of aerosolized medicine that is inhaled by the patient.

Pulsus alternans Alternating between strong and weak heart beats.

Pulsus paradoxus Abnormal decrease in pulse pressure with each inspiratory effort.

Pursed lip breathing The act of exhaling through tightly pressed, puckered lips.

R

Radiolucent Pertaining to a substance or tissue that readily permits the passage of x-rays or other radiant energy; compare with *radiopaque*.

Radiopaque Of or pertaining to a substance or tissue that does not readily permit the passage of x-rays or other radiant energy; compare with *radiolucent*.

Rapid response team A team of health care providers that responds to emergency cases in an effort to decrease the risk of further deterioration.

Reconditioning Physical activity to strengthen essential muscle groups, improve overall oxygen use, and enhance the body's cardiovascular response to physical activity.

Registered Respiratory Therapist (RRT) A certification for respiratory practitioners in the United States; the certificate for the RRT is issued by the National Board for Respiratory Care after passing the NBRC-WRE and NBRC-CSE examinations.

Repolarization Process by which the cell is restored to its resting potential.

Residual volume (RV) Volume of gas remaining in the lungs after a complete exhalation.

Respiratory care practitioner (RCP) A health care professional with special training and experience in the treatment and rehabilitation of patients with respiratory disorders. The respiratory care practitioner typically does not diagnose but must be competent in patient assessment in a variety of clinical settings.

Respiratory care protocols Specification of actions that allows respiratory care practitioners to independently initiate and adjust therapy, within guidelines previously established by medical staff; also called *therapist-driven protocol*.

Respiratory frequency Number of breaths per minute, also called *respiratory rate (RR)*.

Restrictive pulmonary disease A broad category of disorders with widely variable etiologies, but all resulting in a reduction in lung volumes, particularly the inspiratory and vital capacities; categorized according to origin; that is, skeletal or thoracic, neuromuscular, pleural, interstitial, and alveolar.

S

6-minute walk A test generally done at the start of a pulmonary rehabilitation program or to evaluate a patient for lung surgery.

Six rights of medication administration Basic principles to safeguard the medication administration process and prevent errors.

Skilled nursing facility (SNF) An institution or part of an institution that meets criteria for accreditation established by the sections of the Social Security Act that determine the basis for Medicaid and Medicare reimbursement for skilled nursing care. Skilled nursing care includes rehabilitation and various medical and nursing procedures.

Slow vital capacity (SVC) The maximum volume of air that can be expelled at the normal rate of exhalation after maximum inspiration.

Small-volume nebulizer A pneumatically powered device used to aerosolize medications for delivery to patients; can be powered with air or oxygen.

Splinting A process of immobilizing, restraining, or supporting a body part.

Spontaneous breathing trial (SBT) A trial of spontaneous breathing independent of the ventilator.

Static compliance Compliance measurement done under conditions of no gas flow. Compliance is equal to a volume change divided by a pressure change.

Static pressure The pressure exerted by a gas when the bodies on which the pressure is exerted are not in motion.

Subcutaneous emphysema Accumulation of air in subcutaneous tissue due to leakage from the lung.

Sustained maximal inspiration (SMI) A slow, deep inhalation from the FRC up to the total lung capacity, followed by a 5- to 10-second breath-hold.

Swan-Ganz catheter (pulmonary artery catheter) A catheter that is positioned in the pulmonary artery to measure pressures in the heart and pulmonary circulation and can be used to determine the patient's circulatory status.

Synchronized cardioversion Countershock synchronized with the heart's electrical activity.

Synchronized intermittent mandatory ventilation Mode of ventilatory support using periodic assisted ventilation with spontaneous breathing in between. Assisted breaths are responsive to patient demand.

T

Target heart rate Heart rate achieved at 65% of a patient's maximum oxygen consumption during the exercise evaluation, used for aerobic conditioning.

Terminal weaning The process of discontinuing ventilation and liberating the patient from the ventilator.

National Board for Respiratory Care (NBRC) A national credentialing agency for respiratory care practitioners and pulmonary function technologists.

Therapeutic gases Medical gases that are used in respiratory therapy.

Thermodilution A method of cardiac output determination.

Thrombocytes The smallest cells in blood. They are formed in the red bone marrow and some are stored in the spleen. Platelets are disc shaped, contain no hemoglobin, and are essential for the coagulation of blood and in maintenance of hemostasis.

Tidal volume (V_T) The volume of air that is inhaled or exhaled from the lungs during effortless breath.

Total lung capacity (TLC) The total amount of gas in the lungs after a maximum inspiration.

Tracheal stenosis Narrowing of one of the cardiac valves.

Tracheomalacia Softening of the tracheal cartilages.

Transairway pressure The difference between airway pressure and alveolar pressure.

Trismus Motor disturbance of the trigeminal nerve, especially spasm of the masticatory muscles, causing difficulty in opening the mouth (lockjaw).

U

Unipolar leads An array of two electrodes, only one of which transmits potential variation (In a 12-lead ECG, all leads besides the limb leads are unipolar: aVR, aVL, aVF, V_1, V_2, V_3, V_4, V_5, and V_6).

V

Vaccines A biologic preparation that improves immunity to a particular disease.

Venipuncture The process of obtaining intravenous access for the purpose of intravenous therapy or for sampling of venous blood.

Ventilator-associated pneumonia (VAP) Pneumonia that develops 48 hours after a patient has been placed on mechanical ventilation.

Ventilator dependence Continuous or frequent intermittent use of a ventilator.

Vesicular lung sounds The gentle rustling sounds of normal breathing heard by auscultation over most of the lung fields; the inspiratory phase is usually longer than the expiratory phase.

Vital capacity (VC) The total amount of air that can be exhaled after maximum inspiration; the sum of the inspiratory reserve volume, the tidal volume, and the expiratory reserve volume.

Volume control ventilation A mode of ventilatory support in which volume (or flow × time) serves as the cycle variable.

Volume-oriented device Measures volume to achieve result.

W

Water trap A device used for the continuous trapping of liquid from the gas passed by a pressurized breathing circuit of a ventilator or other humidification devices used in respiratory care.

Weaning The process of discontinuing ventilation and liberating the patient from the ventilator.

Note: Some terms have been defined by using http://www.thefreedictionary.com. Accessed April 28, 2013.

Index

Page numbers followed by "f" indicate figures, "t" indicate tables, and "b" indicate boxes.